Multiple myeloma and related disorders

Edited by

Gösta Gahrton MD PhD
Professor, Department of Medicine
Karolinska Institute, Huddinge University Hospital
Stockholm, Sweden

Brian G.M. Durie MD
Departments of Hematology and Oncology
Cedars-Sinai Medical Centre, Los Angeles, CA, USA

and

Diana M. Samson MD
Senior Lecturer in Haematology
Hammersmith Hospital, London, UK

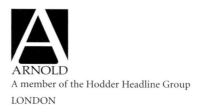

ARNOLD
A member of the Hodder Headline Group
LONDON

First published in Great Britain in 2004 by
Arnold, a member of the Hodder Headline Group,
338 Euston Road, London NW1 3BH

http://www.arnoldpublishers.com

Distributed in the United States of America by
Oxford University Press Inc.,
198 Madison Avenue, New York, NY10016
Oxford is a registered trademark of Oxford University Press

Whilst the advice and information in this book are believed to be true
and accurate at the date of going to press, neither the authors nor the
publisher can accept any legal responsibility or liability for any errors or
omissions that may be made. In particular (but without limiting the
generality of the preceding disclaimer) every effort has been made to
check drug dosages; however, it is still possible that errors have been
missed. Furthermore, dosage schedules are constantly being revised and
new side-effects recognized. For these reasons the reader is strongly
urged to consult the drug companies' printed instructions before
administering any of the drugs recommended in this book.

British Library Cataloguing in Publication Data
A catalogue record for this book is available from the British Library

Library of Congress Cataloging-in-Publication Data
A catalog record for this book is available from the Library of Congress

ISBN   0 340 81010 6
        1 2 3 4 5 6 7 8 9 10

Commissioning Editor: Joanna Koster
Development Editor: Sarah Burrows
Project Editor: Wendy Rooke
Production Controller: Deborah Smith
Cover Design: Lee-May Lim

Typeset in 10/12 pt Minion by Charon Tec Pvt Ltd, Chennai, India.
Printed and bound in UK by Butler & Tanner Ltd

What do you think about this book? Or any other Arnold title?
Please send your comments to **feedback.arnold@hodder.co.uk**

Contents

Contributors

Jutta Ackermann
Department of Medicine I, Clinical Division of Oncology, University Hospital, Vienna, Austria

Michel Attal
Head of Hematological Department, Hôpital Purpan, Toulouse, France

Daniel E. Bergsagel CM MD DPhil
Professor of Medicine, University of Toronto, Department of Medicine, Ontario Cancer Institute/Princess Margaret Hospital, Toronto, Ontario, Canada

P. Leif Bergsagel MD FRCP(C)
Associate Professor of Medicine, Weill Medical College of Cornell University, Department of Medicine, New York Presbyterian Hospital, New York, NY, USA

Joan Bladé MD
Department of Hematology, Institute of Hematology and Oncology, Postgraduate School of Hematology 'Farreras Valenti', Institut d'Investigacions Biomèdiques 'August Pi i Sunyer', Hospital Clínic, University of Barcelona, Barcelona, Spain

Jean-Claude Brouet MD PhD
Service d'Immunologie Clinique, Hôpital Saint-Louis, Paris, France

Ross D. Brown PhD MBA FAIMS
Institute of Haematology, University of Sydney, Royal Prince Alfred Hospital, Camperdown, NSW, Australia

Federico Caligaris-Cappio MD
Professor of Internal Medicine, Università Vita Salute, Istituto Scientifico San Raffaele, Milan, Italy

Raymond L. Comenzo MD
Division of Hematologic Oncology, Department of Medicine, Memorial Sloan-Kettering Cancer Center, New York, NY, USA

William S. Dalton PhD MD
H Lee Moffitt Cancer Center and Research Institute, University of South Florida, Tampa, FL, USA

Faith E. Davies MB BCh MRCP MD
Department of Health Clinician Scientist and Academic SpR, Epidemiology and Genetics Unit, Academic Department of Haematology and Oncology, School of Medicine, University of Leeds, Leeds, UK

Meletios A. Dimopoulos MD
Professor of Therapeutics, Department of Clinical Therapeutics, University of Athens School of Medicine, Athens, Greece

Angela Dispenzieri MD
Consultant, Division of Hematology and Internal Medicine, Mayo Clinic; and Assistant Professor of Medicine, Mayo Medical School, Rochester, MN, USA

Kathleen A. Donovan PhD
Professional Associate in Research, Division of Hematology and Internal Medicine, Mayo Clinic, Rochester, MN, USA

Johannes Drach MD
Department of Medicine I, Clinical Division of Oncology, University Hospital, Vienna, Austria

Brian G.M. Durie MD
Departments of Hematology and Oncology, Cedars-Sinai Medical Centre, Los Angeles, CA, USA

Thierry Facon MD
Service des Maladies du Sang, Hôpital Claude Huriez, CHU, Lille, France

Jean-Paul Fermand MD
Service d'Immunologie Clinique, Hôpital Saint-Louis, Paris, France

Deborah A. Frassica MD
Assistant Professor of Radiation Oncology, Department of Radiation Oncology and Molecular Radiation Sciences, Sidney Kimmel Comprehensive Cancer Center, Johns Hopkins University, Baltimore, MD, USA

Gösta Gahrton MD PhD
Professor, Department of Medicine, Karolinska Institute, Huddinge University Hospital, Stockholm, Sweden

Ramón García-Sanz MD PhD
Department of Hematology, University Hospital of Salamanca, Salamanca, Spain

Deborah Gelbspan MD
UMC, Department of Pathology, University of Arizona, Tucson, AZ, USA

John Gibson MB BS PhD FRACP FRCPA
Institute of Haematology, University of Sydney, Royal Prince
Alfred Hospital, Camperdown, NSW, Australia

Philip R. Greipp MD
Consultant, Division of Hematology and Internal Medicine,
Mayo Clinic, and Professor of Medicine, Mayo Medical School,
Rochester, MN, USA

Thomas M. Grogan MD
UMC, Department of Pathology, University of Arizona,
Tucson, AZ, USA

Jean-Luc Harousseau
Professor, Université de Nantes, Centre Hospitalier Régional,
Hôtel-Dieu, Département d'Hématologie, Nantes, France

P. Joy Ho MB BS DPhil FRACP FRCPA
Institute of Haematology, University of Sydney, Royal Prince
Alfred Hospital, Camperdown, NSW, Australia

Maria C. Jacobs MD
Director, Department of Radiation Oncology, Mercy Medical
Center, Baltimore, MD, USA

Douglas E. Joshua BSc MB BS DPhil FRACP FRCPA
Professor and Head of Institute of Haematology, University of
Sydney, Royal Prince Alfred Hospital, Camperdown, NSW, Australia

Hannes Kaufmann MD
Department of Medicine I, Clinical Division of Oncology,
University Hospital, Vienna, Austria

Robert A. Kyle MD
Consultant, Division of Hematology and Internal Medicine,
Mayo Clinic; and Professor of Medicine and of Laboratory
Medicine, Mayo Medical School, Rochester, MN, USA

Terry H. Landowski PhD
Research Assistant Professor, Department of Medicine, Arizona
Cancer Center, University of Arizona, Tucson, AZ, USA

Xavier Leleu MD
Service des Maladies du Sang, Hôpital Claude Huriez, CHU,
Lille, France

Per Ljungman MD PhD
Department of Medicine, Karolinska Institute, Huddinge
University Hospital, Stockholm, Sweden

Heinz Ludwig MD
Professor, Department of Medicine and Medical Oncology,
Wilhelminenspital, Vienna, Austria

John A. Lust MD PhD
Consultant, Division of Hematology and Internal Medicine,
Mayo Clinic, and Associate Professor of Medicine, Mayo
Medical School, Rochester, MN, USA

Eugene V. McCloskey MB BCh MRCP MD
WHO Collaborating Centre for Metabolic Bone Diseases,
University of Sheffield Medical School, Sheffield, UK

Håkan Mellstedt MD PhD
Professor of Oncologic Biotherapy, Karolinska Institute,
Managing Director, Cancer Centre Karolinska, Department of
Oncology and Hematology, Karolinska Hospital, Stockholm,
Sweden

Giampaolo Merlini MD
Professor of Clinical Biochemistry, Department of Biochemistry,
University of Pavia, and Biotechnology Research Laboratories,
University Hospital Policlinico San Matteo, Pavia, Italy

Gareth J. Morgan PhD FRCP FRCPath
Professor of Haematology, Epidemiology and Genetics Unit,
Academic Unit of Haematology and Oncology, School of
Medicine, University of Leeds, Leeds, UK

Lia A. Moulopoulos MD
Assistant Professor, Department of Radiology, University of
Athens School of Medicine, Athens, Greece

Gregory R. Mundy MD
Departments of Cellular and Structural Biology and
Orthopedics, University of Texas Health Science Center at San
Antonio, San Antonio Cancer Institute, San Antonio, TX, USA

Babatunde O. Oyajobi MD ChB PhD
Departments of Cellular and Structural Biology and Molecular
Medicine, University of Texas Health Science Center at San
Antonio, San Antonio, TX, USA

Dietrich Peest MD
Professor of Medicine and Clinical Immunology, Department
of Hematology and Oncology, Hannover Medical School,
Hannover, Germany

Pamela G. Riches PhD FRCPath
Professor, Protein Reference Unit, Department of Biochemistry
and Immunology, St George's Hospital Medical School,
London, UK

Lisa Rimsza MD
UMC, Department of Pathology, University of Arizona, Tucson,
AZ, USA

Laura Rosiñol MD
Department of Hematology, Institute of Hematology and
Oncology, University of Barcelona, Barcelona, Spain

Diana M. Samson MD
Senior Lecturer in Haematology, Hammersmith Hospital,
London, UK

Jesús F. San Miguel MD PhD
Professor of Hematology, Department of
Hematology, University Hospital of Salamanca,
Salamanca, Spain

Sonja Seidl MD
Department of Medicine I, Clinical Division of Oncology,
University Hospital, Vienna, Austria

Joanna M. Sheldon PhD MRCPath
Protein Reference Unit, Department of Biochemistry
and Immunology, St George's Hospital Medical School,
London, UK

David P. Steensma MD
Fellow in Hematology, Mayo Graduate School of Medicine,
Mayo Clinic, Rochester, MN, USA

Steven P. Treon MD MA PhD
Director, Waldenstrom's Macroglobulinemia Program, Dana
Farber Cancer Institute, Instructor of Medicine, Harvard
University, Boston, MA, USA

Ibrahim Yakoub–Agha MD
Service des Maladies du Sang, Hôpital Claude Huriez, CHU,
Lille, France

Preface

Since the publication of our original book on multiple myeloma in 1996, there has been an enormous increase in knowledge about the disease: more than 5000 articles have been published in scientific journals. The development has been impressive both in the basic knowledge about the disease and in its treatment.

New technologies have made it possible to refine studies on chromosomes and genes and to gain information about gene expression. Microarray is in its early stage, but already there have been pattern descriptions that may have prognostic implications.

We have learned not only that deletions of chromosome 13 are important but also that chromosome 14 translocations involving candidate oncogenes on other chromosomes, such as Cyclin D1 or FGFR3, may be even more important in the pathogenesis of the disease. The prognostic impact of chromosomal abnormalities is now clearer than before, and the complicated interaction between the stroma cells, the myeloma cells, and numerous cytokines and their receptors has been better explained. Most importantly, attempts have been made to utilize this new knowledge to develop targeted therapy and, although results are still modest, improvements have been obtained with thalidomide and analogs, as well as with proteasome inhibitors, such as bortezomib. Many other approaches to targeted therapy are being attempted and are reviewed.

Very important progress has been made in stem-cell transplantation and it is now confirmed in more than one prospective study that high-dose therapy with autologous transplantation is superior to conventional chemotherapy for patients under 65 years of age. It also seems that tandem transplantation may be superior to single autologous transplantation, at least for subgroups of patients. Interesting attempts are being made to decrease the intensity of the conditioning regimen for allogeneic transplantation, and to utilize the immune effect of the donor marrow and donor lymphocytes.

These and other new developments, not only in multiple myeloma, but also in related disorders, such as amyloid light-chain amyloidosis, heavy-chain disease, and Waldenström's macroglobulinemia, are described in this new, expanded book. Each chapter area is able to stand alone; thus, there is some deliberate overlap between chapters.

With this approach, our hope is that the book will be of interest not only for scientists and specialists in the field, but also for practitioners and non-specialists with an interest in basic aspects of treatment of patients with multiple myeloma.

Gösta Gahrton
Brian G.M. Durie
Diana M. Samson

Abbreviations

A	Adriamycin	CALGB	Cancer and Leukaemia Group B
Ab	antibody	CALLA	common acute lymphoblastic leukemia antigen
ABMT	autologous bone marrow transplantation	CAPD	chronic ambulatory peritoneal dialysis
ADCC	antibody-dependent cellular cytotoxicity	CAS	chronic antigenic stimulation
		CC	conventional chemotherapy
ADH	antidiuretic hormone	CCNU	1-(2-chloroethyl)-3-cyclohexyl-1-nitrosourea (lomustine)
Ag	antigen		
AL	amyloid light chain	CCT	combination chemotherapy
ALP	alkaline phosphatase	CDC	complement-dependent cytotoxicity
ALT	alanine aminotransferase	CDR	complementary determining region
AP	acid phosphatase	CEVAD	cyclophosphamide, etoposide, vincristine, Adriamycin, and dexamethasone
AP	anteroposterior		
APC	antigen-presenting cell		
ASCO	American Society for Clinical Oncology	CGH	comparative genomic hybridization
		CI	confidence interval
ASCT	autologous stem-cell transplantation	CIC	circulating immune complexes
		CIDEX	CCNU, idarubicin, and dexamethasone
ASO	allele-specific oligonucleotide	CIDP	chronic inflammatory demyelinating polyradiculopathy
AST	aspartate aminotransferase		
α_1AT	α_1-antitrypsin	CIITA	class II transactivator
ATO	arsenic trioxide	CLL	chronic lymphocytic leukemia
ATTR	mutant transthyretin	CLMTF	Chronic Leukaemia and Myeloma Task Force
β_2M	β_2-microglobulin	CML	chronic myelogenous leukemia
B	BCNU (carmustine)	CMV	cytomegalovirus
bALP	bone-specific alkaline phosphatase	CNTF	ciliary neurotrophic factor
BCNU	1,3-bis(2-chloroethyl)-1-nitrosourea (carmustine)	COX-2	cyclo-oxygenase 2
		CR	complete response/remission
BCCA	British Columbia Cancer Agency	CRP	C-reactive protein
BCSH	British Committee for Standards in Haematology	CT	computed tomography
		CT-1	cardiotrophin-1
BDUR	bromodeoxyuridine	CTL	cytotoxic T lymphocyte
BGP	bone Gla protein	CVP	cyclophosphamide, vincristine, and prednisone
BJP	Bence Jones protein		
Blimp-1	B-lymphocyte-induced maturation protein 1	CZE	capillary zone electrophoresis
BLT-D	clarithromycin, thalidomide, and dexamethasone	D	diversity
		DAP	death-associated protein
BM	bone marrow	DC	dendritic cell
BMD	bone mineral density	DCEP	dexamethasone, cyclophosphamide, etoposide, and cisplatin
BMT	bone marrow transplantation		

DEXA-BEAM	dexamethasone, BCNU, etoposide, cytarabine, and melphalan
DFS	disease-free survival
DHBI	double hemi-body irradiation
DLBCL	diffuse large B-cell lymphoma
DLI	donor lymphocyte infusion
2D-PAGE	two-dimensional polyacrylamide gel electrophoresis
DPD	deoxypyridinoline
DT-PACE	dexamethasone, thalidomide, cisplatin, doxorubicin, cyclophosphamide, and etoposide
DVT	deep vein thrombosis
EAR	excess absolute risk
EBMT	European Group for Blood and Marrow Transplantation
ECM	extracellular matrix
ECOG	Eastern Cooperative Oncology Group
ECV	extracellular fluid volume
EDAP	etoposide, dexamethasone, ara-C (cytosine arabinoside), and cisplatin
EFS	event-free survival
EGFR	epidermal growth factor receptor
ELISA	enzyme-linked immunosorbant assay
ELISPOT	enzyme-linked immune spot analysis
EORTC	European Organisation for Research and Treatment of Cancer
EP	electrophoresis
Epo	erythropoietin
EQA	external quality assurance
ERK	extracellular signal-regulated kinase
FACS	fluorescence-activated cell sorting
FasL	Fas ligand
FDC	follicular dendritic cell
FDG	^{18}F deoxyglucose
FISH	fluorescence *in situ* hybridization
FL	follicular lymphoma
FLC	free light chain
FrC	fragment C of tetanus toxin
FTase	farnesyltransferase
FTI	farnesyltransferase inhibitor
GC	germinal center
G-CSF	granulocyte colony-stimulating factor
GFR	glomerular filtration rate
GGTase I	geranylgeranyltransferase I
GGTI	geranylgeranyltransferase inhibitor
GI	gastrointestinal
GM-CSF	granulocyte macrophage–colony-stimulating factor
GVHD	graft-versus-host disease
GvM	graft versus myeloma

Hb	hemoglobin
HB-EGF	heparin-binding epidermal-like growth factor
HBI	hemi-body irradiation
HCD	heavy-chain disease
HCT	hematocrit
HCV	hepatitis C virus
HDDex	high-dose dexamethasone
HDM	high-dose melphalan
HDT	high-dose therapy
HGF	hepatocyte growth factor
HIV	human immunodeficiency virus
HLA	human leukocyte antigen
HMCL	human myeloma cell line
HPLC	high-performance liquid chromatography
IBMTR	International Bone Marrow Transplant Registry
ICTP	carboxyterminal telopeptide of type I collagen
Id	tumor-derived idiotypic immunoglobulin
IC_{50}	50% inhibitory concentration
I-DOX	4-iodo-4-deoxydoxorubicin
IF	immunofixation
IFCC	International Federation of Clinical Chemists
IFM	Intergroupe Français du Myelome
IFN	interferon
Ig	immunoglobulin
Ig V_L	immunoglobulin light chain variable region
IGF	insulin-like growth factor
IGF-1R	IGF-1 receptor
IgH	immunoglobulin heavy chain
IgL	immunoglobulin light chain
IHC	immunohistochemistry
IL	interleukin
IL-6R	interleukin-6 receptor
IL-15R	interleukin-15 receptor
ImiD	immunomodulatory drug
IMM	indolent multiple myeloma
INR	international normalized ratio
IP	interstitial pneumonitis
IPI	international prognostic index
IPSID	immunoproliferative small-intestinal disease
IRF	interferon-responsive factor
ISH	*in situ* hybridization
ISR	illegitimate switch recombination
ISS	International Staging System
IV	intravenous
IVT	*in vitro* transcription

J	joining
JAK	Janus kinase
KLH	keyhole limpet hemocyanin
LAK	lymphokine-activated killer
LCDD	light-chain deposition disease
LDH	lactic dehydrogenase
LHCDD	light- and heavy-chain deposition disease
LI	labeling index
LIF	leukemia-inhibitory factor
LOD score	log of the ratio of likelihood of linkage to no linkage
LRP	lung-resistant protein
MAb	monoclonal antibody
MAG	myelin-associated glycoprotein
MALDI/TOF	matrix-assisted laser desorption ionization/time of flight
MALT	mucosa-associated lymphoid tissue
MAPK	mitogen-activated protein-kinase
MCL	mantle cell lymphoma
M-CSF	monocyte–macrophage colony-stimulating factor
MD	melphalan and pulsed dexamethasone
MEL-140	melphalan 140 mg/m^2
MEL-200	melphalan 200 mg/m^2
MGB	minor groove binding
MGUS	monoclonal gammopathy of undetermined significance
MHC	major histocompatibility complex
MIDD	monoclonal immunoglobulin deposition diseases
MIP-1α	macrophage inflammatory protein 1α
MM	multiple myeloma
MOPC	mineral-oil-induced plasmacytoma
MP	melphalan and prednisolone
MRC	Medical Research Council
MRD	minimal residual disease
MR	minimal response
MRI	magnetic resonance imaging
MS	mass spectrometry
MSKCC	Memorial Sloan Kettering Cancer Center
MTD	maximum tolerated dose
MTF	Myeloma Task Force
MTC	major translocation cluster
MUC-1	mucin-1 glycoprotein
MVD	microvessel density
NESP	novel erythropoeisis-stimulating protein
NF-κB	nuclear factor κ B
NHL	non-Hodgkin's lymphoma
NK	natural killer

NMSG	Nordic Myeloma Study Group
NNT	number needed to treat
NRTK	non-receptor tyrosine kinase
NSAID	non-steroidal anti-inflammatory drug
NTx	N-terminal telopeptide of type I collagen
OAF	osteoclast-activating factor
OC	osteocalcin
ODN	oligonucleotide
OM	oncostatin M
OPG	osteoprotegerin
OR	odds ratio
OS	overall survival
P	prednisolone
PBL	peripheral blood lymphocyte
PBMC	peripheral blood mononuclear cell
PBPC	peripheral blood progenitor cell
PBSC	peripheral blood stem cell
PBSCT	peripheral blood stem cell transplantation
PC	plasma cell
PCD	plasma cell dyscrasia
PCL	plasma cell leukemia
PCLI	plasma cell labeling index
PCR	polymerase chain reaction
PET	positron emission tomography
PFS	progression-free survival
PFT	pulmonary function test
PgP	P-glycoprotein
PI3-K	phosphatidylinositol 3-kinase
PINP	N-terminal pro-peptide of type I collagen
PKC	protein kinase C
PLT	platelet
PMMA	polymethylmethacrylate
POEMS	polyneuropathy, organomegaly, endocrinopathy, monoclonal gammopathy, and skin changes
P-PCL	primary plasma cell leukaemia
PR	partial response/remission
PTH	parathyroid hormone
PTH-rP	parathyroid hormone-related protein
PYD	pyridinoline
QALY	quality-adjusted life years
QoL	quality of life
Q-TwiST	quality-adjusted time without symptoms or toxicity
RA	rheumatoid arthritis
RAFTK	related adhesion focal tyrosine kinase
RANK	receptor activator of nuclear factor κ B
RANKL	receptor activator of NF-κB ligand
Rb	retinoblastoma

RBC	red blood cell
RFLP	restriction fragment length polymorphism
rhEPO	recombinant human erythropoietin
RIT	radioimmunotherapy
ROTI	related organ or tissue impairment
RRT	regimen-related toxicity
RSV	respiratory syncytial virus
RTK	receptor tyrosine kinase
RTOG	Radiation Therapy Oncology Group
SAP	serum amyloid P component
SBP	solitary bone plasmacytoma
SCF	stem cell factor
scFv	single-chain antibody of VH and VL fragments
SCT	stem cell transplantation
SD	stable disease
SDF-1α	stromal-cell-derived factor 1α
SDS	sodium dodecyl sulfate
SEER	Surveillance, Epidemiology and End Results
SelCID	selective cytokine inhibitory drug
SEP	solitary extramedullary plasmacytoma
SGPG	sulfoglucuronyl paragloboside
s-IL-6R	serum levels of IL-6 receptor
sIL-6R	soluble IL-6 receptor
SKY	spectral karyotyping
SMART	switch mechanism at the 5′-end of RNA transcripts
SMM	smoldering multiple myeloma
SNP	single nucleotide polymorphism
SPEP	serum protein electrophoresis
ST	switch translocation
STAT	signal transducer and activator of transcription
STIR	sagittal T1-weighted inversion recovery
STIR	short inversion-time inversion recovery
SWOG	Southwest Oncology Group
TBI	total body irradiation
^{99m}Tc-MIBI	99m-technetium-2-methoxy-iso-butyl-isonitrile
TCR	T-cell receptor

TD	T-cell-dependent
TD	thanatophoric dysplasia
TdT	terminal deoxynucleotidyl transferase
TGFβ	transforming growth factor β
Th	T helper
TI	T-cell-independent
TK	thymidine kinase
TNFβ	tumor necrosis factor β
TRAIL	TNF-related apoptosis-inducing ligand
TRAP	tartrate-resistant acid phosphatase
TRM	transplant-related mortality
TTF	time to treatment failure
T-TIL	tumor-infiltrating T-lymphocytes
V	variable
V	vincristine
VAD	vincristine, Adriamycin (doxorubicin), and dexamethasone
VAMP	vincristine, doxorubicin, and methylprednisolone
VBAP	vincristine, BCNU (carmustine), Adriamycin (doxorubicin), and prednisone
VBMCP	vincristine, BCNU, melphalan, cyclophosphamide, and prednisone
VCAM-1	vascular cell adhesion molecule 1
VEGF	vascular endothelial growth factor
VGPR	very good partial response
VLA-4	very late antigen 4
VMCP	vincristine, melphalan, cyclophosphamide, and prednisone
VMD	vincristine, mitoxantrone, and dexamethasone
WHO	World Health Organization
WM	Waldenström's macroglobulinemia
WMDA	World Marrow Donor Association
XBP1	X-box-binding protein 1

Notes on reference annotation

The reference lists are annotated, where appropriate, to guide readers to key primary papers and major review articles as follows:

Key primary papers are indicated by a •
Major review articles are indicated by a ◆
Papers that represent the first formal publication of a management guideline are indicated by a *

We hope that this feature will render extensive lists of references more useful to the reader and will help to encourage self-directed learning among both trainees and practicing physicians.

PART 1

History and epidemiology

History of multiple myeloma

ROBERT A. KYLE AND DAVID P. STEENSMA

THE FIRST RECORDED CASES

In 1850, Dr William Macintyre, a 53-year-old Harley Street consultant and physician to the Metropolitan Convalescent Institution and to the Western General Dispensary, St Marylebone,[1] described one of his patients as follows:

> Mr. M, a highly respectable tradesman, aged 45, placed himself under my care on the 30th of October, 1845. He was then confined to the house by excruciating pains of the chest, back and loins, from which he had been suffering, more or less, for upwards to twelve months.[2]

Because edema had been noted, Dr Macintyre examined the urine but found no evidence of sugar. The urine specimen was opaque, acid, and of high density, with a specific gravity of 1.035. When heated, it was found to 'abound in animal matter.' The precipitate dissolved on boiling but again consolidated on cooling. The urine sample and following note were sent by Dr Macintyre and a leading physician of London, Dr Thomas Watson, to Dr Henry Bence Jones, a 31-year-old physician at St George's Hospital, who had already established a reputation as a chemical pathologist.[3]

> Saturday, Nov. 1st, 1845
> Dear Doctor Jones
> The tube contains urine of very high specific gravity. When boiled it becomes slightly opaque. On the addition of nitric acid, it effervesces, assumes a reddish hue, and becomes quite clear; but as it cools, assumes the consistence and appearance which you see. Heat reliquifies it. What is it?[4]

Thomas Alexander McBean, the patient who contributed the urine discussed above, was a highly respectable grocer of 'temperate habits and exemplary conduct.' Having married early, he had numerous offspring, and, with the exception of two or three severe attacks of 'frontal neuralgia,' he had enjoyed good health. His family history was non-contributory: his father had died of the complications of gout and his mother had died suddenly after operation for carcinoma of the breast. For slightly less than a year previous to the onset of symptoms, his family had noted that he fatigued easily and appeared to stoop while walking. He also had urinary frequency, and he was concerned that his 'body linen was stiffened by his urine,' despite the absence of a uretheral discharge.[2] While vaulting out of an underground cavern on a country vacation in September 1844, McBean had 'instantly felt as if something had snapped or given way within the chest, and for some minutes he lay in intense agony, unable to stir.' The pain abated, and he was able to walk to a neighboring inn. Soreness and stiffness of the chest persisted but were relieved by the application of a 'strengthening plaster to the chest.' Three or four weeks later, the pain recurred, and the patient was treated by removal of a pound of blood and the application of leeches. The pain resolved but, as might be expected, the bleeding was followed by considerable weakness for 2 or 3 months.

In the spring of 1845, the pain recurred with an episode of pleuritic pain in the right side, between the ribs and the hip, which was treated by cupping. Therapeutic bleeding produced much greater weakness than before. Wasting, pallor, and slight puffiness of his face and ankles led to

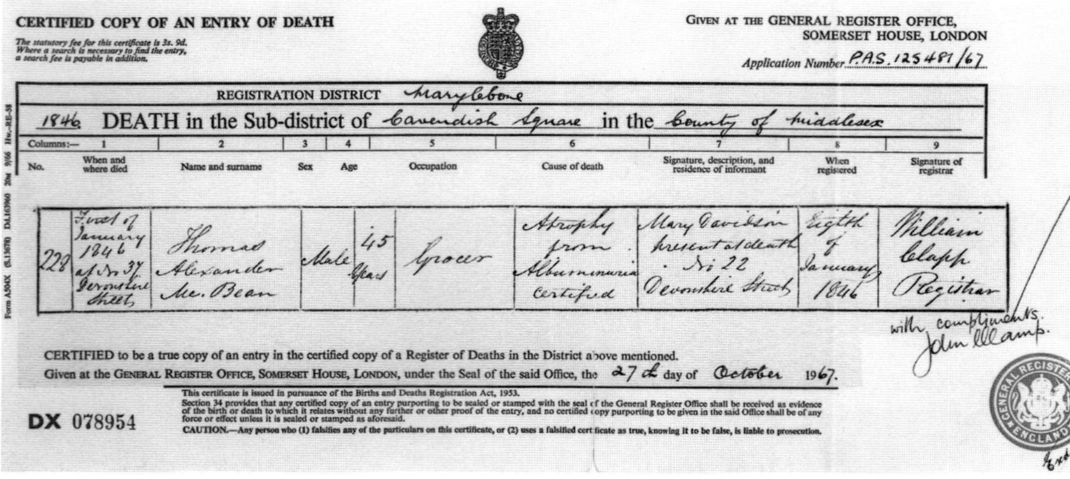

CERTIFIED COPY OF AN ENTRY OF DEATH

The statutory fee for this certificate is 3s. 9d. Where a search is necessary to find the entry, a search fee is payable in addition.

GIVEN AT THE GENERAL REGISTER OFFICE, SOMERSET HOUSE, LONDON

Application Number P.A.S. 125481/67

REGISTRATION DISTRICT Marylebone

1846. DEATH in the Sub-district of Cavendish Square in the County of Middlesex

Columns:— No.	1 When and where died	2 Name and surname	3 Sex	4 Age	5 Occupation	6 Cause of death	7 Signature, description, and residence of informant	8 When registered	9 Signature of registrar
228	First of January 1846 at No 37 Devonshire Street	Thomas Alexander Mc. Bean	Male	45 Years	Grocer	Atrophy from Albuminuria certified	Mary Davidson present at death No 22 Devonshire Street	Eighth of January 1846	William Clapp Registrar

with compliments. John Clamp.

CERTIFIED to be a true copy of an entry in the certified copy of a Register of Deaths in the District above mentioned.

Given at the GENERAL REGISTER OFFICE, SOMERSET HOUSE, LONDON, under the Seal of the said Office, the 27th day of October 1967.

DX 078954

This certificate is issued in pursuance of the Births and Deaths Registration Act, 1953.

Section 34 provides that any certified copy of an entry purporting to be sealed or stamped with the seal of the General Register Office shall be received as evidence of the birth or death to which it relates without any further or other proof of the entry, and no certified copy purporting to be given in the said Office shall be of any force or effect unless it is sealed or stamped as aforesaid.

CAUTION.—Any person who (1) falsifies any of the particulars on this certificate, or (2) uses a falsified certificate as true, knowing it to be false, is liable to prosecution.

GENERAL REGISTER OFFICE ENGLAND

Figure 1.1 *Death certificate of Thomas Alexander McBean. (Courtesy of General Register Office, London, England.)*

consultation with Dr Thomas Watson. Steel and quinine therapy resulted in rapid improvement. By the middle of summer, he was able to travel to Scotland, where on the coast 'he was capable of taking active exercise on foot during the greater part of the day, bounding over the hills, to use his own expression, as nimbly as any of his companions.'[2] His appetite became ravenous – he expressed it as being so much that he dreamed of eating dogs and cats.[4] His recovery was interrupted by an episode of diarrhea, which proved to be obstinate, reducing his strength considerably. In September 1845, he returned to London in a very debilitated state but free of the excruciating pains that he had experienced during the spring and early part of the summer. In October, the lumbar and sciatic pains became severe. Warm baths, Dover's powder (ipecac and opium powder), acetate of ammonia, camphor julap, and compound tincture of camphor did not help.

The pain became 'fixed in the left lumbar and iliac regions, obliging the patient to observe a semi-bent posture, on account of the agony caused by every attempt at movement of the body upon the thighs.'[2] There was intermittent pain involving the chest and shoulders. Great care and cautious maneuvering enabled him to 'get in and out of bed on all-fours.' He became weaker and was confined to his bed. He had considerable flatulence and 'marked fulness and hardness in the region of the liver.'[2] Citrate of iron and quinine produced no benefit. His urine became turbid and thick, like pea soup. This change coincided with improvement, characterized by sleeping well for two nights and the ability to get up and walk around the room with little or no pain. The urine, however, contained the same amount of animal matter. Phlegm in the chest, a cough, and recurrence of the severe pain then developed. He also had an attack of diarrhea, which was precipitated by a dose of rhubarb and soda that had been given to correct the flatulence.

On 15 November, Dr Henry Bence Jones saw the patient in consultation and recommended alum as treatment 'with the view of checking the exhausting excretion of animal matter.' The specific gravity of the urine and animal matter in the urine decreased, and McBean was able to sit up daily for an hour or two and continued to enjoy his food. Unfortunately, on 7 December, he experienced a 'dreadful aggravation of lumbar pains,' which crude opium and morphine failed to relieve. He became weaker and died on 1 January 1846, exhausted, in full possession of his mental faculties (Fig. 1.1).

Postmortem examination revealed emaciation; the ribs, which crumbled under the heel of the scalpel, were soft, brittle, readily broken, and easily cut by the knife. Their interior was filled with a soft 'gelatiniform substance of a blood-red colour and unctuous feel.' The sternum also was involved. The heart and lungs were not remarkable. 'The liver was voluminous, but of healthy structure.' The kidneys appeared to be normal on both gross and microscopic examination. They had 'proved equal to the novel office assigned to them' and had 'discharged the task without sustaining, on their part, the slightest danger.' The thoracic and lumbar vertebrae had the same changes as found in the ribs and sternum, but the humeri and femurs resisted 'all efforts to bend or break them by manual force.'[2]

John Dalrymple, surgeon to the Royal Ophthalmic Hospital, Moorfields, examined two lumbar vertebrae and a rib of Mr McBean. Dalrymple noted that the disease appeared to begin in the cancellous bone, then grew and produced irregularly sized, round, dark-red projections that were visible through the periosteum. Nucleated cells formed the bulk of the gelatiniform mass that filled the cancellous cavities. Most of these cells were round or oval and about one-half to two times as large as an average blood cell. The cells contained one or two nuclei, each with a bright distinct nucleolus. Wood engravings made from the accurate drawings of Mr Dalrymple were consistent with the appearance of myeloma cells (Fig. 1.2).[5]

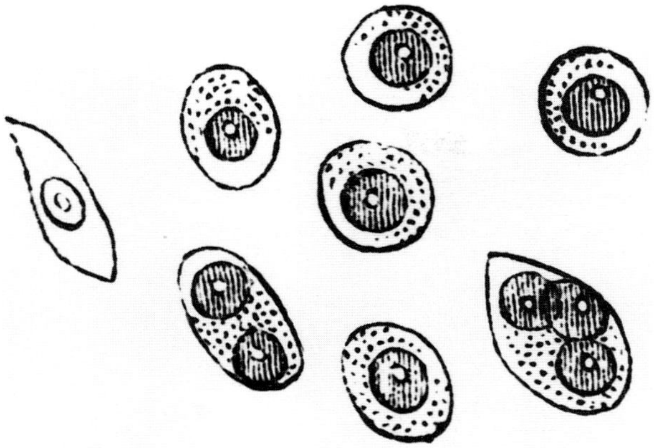

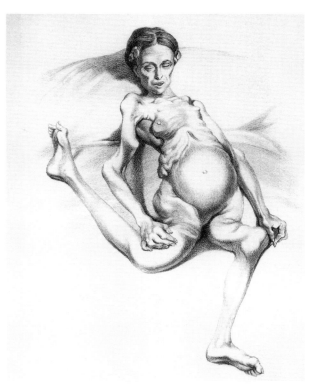

Figure 1.2 *Plasma cells (wood engravings made from drawings by Mr Dalrymple). (Reproduced from Dalrymple.[5])*

Macintyre stated that his 'own share in this part of the inquiry, it must have been seen, was very humble.' He went on to say that the examination and course of the patient seemed to be 'deserving of a detailed account' and that he 'shall be content if I have succeeded in pointing out to future observers, gifted with the requisite qualifications for conducting researches of a higher order, certain definite and distinctive characters by which a peculiar and hitherto unrecorded pathological condition of the urine may be recognized and identified.'[2]

The diarrhea, weakness, emaciation, hepatic enlargement, flatulence, dyspepsia, edema of the ankles, puffiness of the face, and large amount of proteinuria all suggest the possibility of amyloidosis, in addition to multiple myeloma; but the autopsy findings of a normal heart and kidneys and 'voluminous liver of healthy structure' make the presence of amyloidosis unlikely. Because the waxy changes of amyloidosis in the liver were commonly recognized in this era, it is unlikely that amyloidosis would have been overlooked.

As with many so-called first cases, one can find an earlier example. It is almost certain that 39-year-old Sarah Newbury, the second patient described by Dr Solly in 1844, had multiple myeloma.[6] She experienced fatigue and, 4 years before her death, was seized with a violent pain in her back when stooping. Rheumatic pains occurred a year later. Pain in her limbs increased after a fall in February 1842. She felt excruciating pain, 'just as if her thighs were being broken into a thousand pieces,' while her husband was lifting her from the fireplace to carry her to bed. He felt her thighs give way, and she was unable to walk thereafter. Fractures of the clavicles, right humerus, and right radius and ulna occurred (Fig. 1.3). She was hospitalized at St Thomas's Hospital, London, where she was given wine and arrowroot, a mutton chop and a pint of porter daily. She was treated with a rhubarb pill, an infusion of orange peel, and an opiate.[7] She died suddenly on 20 April 1844. Autopsy revealed that the cancellous portion of the sternum (Fig. 1.4) had been replaced by a red substance, which

Figure 1.3 *Sarah Newbury. Fractures of femurs and right humerus. (Reproduced from Solly.[6])*

Macintyre reported was similar to the red substance seen in Mr McBean. The red matter had replaced much of both femurs (Fig. 1.5) and was examined by Dr Solly and Mr Birkett of Guy's Hospital. Most of the nucleated cells had a clear, oval outline and one or, rarely, two bright central nucleoli. Solly believed that the process was inflammatory and that it had begun with a 'morbid action of the blood-vessels' in which the 'earthy matter of the bone is absorbed and thrown out by the kidneys in the urine.' Little did he know that more than one and a half centuries later, anti-angiogenesis drugs would be used for the treatment of multiple myeloma.[7]

Examining the specimen of McBean's urine received from Watson and Macintyre on 1 November, Bence Jones corroborated Macintyre's finding that the addition of nitric acid produced a precipitate that was redissolved by heat and formed again on cooling. He calculated that the patient excreted 67 g/day and concluded that the protein was an oxide of albumin, specifically 'hydrated deutoxide of albumen.'[8]

There is some justification for changing the name 'multiple myeloma' to 'McBean's disease with Macintyre's proteinuria.' Although Macintyre described the heat properties of the urine, Bence Jones emphasized its place in the diagnosis of myeloma, for he said, 'I need hardly remark on the importance of seeking for this oxide of albumen in other cases of mollities ossium' (softening of the bone).[4]

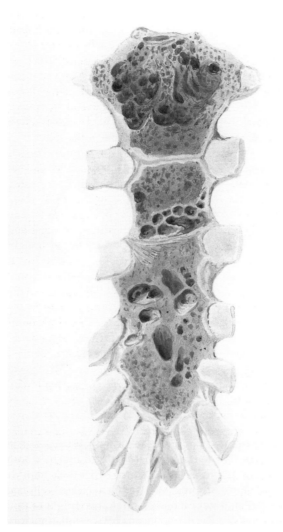

Figure 1.4 *Sternum of Sarah Newbury, showing destruction of bone. (Reproduced from Solly.[6])*

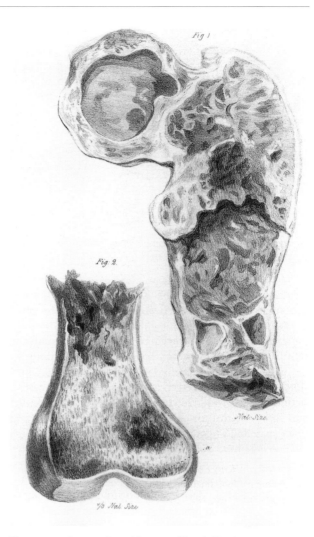

Figure 1.5 *Destruction of femurs of Sarah Newbury by myeloma tumor. (Reproduced from Solly.[6])*

Henry Bence Jones

Henry Bence Jones was born on 31 December 1813, at Thorington Hall, Yoxford, Suffolk, England, at the home of his maternal grandfather, the Reverend Mr Bence Sparrow, Rector of Beccles. The Bence family was related to the Winthrops of colonial America, including John Winthrop, the first governor of Connecticut, and also to the Bowdoins, including James Bowdoin, the first president of the American Academy of Arts and Sciences. Jones' father, William, originated from Cork, Ireland, and served in the Fifth Dragoon Guards and fought in the Peninsular War at Salamanca.[9] Henry Bence Jones attended Harrow, where he excelled in sports and was on the cricket team. Proceeding from Harrow to Cambridge, he entered Trinity College, where he was a member of the boating crew. He attended the Divinity Lectures in preparation for ordination but decided against the career of a clergyman[10] after obtaining his arts degree in January 1836. Instead, he became a pupil of Mr John Hammerton, apothecary at St George's Hospital. Bence Jones prepared medicines in the apothecary shop for 6 months and later said that this 'was of the utmost use to me all my life.'[11]

He enrolled as a full-time medical student after 18 months. During this time, he learned the use of the stethoscope, a relatively new instrument. Bence Jones remarked that 'the glorious discoveries of Dr Bright were not valued by any of our medical men.'[11] To acquire a knowledge of chemistry, he became a private pupil of Professor Thomas Graham at University College, London. As a part of his studies, he was required to examine a calculus from the University College Museum. This stone consisted of cystine and led to his first publication. After 6 months during 1841 spent studying chemistry with Justus von Liebig at Giessen, Germany, he returned to St George's Hospital,

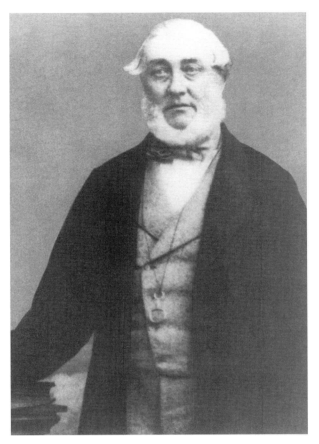

Figure 1.6 *Dr Henry Bence Jones. (From Snapper I, Kahn A (ed.)* Myelomatosis: fundamentals and clinical features. *Baltimore: University Park Press, 1971. By permission of S Karger AG Basel.)*

best 'chemical doctor' in London. He served as one of the original members of the Council of the Nightingale Fund and was also influential in the establishment of the Hospital for Sick Children on Great Ormond Street, on whose board he served. As a student, Bence Jones attended lectures of the physicist Michael Faraday at the Royal Institution. He subsequently became a friend and physician to Faraday and, in 1870, he published a well-received two-volume biography of the prominent physicist.

Bence Jones was the first to describe xanthine crystals in the urine.[14] He emphasized the frequency of diabetes in the older population – 11 of his 29 patients were more than 60 years of age,[15] and noted that sugar was still found in the urine despite the withholding of sugar-containing foods.[16] He recommended small meals free of sugar and acid as the best diet for diabetes.[15] Bence Jones thought that medication must diffuse through tissue before it could produce a medical effect. He believed that it would be worthwhile to determine the rates of diffusion and the amount of time that the medication was present in the body. He and August Dupré gave guinea pigs small doses of lithium carbonate, orally or subcutaneously, and sacrificed them at intervals of a few minutes to several days. Lithium was detected in vascular tissues, the cartilage of the hip joint, and the humors of the eye within 15 minutes. In a half-hour, it appeared in the lens of the eye. They then studied quinine and reported that it '… passed into all the vascular, and most probably into the extra-vascular textures'[17] of guinea pigs within 15 minutes of ingestion of the drug. They extended their studies to humans and found that quinine was detectable in the urine 10–20 minutes after ingestion. It attained a maximal level in tissues at 3 hours. Thus, Bence Jones introduced the use of biochemical tracers in medicine.[9]

Jones published a series of lectures on the 'applications of chemistry and medicine to pathology and therapeutics.' He became secretary of the Royal Institution in 1860 and subsequently wrote a history of it, including its first founders and first professors. He served as editor of the *Manual of Chemistry*. He believed that medical men would be better served if they spent time acquiring knowledge about chemistry and physics rather than learning Latin and Greek. Bence Jones began his laboratory work each day at dawn, and spent the afternoons and evenings doing hospital rounds. Medical students did not seek his clerkship because he was not adept at clinical teaching and had a well-known lack of punctuality. He made his diagnoses quickly and briefly. Irritable in manner and at times impetuous, he was sometimes too quick with criticism for those with opposing views. He was self-reliant and strong-willed, and his chief characteristics were scientific truth, accuracy, and a dislike of empiricism. He always called for the 'medical facts.' Bence Jones taught students to 'be as long as you like in forming your opinion on a case, but when you have thoroughly formed it, stick to

where he subsequently advanced rapidly to assistant physician and then to physician. In 1846, he was elected a Fellow of the Royal Society.

Dr Bence Jones was an accomplished physician and soon acquired a large and remunerative practice (Fig. 1.6). His patients included the German chemist, August Wilhelm Hofmann, and the English biologist, Thomas Huxley. Charles Darwin, the great naturalist, was another of his patients, whom he treated with a diet that 'half starved him to death.' His profits reached £7400 from 5 April 1864 to 5 April 1865.[12] Bence Jones stated that 'each year my practice gradually increased and I endeavoured to let no year pass without doing something original in natural science as applied to medicine.'[11,13]

Hermann von Helmholtz, the inventor of the ophthalmoscope, had great respect for Bence Jones, whom he described as a charming man, simple, harmless, cordial as a child, and extraordinarily kind. Bence Jones was also well acquainted with Florence Nightingale and had a high opinion of her, seeking her advice about a project that he was considering for reform of nurses' training in the hospitals of London. She, in turn, regarded him as the

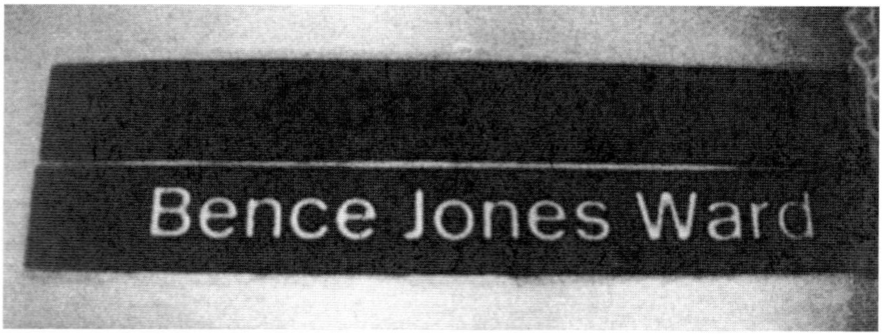

Figure 1.7 *Bence Jones ward at St George's Hospital, Tooting. (From Kyle.[68] By permission of Churchill Livingstone, New York.)*

it.'[12] He was unwilling to mix several chemicals together. His prescriptions were said to be simple and precise.[9] He is quoted as saying that there is scarcely a drug '... which may not under different conditions produce opposite effects.'[13]

In 1861, Bence Jones experienced frequent heart palpitations and diagnosed rheumatic heart disease with his stethoscope on hearing a mitral systolic murmur. He had had an episode of rheumatic fever in 1839. He resigned as physician at St George's Hospital in early 1862. He also gave up attending at the Institution for Invalid Ladies in Harley Street. A pleural effusion developed in 1866, and he again examined himself and stated, 'I fancied that one side was half-full of fluid.'[11] Despite his illness, he went to Nottingham as the chairman of the Chemical Section of the British Association for the Advancement of Science. He was the first physician to hold this prestigious position. He returned to his home in Folkestone on 1 September and was taken 'dangerously ill.' He returned to London at the beginning of winter, but his disease exacerbated and he almost died in January 1867. He improved slowly and was able to leave the house in May. The following year, he delivered the Croonian Lectures on 'Matter and Force' at the College of Physicians.[9] From then on, his energy decreased, although he traveled to Oxford in 1870 to receive an honorary degree of Doctor of Civil Letters. In a letter to John Tyndall, in August 1870, he stated: 'I am very lazy and feel unfit for any work and as neither eating, drinking nor sleeping come pleasantly to me I am a useless mortal and had better be helping the worms and the grass to grow faster than they otherwise would do ...'[18] He gave up his practice in early 1873 because of congestive hepatomegaly, ascites and anasarca. He resigned as secretary of the Royal Institution on 3 March 1873. He wrote, 'I cannot end this letter without expressing to you again my report that I must cease to be your secretary, but my health forbids me to ... continue to be your most earnest servant. Signed – Henry Bence Jones.'[19]

Bence Jones died at home at 84 Brook Street in London of congestive heart failure on 20 April 1873 at the age of 59 years and was buried at Kensal Green Cemetery.[12] Interestingly, although Bence Jones's obituary described his work on renal stones, diabetes mellitus, and malignant and tuberculous involvement of the kidney, and his emphasis on the value of microscopic analysis of the urine, there was no mention of his articles on the unique urinary protein that bears his name.[16]

Incidentally, Henry Bence Jones did not use the hyphen in his name, and it does not appear in any of his more than 40 papers and books; books published during his lifetime enter him under Jones. The hyphen was added by his descendants over half a century after his death.[20] The Bence Jones Ward still exists at St George's Hospital in Tooting (Fig. 1.7).

Other players in the history of Bence Jones proteinuria

Several other persons were involved in the story of Bence Jones proteinuria. J.F. Heller (Fig. 1.8) in 1846 described a protein in the urine that precipitated when warmed a little above 56 °C and then disappeared on further heating. Although Heller did not recognize the precipitation of the protein when the urine was cooled, it is nearly certain that this was Bence Jones protein. He distinguished this new protein from albumin and casein.[21] Bradshaw, in 1898, found that meals had little or no influence on the amount of Bence Jones proteinuria.[22] There was no nocturnal variation and he believed that the rate of excretion was 'pretty constant throughout the 24 hours.' This finding was supported by Walters, who reported that the amount of protein in a patient's diet had no effect on the amount of Bence Jones proteinuria.[23]

Two distinct groups of Bence Jones proteins were recognized by Bayne-Jones and Wilson in 1922.[24] In 1956, Korngold and Lipari demonstrated a relationship between Bence Jones protein and the serum proteins of multiple myeloma.[25] It is in tribute to Korngold and Lipari that the two major classes of Bence Jones protein have been designated κ and λ.

In 1962, 117 years after the description of the unique heat properties, Edelman and Galley[26] demonstrated that the light chains prepared from a serum immunoglobulin G (IgG) myeloma protein and the Bence Jones protein from the same patient's urine had the same amino acid

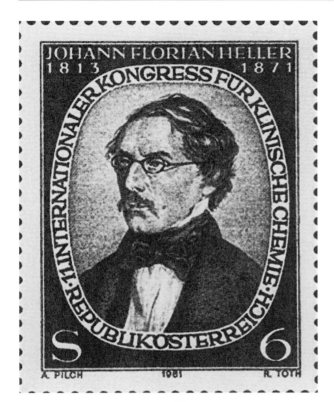

Figure 1.8 *J.F. Heller. (From Kyle.[68] By permission of Churchill Livingstone, New York.)*

sequence, similar spectrofluorometric behavior, the same molecular weight, identical appearance on chromatography with carboxymethylcellulose and on starch-gel electrophoresis after reduction and alkylation, and the same ultracentrifugal pattern – as well as the same thermal solubility. The light chains precipitated when the protein was heated to between 40 °C and 60 °C, dissolved on boiling, and reprecipitated when cooled to between 40 °C and 60 °C.

MULTIPLE MYELOMA – SOME FURTHER EARLY CASES

In 1867, Hermann Weber described a 40-year-old man with myeloma who suffered frequent colds in the spring and experienced sternal pain in May.[27] The sternum was tender and then became deformed. The patient also had severe pain in the lumbar region. Movement of his head produced pain in his neck and arms. He died 3.5 months after the onset of pain. Postmortem examination revealed that the sternum was almost entirely replaced by a grayish-red substance that had the microscopic appearance of a sarcoma. There were also two fractures of the sternum. Several round defects in the skull were

replaced by the same morbid substance as found in the sternum. Many of the ribs, several vertebrae, and parts of the pelvis were involved. Amyloid was found in the kidneys and spleen. Five years later, William Adams described a patient with 'acute rheumatism' characterized by bone pain, fractures, and fever.[28] The left humerus and femur fractured while placing the body on the autopsy table. Lardaceous changes were found in the liver and kidneys. The cancellous portion of the bones was replaced by a homogeneous, soft, gelatinoid substance. Examined microscopically, the colloid substance filling the hollowed bone consisted of small, spherical and oval cells that contained one oval nucleus (rarely, two) with a bright nucleolus.

The term 'multiple myeloma' was introduced in 1873 by von Rustizky[29] (working in von Recklinghausen's laboratory) when, during autopsy, he found eight separate tumors of bone marrow and designated them as multiple myeloma. The patient, a 47-year-old man, had presented with a gradually enlarging tumor in the right temple. Subsequently, thickening of the manubrium and seventh rib developed. This was followed by paraplegia. At autopsy, it was revealed that an apple-sized tumor in the right frontal region extended into the orbit and had produced ophthalmoplegia. Other findings included an apple-sized tumor in the right fifth rib, a tumor in the left seventh rib (producing a fracture), a tumor of the sternum, a tumor of the sixth to the eighth thoracic vertebrae (producing paraplegia), and three tumors of the right humerus. He did not mention the presence of abnormal urine protein. Although von Rustizky's description of the tumor cells is vague, he described round cells the size of white cells whose nucleus was located in the periphery near the cell membrane. In Russia, the term 'Rustizky's disease' is often used.

Willy Kühne, in 1883, described a 40-year-old man from Amsterdam who he thought had acute osteomalacia.[30] He had marked tenderness of the cervical and thoracic spine and had trouble sleeping at night because of pain and curvature of the spine. He was unable to lie on his back. His head was flexed forward. During the last weeks of his life, dysphasia and paralysis of the seventh cranial nerve developed, probably from an extradural plasmacytoma. He died on 27 August 1869, 9 months after the onset. There was no autopsy report. His brother is thought to have died of the same disease. The patient's urine precipitated on warming to between 40 °C and 50 °C and cleared at 100 °C. Kühne isolated the protein and found that the carbon, hydrogen, and nitrogen levels were similar to those described by Bence Jones. Kühne attributed any differences to the fact that his preparation was more pure than Bence Jones' preparation. He labeled the protein 'albumosurie.'

There was little further interest in the disease until 1889, when Otto Kahler described a striking case involving a 46-year-old physician named Dr Loos.[31] His first symptom, noted in July 1879, consisted of sudden severe pain in the right upper thorax, which was aggravated by taking a deep breath. Six months later, the pain recurred and became localized to the right third rib, which was tender to pressure. During the next 2 years, intermittent pain, aggravated by exercise, occurred in the ribs, spinal column, left shoulder, upper arm, and right clavicle. Albuminuria was first noticed in September 1881. Skeletal pain, made worse by movement, continued to occur intermittently. Pallor was noted in 1883. In December 1885, Dr Loos was first seen by Kahler, who noted anemia, severe kyphosis and tenderness of many bones, and albumosuria. The urinary protein had the same characteristics as that described by Bence Jones. When Dr Loos stood, the lower ribs touched the iliac crest. He had recurrent bronchial infections and intermittent hemoptysis. During the following year, kyphosis increased and his height decreased monthly. He became dwarf-like. The kyphosis of the upper thoracic spinal column increased and his chin pressed against the sternum, producing a decubitus ulcer.

On 26 August 1887, Dr Loos died, 8 years after the onset of symptoms. Autopsy revealed hepatosplenomegaly. The ribs were soft and could be broken with minimal effort. Soft gray-reddish masses were noted in the ribs and thoracic vertebrae. Microscopic examination showed large, round cells consistent with myeloma. It is interesting to note that the patient had a high fluid intake and took sodium bicarbonate on a regular basis. This may have helped prevent renal failure.

Otto Kahler

Otto Kahler, born in 1849, was the son of a well-known physician in Prague (Fig. 1.9). He received his MD degree from the University of Prague in 1871 and then worked as an assistant in Professor Halla's clinic. During a sabbatical in Paris, he met two French neurologists, Jean Martin Charcot and G.B.A. Duchenne (Duchenne de Boulogne). Kahler became interested in neurology and particularly in anatomy. He contributed to the pathologic anatomy of the central nervous system and to the anatomy of tabes dorsalis, localization of central oculomotor paralysis, and slow compression of the spinal cord. He became professor of medicine in Prague and, after Halla's resignation, became head of the Second Medical Clinic at the German University of Prague. In 1889, Kahler was invited to succeed the famous physician Heinrich Bamberger as professor at the University of Vienna.[32] In his inaugural address on 13 May 1889, Kahler paid tribute to Professor Bamberger and finished his lecture with one of Bamberger's quotes: 'Ars longa, vita brevis' (the art of medicine is long, life is short).[33] Little did he realize

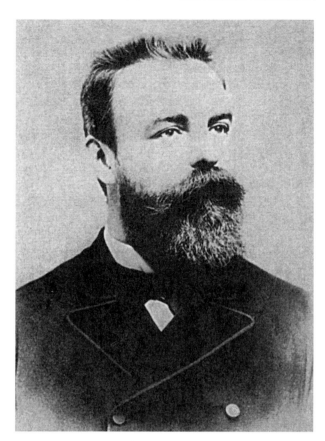

Figure 1.9 *Otto Kahler. (Courtesy of Dr Heinz Ludwig, Vienna.)*

that the tumor on his tongue biopsied in the summer of 1889 was malignant. The carcinoma recurred the following year and a huge tumor developed, causing paralysis of the vagus nerve and compression of the esophagus and main bronchus. Kahler died on 24 January 1893, shortly after his forty-fourth birthday.[34]

Kahler was extremely kind to his patients and was an excellent teacher. He emphasized that it was important to cover the entire field of general internal medicine. His obituaries and eulogies made no mention of his famous case report. It is of interest to note that the landmark contributions by Henry Bence Jones and Otto Kahler were not recognized during their lifetimes.

MULTIPLE MYELOMA IN THE NINETEENTH AND TWENTIETH CENTURIES

The first case of multiple myeloma in the United States was reported by Herrick and Hektoen in 1894.[35] The patient, a 40-year-old white woman, had lumbar pain and a nodule on the lower end of the sternum. At autopsy, multiple nodules attached to the sternum, right clavicle, and ribs were found. The sternum was thickened, irregular and covered with tumor masses, but it was soft and flexible. Multiple nodules were found on the ribs, which bent readily without cracking. Two of the dorsal vertebral bodies were largely replaced by soft tumor masses. Fungoid masses were seen in the skull. Microscopic examination revealed round, lymphoid cells with large nuclei.

Just 3 years after the discovery of X-rays by Roentgen, Weber reported a case of multiple myeloma and stated that the diagnosis of such cases would be greatly facilitated by the use of X-rays. He concluded that Bence Jones protein was produced by the bone marrow. He also believed that the presence of Bence Jones protein was of 'fatal significance' and nearly always indicated that the patient had multiple myeloma.[36] Weber and Ledingham later suggested that Bence Jones protein came from the cytoplasmic residua of karyolyzed plasma cells.[37]

In 1900, Wright described a 54-year-old man with multiple myeloma and pointed out that the tumor consisted of plasma cells.[38] He emphasized that the neoplasm originated not from red marrow cells collectively but from only one type of cell, the plasma cell. (This patient was one of the first in whom roentgenograms revealed changes in the ribs and thus contributed to the diagnosis.) The term 'plasma cell' was coined by Waldeyer in 1875,[39] but his description is not characteristic of plasma cells, and he most likely was describing tissue mast cells. Plasma cells were described accurately by Ramón y Cajal in 1890 during study of syphilitic condylomas; he stated that the unstained perinuclear area (hof) contained the Golgi apparatus.[40] In 1891, Unna used the term 'plasma cell' while describing cells seen in the skin of patients with lupus erythematosus.[41] However, it is not known whether he actually saw plasma cells. In 1895, Marschalkó described the essential characteristics of plasma cells, including blocked chromatin, eccentric position of the nucleus, a perinuclear pale area (hof), and spherical or irregular cytoplasm.[42]

Geschickter and Copeland in 1928 presented an analysis of all 425 cases of multiple myeloma reported since 1848.[43] They called attention to six cardinal features of the disease: back pain, anemia, chronic renal disease, Bence Jones proteinuria, pathologic fractures, and multiple involvement with tumors of the skeletal trunk. Sternal aspiration of the bone marrow, described in 1929 by Arinkin,[44] greatly increased the antemortem recognition of multiple myeloma.[45] Bayrd and Heck described 83 patients with histologic proof of multiple myeloma seen at the Mayo Clinic through December 1945.[46] The duration of survival ranged from 1 to 84 months (median 15 months).

Although Jacobson had reported Bence Jones protein in the serum and urine in 1917,[47] it was not until 1928 that Perlzweig et al. reported hyperproteinemia when they described a patient with multiple myeloma who had 9–11 g of globulin in his serum.[48] The patient also had Bence Jones proteinuria and probably a small amount of Bence Jones protein in the plasma. They also noted that it was almost impossible to obtain serum from the clotted blood because the clot failed to retract, even on prolonged centrifugation. Cryoglobulinemia was recognized by Wintrobe and Buell[49] in 1933 and named 'cryoglobulin' by Lerner and Watson in 1947.[50] In 1938, von Bonsdorff et al. described a patient with cryoglobulinemia in which the globulins crystallized after exposure to the cold for 24 hours.[51]

In 1890, von Behring and Kitasato described a specific neutralizing substance in the blood of animals immunized with diphtheria and tetanus toxin.[52] These antibodies were found after the injection of most foreign proteins. In 1937, Tiselius used an electrophoretic technique to separate serum globulins into three components, which he designated α, β and γ.[53] Interestingly, this article, which led to his Nobel Prize and later to the presidency of the Nobel Foundation, was rejected initially by Biochemical Journal.[54] Two years later, Tiselius and Kabat localized antibody activity in the gamma globulin fraction of the plasma proteins.[55] They noted that antibodies to albumin or pneumococcus type I were found in the area of γ mobility in rabbit serum and antibodies to pneumococcal organisms migrated between β and γ in horse serum. Later, it was recognized that some antibodies migrate in the fast γ region and others in the slow, and some sediment in the ultracentrifuge as 7S and others as 19S molecules; but the concept of a family of proteins with antibody activity was not proposed until late in the 1950s.[56] Before 1960, the term 'gamma globulin' was used for any protein that migrated in the γ mobility region of the electrophoretic pattern. Now these proteins are referred to as immunoglobulins – IgG, IgA, IgM, IgD, and IgE.

In 1939, Longsworth et al. applied electrophoresis to the study of multiple myeloma and demonstrated the tall, narrow-based 'church-spire' peak.[57] The electrophoresis apparatus was cumbersome and difficult to use; the original commercial models were 20 feet long and 5 feet high, and often occupied a separate laboratory room. A single electrophoresis run required a full day and the interpretation of an experienced operator.[18] The use of filter paper as a support permitted the separation of protein into discrete zones that could be stained with various dyes.[58] Cellulose acetate then supplanted filter paper.[59] Electrophoresis on agarose gel is now used in most laboratories. In 1953, Grabar and Williams described immunoelectrophoresis, which has facilitated the diagnosis of multiple myeloma.[60] Immunofixation or direct immunoelectrophoresis was described by Wilson in 1964, when he applied antisera on the surface of the agar immediately after the completion of electrophoresis.[61]

Alwall, in 1947, reported that a patient with typical multiple myeloma had a reduction in globulin from

5.9 to 2.2 g/dl, an increase in hemoglobin from 60% to 87%, disappearance of proteinuria, and a reduction in bone marrow plasma cells from 33% to 0% when treated with urethane.[62] For almost 20 years, urethane was commonly used for the treatment of myeloma. Holland *et al.* randomized 83 patients with treated or untreated multiple myeloma to receive urethane or a placebo consisting of cherry and cola-flavored syrup.[63] There was no difference in objective improvement nor in survival of the two treatment groups. In fact, the urethane-treated patients died earlier on average than those treated with placebo. This difference was ascribed to the increased mortality of urethane-treated patients who were azotemic. The patients with poorer prognostic features had a significantly shorter survival with urethane therapy.

In 1958, Blokhin *et al.* reported benefit in three of six patients with multiple myeloma who were treated with sarcolysin.[64] Four years later, Bergsagel *et al.* found significant improvement in eight of 24 patients with multiple myeloma who were treated with DL-phenylalanine mustard (melphalan, Alkeran).[65] Six other patients obtained improvement in one or more objective factors. Cyclophosphamide-treated patients with myeloma had a median survival of 24.5 months, whereas an ancillary myeloma group had a median survival of 9.5 months.[66] Objective improvement occurred in 81 of 207 patients. Various combinations of alkylating agents have since been used for the treatment of multiple myeloma, but there is no evidence that they are superior to melphalan and prednisone.[67,68]

KEY DATES

- 1844 First case report of multiple myeloma (Sarah Newbury).
- 1847 Description of Bence Jones proteinuria.
- 1850 Case report of Thomas Alexander McBean.
- 1873 Introduction of term 'multiple myeloma.'
- 1875 The term 'plasma cell' was coined by Waldeyer.
- 1900 First description of abnormal radiographs in multiple myeloma.
- 1928 Hyperglobulinemia noted in multiple myeloma.
- 1937 Electrophoresis delineates α, β and γ globulins.
- 1939 Tall, narrow-based, 'church-spire' peak described in multiple myeloma.
- 1958 Report of sarcolysin (melphalan) for therapy by Blokhin.

ACKNOWLEDGMENTS

This was supported in part by grant CA62242 from the National Cancer Institute. Parts of this chapter have been previously published in Kyle.[3] This source is copyrighted by the authors and used with permission.

REFERENCES

- = Key primary paper
◆ = Major review article
* = Paper that represents the first formal publication of a management guideline

1. Clamp JR. Some aspects of the first recorded case of multiple myeloma. *Lancet* 1967; **2**:1354–6.
●2. Macintyre W. Case of mollities and fragilitas ossium, accompanied with urine strongly charged with animal matter. *Medico-Chir Trans Lond* 1850; **33**:211–32.
◆3. Kyle RA. History of multiple myeloma. In: Wiernik PH, Canellos GP, Kyle RA, Schiffer CA (eds) *Neoplastic diseases of the blood*, 2nd edn. New York: Churchill Livingstone, 1991:325–32.
4. Bence Jones H. Chemical pathology. *Lancet* 1847; **2**:88–92.
5. Dalrymple J. On the microscopical character of mollities ossium. *Dublin Q J Med Sci* 1846; **2**:85–95.
6. Solly S. Remarks on the pathology of mollities ossium: with cases. *Medico-Chir Trans Lond* 1844; **27**:435–61.
◆7. Kyle RA. Multiple myeloma: an odyssey of discovery (historical article). *Br J Haematol* 2000; **111**:1035–44.
8. Bence Jones H. On a new substance occurring in the urine of a patient with mollities ossium. *Phil Trans R Soc Lond Biol* 1848; 55–62.
◆9. Kyle RA. Henry Bence Jones: physician, chemist, scientist and biographer: a man for all seasons. *Br J Haematol* 2001; **115**:13–18.
10. Coley NG. Henry Bence-Jones, M.D., F.R.S. (1813–1873). *Notes Rec R Soc Lond* 1973; **28**:31–56.
●11. Bence Jones H. *An autobiography (with elucidations at later dates by his son, A. B. Bence-Jones)*. London: Crusha & Sons Limited (privately printed), 1929.
12. Obituary. Henry Bence Jones, M.D., M.A., F.R.C.P., F.R.S. *Med Times Gaz* 1873; **1**:505.
13. Rosenbloom J. An appreciation of Henry Bence Jones, M.D., F.R.S. (1814–1873). *Ann Med Hist* 1919; **2**:262–4.
14. Bence Jones H. On a deposit of crystallized xanthin in human urine. *J Chem Soc Lond* 1862; **15**:78–80.
15. Bence Jones H. On intermitting diabetes, and on the diabetes of old age. *Medico-Chir Trans Lond* 1853; **36**:403.
16. Obituary. Dr Henry Bence Jones. *Lancet* 1873; **1**:614–15.
17. Bence Jones H, Dupré A. On a fluorescent substance, resembling quinine, in animals; and on the rate of passage of quinine into the vascular and non-vascular textures of the body. *Proc R Soc Lond Ser B Biol Sci* 1866; **15**:73–93.
◆18. Putnam FW. Henry Bence Jones: the best chemical doctor in London. *Perspect Biol Med* 1993; **36**:565–79.
19. Bence Jones H. Letter of resignation of office of Secretary of the Royal Institution. 3 March, 1873.

20. Rosenfeld L. Henry Bence Jones (1813–1873): the best 'chemical doctor' in London. *Clin Chem* 1987; **33**:1687–92.

21. Heller JF. Die mikroskopisch-chemisch-pathologische Untersuchung. In: von Gaal G. (ed.) *Physikalische Diagnostik und deren Anwendung in der Medicin, Chirurgie, Oculistik, Otiatrik und Geburtshilfe, enthaltend: Inspection, Mensuration, Palpation, Percussion und Auscultation, nebst Einer Kurzen Diagnose der Krankheiten der Athmungsund Kreislaufsorgane.* Vienna: Braumüller and Seidel, 1846:576–97.

22. Bradshaw TR. Cited in Bryant T. A case of albumosuria in which the albumose was spontaneously precipitated. *Br Med J* 1898; **1**:1136.

23. Walters W. Bence-Jones proteinuria: a report of three cases with metabolic studies. *J Am Med Assoc* 1921; **76**:641–5.

●24. Bayne-Jones S, Wilson DW. Immunological reactions of Bence-Jones proteins. II. Differences between Bence-Jones proteins from various sources. *Bull Johns Hopkins Hosp* 1922; **33**:119–25.

25. Korngold L, Lipari R. Multiple-myeloma proteins. III. The antigenic relationship of Bence Jones proteins to normal gamma-globulin and multiple-myeloma serum proteins. *Cancer* 1956; **9**:262–72.

26. Edelman GM, Galley JA. The nature of Bence-Jones proteins: chemical similarities to polypeptide chains of myeloma globulins and normal γ-globulins. *J Exp Med* 1962; **116**:207–27.

27. Weber H. Mollities ossium, doubtful whether carcinomatous or syphilitic. *Trans Pathol Soc Lond* 1867; **18**:206–9.

28. Adams W. Mollities ossium. *Trans Pathol Soc Lond* 1872; **23**:186–7.

29. Von Rustizky J. Multiples myelom. *Deutsche Zeitschrift Chir (Berlin)* 1873; **3**:162–72.

30. Kühne W. Ueber Hemialbumose im Harn. *Zeitschrift Biol (Munich)* 1883; **19**:209–27.

●31. Kahler O. Zur Symptomatologie des multiplen Myeloms: Beobachtung von Albumosurie. *Prager Med Wochenschr (Prague)* 1889; **14**:33; 45.

32. Kraus F. Gedächtnisrede auf Otto Kahler. *Wiener Klin Wochenschr (Wien)* 1894; **27**:110.

33. Sigmund CL. Zur örtlichen Behandlung: syphilitischer Mund-Nasen- und Rachenaffektionen. *Wiener Klin Wochenschr (Wien)* 1870; **20**:781.

34. Nothnagel. Hofrath Otto Kahler. *Wiener Klin Wochenschr (Wien)* 1893; **6**:79–80.

35. Herrick JB, Hektoen L. Myeloma: report of a case. *Med News* 1894; **65**:239–42.

36. Weber FP, Hutchison R, Macleod JJR. Multiple myeloma (myelomatosis), with Bence-Jones protein in the urine (myelopathic albumosuria of Bradshaw, Kahler's disease). *Am J Med Sci* 1903; **126**:644–65.

37. Weber FP, Ledingham JCG. A note on the histology of a case of myelomatosis (multiple myeloma) with Bence-Jones protein in the urine (myelopathic albumosuria). *Proc R Soc Med Lond* 1909; **2**:193–206.

38. Wright JH. A case of multiple myeloma. *Johns Hopkins Hosp Rep* 1900; **9**:359–66.

39. Waldeyer W. Ueber Bindegewebszellen. *Arch mikrosk Anat (Bonn)* 1875; **11**:176–94.

40. Ramón y Cajal S. Estudios histológicos sobre los tumores epiteliales. *Rev Trimest Microgr* 1896; **1**:83–111.

41. Unna PG. Über plasmazellen, insbesondere beim Lupus. *Monatsschrift Praktische Dermatol (Hamburg)* 1891; **12**:296.

42. Marschalkó T. Ueber die sogenannten Plasmazellen, ein Beitrag zur Kenntniss der Herkunft der entzündlichen Infiltrationszellen. *Arch Dermatol Syphilis (Wien)* 1895; **30**:241.

43. Geschickter CF, Copeland MM. Multiple myeloma. *Arch Surg* 1928; **16**:807–63.

44. Arinkin MI. Die intravitale Untersuchungsmethodik des Knochenmarks. *Folia Haematol (Leipzig)* 1929; **38**:233–40.

45. Rosenthal N, Vogel P. Value of the sternal puncture in the diagnosis of multiple myeloma. *Mt Sinai J Med* 1938; **4**:1001–19.

46. Bayrd ED, Heck FJ. Multiple myeloma: a review of eighty-three proved cases. *J Am Med Assoc* 1947; **133**:147–57.

47. Jacobson VC. A case of multiple myelomata with chronic nephritis showing Bence-Jones protein in urine and blood serum. *J Urol* 1917; **1**:167–78.

48. Perlzweig WA, Delrue G, Geschickter C. Hyperproteinemia associated with multiple myelomas: report of an unusual case. *J Am Med Assoc* 1928; **90**:755–7.

49. Wintrobe MM, Buell MV. Hyperproteinemia associated with multiple myeloma: with report of a case in which an extraordinary hyperproteinemia was associated with thrombosis of the retinal veins and symptoms suggesting Raynaud's disease. *Bull Johns Hopkins Hosp* 1933; **52**:156–65.

50. Lerner AB, Watson CJ. Studies of cryoglobulins. I. Unusual purpura associated with the presence of a high concentration of cryoglobulin (cold precipitable serum globulin). *Am J Med Sci* 1947; **214**:410–15.

51. Von Bonsdorff B, Groth H, Packalén T. On the presence of a high-molecular crystallizable protein in the blood serum in myeloma. *Folia Haematol (Leipzig)* 1938; **59**:184–208.

52. Von Behring S, Kitasato TI. Aus dem hygienischen Institut des Herrn Geheimerath Koch in Berlin. Ueber das Zustandekommen der Diphtherie-Immunität und der Tetanus-Immunität bei Thieren. *Deutsche Med Wochenschr (Leipzig)* 1890; **49**:1113–45.

●53. Tiselius A. Electrophoresis of serum globulin. II. Electrophoretic analysis of normal and immune sera. *Biochem J* 1937; **31**:1464–77.

◆54. Putnam FW. From the first to the last of the immunoglobulins: perspectives and prospects. *Clin Physiol Biochem* 1983; **1**:63–91.

55. Tiselius A, Kabat EA. An electrophoretic study of immune sera and purified antibody preparations. *J Exp Med* 1939; **69**:119–31.

56. Heremans JF. Immunochemical studies on protein pathology: the immunoglobulin concept. *Clin Chim Acta* 1959; **4**:639–46.

57. Longsworth LG, Shedlovsky T, MacInnes DA. Electrophoretic patterns of normal and pathological human blood serum and plasma. *J Exp Med* 1939; **70**:399–413.

58. Kunkel HG, Tiselius A. Electrophoresis of proteins on filter paper. *J Gen Physiol* 1951; **35**:89–118.

59. Kohn J. A cellulose acetate supporting medium for zone electrophoresis. *Clin Chim Acta* 1957; **2**:297–303.

60. Grabar P, Williams CA. Méthode permettant l'étude conjuguée des proprieteés électrophorétiques et

immunochimiques d'un mélange de protéines. Application au sérum sanguin. *Biochem Biophys Acta* 1953; **10**:193–4.

61. Wilson AT. Direct immunoelectrophoresis. *J Immunol* 1964; **92**:431–4.

62. Alwall N. Urethane and stilbamidine in multiple myeloma: report on two cases. *Lancet* 1947; **2**:388–9.

*63. Holland JF, Hosley H, Scharlau C, Carbone PP, Frei E III, Brindley CO, *et al*. A controlled trial of urethane treatment in multiple myeloma. *Blood* 1966; **27**:328–42.

◆64. Blokhin N, Larionov L, Perevodchikova N, Chebotareva L, Merkulova N. Clinical experiences with sarcolysin in neoplastic diseases. *Ann N Y Acad Sci* 1958; **68**:128–32.

65. Bergsagel DE, Sprague CC, Austin C, Griffith KM. Evaluation of new chemotherapeutic agents in the treatment of multiple myeloma. IV. L-phenylalanine mustard (NSC-8806). *Cancer Chemother Rep* 1962; **21**:87–99.

66. Korst DR, Clifford GO, Fowler WM, Louis J, Will J, Wilson HE. Multiple myeloma: II. Analysis of cyclophosphamide therapy in 165 patients. *J Am Med Assoc* 1964; **189**:758–62.

67. Myeloma Trialists' Collaborative Group. Combination chemotherapy versus melphalan plus prednisone as treatment for multiple myeloma: an overview of 6,633 patients from 27 randomized trials. *J Clin Oncol* 1998; **16**:3832–42.

◆68. Kyle RA. History of multiple myeloma. In: Wiernik PH, Canellos GP, Kyle RA, Schiffer CA (eds) *Neoplastic diseases of the blood,* 3rd edn. New York: Churchill Livingstone, 1996:411–22.

2

Epidemiology and etiology of plasma cell neoplasms

DANIEL E. BERGSAGEL AND P. LEIF BERGSAGEL

INTRODUCTION

Plasma cell neoplasms are distinguished by an idiotypic rearrangement of the immunoglobulin gene, which occurs prior to the malignant transformation of an early plasma cell precursor. The clone that develops must increase to about 5×10^9 cells before it produces enough of the idiotypic immunoglobulin to be recognized as a monoclonal 'spike' (M-protein or paraprotein) in a serum electrophoresis pattern. Most subjects with a serum M-protein are asymptomatic; if other causes of an M-protein can be ruled out, they are labeled as monoclonal gammopathies of undetermined significance (MGUS). By definition, the monoclone in MGUS is stable and the serum M-protein concentration remains level for many years. However, prolonged follow-up of a large group of MGUS subjects at the Mayo Clinic has shown that about 2% of these patients progress per year to develop symptomatic multiple myeloma (MM), macroglobulinemia, malignant lymphoma, chronic lymphocytic leukemia or amyloidosis (Chapter 24).[1] MGUS is considered to be a premalignant lesion because the clone does not grow progressively but is stable and asymptomatic. Almost all of the genetic aberrations identified in MM (aneuploidy, monosomy 13, 14q32 chromosome translocations) are also present in MGUS.[2] Additional neoplastic changes are required to convert this large stable clone into MM, a progressively expanding tumor with malignant characteristics.

THE FREQUENCY OF MGUS AND MM

Prevalence of MGUS

The *prevalence* of an M-protein (i.e. the number of cases in a defined population at a certain time) in people over the age of 25 years was determined in the spring of 1964 in the Värmland district of Sweden by performing paper electrophoresis on 6995 consecutive serum samples. The sera of 64 subjects in this sample (0.9%) contained an M-protein.[3] Only one of these subjects was found to have MM; 63 were classified as MGUS. Among the 6931 subjects without serum M-components in 1964, two were diagnosed as MM (one had light-chain myeloma) within 3 years.[4] The population of Värmland in 1964 was about 100 000. In the 70% of the adult population of this district who had a serum electrophoresis done in the spring of 1964, the prevalence of MGUS was 901/100 000 (0.9%), and of MM 43/100 000 (0.04%). MGUS is encountered much more frequently than MM because these subjects are well; in contrast to MM patients, who have a median survival of only 32 months from the onset of treatment with conventional chemotherapy, MGUS cases tend to survive for prolonged periods and thus accumulate in the population.

Incidence of MGUS

The *incidence* of MGUS (i.e. the number of new cases developing in a defined population over a defined period of time) has not been determined. Two recent registry studies help to provide a rough estimate. In the Comprehensive Cancer Center West Netherlands, the registry collected information from 15 hospitals in a region with 1.7 million inhabitants. They found a frequency of newly discovered paraproteinemias of 31/100 000, and 189/100 000 in those over 70, and 56% of these were classified as MGUS. In Iceland, a database was constructed of the 713 people with monoclonal gammopathy diagnosed between 1976 and 1997, and compared with the Icelandic Cancer Registry. The authors estimated an age-standardized (world standard) incidence of monoclonal gammopathy per 100 000 of 14.7 (men) and 12.5 (women) for the period 1992–97. Of these, approximately 71% were MGUS.[5]

Incidence of MM

The frequency of MM in a population is strongly influenced by age, race and the availability of good medical care. In the USA, the Surveillance, Epidemiology, and End Results (SEER) program has provided MM incidence data since 1973. Traditionally it has adjusted rates to the

1970 US standard population. Starting in 2002, it is using the 2000 US standard population, which places more emphasis on older persons, in whom MM rates are more common, so that the rates are not directly comparable with rates reported in previous years. For the 1995–99 period, the average, annual, age-adjusted (2000 US standard) incidence rates per 100 000 for all races in the USA was 5.6 for both sexes, 6.9 for males, and 4.6 for females.[6] In a disease like MM, *mortality rates* are very similar to the incidence rates because almost all of the people who develop the disease die from it. Reported mortality rates for MM, however, are usually somewhat lower than incidence rates. For 1995–99, they were 3.9 for both sexes, 4.9 for males, and 3.3 for females.

MM is slightly more common in men than in women, and in blacks than in whites. The incidence of MM appeared to increase markedly in many parts of the world between 1950 and 1980. In the USA, the incidence rate appeared to increase 0.9% per year up until the early 1990s. This apparent increase has stopped, and in the period from 1997 to 1999 the incidence rate has decreased

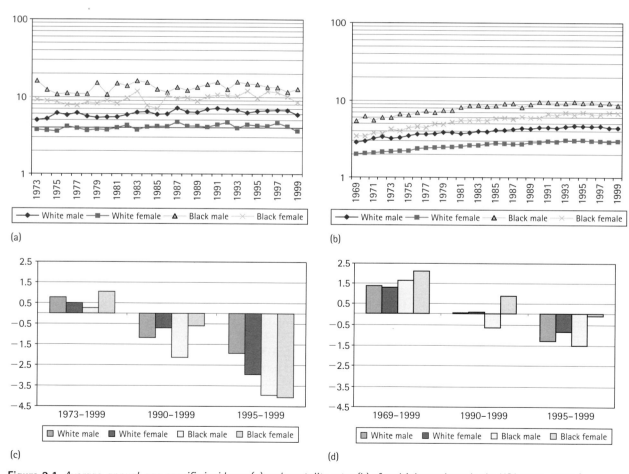

Figure 2.1 *Average, annual, age-specific incidence (a) and mortality rates (b) of multiple myeloma in the USA 1973–1999 (cases per 100 000), and estimated annual percentage change in these rates (c, incidence; d, mortality). Age-adjusted rates refer to the 2000 US (total) population.[6]*

at 7.6% per year. This figure seems quite high and no doubt longer follow-up is required to obtain an accurate estimate. It is safe to say, however, that over the past 10 years, the incidence rate in the USA is no longer increasing but is decreasing slightly. The incidence rates over times are summarized by race and gender in Fig. 2.1. The lifetime risk for being diagnosed with MM is 0.66% for men and 0.55% for women.[6]

Age

The median age of diagnosis of MM in the USA is 71 years, with a high of 73 years for white women and a low of 66 years for black men. The age-specific incidence rates for MM in the USA for 1995–99 are shown in Fig. 2.2. Myeloma was not detected in patients under the age of 35 in this sample. The incidence increases progressively with age, to reach $40.3/10^5$ in the population aged 80–84.[6] A similar study in Malmö, Sweden, in 1970–79 determined an incidence of $64.5/10^5$ in males and $36.6/10^5$ in females over the age of 80 years.[7] The median age of MM patients

eligible for admission to large clinical group studies in North America is about 62 years[8] but, when the total population of myeloma patients in an area is determined, with no exclusions, as was done in the Health Care Region of Western Sweden, the median age at diagnosis was 72 years, and the male/female ratio 1.1.[9]

The frequency of MGUS also increases with age. Axelsson et al. detected an M-protein in 0.2% of subjects aged 30–49, in 1.4% between the ages of 40 and 69, and in 4.0% of subjects aged 70–89.[3] Two surveys of the serum electrophoresis patterns of non-agenarians both reported that a surprising 19% of these sera contain M-proteins.[10,11] In the population aged 80–84 in Iceland, they estimated an incidence per 100 000 of 169 and 119 in men and women, respectively.

Race

The age-adjusted incidence (world standard population) of MM from selected population-based cancer registries

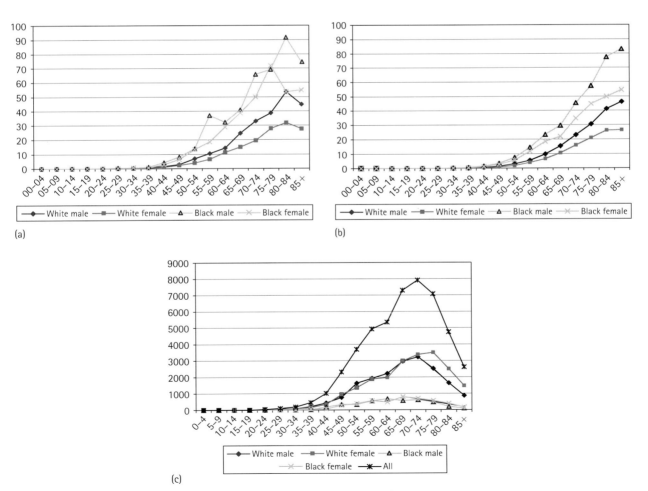

(a)

(b)

(c)

Figure 2.2 *Age-specific incidence (a) and mortality rates (b) per 100 000 (2000 US standard) for (1995–1999) and age-specific prevalence (c, 1999).*[6]

around the world range from 0.5 in Hawaiian Japanese males to 8.2 in US Bay Area black males per 100 000 person-years.[12] The incidence of MM is distinctly lower (1.4/10[5], or less, world standard population) for the Chinese of Shanghai and Singapore, and the Japanese of Osaka and Hawaii, than in the Caucasian populations of North America and Europe. Comparisons between incidence rates from cancer registries in different countries must be made cautiously, since the populations served may vary in terms of the availability of medical care and diagnostic services, the completeness of case ascertainment and the calculation of age-adjusted incidence rates. Still, there do appear to be real differences in the incidence of MM in different races. The observation that the incidence of MM, age-adjusted to the 1970 US standard, in male Chinese (2.3/10[5]) and Japanese (1.7/10[5]) living in San Francisco–Oakland and Hawaii are distinctly lower than for white males (4.6/10[5]) in the same regions support this view.[13] Surprisingly, the incidence in Filipino males (4.7/10[5]) is almost the same as that of white males in these regions.

The average annual age-adjusted (2000 US standard) incidence rates for blacks in America are more than double the rates in whites, at 13.1/10[5] for black males and 10.3/10[5] for black females.[6] The increased incidence of MM in blacks makes this disease the most common cause of hematologic malignancy mortality in the black population of the USA (Fig. 2.3). The proportion of patients who die from leukemia is similar in the two groups, while MM accounts for 37% of hematologic malignancy deaths in blacks and only 17% in whites. Hodgkin and non-Hodgkin lymphoma deaths are reduced to 30% in blacks versus 45% in whites.[6] Lower socioeconomic status may account for less then half of the increased incidence of MM in American blacks.[14] Comprehensive MM incidence data are not available for African populations, but it does appear to be high among Jamaicans and in the West Indies.[15,16] Valuable insights into the reasons for the increased incidence of MM in blacks in America might be gained if variations were to be found among black populations around the world.

A comparison of the prevalence of MGUS in subjects over the age of 60 years in retirement communities in Japan and the USA revealed an M-protein in 4/146 Japanese (2.7%) versus 11/111 American (10%).[17] The reduced prevalence of MGUS in Japan is in keeping with the lower incidence of MM in Japan. Measurements of normal immunoglobulins in these subjects by laser nephelometry provided the surprising observation that, for unknown reasons, IgG and IgA levels were significantly higher in the elderly Japanese. The frequency of MGUS in sera submitted for electrophoresis at the Houston Veterans Administration Hospital in Texas was found to be much higher in blacks than in whites, especially in the group over the age of 79.[18] Also, community screening of 1732 subjects over the age of 70 years in North Carolina identified a greater than twofold difference in prevalence between blacks (8.4%) and whites (3.8%),[19] again in agreement with the increased incidence of MM in blacks.

Prevalence of MM

In 1999, it is estimated that there were 47 709 people in the USA who had been diagnosed with MM: 18 530 white men, 20 618 white women, 4066 black men and 4495 black women. At first glance, it seems surprising that white women have the lowest incidence of MM but are most prevalent, and that black men have the highest incidence and are least prevalent. This is explained by the increased frequency of white women in the older population most at risk, and can be seen graphically when the age-specific prevalence is plotted by age and sex (Fig. 2.2).

Increasing mortality rates for MM

Trends in the MM mortality rates in the USA between 1969 and 1999 are shown in Fig. 2.1. A striking increase occurred in these rates during this period up to the early 1990s, especially in the older age groups. Similar increases were noted in the reported myeloma death rates from the UK, France, Germany, Japan, and Italy.[20] The rate of increase is largest in the group over the age of 85 years

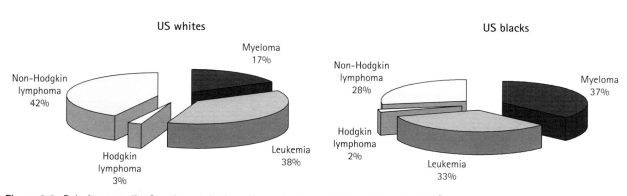

Figure 2.3 *Relative mortality from hematologic malignancies in US whites and blacks, 1999.*[6]

and falls continuously with decreasing age. The rate of increase is substantial by age 70, more than doubling in both sexes in all countries between 1968 and 1986. There has been much debate about whether this increasing mortality rate is real or the result of steadily improving case ascertainment. Since the early 1990s, the increase seems to have stopped and, if anything, mortality rates appear to be declining in the USA.

Myeloma mortality rates did not increase in Olmsted County, Minnesota, during the 33-year period from 1945 to 1977.[21] The Mayo Clinic, where there has been a continuing interest in detecting and diagnosing all plasma cell neoplasms accurately, provides most of the medical care for Olmsted County. Linos et al. suggest that all of the cases of MM have been detected and reported in Olmsted County since 1945, and since an increasing incidence has not been observed there, the reported increase in other parts of the USA is probably due to improving case ascertainment, and more apparent than real.[21] Other regions with a high standard of medical care and an interest in myeloma, such as Malmö, Sweden, and the canton of Vaud, Switzerland, also have not observed an increased incidence of myeloma.[7,22] The authors of these reports agree with the Mayo Clinic interpretation that they represent the asymptote of myeloma detection that may be matched in other areas as their case ascertainment becomes complete. In Denmark, there was a two- to three-fold increase in the incidence of MM in both men and women between 1943 and 1962 but, since then, the incidence has been stable.[23] According to the SEER database in the USA, the MM mortality rate increased at 3.8% per year from 1973 to 1976 and 1.4% from 1976 to 1994, and has decreased at 0.7% per year from 1994 to 1999.[6]

Caution must be exercised in accepting this interpretation of the worldwide increase in the incidence and mortality rates for MM, for the increases may be real. Similar patterns of increase in both men and women suggest a ubiquitous, possibly environmental factor, rather than occupational exposure. Cuzick notes that the increasing trends appear to have slowed since 1980 and are even more confined to the oldest age groups. If this increase is due to an environmental factor, then its introduction is now largely complete, suggesting that any such factor was introduced at least 20 years ago.[24] The mortality rates in the US population over 75 have been stable since 1993, with no further evidence of increase.[6]

ETIOLOGY

Radiation exposure

In 1979, Ichimaru et al. concluded that there was a statistically significant increased incidence of MM between 1950 and 1976 among the survivors exposed to radiation dose estimates of more than 1 Gy after the atomic bombs at Hiroshima and Nagasaki.[25] The increased incidence of MM became apparent about 20 years after radiation exposure. The Life Span Study of Atomic Bomb Survivors by the Radiation Effects Research Foundation has added 12 years of follow-up for the occurrence of MM. A reanalysis of the data, using Dosimetry System 1986 dose estimates, re-evaluation of all of the cases included in previous studies, and an estimation of the excess absolute risk (EAR) has changed the conclusions about the effect of radiation on the incidence of MM.[26] The increased EAR for acute lymphocytic leukemia, acute myelogenous leukemia, and chronic myelogenous leukemia was confirmed. There was some evidence of an increased risk of lymphoma in males but not in females. The risk of developing chronic lymphocytic leukemia and MM was not increased.

Also, the frequency of a monoclonal gammopathy does not appear to have increased in the survivors of the atomic bombs.[27] Cellulose acetate electrophoresis was done on an aliquot of serum from all persons examined in the Adult Health Study in Hiroshima and Nagasaki between October 1979 and September 1981, and in a second survey between June 1985 and May 1987. In the first study an M-protein was found in 31 of 8796 (0.35%), and in the second in 68 of 7350 subjects (0.93%). The relative risk of having an M-protein detected in the two surveys was not significantly increased with increasing radiation dose.

An increased risk of MM has also been reported among workers at nuclear processing plants at Hanford, Washington, and Windscale, UK, and in radium-dial painters.[28] Other studies have not noted an increased incidence of MM in radiation-exposed groups, most notably among the atomic bomb survivors.[26] An update of the National Registry of Radiation Workers in the UK has released an update on a cohort of 124 743 workers. There was no increased incidence of MM observed (40 expected, 40 observed).[29] A case-control study of 115 143 workers at three US nuclear power sites (Hanford, Oak Ridge National Laboratories and Savannah River) did not find an association of multiple myeloma with cumulative radiation dose across all ages, although it did notice a positive association with doses received at older ages.[30]

The search for other causes of plasma cell neoplasms

When a sleuth begins to hunt for a criminal, they look first for clues associated with the crime, which they try to organize into a pattern that associates one, or more, of the suspects with the felony. When enough useful clues have been collected, a testable hypothesis is formulated for the identification of the guilty person and the search moves on. The problem becomes much more complicated when there is more than one criminal. The most blatant, but not necessarily the major, culprit is usually caught first, leaving the defenders of society with the daunting task of tracking down the more devious collaborators. Since we have no promising leads, we are still in the tiresome phase of looking for clues in the dark.

The induction of plasma cell neoplasms is probably a multistep process. Genetic factors probably play a role in making a person susceptible to a change that results in the proliferation of an early B-cell precursor, to form a stable clone of plasma cells producing a monoclonal protein, as in MGUS. The conversion of the controlled stable monoclone of MGUS into the uncontrolled, progressive, malignant tumor of MM probably requires one, or more, additional changes.

COHORT STUDIES

The major tools employed by epidemiologic detectives in looking for the causes of cancer are cohort studies and case-control studies.[31] A cohort study is often the first broad-ranging attempt to detect an exposure that may be responsible for causing a cancer. Suspicious exposures are then investigated in more detail, perhaps with the aid of a hypothesis about the biologic mode of action of the agent in question. Cohort studies are not very sensitive, and they are rarely specific enough to identify the causative agent.

In a cohort study, defined populations exposed to factors suspected of increasing or decreasing the incidence of a cancer, and a control group not so exposed, are followed for an interval long enough for a number of cancers to develop. The incidence of cancer in the two groups is then compared. Of course, the exposed and unexposed groups must be as alike as possible. In an experimental trial, the exposure under investigation can be randomly assigned, and the subjects followed for the development of cancer according to a predetermined schedule and examination routine. This type of experimental trial is rarely possible in the investigation of the causes of cancer and so an observational cohort study is substituted in which the allocation of the exposure is not under the control of the investigators.

Cohort studies compare the cancer incidence in the exposed and unexposed groups. The contribution of the exposure to cancer risk is examined by calculating the ratio of the risks in the two groups, i.e. the relative risk. These studies require very large numbers of subjects, and prolonged observation, in order to have a reasonable chance of detecting a change in the incidence of cancer following exposure.

CASE-CONTROL STUDIES

Case-control studies begin with a group of patients with a cancer, e.g. myeloma, and compare the exposure to various agents of these cases with the exposure of a control group, selected to match the cases in terms of important confounding variables, such as age, race, sex, smoking history, etc. The exposure in question is assessed by a questionnaire administered to both the cases and controls; this is one of the problems with case-control studies, for exposure requires recall, which may differ in cases and controls.

The influence of the exposure being investigated on the occurrence of myeloma is assessed with the odds ratio: the number of cases exposed multiplied by the number of controls not exposed divided by the number of controls exposed multiplied by the number of cases not exposed.[31]

Case-control studies can be done quickly and require fewer subjects to detect a given level of risk. However, they are dependent on the ability of the cases and the controls to remember their exposures, and there are many potential biases in the selection of subjects and the measurement of exposure. Despite these disadvantages, case-control studies may be the best that can be done to investigate the validity of new theories about cancer risk in humans.

Socioeconomic status

In earlier times, myeloma was reported to cause increased mortality rates in members of the higher levels of society.[32] This association probably occurred because the disease was underascertained in the poor and uneducated. The reduced detection of myeloma in lower socioeconomic groups has gradually decreased with time, until the 1970s, when it disappeared.[33] A case-control study at Duke University in North Carolina failed to demonstrate any association of myeloma with family income, education, occupation, dwelling size, or an index of crowding in the home.[34]

Socioeconomic factors such as occupation, income and education have been reported to account for a fraction (49%, 28%, and 17%, respectively) of the excess risk in blacks.[14] In an earlier study, the incidence in blacks remained twice that of whites after adjustment for incomes below and above the poverty level.[35] No occupational or environmental factors have been discovered to explain the marked difference in the incidence of myeloma in blacks and whites.

Smoking

A prospective cohort study of 34 000 US Seventh Day Adventists followed for 6 years detected nine cases of myeloma in ex-smokers and two in current smokers. The risk of developing myeloma was threefold greater in subjects who had ever smoked than in those who had never smoked; a dose–response trend was also noted.[36] This group will have to be followed for longer because this positive result differs from the negative association observed in most other studies. In a cohort study done on the use of tobacco and the occurrence of leukemia, lymphoma or myeloma, Adami et al. followed 334 957 Swedish construction workers from 1971 to 1991. A total of 1322 incident cancers were identified, with no increased risk of developing leukemia, lymphoma, or myeloma.[37] Heineman et al. followed 250 000 US veterans for 26 years.[38] Myeloma deaths occurred in 582 patients in this study, but the relative risk of dying of myeloma was the same for both the smokers and those who had never smoked. Similarly, a smaller prospective cohort study of 17 633 male holders of Lutheran Brotherhood insurance, who completed a self-administered questionnaire about their use of tobacco in 1966, did not observe a significantly increased risk of death from myeloma among those who were smokers. Strangely, and in contrast, the risk of death from non-Hodgkin's lymphoma in this study was increased among men who had ever smoked, and was almost fourfold greater among the heaviest smokers.[39]

Occupations

Riedel et al. have reviewed reports of positive associations between specific occupations/industries and myeloma reported in 53 case-control, prospective and proportionate incidence/mortality studies.[12]

Employment in agriculture (predominantly farming) is the occupation most frequently associated with myeloma. Most studies have detected this association, but a few have not.[40–42] These studies have not been able to identify the aspect of agricultural work, be it contact with animals, grains, dust, fertilizers, pesticides, or engines, which increases the risk of farmers for myeloma.

Statistical associations have been made between employment as metal workers and an increased risk of myeloma. Small numbers of cases and a lack of information on actual exposures make it difficult to determine whether particular metal dusts or fumes, or other occupational exposures, are responsible for the elevated risks observed.

Five reports of increased myeloma mortality in workers employed in rubber manufacturing are included in a review by Riedel et al.,[12] but only one of these studies reported a statistically significant increase, and that was in white male union rubber reclaim workers in the USA.[43] An evaluation of British rubber reclaim workers did not find an increased risk of myeloma mortality.[44]

There have been several case reports of myeloma in subjects exposed to benzene.[45] A cohort analysis of workers (predominantly white males) employed in the manufacture of rubber hydrochloride in Pliofilm plants, by a process that includes the dissolution of natural rubber in benzene, detected four deaths from myeloma. The expected number of myeloma deaths in an unexposed normal population of the same age, sex, and race was one. However, three of the workers who developed myeloma in this study had had minimal exposure to benzene (one had worked at the plant for only 4 days) and there was no trend toward an increasing myeloma incidence with greater exposure.[46] An update of this study has added 7 years of follow-up.[47] No new cases of myeloma have developed and the standardized mortality ratio for this disease is no longer elevated significantly.

Workers in petroleum refining and petroleum production, and those exposed to fuel combustion products (e.g. truck drivers), may also be exposed to benzene, among other petroleum products. A meta-analysis of close to 100 published and unpublished reports of epidemiologic surveys of petroleum industry employees found that the risk of developing myeloma was the same as the risk in the general population.[48] Two recent, large studies of exposure to exhaust fumes have reached different conclusions. In Denmark, a historical cohort study compared the cancer-specific mortality of 14 225 exposed truck drivers with an unexposed group of 43 024 unskilled laborers, both followed for 10 years.[49] There were five deaths from myeloma among the truck drivers, where 1.25 were expected. This was an unexpected finding and the author cautions that, although it is statistically significant, it may still be due to chance. In contrast, a study of the cancer risk of 160 230 members of a prepaid health care plan who reported their exposure to engine exhaust during a routine health examination, failed to detect an increased risk of myeloma among exposed workers.[50] Two recent meta-analyses of cohort studies encompassing more than 250 000 petroleum workers[51] and case-control studies[52] did not identify an increased incidence with exposure to benzene or petroleum products. This latter study also noted a significant positive association with engine exhaust, with a summary odds ratio of 1.34, 95% confidence intervals 1.14–1.57.

An association of an increased risk of myeloma with workers in the wood, leather and textile industries has been found in some studies, but the results are inconsistent, for the association has not been detected by others.[53]

An increased risk of myeloma has been reported among painters.[54–59] The exposure of painters to chemical compounds is complex, for there are various dyes, pigments, and solvents that are known to be mutagenic in their environments. The specific agent(s), if there are any, associated with the increased risk of myeloma in painters have not been identified.

The use of hair dye has been associated with an increased risk of myeloma in several[60–63] but not all[64] studies. A prospective study conducted by the American

Cancer Society of 547 586 women who provided information on hair dye use in 1982 identified a marginally increased incidence only in women who used black dye for 10 or more years.[65] Hair coloring agents are known to contain constituents, including aromatic, nitro, and amino compounds, that are carcinogenic or mutagenic in animal or laboratory tests. Again, suspicion has not focused on any specific component of hair dyes.

Exposure to *asbestos* has been linked to an increased risk of myeloma in at least two case-control studies.[55,66] In contrast, other case-control studies have not detected this association;[67-69] it will take further work to determine whether asbestos plays a role in the etiology of myeloma.

Chronic antigenic stimulation

Clinicians have long wondered whether chronic antigenic stimulation (CAS) plays a role in the pathogenesis of myeloma.[70] The hypothesis is that CAS stimulates a proliferative response in the immune system, and that myeloma develops in one of the responding cells. There have been several attempts to correlate the occurrence of myeloma with a past history of exposure to viral or bacterial infections, immunizations, allergies, allergy desentitization therapy and autoimmune disease, but the results are inconsistent.[53] There does, however, appear to be an association between *rheumatoid arthritis* and myeloma. At least two follow-up studies of patients with rheumatoid arthritis have detected a subsequent increased incidence of myeloma,[71-73] and an excess of rheumatoid arthritis has been detected in case-control studies of myeloma in New Zealand and northern Sweden.[74,75] An examination of the frequency of autoimmune diseases among first-degree relatives of myeloma patients discovered a significantly increased risk of rheumatoid arthritis, as compared with the incidence in first-degree relatives of the controls.[76] If this finding is confirmed in larger studies, it will suggest that genetic factors underlie the association.

A case-control study of patients with *Gaucher's disease* in Israel found that these cases have an increased risk of developing hematologic malignancies, including myeloma.[77] A possible mechanism is that the accumulating glucocerebroside acts as a chronic antigenic stimulant of the immune system, as was first suggested by Shoenfeld *et al.*[78] These authors found that patients with Gaucher's disease had elevated levels of serum immunoglobulins and that these levels increased with age. In addition, Marti *et al.* detected diffuse polyclonal hyperglobulinemia in ten, oligoclonal hyperglobulinemia in six and monoclonal gammopathy (MGUS) in two of 23 patients with Gaucher's disease.[79] The sequence could be that CAS leads to a polyclonal, followed by an oligoclonal lymphocytosis and then a monoclonal proliferation, resulting in MGUS, myeloma, a lymphoma, or leukemia.

The discovery of a *human immunodeficiency virus 1 (HIV-1)-seropositive* patient with myeloma, whose IgG/kappa M-protein specifically recognized the HIV-1 p24 *gag* antigen, suggests that the antigen-driven response to the viral infection did play a role in the pathogenesis of myeloma in this patient.[80] In a prospective study of 239 patients with *hepatitis C virus* (HCV)-positive chronic liver disease and 98 patients with HCV-negative chronic liver disease, a monoclonal gammopathy was detected in 11% of the HCV-positive patients and in only 1% of the HCV-negative patients.[81]

Genetic factors

Striking differences in the incidence of plasmacytomas in inbred strains of mice, racial differences in the incidence of plasma cell neoplasms, the association of an increased risk of developing myeloma with certain human leukocyte antigens (HLA) and the occurrence of familial myeloma all suggest that genetic factors play an important role in the pathogenesis of these neoplasms.

MOUSE PLASMACYTOMAS

There are striking differences in the incidence of monoclonal gammopathy in different inbred strains of mice. About 60% of *C57BL/Ka* mice develop one or more M-proteins (usually IgG) by 24 months of age.[82] In *C3H* and *NZB* mice, 40% develop M-proteins of the IgM type, while the incidence in *BALB/c* and *CBA/Rij* mice is low.[82] The specific genes responsible for the high incidence of monoclonal gammopathy in these mice have not been identified. Few mice progress to develop a malignant plasma cell neoplasm. There is no correlation between the development of spontaneous gammopathy and susceptibility to the induction of plasmacytomas (usually IgA) by the intraperitoneal injection of mineral oil. *BALB/c* is the strain that is most susceptible to oil-induced plasmacytomas, while *C57BL/Ka* are relatively resistant.[83]

RACIAL DIFFERENCES IN THE INCIDENCE OF MM AND MGUS

As mentioned earlier, there appear to be real differences in the incidence of MM and MGUS among different races. The incidence of MM is lowest among the Japanese of Hawaii and Osaka, and the Chinese of Shanghai and Singapore, and highest in the blacks of the Bay Area and Connecticut in the USA.[12] The low incidence of MM in Japanese and Chinese populations has moved with them to Hawaii and the USA,[13] suggesting that the incidence of the disease in these populations is determined more by genetic rather than by environmental factors. The prevalence of MGUS in persons over the age of 60 years is also distinctly lower in Japan (2.7%) than in America (10%).[17]

ASSOCIATION BETWEEN MYELOMA AND HLA TYPE

A large population-based study of 46 black male MM cases (with 88 black male controls) and 85 white male MM cases (with 122 white male controls) was carried out to determine whether there is any association of human leukocyte antigens of class I (HLA -A, -B, -C) and class II (HLA-DR, HLA-DQ) with the disease.[84] Black cases had significantly higher gene frequencies than their controls for Bw65, Cw2, and DRw14, while white cases had higher gene frequencies than controls for A3 and Cw2, and blanks at the DR and DQ loci. The frequency of Cw2 in the black and white controls was similar. These findings suggest that the Cw2 allele, or a gene close to the C loci, confers susceptibility to the development of MM, but does not explain the higher risk among blacks. A more recent study among 62 South African blacks identified an association with HLA B18 (odds ratio 6.3, 95 per cent confidence interval 1.013–39.727).[85]

FAMILIAL PLASMA CELL NEOPLASIA

Several families have been reported with multiple cases of MM and MGUS (of the IgG, IgA, light chain, and IgD variety). To the 41 families reviewed by Loth et al.[86] can be added two brothers who developed IgG/k myeloma,[87] and another family in which a female patient with IgG MM was found to have two sisters and two brothers with IgG MGUS.[88] In these 43 families, MM or MGUS was detected in seven first-degree relations (parent and child), was most frequent in 32 second-degree relatives (siblings), and was much less frequent in more distant relatives, with occurrences in only one third-degree (aunt–niece) and three fourth-degree (first cousins) relations. Similar results were noted in two recent studies that add another 16 families.[89,90] Among 25 families with IgM M-proteins (Waldenström's macroglobulinemia, WM, or asymptomatic monoclonal IgM) reviewed by Renier et al.,[91] nine were first-degree and 16 were second-degree relatives.

It is of interest that the M-protein may have the same heavy and light chain in two relatives with MM or MGUS, or the light chains may differ, or the relative's M-protein may be of the IgG, IgA, or IgD variety, but no relative with an IgM M-protein has been reported. Similarly, relatives of patients with WM have been found to have an IgM M-protein but not one with any of the other heavy chains.

Although the heavy and light chains of the M-proteins in the relatives may be of the same heavy and light chain type, not surprisingly, the proteins in some of these patients have been clearly shown to be different. A rabbit antiserum to a purified urinary lambda light chain of a patient with IgA/λ myeloma did not react with the M-protein of her sister's IgA/λ M-protein.[86] In another family, idiotypic rabbit

antisera prepared against each of the IgM M-proteins of four brothers with WM failed to cross-react, showing that they do not share idiotypes.[91] The occurrence of multiple cases of a malignancy in a family without a clear Mendelian pattern of inheritance suggests that the family members may be exposed to the same environmental hazard, but no hazardous factor has been recognized in any of the MM and WM families that have been investigated.

On the other hand, the discovery that several affected family members have inherited identical HLA haplotypes[74,75,78] suggests that the tendency to develop these B-cell neoplasms may be inherited. A LOD score (the log of the ratio of likelihood of linkage to no linkage) was calculated by the LIPED Program to test whether the occurrence of Waldenström's macroglobulinemia and autoimmune manifestations in a family was segregating with the HLA region on chromosome six. The LOD score was 4.86; this favors chromosomal linkage of a postulated susceptibility gene to the HLA complex.[92]

KEY POINTS

- The frequency of multiple myeloma (MM) in a population is strongly influenced by age and race.
- The frequency is also influenced by the availability of good medical care, as this increases the likelihood of diagnosis.
- The incidence of MM increases with age; it is rare below 40 years and the median age at diagnosis is 71.
- The incidence of MM appeared to increase up until the early 1990s but is no longer increasing.
- MM is twice as common in black Americans as in whites and is less frequent in oriental races.
- No firm linkage exists between exposure to environmental factors (e.g. radiation, benzene) and the development of MM.
- Genetic changes presumably underlie the different susceptibility to MM among strains of inbred mice and some of the gender and racial differences in humans.
- Familial MM has been described but is uncommon.

REFERENCES

● = Key primary paper
◆ = Major review article

●1. Kyle RA, Therneau TM, Rajkumar SV, Offord JR, Larson DR, Plevak MF, et al. A long-term study of prognosis in monoclonal gammopathy of undetermined significance. N Engl J Med 2002; **346**:564–9.

●2. Avet-Loiseau H, Facon T, Daviet A, Godon C, Rapp MJ, Harousseau JL, et al. 14q32 translocations and monosomy 13 observed in monoclonal gammopathy of undetermined significance delineate a multistep process for the oncogenesis of multiple myeloma. Intergroupe Francophone du Myelome. Cancer Res 1999; 59:4546–50.

3. Axelsson U, Bachmann R, Hallen J. Frequency of pathological proteins (M-components) in 6,995 sera from an adult population. Acta Med Scand 1966; 179:235–47.

4. Axelsson U, Hallen J. A population study on monoclonal gammapathy. Follow-up after 5 and one-half years on 64 subjects detected by electrophoresis of 6995 sera. Acta Med Scand 1972; 191:111–13.

5. Ogmundsdottir HM, Haraldsdottir V, Johannesson G, Olafsdottir G, Bjarnadottir K, Sigvaldason H, et al. Monoclonal gammopathy in Iceland: a population-based registry and follow-up. Br J Haematol 2002; 118:166–73.

●6. Ries LAG, Eisner MP, Kosary CL, Hankey BF, Miller BA, Clegg L, et al. SEER Cancer Statistics Review, 1973–1999. Bethesda, MD: National Cancer Institute, 2002.

7. Turesson I, Zettervall O, Cuzick J, Waldenstrom JG, Velez R. Comparison of trends in the incidence of multiple myeloma in Malmo, Sweden, and other countries, 1950–1979. N Engl J Med 1984; 310:421–4.

8. Belch A, Shelley W, Bergsagel D, Wilson K, Klimo P, White D, et al. A randomized trial of maintenance versus no maintenance melphalan and prednisone in responding multiple myeloma patients. Br J Cancer 1988; 57:94–9.

9. Hjorth M, Holmberg E, Rodjer S, Westin J. Impact of active and passive exclusions on the results of a clinical trial in multiple myeloma. The Myeloma Group of Western Sweden. Br J Haematol 1992; 80:55–61.

10. Englisova M, Englis M, Kyral V, Kourilek K, Dvorak K. Changes of immunoglobulin synthesis in old people. Exp Gerontol 1968; 3:125–7.

11. Radl J, Sepers JM, Skvaril F, Morell A, Hijmans W. Immunoglobulin patterns in humans over 95 years of age. Clin Exp Immunol 1975; 22:84–90.

12. Riedel DA, Pottern LM, Blattner WA. Epidemiology of multiple myeloma. In: Wiernik PH, Canellos GP, Kyle RA, Schiffer CA (eds) Neoplastic diseases of the blood, 2nd edn. Edinburgh: Churchill Livingstone, 1991:347–72.

13. Devesa SS. Descriptive epidemiology of multiple myeloma. In: Obrams GI, Potter M (eds) Epidemiology and biology of multiple myeloma. Berlin: Springer-Verlag, 1991:3–12.

14. Baris D, Brown LM, Silverman DT, Hayes R, Hoover RN, Swanson GM, et al. Socioeconomic status and multiple myeloma among US blacks and whites. Am J Public Health 2000; 90:1277–81.

15. Talerman A. Clinico-pathological study of multiple myeloma in Jamaica. Br J Cancer 1969; 23:285–93.

16. Besson C, Gonin C, Brebion A, Delaunay C, Panelatti G, Plumelle Y. Incidence of hematological malignancies in Martinique, French West Indies, overrepresentation of multiple myeloma and adult T cell leukemia/lymphoma. Leukemia 2001; 15:828–31.

17. Bowden M, Crawford J, Cohen HJ, Noyama O. A comparative study of monoclonal gammopathies and immunoglobulin levels in Japanese and United States elderly. J Am Geriatr Soc 1993; 41:11–14.

18. Singh J, Dudley AW Jr, Kulig KA. Increased incidence of monoclonal gammopathy of undetermined significance in blacks and its age-related differences with whites on the basis of a study of 397 men and one woman in a hospital setting. J Lab Clin Med 1990; 116:785–9.

19. Cohen HJ, Crawford J, Rao MK, Pieper CF, Currie MS. Racial differences in the prevalence of monoclonal gammopathy in a community-based sample of the elderly. Am J Med 1998; 104:439–44.

20. Schwartz J. Multinational trends in multiple myeloma. Ann N Y Acad Sci 1990; 609:215–24.

21. Linos A, Kyle RA, O'Fallon WM, Kurland LT. Incidence and secular trend of multiple myeloma in Olmsted County, Minnesota: 1965–77. J Natl Cancer Inst 1981; 66:17–20.

22. Levi F, Te VC, La Vecchia C. Changes in cancer incidence in the Swiss Canton of Vaud, 1978–87. Ann Oncol 1990; 1:293–7.

23. Hansen NE, Karle H, Olsen JH. Trends in the incidence of multiple myeloma in Denmark 1943–1982: a study of 5500 patients. Eur J Haematol 1989; 42:72–6.

24. Cuzick J. International time trends for multiple myeloma. Ann N Y Acad Sci 1990; 609:205–14.

25. Ichimaru M, Ishimaru T, Mikami M, Matsunaga M. Multiple myeloma among atomic bomb survivors in Hiroshima and Nagasaki, 1950–76: relationship to radiation dose absorbed by marrow. J Natl Cancer Inst 1982; 69:323–8.

26. Preston DL, Kusumi S, Tomonaga M, Izumi S, Ron E, Kuramoto A, et al. Cancer incidence in atomic bomb survivors. Part III. Leukemia, lymphoma and multiple myeloma, 1950–1987. Radiat Res 1994; 137(2 Suppl):S68–97.

27. Neriishi K, Yoshimoto Y, Carter RL, Matsuo T, Ichimaru M, Mikami M, et al. Monoclonal gammopathy in atomic bomb survivors. Radiat Res 1993; 133:351–9.

28. Cuzick J. Radiation-induced myelomatosis. N Engl J Med 1981; 304:204–10.

29. Muirhead CR, Goodill AA, Haylock RG, Vokes J, Little MP, Jackson DA, et al. Occupational radiation exposure and mortality: second analysis of the National Registry for Radiation Workers. J Radiol Prot 1999; 19:3–26.

30. Wing S, Richardson D, Wolf S, Mihlan G, Crawford-Brown D, Wood J. A case control study of multiple myeloma at four nuclear facilities. Ann Epidemiol 2000; 10:144–53.

31. Boyd NF. The epidemiology of cancer: Principles and Methods. In: Tannock IF, Hill RP (eds) The basic science of oncology, 2nd edn. Toronto: Pergamon Press, 1992.

32. MacMahon B. Epidemiology of Hodgkin's disease. Cancer Res 1966; 26:1189–201.

33. Velez R, Beral V, Cuzick J. Increasing trends of multiple myeloma mortality in England and Wales; 1950–79: are the changes real? J Natl Cancer Inst 1982; 69:387–92.

34. Johnston JM, Grufferman S, Bourguet CC, Delzell E, Delong ER, Cohen HJ. Socioeconomic status and risk of multiple myeloma. J Epidemiol Commun Health 1985; 39:175–8.

35. McWhorter WP, Schatzkin AG, Horm JW, Brown CC. Contribution of socioeconomic status to black/white differences in cancer incidence. Cancer 1989; 63:982–7.

36. Mills PK, Newell GR, Beeson WL, Fraser GE, Phillips RL. History of cigarette smoking and risk of leukemia and myeloma: results from the Adventist health study. J Natl Cancer Inst 1990; 82:1832–6.

37. Adami J, Nyren O, Bergstrom R, Ekbom A, Engholm G, Englund A, et al. Smoking and the risk of leukemia, lymphoma, and multiple myeloma (Sweden). Cancer Causes Control 1998; 9:49–56.

38. Heineman EF, Zahm SH, McLaughlin JK, Vaught JB, Hrubec Z. A prospective study of tobacco use and multiple myeloma: evidence against an association. Cancer Causes Control 1992; 3:31–6.

39. Linet MS, McLaughlin JK, Hsing AW, Wacholder S, Co Chien HT, Schuman LM, et al. Is cigarette smoking a risk factor for non-Hodgkin's lymphoma or multiple myeloma? Results from the Lutheran Brotherhood Cohort Study. Leuk Res 1992; 16:621–4.

40. Brownson RC. Cigarette smoking and risk of myeloma. J Natl Cancer Inst 1991; 83:1036–7.

41. Reif JS, Pearce NE, Fraser J. Cancer risks among New Zealand meat workers. Scand J Work Environ Health 1989; 15:24–9.

42. Tollerud DJ, Brinton LA, Stone BJ, Tobacman JK, Blattner WA. Mortality from multiple myeloma among North Carolina furniture workers. J Natl Cancer Inst 1985; 74:799–801.

43. Delzell E, Monson RR. Mortality among rubber workers: X. Reclaim workers. Am J Ind Med 1985; 7:307–13.

44. Sorahan T, Parkes HG, Veys CA, Waterhouse JA, Straughan JK, Nutt A. Mortality in the British rubber industry 1946–85. Br J Ind Med 1989; 46:1–10.

45. Aksoy M, Erdem S, Dincol G, Kutlar A, Bakioglu I, Hepyuksel T. Clinical observations showing the role of some factors in the etiology of multiple myeloma. A study in 7 patients. Acta Haematol 1984; 71:116–20.

46. Rinsky RA, Smith AB, Hornung R, Filloon TG, Young RJ, Okun AH, et al. Benzene and leukemia. An epidemiologic risk assessment. N Engl J Med 1987; 316:1044–50.

47. Paxton MB, Chinchilli VM, Brett SM, Rodricks JV. Leukemia risk associated with benzene exposure in the pliofilm cohort: I. Mortality update and exposure distribution. Risk Anal 1994; 14:147–54.

48. Wong O, Raabe GK. A critical review of cancer epidemiology in the petroleum industry, with a meta-analysis of a combined database of more than 350,000 workers. Regul Toxicol Pharmacol 2000; 32:78–98.

49. Hansen ES. A follow-up study on the mortality of truck drivers. Am J Ind Med 1993; 23:811–21.

50. Van Den Eeden SK, Friedman GD. Exposure to engine exhaust and risk of subsequent cancer. J Occup Med 1993; 35:307–11.

51. Wong O, Raabe GK. Multiple myeloma and benzene exposure in a multinational cohort of more than 250 000 petroleum workers. Regul Toxicol Pharmacol 1997; 26:188–99.

52. Sonoda T, Nagata Y, Mori M, Ishida T, Imai K. Meta-analysis of multiple myeloma and benzene exposure. J Epidemiol 2001; 11:249–54.

53. Riedel DA, Pottern LM. The epidemiology of multiple myeloma. Hematol Oncol Clin North Am 1992; 6:225–47.

54. Bethwaite PB, Pearce N, Fraser J. Cancer risks in painters: study based on the New Zealand Cancer Registry. Br J Ind Med 1990; 47:742–6.

55. Cuzick J, De Stavola B. Multiple myeloma – a case-control study. Br J Cancer 1988; 57:516–20.

56. Demers PA, Vaughan TL, Koepsell TD, Lyon JL, Swanson GM, Greenberg RS, et al. A case-control study of multiple myeloma and occupation. Am J Ind Med 1993; 23:629–39.

57. Friedman GD. Multiple myeloma: relation to propoxyphene and other drugs, radiation and occupation. Int J Epidemiol 1986; 15:424–6.

58. Lundberg I. Mortality and cancer incidence among Swedish paint industry workers with long-term exposure to organic solvents. Scand J Work Environ Health 1986; 12:108–13.

59. Lundberg I, Milatou-Smith R. Mortality and cancer incidence among Swedish paint industry workers with long-term exposure to organic solvents. Scand J Work Environ Health 1998; 24:270–5.

60. Brown LM, Everett GD, Burmeister LF, Blair A. Hair dye use and multiple myeloma in white men. Am J Public Health 1992; 82:1673–4.

61. Guidotti S, Wright WE, Peters JM. Multiple myeloma in cosmetologists. Am J Ind Med 1982; 3:169–71.

62. Spinelli JJ, Gallagher RP, Band PR, Threlfall WJ. Multiple myeloma, leukemia, and cancer of the ovary in cosmetologists and hairdressers. Am J Ind Med 1984; 6:97–102.

63. Zahm SH, Weisenburger DD, Babbitt PA, Saal RC, Vaught JB, Blair A. Use of hair coloring products and the risk of lymphoma, multiple myeloma, and chronic lymphocytic leukemia. Am J Public Health 1992; 82:990–7.

64. Teta MJ, Walrath J, Meigs JW, Flannery JT. Cancer incidence among cosmetologists. J Natl Cancer Inst 1984; 72:1051–7.

65. Altekruse SF, Henley SJ, Thun MJ. Deaths from hematopoietic and other cancers in relation to permanent hair dye use in a large prospective study (United States). Cancer Causes Control 1999; 10:617–25.

66. Linet MS, Harlow SD, McLaughlin JK. A case-control study of multiple myeloma in whites: chronic antigenic stimulation, occupation, and drug use. Cancer Res 1987; 47:2978–81.

67. Boffetta P, Stellman SD, Garfinkel L. A case-control study of multiple myeloma nested in the American Cancer Society prospective study. Int J Cancer 1989; 43:554–9.

68. Eriksson M, Karlsson M. Occupational and other environmental factors and multiple myeloma: a population based case-control study. Br J Ind Med 1992; 49:95–103.

69. Schwartz DA, Vaughan TL, Heyer NJ, Koepsell TD, Lyon JL, Swanson GM, et al. B cell neoplasms and occupational asbestos exposure. Am J Ind Med 1988; 14:661–71.

70. Isobe T, Osserman EF. Pathologic conditions associated with plasma cell dyscrasias: a study of 806 cases. Ann N Y Acad Sci 1971; 190:507–18.

71. Hakulinen T, Isomaki H, Knekt P. Rheumatoid arthritis and cancer studies based on linking nationwide registries in Finland. Am J Med 1985; 78:29–32.

72. Isomaki HA, Hakulinen T, Joutsenlahti U. Excess risk of lymphomas, leukemia and myeloma in patients with rheumatoid arthritis. J Chronic Dis 1978; 31:691–6.

73. Katusic S, Beard CM, Kurland LT, Weis JW, Bergstralh E. Occurrence of malignant neoplasms in the Rochester, Minnesota, rheumatoid arthritis cohort. Am J Med 1985; 78:50–5.

74. Eriksson M. Rheumatoid arthritis as a risk factor for multiple myeloma: a casecontrol study. Eur J Cancer 1993; 2:259–63.

75. Pearce NE, Smith AH, Howard JK, Sheppard RA, Giles HJ, Teague CA. Case-control study of multiple myeloma and farming. Br J Cancer 1986; 54:493–500.

76. Linet MS, McLaughlin JK, Harlow SD, Fraumeni JF. Family history of autoimmune disorders and cancer in multiple myeloma. *Int J Epidemiol* 1988; **17**:512–13.

77. Shiran A, Brenner B, Laor A, Tatarsky I. Increased risk of cancer in patients with Gaucher disease. *Cancer* 1993; **72**:219–24.

78. Shoenfeld Y, Gallant LA, Shaklai M, Livni E, Djaldetti M, Pinkhas J. Gaucher's disease: a disease with chronic stimulation of the immune system. *Arch Pathol Lab Med* 1982; **106**:388–91.

79. Marti GE, Ryan ET, Papadopoulos NM, Filling-Katz M, Barton N, Fleischer TA, *et al.* Polyclonal B-cell lymphocytosis and hypergammaglobulinemia in patients with Gaucher disease. *Am J Hematol* 1988; **29**:189–94.

●80. Konrad RJ, Kricka LJ, Goodman DB, Goldman J, Silberstein LE. Brief report: myeloma-associated paraprotein directed against the HIV-1 p24 antigen in an HIV-1-seropositive patient. *N Engl J Med* 1993; **328**:1817–19.

81. Andreone P, Zignego AL, Cursaro C, Gramenzi A, Gherlinzoni F, Fiorino S, *et al.* Prevalence of monoclonal gammopathies in patients with hepatitis C virus infection. *Ann Intern Med* 1998; **129**:294–8.

82. Radl J, Hollander CF, van den Berg P, de Glopper E. Idiopathic paraproteinaemia. I. Studies in an animal model–the ageing C57BL/KaLwRij mouse. *Clin Exp Immunol* 1978; **33**:395–402.

83. Potter M, Pumphrey JG, Bailey DW. Genetics of susceptibility to plasmacytoma induction. I. BALB/cAnN (C), C57BL/6N (B6), C57BL/Ka (BK), (C times B6)F1, (C times BK)F1, and C times B recombinant-inbred strains. *J Natl Cancer Inst* 1975; **54**:1413–17.

84. Pottern LM, Gart JJ, Nam JM, Dunston G, Wilson J, Greenberg R, *et al.* HLA and multiple myeloma among black and white men: evidence of a genetic association. *Cancer Epidemiol Biomarkers Prev* 1992; **1**:177–82.

85. Patel M, Wadee AA, Galpin J, Gavalakis C, Fourie AM, Kuschke RH, *et al.* HLA class I and class II antigens associated with multiple myeloma in southern Africa. *Clin Lab Haematol* 2002; **24**:215–19.

86. Loth TS, Perrotta AL, Lima J, Whiteaker RS, Robinson A. Genetic aspects of familial multiple myeloma. *Mil Med* 1991; **156**:430–3.

87. Grosbois B, Gueguen M, Fauchet R, Lebouc H, Guenot A, Lancelin F, *et al.* Multiple myeloma in two brothers. An immunochemical and immunogenetic familial study. *Cancer* 1986; **58**:2417–21.

88. Bizzaro N, Pasini P. Familial occurrence of multiple myeloma and monoclonal gammopathy of undetermined significance in 5 siblings. *Haematologica* 1990; **75**:58–63.

89. Lynch HT, Sanger WG, Pirruccello S, Quinn-Laquer B, Weisenburger DD. Familial multiple myeloma: a family study and review of the literature. *J Natl Cancer Inst* 2001; **93**:1479–83.

90. Grosbois B, Jego P, Attal M, Payen C, Rapp MJ, Fuzibet JG, *et al.* Familial multiple myeloma: report of fifteen families. *Br J Haematol* 1999; **105**:768–70.

91. Renier G, Ifrah N, Chevailler A, Saint-Andre JP, Boasson M, Hurez D. Four brothers with Waldenstrom's macroglobulinemia. *Cancer* 1989; **64**:1554–9.

92. Blattner WA, Garber JE, Mann DL, McKeen EA, Henson R, McGuire DB, *et al.* Waldenstrom's macroglobulinemia and autoimmune disease in a family. *Ann Intern Med* 1980; **93**:830–2.

PART 2

Biology and pathophysiology

3

The immune system in myeloma

DOUGLAS E. JOSHUA, P. JOY HO, JOHN GIBSON AND ROSS D. BROWN

NORMAL B–CELL DEVELOPMENT

Lymphoid cells are derived from a common lymphoid progenitor, which has the capacity to develop into T, B, or natural killer (NK) cells.[1] Subsequently, a B-cell precursor, which differs from the T-, NK-, and dendritic cell precursor, leads to the development of the first recognizable B-cell type, a *pro B cell* (Fig. 3.1). At least three transcription factors have been identified as being essential for B-cell commitment. These include E_2A[2] and EBF,[3] both basic helix–loop–helix proteins, in the absence of which no B-cell progenitors develop. A third factor, Pax 5, is also essential

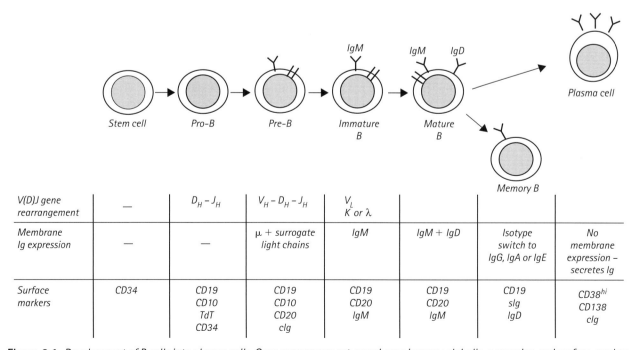

V(D)J gene rearrangement	—	$D_H - J_H$	$V_H - D_H - J_H$	V_L K or λ		
Membrane Ig expression	—	—	μ + surrogate light chains	IgM	IgM + IgD	Isotype switch to IgG, IgA or IgE	No membrane expression – secretes Ig
Surface markers	CD34	CD19 CD10 TdT CD34	CD19 CD10 CD20 cIg	CD19 CD20 IgM	CD19 CD20 IgM	CD19 sIg IgD	CD38^{hi} CD138 cIg

Figure 3.1 *Development of B cells into plasma cells. Gene rearrangement, membrane immunoglobulin expression and surface marker state of each cell type is documented.*

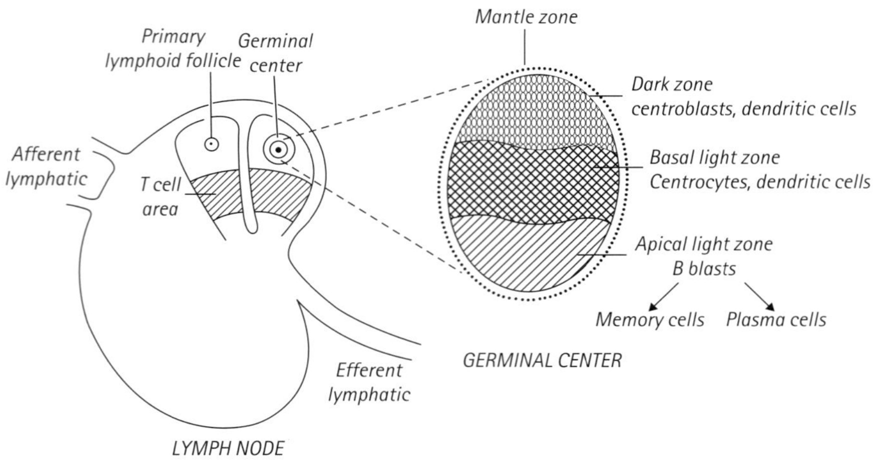

Figure 3.2 *Diagrammatic representation of lymph node and germinal center where cognate interaction between dendritic cells, T cells and B cells takes place.*

for B commitment.[4] B-cell development takes place in the bone marrow from mid-gestation onwards. The *pro B* cell, which expresses cell surface CD19 but not cytoplasmic μ immunoglobulin, undergoes rearrangement of its immunoglobulin heavy chain. This is then associated with the products of variable pre-beta and lambda 5 genes, which encode proteins that associate with each other to form the surrogate light chain.[5] Covalently bound μ and surrogate light chains are only expressed on the surface of B-lineage precursors. The surrogate light chain expression disappears with more mature B-cell development. Its expression early in B-cell ontogeny allows the variable regions of the heavy chain (in conjunction with the surrogate light chain) to be exposed to stromal cells, a requirement for the production of cytokines involved in B-cell development.[6] Subsequent rearrangement of the true light chain gene enables the cell (the immature B cell) to formally express surface IgM. The *immature B cell* thus expresses CD19 as well as cell-surface IgM associated with kappa or lambda light chains, i.e. the B-cell receptor. *Immature B lymphocytes* are able to leave the bone marrow, circulate in the blood and develop the ability to express surface IgD. A *virgin B cell* is an IgM, IgD + peripheral blood cell, which is in G_0 phase of the cell cycle. Such cells may be activated, proliferate and give rise to both plasma cells and *memory B cells*. Such activation requires contact with T cells.

Sites of specific cognate interaction with T cells include the extra follicular T zones of lymph nodes, in which stimulation of B cells to undergo Ig class switch and/or differentiation into mature, short-lived plasma cells occurs (Fig. 3.2).[7] Short-lived plasma cells may not undergo somatic mutation and are the origin of the primary immune response. In contrast, B cells that travel from the extrafollicular areas of the lymph node to the germinal center are exposed to antigen and co-stimulatory molecules on dendritic cells and develop a secondary response. These cells differentiate into centroblasts and undergo isotype switching and somatic mutation with the generation of high-affinity antibodies. Cells that do not receive viable antigenic signals from follicular dendritic cells undergo apoptosis.[8,9]

Centroblasts that have received antigenic stimulation progress through a centrocytic stage and re-express surface immunoglobulin. Morphological changes associated with this process are visible and the collection of centroblasts next to the T zone forms a characteristic dark zone of a germinal center, whereas the characteristic light zone of the germinal center is due to centrocytes, which are not in the cell cycle. B cells with high-affinity receptors receive survival signals from antigen on dendritic cells, and differentiate into either memory B cells or plasmablasts, which subsequently move to the bone marrow and develop into plasma cells. These bone marrow plasma cells have a long life span and produce the majority of secreted immunoglobulin in the plasma.[10]

The life span of long-lived plasma cells is in the order of 1–2 months. As antibody responses can persist for years, it follows that there must be continued generation of antigen-specific plasma cells. This phenomenon is the result of the ongoing interaction with antigen remaining on follicular dendritic cells.

IMMUNOGLOBULIN HEAVY CHAIN (IgH) GENE REARRANGEMENTS AND V GENE USAGE IN MYELOMA

IgH Gene rearrangements and V gene usage in myeloma

The normal immunoglobulin molecule consists of two heavy chains and two light chains (Fig. 3.3). Maturation of normal B-cell precursors to mature plasma cells that secrete immunoglobulin involves rearrangement of the immunoglobulin genes with subsequent somatic mutation of the variable (V) region of the immunoglobulin gene. The variable region of the immunoglobulin heavy chain

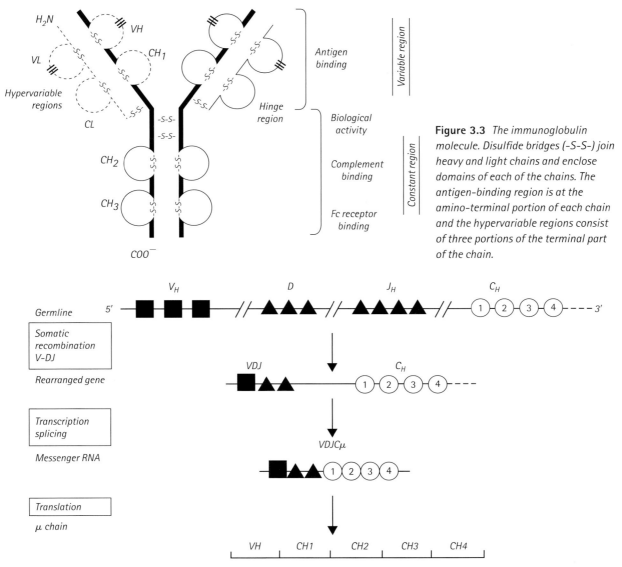

Figure 3.3 *The immunoglobulin molecule. Disulfide bridges (-S-S-) join heavy and light chains and enclose domains of each of the chains. The antigen-binding region is at the amino-terminal portion of each chain and the hypervariable regions consist of three portions of the terminal part of the chain.*

Figure 3.4 *DNA gene rearrangements resulting in the production of a heavy chain. The first DNA rearrangement results in a unique VDJ segment, which is subsequently joined to the CH segments. This is transcribed into messenger RNA, followed by translation into protein.*

is derived from three distinct gene segments encoded by the variable, diversity (D), and joining (J) region sequences, whereas the light-chain segments, variable kappa or lambda, and the joining segment genes encode the variable fraction of the immunoglobulin light chain. Rearrangement of the V-gene sections is dependent on the protein products of recombinase activating genes. Immunoglobulin heavy and light chain genes also contain three hypervariable or complementary determining regions (CDR segments). These segments can be used as a marker to detect minimal residual disease in B-cell tumors. CDR3 or the third CDR fragment is the most variable portion of the immunoglobulin molecule, and is the principal site for somatic mutation and antibody affinity maturation of the immunoglobulin molecule (Fig. 3.4).[11]

Rearrangement of immunoglobulin genes during B-cell development is sequential and ordered, occurring in distinct sites at distinct stages of development. Heavy-chain genes undergo rearrangement before the light-chain genes. The product of a successful heavy-chain VDJ joining activates rearrangements of the kappa locus, which precedes any lambda rearrangement.[12]

The mu heavy chain is first expressed during B-cell differentiation followed by the delta chain. As the immune response proceeds, class switching to alternate heavy chains is the result of the deletion of the unwanted heavy chain, and constant region genes between the VH and CK regions. A deletional recombination mechanism involving distinct switch region segments in the JHC mu intron is the key functional element. Many of the gene translocations seen in multiple myeloma occur in these switch regions.[13] The process of VDJ rearrangement and class switching allows a single B-cell clone to produce antibodies of different heavy-chain classes to the same antigenic epitope.

In myeloma, the malignant plasma cells have already undergone somatic mutation within the germinal centre and no ongoing mutation occurs with progressive disease.[14,15] Thus, the mutation mechanism is no longer active in the malignant clone. Analysis of the variable gene has indicated that the overwhelming majority of the malignant population is derived from a post-antigen-selected plasma cell. However, it is also recognized that less mature but minor B-cell populations of identical variable gene sequences may coexist both in the post-switch and pre-switch populations in the circulation.[16]

VH families

Sequence analysis of the variable genes and the immunoglobulin families in patients with malignancies of B cells reveals biases compared with normal usage of the VH repertoire. It has been suggested that this observation may indicate a possible role for specific antigens and certain B cells in the pathogenesis of these malignancies.

The VH gene segments, encoding for the first 95 amino acids of the heavy chain, are subdivided into six families, VH1–6, on the basis of regions of DNA homology. There are approximately 25 VH1, five VH2, 28 VH3, 14 VH4, three VH5, and one VH6 gene segments. VH gene families have been shown to have a developmentally regulated pattern of use in B cells. Rearranged VH3 genes are rarely found in the germinal center but are abundant in blood. Low-affinity IgM antibody in the primary state is predominantly of the VH3 subfamily, whereas high-affinity antibodies produced after immunization contain all families.[17]

Apparent non-stochastic use of certain VH families occurs in a variety of conditions. For example, the preferential use of VH5 has been reported in chronic lymphatic leukemia and in acute lymphoblastic leukemia.[18] In myeloma there is conflicting evidence of preferential use of VH families. Some reports indicate non-preferential use of VH5,[19] while others have found preferential non-stochastic usage of the families VH4–VH6.[20]

ORIGIN OF THE MALIGNANT PLASMA CELL

The precise nature of the myeloma stem cell remains elusive. Current evidence, however, suggests that it is likely to be a long-lived plasma cell that homes to the bone marrow and that has already undergone somatic hypermutation.

Molecular analysis of peripheral blood mononuclear cells in myeloma has clearly demonstrated the presence of circulating B cells that are clonally identical CDR3 mutations related to the bone marrow plasma cells. However, surprisingly, as noted before, both pre- and post-switch clonal isotypes are present in myeloma, and these cells appear to lack clonal diversity.[16,21,22] For example, IgM-positive cells with the same CDR3 sequence as the dominant clone can be found in IgG myeloma. The role that such pre-switch clonotypic cells play in the progression of the disease remains unknown, although recent data have suggested their presence may have prognostic significance and that they may be a reservoir of drug-resistant cells.[22]

It has been suggested that myeloma progenitors are pre-switched cells that have gained the ability to respond selectively to cytokines, which regulate switching and which result predominately in one specific isotype switch. Pre-switch clonogenic cells may, therefore, represent precursor cells in the context of neoplastic transformation. This is supported by data showing both pre- and post-switched isotypes are able to engraft SCID-NOD mice.[22] It is also possible, and supported by recent murine data, that there could be a dynamic equilibrium between neoplastic memory cells, neoplastic plasmablasts and pre-switch B cells, and that changes can occur between these cell types.[23] It is, however, extremely rare to find more than one neoplastic clone in myeloma and pathogenic consequences of the disease remain in the post-switch cells. Molecular change that is already present in an isotype pre-switched cell is, therefore, unlikely to cause disease. Experiments using murine myeloma models have suggested that isotype switch variants originate from the major tumor clone, either by downstream switching or *trans* switching to sister chromatids. This suggests that isotype switch variants originate from the major tumor clone and that IgM-expressing clonotypic cells do not play a role as a pre-switch precursor to myeloma. It has thus been suggested that the appearance of such cells could be considered a rare but normal event, which is visible due to the high numbers of clonotypic cells present in myeloma.[23] The persistent expression of clonotypic IgM would then merely reflect tumor bulk and thus be correlated with a poor prognosis, as has been reported.

In summary it seems far more likely that neoplastic change occurs after the germinal center stage of B-cell development and that the post-germinal center blast or memory B cell is the most likely candidate for the genetic change that leads to malignancy.

IgH SWITCH TRANSLOCATIONS IN MYELOMA

Isotype switch recombination

As previously mentioned, during B-cell maturation, the IgH genes undergo the processes of variable region (VDJ) recombination, followed by isotype switching and somatic hypermutation after exposure to antigen. Isotype switching is the process by which a given Ig variable region can be associated with different isotype classes, thus conferring different physiological functions. Its particular relevance in myeloma lies in the fact that the majority of translocations affecting the IgH locus on chromosome 14q32 occur at the regions in which normal switch recombinations occur. These are known as switch translocations (STs).[13] The IgH genes are arranged in the order of 5′–Cμ, Cδ, Cγ3, Cγ1, Cψε, Cα1, Cγ2, Cδ4, Cε, Cα2–3′. Switch regions, consisting of repeat sequences, are located in front of each constant region gene except Cδ. The first heavy-chain isotype, IgM, is expressed by RNA splicing from the end of the rearranged variable region to the Cμ gene. During isotype switch recombination the μ isotype changes to another isotype class by recombination of the respective switch regions. For instance, $S\mu$ recombines with $S\alpha$ for the μ to α switch, with the deletion of the intervening DNA in an excision circle (Fig. 3.5). Switch recombination mostly involves switch regions on the same chromosome (in *cis*). *Trans*-switching involving

switch regions on both alleles may also rarely occur. The fact that switch regions are physiological recombination hotspots may account for their propensity to be involved in chromosomal translocation. The retention of Ig production by the myeloma plasma cell would imply that the STs are most likely to occur on the non-productive allele.

Switch translocations in myeloma

Apart from monosomy 13, the most common cytogenetic abnormality in myeloma is chromosomal translocation into the switch regions of the IgH genes on chromosome 14q32. These translocations were initially detected by conventional cytogenetics at a rate of 20–40%.[24–26] The partner chromosome was often not elicited and the karyotypic abnormality was denoted 14q+. Using a Southern blot technique to look for illegitimate switch recombinations (ISRs) as candidates for switch translocations in human myeloma cell lines (HMCLs), it became evident that STs were much more common than previously suspected.[13] It is estimated that approximately 90% of HMCLs have either IgH or IgL

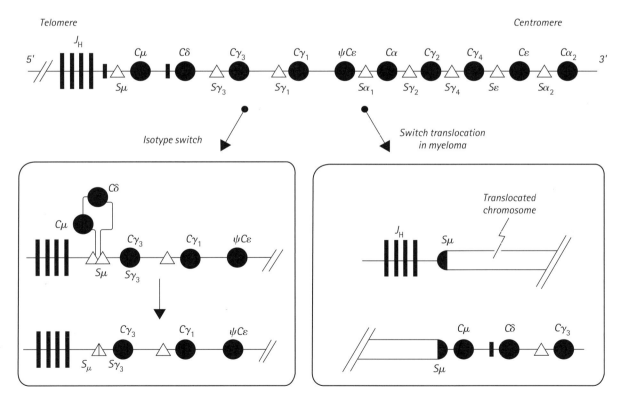

Figure 3.5 *The structure of the IgH locus (chromosome 14q32) with the arrangement of the constant genes shown at the top of the figure. The constant genes are represented by circles and denoted 'C;' the switch regions are represented by triangles and denoted 'S'. The small rectangles upstream of Sμ: and Cδ represent the σμ and σδ sequences, which are involved in the μ to δ switch. Physiological isotype recombination is shown in the lower left panel, with recombination of the switch regions and deletion of the intervening DNA sequence. Switch translocations are shown in the lower right panel, with a non-Ig sequence translocated to the IgH genes, with the breakpoints predominantly located at the switch regions.*

(immunoglobulin light-chain) translocation. Cloning of breakpoints and molecular cytogenetic studies have revealed a large array of chromosomal partners for the STs, the most common being chromosomes 11q, 4p, and 16q, with candidate oncogenes characterized on each partner. The translocation breakpoints are mostly centromeric to the candidate oncogenes, which are translocated to der(14) and placed under the control of one of the 3′ IgH enhancers (Eα1 or Eα2). In addition, in cases such as chromosome 4p, a second putative oncogene is also overexpressed on der(4), presumably dysregulated by the 5′ intronic enhancer (Eμ) translocated to der(4). The role of these candidate genes in the pathogenesis of myeloma has been examined by assessing their level of expression and their oncogenicity in both *in vitro* and *in vivo* models.

Translocation partner chromosomes

The common translocation partners and candidate oncogenes in switch translocations in myeloma are illustrated in Table 3.1.

CHROMOSOME 11q

Chromosome 11q has been identified as a partner chromosome in 15–20% of myeloma,[27,28] with translocations located at 11q13. Early studies using conventional cytogenetics suggested that this translocation was associated with a poorer prognosis.[28,29] However, conventional cytogenetic analysis requires metaphases from actively dividing cells, thus possibly 'selecting' for more aggressive disease. Subsequent studies by interphase fluorescence *in situ* hybridization (FISH) have not confirmed a prognostic relationship.[27]

Chromosome 11 ST breakpoints are not as telomeric compared with other partner chromosomes, such as chromosome 4p, and are, therefore, more amenable to detection by conventional cytogenetics. Mantle cell lymphoma (MCL) also bears a characteristic t(11;14)(q13;q32) translocation, with the majority of MCL breakpoints located within the major translocation cluster (MTC) region 110 kb upstream of *cyclin D1* (*CD1*, a candidate oncogene for both MCL and myeloma). In contrast, the breakpoints in myeloma are more widely scattered over a region 100–330 kb centromeric to *CD1*. In myeloma, except for several breakpoints in the J_H region, most of the known IgH breakpoints occur in the switch regions. In MCL in contrast, they are located in the J_H region, indicating the involvement of the VDJ recombination mechanism at an earlier stage of B-cell development.

The finding of *CD1* upregulation in myeloma tumors and cell lines bearing t(11;14) supports its role as a candidate oncogene in myeloma.[30–32] The cyclins are a family of cell-cycle regulators, of which the members *CD2* and *CD3* are normally expressed in lymphoid cells. The expression of *CD1* is, therefore, ectopic in t(11;14)-bearing myeloma cells. All the cyclin proteins interact with CD-dependent kinases, phosphorylating and inactivating the retinoblastoma protein (Rb), thus promoting the G_1/S phase transition.[33]

A second candidate oncogene named *myeov* (myeloma overexpressed gene) has been characterized on chromosome 11q, 360 kb centromeric to *cyclin D1*. All known myeloma breakpoints are situated in the region between *CD1* and *myeov*.[34] *Myeov* was originally isolated from gastric carcinoma by a tumorigenicity assay. In myeloma, *myeov* was upregulated in three of seven cell lines carrying t(11;14), indicating that not all myeloma lines carrying the translocation overexpressed *myeov*. The variation is presumably related to the site of the breakpoint, the orientation of the translocation and the placement of enhancers. Surprisingly, some cell lines not carrying t(11;14) express

Table 3.1 *Common chromosomal partners and candidate oncogenes in switch translocations in myeloma*

Chromosomal partner	Candidate oncogenes		Distance between breakpoints and telomeric oncogenes	Function
	Candidate oncogene	Localization		
11q13	1. *Cyclin D1*	der(14)	100–330 kb	Cell-cycle regulator
	2. *myeov*	der(11)		Unknown
4p16	1. *FGFR3*	der(14)	50–100 kb	Growth factor receptor tyrosine kinase
	2. *MMSET/WHSC1*			Epigenetic regulator of transcription (chromatin remodeling)
16q32	c-*maf*	der(14)	550–1350 kb	Transcription factor
6p21	*Cyclin D3*	der(14)	65 kb	Cell-cycle regulator
6p25	*MUM1/IRF4*	der(14)	Immediately adjacent	Transcriptional regulator of IFN and IFN-stimulated genes

IFN, interferon; see text for references.

moderate levels of *myeov*.[34] Hence the role of *myeov* in myeloma is still not clear.

CHROMOSOME 4p

The t(4;14)(p16;q32) translocation is difficult to detect by conventional cytogenetics or spectral karyotyping (SKY),[35–37] owing to the extreme telomeric localization of the breakpoints. The cloned breakpoints were located 50–100 kb centromeric of the fibroblast growth factor receptor 3 gene (*FGFR3*), one of the two candidate oncogenes on chromosome 4.[38,39] The translocation can be detected by FISH, with the reported incidence varying from 12%[27] to 17%.[40] It is also detected in 2–6% of patients with MGUS.[41,42] The latter estimate was obtained by the demonstration of a fusion transcript derived from chromosomes 4 and 14.

FGFR3 is one of a family of fibroblast growth factor receptor tyrosine kinases, mutations of which cause several forms of dwarfism, including thanatophoric dysplasia (TD).[43,44] *FGFR3* can be dysregulated in myeloma by translocation to the vicinity of IgH enhancers, activating mutations or both. It is overexpressed in several myeloma cell lines and tumors, with selective expression of the mutant allele found in all three cell lines examined carrying *FGFR3* mutations.[45] The frequency and role of *FGFR3* mutations in primary myeloma tumor samples is much debated, owing to the apparent low incidence in primary tumor. In analysis of *FGFR3* genomic DNA, a single nucleotide change was found in one of 80 primary myeloma tumors.[46] A low incidence was also detected in cDNA from the expressed allele – only one of 11 cases overexpressing FGFR3 demonstrated an activating mutation.[47] It was concluded from these studies that the incidence of activating mutations of *FGFR3* in myeloma was 10% in cases bearing t(4;14), which constitutes only 2% of all myeloma primary tumors. The tumorigenicity of FGFR3 has also been examined. By retroviral transduction of wild-type and mutant *FGFR3* into a murine interleukin-6 (IL-6)-dependent plasmacytoma cell line, increased *FGFR3* expression (both wild type and mutant) promoted cellular proliferation and survival, with an enhanced response to IL-6 and IL-6-independence.[48] The oncogenicity of mutant *FGFR3* has also been demonstrated in an *in vivo* animal model using a mutant *FGFR3*-transfected fibroblast cell line.[45] Mutant FGFR3 has been found to cause transformation in hemopoietic cells, but whether upregulated levels of non-mutated FGFR3 have the same effect is presently unclear.[49]

A second candidate gene for t(4;14) was localized on the reciprocal chromosome [der(4)]. The chromosome 4p breakpoints are telomeric to or within the 5′ introns of *MMSET/WHSC1*, characterized as a candidate gene for a multiple malformation syndrome known as Wolf–Hirschhorn sydrome.[50] *MMSET* is a member of the trithorax nuclear proteins, which includes *MLL*, one of the most common genes involved in human acute leukemia. *MLL* is involved in the epigenetic regulation of gene expression through chromatin remodeling, and consists of PHD (zinc finger) and SET domains. The latter has been shown to cause transformation in fibroblasts.[51] In t(4;14) MMSET is placed in close proximity to and presumably upregulated by the 5′ intron IgH enhancer. Hybrid transcripts of 5′IgH joined to MMSET are produced, initiating either from the J_H or $I\mu$ exons.[52] However, few of the fusion transcripts are expected to produce functional proteins owing to premature stop codons or the absence of the amino terminal as a result of splicing. The size of proteins could also vary according to the use of different promoters, alternative splicing, specific mRNA degradation, and variation in the site of polyadenylation. Although it has been proposed that such variations may modulate the phenotypic diversity of MM,[50] so far there has been no evidence for a correlation with clinicopathological characteristics.

CHROMOSOME 16q

The t(14;16)(q32;q23) translocation has been found in approximately 5–12% of myeloma patients.[36,37] The chromosome 16q23 breakpoints were localized to a region 550–1350 kb centromeric of c-*maf*, although a breakpoint telomeric to c-*maf* was also found in a t(16;22) translocation.[53,54] C-*maf* is a basic zipper transcription factor involved in cellular differentiation, proliferation, and the IL-6 response and is capable of oncogenic transformation in a model system.[55] Its role in myelomagenesis is supported by the finding of upregulated expression in five HMCLs carrying the (14;16) translocation, including the tumor of origin of one cell line, with selective expression of one c-*maf* allele in two informative lines.[53] The cloned breakpoints are located in a common fragile site (FRA16D) on chromosome 16, within the newly characterized *WWOX* gene, a candidate tumor suppressor gene in breast cancer.[56] Although this region is susceptible to allelic deletion in several non-hematological cancers, no mutations have been found in the remaining allele of WWOX and its possible role as a tumor suppressor gene is not yet known. Similarly, its role in myeloma is unclear, as breakpoints occurring within *WWOX* would inactivate only one of the two alleles.

CHROMOSOME 6p

The t(6;14) (p25;q32) translocation was one of the first STs reported in a myeloma cell line,[57] in which *MUM1/IRF4*, an interferon (IFN)-responsive factor (IRF), was proposed as a candidate oncogene. IRFs are involved in transcriptional control, can be rapidly induced by T- and B-receptor cross-linking, and regulate the IFNs and IFN-stimulated genes. They, therefore, have a critical role in plasma cell development.[58] IRF4 was overexpressed in HMCLs and demonstrated transforming ability in fibroblasts.[57] Molecular cytogenetics have revealed an incidence of this ST of 18% in HMCLs[59] but a low frequency of approximately 5% in primary myeloma,[36,37] and its role in myeloma pathogenesis is as yet unclear.

More recently, a second translocation affecting chromosome 6p – t(6:14) (p21;q32) – was identified. *Cyclin D3* (*CD3*), located approximately 65 kb telomeric of the breakpoint at 6p21, has been proposed as the candidate oncogene.[60] This translocation was originally found in one of 30 myeloma cell lines, and then in 4% of 150 primary tumors by metaphase FISH and SKY. *CD3* overexpression was further detected by microarray analysis in three of 53 primary tumors, in which t(6;14) breakpoints were subsequently confirmed, one other tumor having a variant t(6;22) translocation. As noted earlier, all the cyclin D proteins are known to phosphorylate Rb, facilitating the G_1/S phase transition. Unlike *CD1*, *CD3* is normally expressed in lymphoid cells and upregulated expression would be expected to promote proliferation.

OTHER CHROMOSOMAL PARTNERS

C-*myc* on chromosome 8q24 is the oncogene characteristically dysregulated in murine plasmacytoma and human Burkitt's lymphoma. Reciprocal translocations involving chromosome 8q24 and the Ig genes account for only 25% of the c-*myc* rearrangements in myeloma,[61] with the majority involving non-Ig loci.

Apart from the more common STs already discussed, a large number of other chromosomal partners have been reported, many detected only once. Reciprocal translocations with chromosome 1q have been detected by SKY, occurring in up to 4–5% of primary tumors.[36] Possible candidate oncogenes on chromosome 1q are IRTA1 and 2, two novel B cell surface receptors. IRTA2 has been found to be upregulated in t(1;14)-carrying tumor cell lines.[62] Other infrequent partners found in myeloma cell lines include 3q, 4q, 20q, 21q, and 22q. The non-recurrent nature of some of these aberrations makes elucidation of a potential role in multiple myeloma pathogenesis difficult to define.

Switch translocations – implications for pathogenesis

Whether STs are an early oncogenic change, a late 'trigger' of disease progression or a non-pathogenic marker of genetic instability has been an interesting question with important implications in our understanding of myeloma pathogenesis. If STs contribute to oncogenesis, their presence in 50–75% of primary myeloma tumors[27,36,63,64] and the heterogeneity of chromosomal

partners and partner oncogenes would imply that STs cannot be the only oncogenic factor; a number of mechanisms must be involved. The heterogeneity of chromosomal partners has been proposed as one of the arguments against STs being a unifying oncogenic change.[27] However, the 'final common pathway' of myeloma development from multiple mechanisms could simply reflect the single possible phenotype of the transformed plasma cell.[54]

The concept of primary and secondary translocations has been introduced to distinguish translocations that occur early in disease and may be oncogenic from late changes that may play a role in disease progression.[54]

Translocations such as STs, which involve B-cell recombination mechanisms, occur in some cases of MGUS and demonstrate little heterogeneity within the myeloma cell population, are more likely to represent primary changes. Conversely, changes that do not involve the Ig loci, which are not present in MGUS and which demonstrate heterogeneity within a given tumor, are more likely to represent late secondary changes. These may include the complex c-*myc* translocations, which do not occur at the Ig recombination sites and demonstrate intratumor heterogeneity.

An interesting consideration of the role of STs in the causation of myeloma is their occurrence in MGUS. Not all MGUS are pre-malignant, and there are presently no clearly defined molecular or other phenotypic features that enable us to predict the risk of myeloma development. If STs are an oncogenic change, the presence of STs may distinguish the benign and pre-malignant forms of MGUS. In the largest series of MGUS patients assessed by FISH so far,[41] chromosome 14q32 translocations have been found to occur in 47%. In intramedullary myeloma (stage III), the frequency was 60% and in plasma cell leukemia (PCL) 70–80%.[65]

The study of when STs occur in the ontogeny of the myeloma plasma cell can help to elucidate the cell of origin of the myeloma clone. Such studies have suggested that myeloma may originate in a pre-switch B cell or pre-plasma cell.[21,22] As STs are commonly thought to occur during isotype switch recombination, the finding of pre-switch clonotypic cells raises the interesting question of whether these presumed myeloma precursors contain STs.

Prognostic significance of switch translocations and interactions with other abnormalities

By conventional cytogenetics, the most consistent chromosomal abnormality associated with a poor patient outcome is del 13 – either complete or partial deletions.[29,66] However, this could not be confirmed in the original study when FISH was used,[29] as there was a much higher frequency of deletions (60–70%), with no impact on outcome attributed to chromosome 13 deletions detected by FISH alone, in contrast to other FISH series, which show adverse prognostic associations to chromosome 13 deletions.[6,7] Conventional karyotyping has also demonstrated a poor prognostic significance of chromsome 11q translocations including t(11;14) translocation and reciprocal translocations with chromosomes 8, 9, and 12.[28,29] However, this was not confirmed by molecular cytogenetics.[27] The possibility that conventional karyotypes have 'selected' out cases that are 'hyperproliferative' must be considered, especially when long-term cultures were used. The combination of aberrations of both chromosomes 11 and 13 has been found to produce a dismal outcome.[29]

In a study utilizing the detection of illegitimate switch recombinations as an indication of STs, in general no relationship with parameters of disease activity or prognosis was found in patients with progressive disease.[64] It was concluded that as a single entity, STs *per se* were unlikely to be a feature of disease progression or have prognostic significance, but subgroup analysis according to translocation partner is obviously required. This has been most efficiently examined by molecular cytogenetics. No correlation was found between the presence of chromosome 14q32 translocations and disease stage or β_2 microglobulin in a study of 127 myeloma and 14 PCL patients.[27] In another analysis,[67] 89 patients were divided into three risk categories according to three chromosomal abnormalities – del 13q, abnormalities of chromosomes 11 and del 17q. When assessed separately, the only independent prognostic feature was del 13, with increased prognostic significance seen with the addition of β_2 microglobulin levels. A recent study of PCL and late-stage myeloma demonstrated a higher incidence of t(11;14), t(14;16) and monosomy 13 in patients with high tumor mass, but no difference in t(4;14). Paradoxically, a longer survival was observed in patients with t(11;14) in this group.[65] Thus, further investigation is obviously still required to elucidate the prognostic significance of specific ST subgroups.

THE NORMAL IMMUNE SYSTEM IN MYELOMA

B cells

Patients with myeloma have a primary immune defect, which results in an increased incidence of infection. Such infections are predominantly bacterial and a number of reports have stressed the frequency of infections, such as pneumococcal pneumonia, as a presenting feature of multiple myeloma.[68] The etiology of the primary immune deficit in myeloma is unclear. Early murine studies have

suggested a relationship to a macrophage processing defect, rather than a defect in normal B cells.[69] Supporting these observations are recent reports, in human myeloma, of a defect in dendritic cell function, which may in part be responsible for the impaired primary immune deficit.[70] Reduction of the synthesis of normal residual immunoglobulin frequently results in severe hypogammaglobulinemia, which clearly is a major contribution to the high incidence of infection. It is well recognized that this, together with the additional immunosuppressive chemotherapy, leads to a high incidence of infection, especially in the first 6 months of treatment.[71] Although pneumococci and *Haemophilus influenzae* were initially identified as major causes of early infection, it is now clear that enteric Gram-negative organisms are also frequent causes of infection, especially after aggressive chemotherapy.[68] Fungal and *Mycobacterium tuberculosis* infections are relatively uncommon, although varicella zoster is well recognized, usually in association with the immunosuppression of chemotherapy. A number of studies evaluated the use of prophylactic intravenous immunoglobulin preparations in myeloma but there did not appear to be a significant reduction in the incidence of infection and, therefore, they cannot be recommended as a routine prophylactic measure. In contrast, specific patients with documented (bacterial) infections may benefit from regular immunoglobulin replacement. In addition, there is no suggestion that routine immunoglobulin replacement during plateau phase is beneficial. Plateau-phase myeloma itself is usually associated with a fairly low incidence of infections.[72] It has, however, been reported that routine prophylactic antibiotics, especially in the first 6 months of chemotherapy, may be beneficial.[73]

T cells and T–cell clonal expansions

T CELLS IN MYELOMA

Although multiple myeloma is a B-cell malignancy, there are a number of phenotypic and functional abnormalities within the T-cell compartment of patients with this disease. In addition, the immunoregulatory role of T cells and the possibility of enhancing the immune response against tumor cells have become important issues for designing effective immunotherapy programmes. Thus, there is now considerable interest in understanding the nature and antitumor potential of the T cells in patients with myeloma.[74]

The absolute peripheral blood lymphocyte and T-cell count are often decreased in patients with myeloma primarily owing to a reduction in the absolute number of $CD4^+$ cells. Since the absolute number in the $CD8^+$ T-cell compartment often remains normal, the relative number of $CD8^+$ T cells may be increased, causing a significantly reduced CD4/CD8 ratio.[75] This depression of the CD4/CD8 ratio is usually more obvious in patients with progressive disease. Within the CD4[+] T-cell compartment, there is a selective loss of cells in the naive CD4[+] CD45R[+] subset, suggesting a relative enrichment of memory CD4[+] cells and a failure in the differentiation pathway to give rise to new naive CD4[+] T cells. Conversely, in patients with myeloma at diagnosis, a reduction in total and activated CD4[+] T cells but not naive CD4[+] subsets has also been reported.[76] Various changes in T-cell subsets and tumor-induced inhibition of a T-cell response may provide another explanation for the defect in the primary immune response, in addition to defects in macrophage and dendritic cell function described previously.[69,70]

FUNCTIONAL CHARACTERISTICS OF T CELLS IN MYELOMA

A variety of observations have demonstrated functional abnormalities in the T cells of myeloma patients. One series of observations found a significantly increased activation state as demonstrated by an increase in the expression of the activation markers CD37 and HLA-DR,[77] serum neopterin,[78] serum thymidine kinase,[79] and Ki67.[80] These hyperactive T cells produce high levels of IL-2 and IFNβ. In addition, the high expression of CD95 (Fas) and a low expression of Bcl-2 on HLA-DR[+] T cells in myeloma suggests a state of chronic activation and is associated with an enhanced susceptibility to apoptosis.[81]

Although these T cells manifest upregulation of various markers of 'activation,' the generation of cytotoxic T lymphocytes and IL-2 induction of lymphokine-activated killer (LAK) cells has been shown to be defective, and this correlates with disease status.[82,83] Other studies have demonstrated that T cells from patients with myeloma display an impaired response to mitogens,[84] while abnormal immunoregulatory functions, such as T-suppressor cell dysfunction and suppression of polyclonal immunoglobulin synthesis,[85] and a decreased cloning efficiency of CD8[+] T cells have also been demonstrated.[86]

A number of studies have reported the presence of expanded populations of T cells in myeloma.[87] Expanded T-cell populations have been detected by Southern blotting, T-cell receptor (TCR) CDR3 fragment length analysis, determination of V beta gene usage and nucleotide sequencing.[88–92] TCR CDR3 fragment length analysis and nucleotide sequencing have demonstrated that it is the CD8[+] CD57[+] cells within the expanded TCRVβ family that are clonal.[93] While age-matched normal controls also contain expanded T-cell populations, these are predominantly CD4[+] T cells.[93] The functional capacity of CD8[+] T-cell expansions in patients with myeloma and their specificity to malignant plasma cells are key issues that require further study. Flow cytometric analysis of these expanded T-cell populations has demonstrated the phenotype of cytotoxic T cells, i.e. CD8[+], CD45RA[+], CD57[+], CD28-, and perforin positive.[91] The most significant

observation concerning expanded T-cell clones is that their presence is associated with a prolonged overall survival compared with patients without such populations.[88] However, it is still unknown whether the function of such cells is directly tumor-specific or whether they merely indicate the patients in whom the ability to mount an immune response to other non-myeloma antigens remains intact.

IDIOTYPE REACTIVITY

It has been reported that stimulation of peripheral blood T cells with F(ab')$_2$ fragments of autologous idiotype results in T-cell responses. Such responses were observed in both proliferation and cytokine secretion assays.[94] It was predominantly Th$_1$-type T-cell response (IFNγ- and IL-2-secreting T-helper cells) and was inhibited by an anti-HLA-DR antibody, suggesting that the idiotype-induced T-cell stimulation is MHC class II restricted.[95] Idiotype-induced T-cell stimulation was shown to require the presence of antigen presenting cells, such as B cells or monocytes, indicating that the idiotype alone is not sufficient to elicit a response.[96] Myeloma plasma cells function poorly as antigen-presenting cells, but the idiotype could potentially be transferred to other types of antigen-presenting cells, thus facilitating MHC class II reduced antigen presentation to CD4[+] T cells.[97]

Evidence that idiotypic protein can bind also to T-cell populations in a non-MHC restricted manner comes from panning experiments and from incubation with fluorescent labelled F(ab')$_2$ fragments. In the latter study using fluorescent labeled F(ab')$_2$ and flow cytometry, a close correlation was observed between the idiotype-binding T cells and the presence of T-cell populations in peripheral blood.[88] However, when idiotype-induced reactivity was studied in patients with restricted TCRVβ expansions, idiotype recognition was not confined to the expanded populations.[98] Thus, the exact nature of the idiotype-induced effects on T cells remains obscure.

The identification of the immunodominant peptides is an important goal if tumor specific peptides are to be used in vaccination strategies. The strength of the T-cell response depends on the binding affinity of the peptide (antigen) to the HLA molecule, the stability of the HLA-bound peptide, and the avidity of the TCR for the peptide–HLA complex. Bioinformatics can be used to predict which human immunoglobulin-derived peptides are capable of inducing a T-cell response. This process has demonstrated that CD8[+] cells can recognize immunoglobulin-derived peptides bound to MHC class I molecules.[99,100] We have recently used this method to predict immunodominant peptides from the sequence of the CDR3 region of the IgH gene of 16 patients with myeloma. CDR3 sequence-derived peptides from most patients failed to achieve a 'high score,' indicating a poor affinity between the unique peptides and the patient's HLA. It would then be predicted that such peptides would fail to generate a significant T-cell response.[101] In other B-cell malignancies, the majority of immunodominant peptides have been found outside the CDR3 region, more often in framework regions. Future studies in patients with myeloma should, therefore, not expect that immunodominant peptides with the potential to stimulate antitumor T-cell activity will be found only in the CDR3 region.[101]

TUMOR–DERIVED SUPPRESSION/INHIBITION OF T CELLS

Tumor cells may interfere with the immune response by secreting suppressive factors or by promoting apoptosis of the immunoregulatory cells. Transforming growth factor 1 (TGFβ) produced by multiple myeloma cell lines has been shown to suppress T-cell proliferation by inhibiting responses to IL-2 in stimulated peripheral blood T lymphocytes.[102] In addition, it has been shown that TGFβ is responsible for the failure of normal maturation of dendritic cells in myeloma.[70] Fas ligand, which induces programmed cell death in Fas-positive and Fas-sensitive target cells, is expressed on myeloma cell lines, suggesting a possible mechanism for the tumor to escape from immune surveillance.[103] Even though myeloma cells also express Fas antigen, not all myeloma cells undergo apoptosis in response to anti-Fas antibodies. In line with this observation, mutations in the Fas antigen have also been reported from patients with multiple myeloma, suggesting a loss of death control in these cells rather than a lack of growth control.[104]

ANTI–MYELOMA ACTIVITY BY T CELLS

In murine models, T cells with a specificity for myeloma proteins have been detected and antitumor responses involving both T-cell cytotoxicity and productive immunity have been demonstrated.[105–107] Tumor immunity was shown to be ablated by post-immunization thymectomy, suggesting a short-lived regulatory effector cell rather than a conventional cytotoxic T cell as the tumor suppressor cell. Anti-idiotypic antibodies to MOPC-315 tumor cells were shown to mediate a reduction of surface membrane expression of M315, but did not influence M315 secretion or MOPC-315 growth. In contrast, anti-idiotypic T cells blocked the secretion of the M315 protein by the tumor cells without effects on cell growth, viability or surface membrane M315 expression.[108]

The murine model has demonstrated that idiotype-specific T cells recognize a CDR3 peptide produced owing to somatic mutation. These idiotype-specific T cells demonstrate TCR diversity, suggesting that there is more than one T-cell clone with tumor specificity.[109,110] In human studies, T cells have been shown to have suppressive effects on polyclonal immunoglobulin production in patients with myeloma.[111] Peripheral blood lymphocytes from patients with myeloma have demonstrated direct antimyeloma activity by proliferative and cytotoxic responses to

autologous and allogeneic myeloma plasma cells.[85] However, the identification of tumor specific T cells in patients with myeloma has been less convincing than in murine studies. The use of a new technology such as the tetramer method, where four class 1 MHC molecules are complexed to specific peptides and allow direct binding to TCRs, may offer the potential to detect and enumerate CD8[+] antigen-specific T cells, and such studies need to be performed with tetramers prepared with idiotype-specific and immunodominant peptides.

ADOPTIVE IMMUNITY AND T CELLS IN MYELOMA

Adoptive immunotherapy, the transfer of immunocompetent cells, such as donor-derived lymphocytes, has been demonstrated to have antitumor activity in some patients who have relapsed following allogeneic bone marrow transplantation.[112] It has also been shown that infusion of selected CD3[+] T cells can induce a graft-versus-myeloma effect, although not without the risk of exacerbating graft-versus-host disease (Chapter 17).[113]

Specific immunization of potential donors with recipient idiotype prior to allogeneic transplantation has also been reported.[114] Two years after transplantation, the monoclonal protein remained low. In another study, the donor was immunized against the recipient monoclonal protein before the infusion of donor T lymphocytes given to treat relapse after bone marrow transplantation. Nineteen months after donor lymphocyte infusion, the patient remained in remission.[115]

The mechanisms involved in the killing of myeloma cells by donor T cells have been shown to include CD4[+] T cells with specificity for myeloma idiotype and CD8[+] allospecific T cells that mediate the cytotoxicity through the perforin-mediated pathway.[116] Recent studies showing that the T-cell repertoire of graft-versus-myeloma differs from that of graft-versus-host disease have encouraged investigation into strategies that will stimulate a graft-versus-myeloma effect, while ameliorating a graft-versus-host toxicity.[117]

Restoration of T-cell function by either active or passive immunotherapy holds some promise for the future therapy of not only patients with multiple myeloma but also many other malignancies. The role of tolerogenic antigen-presenting cells (APCs) is currently under study as they may present a critical barrier for T-cell adoptive immunotherapy. Further studies are needed, however, to understand how T cells and other players of the immune system can be induced to a higher functional antitumor capacity in patients with myeloma.

Natural killer cells

The role of natural killer cells in antitumor immunity remains unclear. A significant increase in both absolute and relative numbers of CD57[+] cells in myeloma patients, especially in the early stages of disease, suggests a possible surveillance mechanism in response to the emerging malignant clone. CD57[+] CD16[+] cells have been reported to be lower in myeloma than MGUS.[118] Studies have shown an increase in CD16[+] CD3[+] cells, indicating that T cells with NK phenotype were expanded in a subset of patients. However, despite the increased frequency of cells with NK phenotype, the assays of NK function were shown to be comparable in patients with MGUS and multiple myeloma with that in normal individuals.[119] There is evidence that an increase in CD56[+] CD3[-] cells is associated with progressive disease and poor prognosis, while patients with an increased number of CD57[+] CD8[-] cells have a better prognosis.[120] Other studies have shown lack of correlation of either the percentage or absolute number of any subpopulation of NK cells or CD56[+] T cells with disease activity.[121]

Thalidomide and related analogs mediate an antimyeloma effect by modulating NK cell number and function.[122] Thalidomide increases NK cell numbers *in vivo* and increases lysis of myeloma cell lines *in vitro*, a factor that is CD56[+] cell specific. The role of circulating non-MHC-restricted cytotoxic lymphocytes in maintaining disease activity in patients with myeloma has yet to be determined.

HOST–TUMOR INTERACTIONS

Clinical observations over a number of years have suggested the presence of beneficial host–tumor interactions and immune surveillance in certain situations in patients with myeloma. For instance, the phenomenon of plateau phase after chemotherapy, the stability of protein levels in patients who have MGUS and the non-progressive nature of smoldering myeloma all suggest the presence of immunoregulatory mechanisms.[123] Recent observations relating to the presence and improved prognosis associated with clonal expansions of T cells in this disease, the abnormalities and restriction of the T-cell repertoire also suggest immunoregulatory mechanisms.[88] Antitumor activity has been suggested to be a possible role of gamma–delta T cells and it has also been suggested that this role may be stimulated by aminobisphosphonates.[124]

Myeloma-specific cytotoxic lymphocytes can be generated *in vitro* by pulsing dendritic cells with autologous myeloma lysates, but the specific antigens involved and the immunodominant peptides responsible for this cytotoxicity are unclear. CD80[+] T cells are increased in myeloma and it is possible that they represent anergic T-cell clones.[125] CD80 and CD86 expression on CD3[+] cells is not endogenously upregulated but rather is acquired when lymphocyte-bound CD28 binds to these co-stimulatory molecules during antigen presentation. CD80[+] T cells are almost exclusively CD45 RO[+] cells, i.e. suggestive of memory T cells. CD45 RA[+] cells, i.e. naive T cells, are limited to the CD80[-] T-cell population. These studies suggest that CD80[+] T cells are common in patients with myeloma and may constitute a population of post-antigen presentation and unresponsive memory T cells, which may have tumor specificity. While it is possible that the antigen responsible in myeloma is a tumor antigen, whether this is the idiotype has yet to be resolved.

Reversing of T-cell unresponsiveness may be a key factor in the development of immunotherapy strategies in patients with myeloma. Possible enhancement of this immunoregulatory process by idiotypic or other vaccination is currently being studied in depth and, although clinical results may not be encouraging at present, demonstration of cytotoxic T cells stimulated by tumor lysates and the documentation of idiotype-specific cytotoxic T cells both in mature plasmacytomas and human myeloma demonstrates, in principle, that enhancement of these processes may be possible.

OPTIONS FOR IMMUNOTHERAPY

Vaccines

Naturally occurring responses against idiotypic antigens and other tumor antigens have been demonstrated in patients with low tumor burden, and the optimal clinical setting for vaccination and the methods of vaccination need further exploration. Tumor vaccination, either based on immunization against specific tumor antigens or adoptive transfer of *ex vivo* generated lymphocytes, is an attractive proposition in many malignancies. In myeloma the idiotypic specific marker has most frequently been used for immunotherapy. However, the results of vaccination with idiotypic protein-pulsed dendritic cells have so far been somewhat disappointing. Other potentially more effective approaches need analysis. Under active consideration are the use of more mature dendritic cells, tumor DNA vaccines, and neutralizing a tumor-generated inhibitor, which may impair the efficacy of vaccination.

The role of high-potency dendritic cell vaccination in myeloma, as opposed to the use of cytokine or lymphoid dendritic cells, has yet to be analyzed. It is not clear whether the relatively poor clinical responses seen to date are the result of poor idiotypic presentation by dendritic cells and T cells, as suggested by bioinformatic analysis, or the use of low-potency dendritic cells. As mentioned, the presence of CD57[+] CD8[+] T-cell clones and that their presence is correlated with an improved prognosis, does suggest that immune responses are available to be utilized. A number of phase II studies have demonstrated that dendritic cells together with idiotypic protein produce cytotoxic idiotypic T-cell responses *in vitro*. Such responses may be augmented by the use of single-chain

DNA vaccinations.[126] Bioinformatic data, which suggest that less than 20% of patients will have CDR3 fragments with high binding to T-cell receptors,[101] have led to the use of tumor lysates as immunizing agents, as well as the evaluation of other tumor antigens.[127,128]

Other potential tumor antigen candidates that have been identified in multiple myeloma include MUC-1 and the cancer germ-line genes MAGE, NY-ESO-1. Muc-1 is a glycosolated transferinase protein expressed on human adenocarcinoma and in hematological malignancies, including myeloma. Cytotoxic T cells specific for idiotypes present on Muc 1 have been described. The induction of MHC unrestricted CTLs against Muc 1 from patients with myeloma has also been reported.[128] However, vaccination strategy to treat multiple myeloma has, at this stage, been largely disappointing. Selection of immunodominant idiotypes will require further study. In addition, the time of vaccination, especially in view of the immune deficit associated with myeloma, may be a key and, as yet, only superficially evaluated variable.

Adoptive immunity and T cells in myeloma

Antibody-mediated immunotherapy with chimeric anti-CD-20 monoclonal antibodies has also been extensively evaluated. CD20+ bone marrow plasma cells are present in approximately 50% of patients who could thus theoretically benefit from CD20 antibody administration. Preliminary data have been presented showing partial response in some patients. Anti-CD20 monoclonal antibody therapy has also be used following high-dose therapy, where it has been reported to be safe with some clinical efficacy.[129]

Other cell-surface markers, such as syndecan CD138, and the protein recognized by the monoclonal antibody HM124, are additions to potentially new targets for adoptive serotherapy.[130]

KEY POINTS

- The malignant plasma cell has undergone somatic mutation of the immunoglobulin gene, placing its ontogeny after the germinal center reaction of B-cell development.
- Translocations into the immunoglobulin gene in myeloma occur predominantly into the switch regions.
- Translocation partner chromosomes are varied but are most commonly chromosomes 11q, 4p, 16q, and 6p.
- Switch translocations are almost universal in plasma cell lines and occur in at least 50% of primary tumors.

- Myeloma is associated with a defect in the primary immune response, leading to high-grade bacterial infections.
- T-cell clones exist in myeloma and are predominantly CD8+ expansions with the phenotype of cytotoxic T cells.
- The presence of T-cell clones is associated with a good prognosis.
- Idiotypic vaccination can stimulate cytotoxic T-cell clones and the potential clinical effects of vaccination are under investigation.

REFERENCES

● = Key primary paper
◆ = Major review article

1. Konde M, Weissman IL, Akashi K. Identification of clonogenic common lymphoid progenitors in mouse bone marrow. *Cell* 1997; **91**:61–72.
2. Bain G, Maandag EC, Izon DJ, Amsen D, Kruisbeek AM, Weintraub BC, *et al.* E2A proteins are required for proper B cell development and initiation of immunoglobulin gene rearrangements. *Cell* 1994; **79**:885–92.
3. Lin H, Grosschedl R. Failure of B-cell differentiation in mice lacking the transcription factor EBF. *Nature* 1995; **376**:263–7.
4. Nutt SL, Morrision AM, Dorfler P, Rolink AG, Busslinger M. Commitment to the B lymphoid lineage depends on the transcription factor Pax5. *Nature* 1999; **401**:556–62.
●5. Karasuyama H, Kado A, Melchers F. The proteins encoded by the VpreB and lambda 5 pre-B cell-specific genes can associate with each other and with mu heavy chain. *J Exp Med* 1990; **172**:969–72.
6. Kitamura D, Kudo A, Schaal S, Muller W, Melchers F, Rajewsky K. A critical role of lambda 5 protein in B cell development. *Cell* 1992; **69**:823–31.
●7. Liu Y-J, Zhang J, Zhang J, Lane PJL, Chan E-Y-T, MacLennan ICM. Sites of B cell activation in primary and secondary responses to T cell-dependent and T cell-independent antigens. *Eur J Immunol* 1991; **21**:2951–62.
8. Liu Y-J, Malisan F, de Bouteiller O, Guret C, Lebecque L, Banchereau J, *et al.* Within germinal centers, isotype switching of immunoglobulin genes occurs after the onset of somatic mutation. *Immunity* 1995; **4**:241–50.
●9. Liu Y-J, Joshua DE, Williams GT, Smith CA, Gordon J, MacLennan ICM. Mechanisms of antigen-driven selection in germinal centres. *Nature* 1989; **342**:929–31.
◆10. MacLennan ICM. Antibody-secreting cells and their origins. In: Malpas J, Bergsagel D, Kyle R, Anderson K (eds) *Myeloma: biology and management.* Oxford: Oxford University Press, 1998:29–47.
11. Bakkus MH, Van Reit I, De Greef C, Van Camp B, Thielemans K. The clonogenic precursor cell in multiple myeloma. *Leukemia Lymphoma* 1995; **18**:21.
◆12. Blackwell TK, Alt FW. Immunoglobulin genes. In: Hames BD, Glover DM (eds) *Molecular immunology.* Oxford: IRL Press, 1989:1–600.

●13. Bergsagel PL, Chesi MC, Nardini E, Brents LA, Kirby SL, Kuehl WM. Promiscuous translocations into immunoglobulin heavy chain switch regions in multiple myeloma. *Proc Natl Acad Sci USA* 1996; **93**:13931–6.

●14. Bakkus MHC, Heirman C, Van Reit IV, Van Camp B, Theilmans K. Evidence that multiple myeloma Ig heavy chain VDJ genes contain somatic mutations but show no intraclonal variation. *Blood* 1992; **80**:2326.

●15. Ralph Q, Brisco M, Joshua DE, Brown RD, Gibson J, Morley AA. Advancement of multiple myeloma from diagnosis through plateau phase to progressive does not involve a new B cell clone: evidence from the immunoglobulin heavy chain gene. *Blood* 1993; **82**:202–6.

●16. Bakkus MHC, Van Riet I, Van Camp B, Thielemans K. Evidence that the clonogenic cell in multiple myeloma originates from a pre-switched but somatically mutated B cell. *Br J Haematol* 1994; **87**:68–74.

◆17. Walter M, Surti V, Hofker M, Cox D. The physical organization of the human immunoglobulin heavy chain gene complex. *EMBO J* 1990; **9**:3303.

18. Humphries CG, Shen A, Kuzel A, Capra JD, Blattner FR, Tucker PW. A new human immunoglobulin VH family preferentially rearranged in immature B cell tumours. *Nature* 1988; **331**:446.

19. Clofent G, Brockly F, Commes T, Lefranc M, Bataille R, Klein B. No preferential use of VH5 family in human multiple myeloma. *Br J Haematol* 1989; **73**:486.

20. Rettig MB, Vescio RA, Cas J, Wa CH, Lee JC, Han E, *et al.* VH gene usage in multiple myeloma in complete absence of the VH4.21 (VH4.34) gene. *Blood* 1996; **87**:2846–52.

●21. Szczepak AJ, Seeberger K, Wizniak J, Mant MJ, Belch AR, Pilarski LM. A high frequency of circulating B cells share clonotypic Ig heavy-chain VDJ rearrangements with autologous bone marrow plasma cells in multiple myeloma, as measured by single-cell and in situ reverse transcriptase-polymerase chain reaction. *Blood* 1998; **92**:2844–55.

22. Reiman T, Seeberger K, Taylor BJ, Szczepek AJ, Hanson J, Mant MJ, *et al.* Persistent preswitch clonotypic myeloma cells correlate with decreased survival: evidence for isotype switching within the myeloma clone. *Blood* 2001; **98**:2791–9.

23. Bakkus MH, Asosingh K, Vanderkerken K, Thielemans K, Hagemeijer A, De Raeve H, *et al.* Myeloma isotype-switch variants in the murine 5T myeloma model: evidence that myeloma IgM and IgA expressing subclones can originate from the IgG expressing tumour. *Leukemia* 2001; **15**:1127–32.

24. Taniwaki M, Nishida K, Takashima T, Nakagawa H, Fujii H, Tamaki T, *et al.* Nonrandom chromosomal rearrangements of 14q32.3 and 19p13.3 and preferential deletion of 1p in 21 patients with multiple myeloma and plasma cell leukemia. *Blood* 1994; **84**:2283–90.

25. Lai JL, Zandecki M, Mary JY, Bernardi F, Izydorczyk V, Flactif M, *et al.* Improved cytogenetics in multiple myeloma: a study of 151 patients including 117 patients at diagnosis. *Blood* 1995; **85**:2490–7.

26. Taniwaki M, Nishida K, Ueda Y, Takashima T. Non-random chromosomal rearrangements and their implications in clinical features and outcome of multiple myeloma and plasma cell leukemia. *Leukemia Lymphoma* 1996; **21**:25–30.

27. Avet-Loiseau H, Li J, Facon T, Brigadeau C, Morineau N, Maloisel F, *et al.* High incidence of translocations t(11;14)(q13;q32) and t(4;14)(p16;q32) in patients with plasma cell malignancies. *Cancer Res* 1998; **58**:5640–5.

28. Fonseca R, Witzig TE, Gertz MA, Kyle RA, Hoyer JD, Jalal SM, *et al.* Multiple myeloma and the translocation t(11;14) (q13;q32): a report on 13 cases. *Br J Haematol* 1998; **101**:296–301.

●29. Tricot G, Barlogie B, Jagannath S, Bracy D, Mattox S, Vesole DH, Naucke S, Sawyer JR. Poor prognosis in multiple myeloma is associated only with partial or complete deletions of chromosome 13 or abnormalities involving 11q and not with other karyotype abnormalities. *Blood* 1995; **86**:4250–6.

30. Chesi M, Bergsagel PL, Brents LA, Smith CM, Gerhard DS, Kuehl WM. Dysregulation of cyclin D1 by translocation into an IgH gamma switch region in two multiple myeloma cell lines. *Blood* 1996; **88**:674–81.

31. Hoyer JD, Hanson CA, Fonseca R, Greipp PR, Dewald GW, Kurtin PJ. The (11;14)(q13;q32) translocation in multiple myeloma. A morphologic and immunohistochemical study. *Am J Clin Pathol* 2000; **113**:831–7.

32. Pruneri G, Fabris S, Baldini L, Carboni N, Zagano S, Colombi MA, *et al.* Immunohistochemical analysis of cyclin D1 shows deregulated expression in multiple myeloma with the t(11;14). *Am J Pathol* 2000; **156**:1505–13.

33. Sherr CJ. The Pezcoller lecture: cancer cell cycles revisited. *Cancer Res* 2000; **60**:3689–95.

34. Janssen JWG, Vaandrager JW, Jeuser T, Jauch A, Kluin PM, Geelen E, *et al.* Concurrent activation of a novel putative transforming gene, myeov, and cyclin D1 in a subset of multiple myeloma cell lines with t(11;14)(q13;q32). *Blood* 2000; **95**:2691–8.

35. Rao PH, Cigudosa JC, Ning Y, Calsanz MJ, Iida S, Tagawa S, *et al.* Multicolor spectral karyotyping identifies new recurring breakpoints and translocations in multiple myeloma. *Blood* 1998; **92**:1743–8.

36. Sawyer JR, Lukacs JL, Munshi N, Desikan KR, Singhal S, Mehta J, *et al.* Identification of new nonrandom translocations in multiple myeloma with multicolor spectral karyotyping. *Blood* 1998; **92**:4269–78.

37. Sawyer JR, Lukacs JL, Thomas EL, Swanson CM, Goosen LS, Sammartino G, *et al.* Multicolour spectral karyotyping identifies new translocations and a recurring pathway for chromosome loss in multiple myeloma. *Br J Haematol* 2001; **112**:167–74.

38. Chesi M, Nardini E, Brents LA, Schrock E, Ried T, Kuehl WM, *et al.* Frequent translocation t(4;14)(p16.3;q32.3) in multiple myeloma is associated with increased expression and activating mutations of fibroblast growth factor receptor 3. *Nat Genet* 1997; **16**:260–4.

39. Richelda R, Ronchetti D, Baldini L, Cro L, Viggiano L, Marzella R, *et al.* A novel chromosomal translocationt (4;14) (p16.3;q32) in multiple myeloma involves the fibroblast growth-factor receptor 3 gene. *Blood* 1997; **90**:4062–70.

40. Finelli P, Fabris S, Zagona S, Baldini L, Intini D, Nobili L, *et al.* Detection of t(4;14)(p16;q32) chromosomal translocation in multiple myeloma by double-color fluorescent in situ hybridization. *Blood* 1999; **94**:724–32.

41. Avet-Loiseau H, Facon T, Daviet A, Godon C, Rapp M, Harousseau J, *et al.* 14q32 translocations and monosomy 13 observed in monoclonal gammopathy of undetermined significance delineate a multistep process for the oncogenesis of multiple myeloma. *Cancer Res* 1999; **59**:4546–50.

42. Malgeri U, Baldini L, Perfetti V, Fabris S, Vignarelli MC, Colombo G, et al. Detection of t(4:14)(p16.3;q32) chromosomal translocation in multiple myeloma by reverse transcription-polymerase chain reaction analysis of IGH-MMSET fusion transcripts. *Cancer Res* 2000; **60**:4058–61.

43. Naski MC, Wang Q, Xu J, Ornitz DM. Grades activation of fibroblast growth factor receptor 3 by mutations causing achondroplasia and thanatophoric dysplasia. *Nat Genet* 1996; **13**:233–7.

44. Webster MK, D'Avis PY, Robertson SC, Donoghue DJ. Profound ligand-independent kinase activation of fibroblast growth factor receptor 3 by the activation loop mutation responsible for a lethal skeletal dysplasia, thanatophoric dysplasia type II. *Mol Cell Biol* 1996; **16**:4081–87.

●45. Chesi M, Brents LA, Ely SA, Bais C, Robbiani DF, Mesri EA, et al. Activated fibroblast growth factor receptor 3 is an oncogene that contributes to tumor progression in multiple myeloma. *Blood* 2001; **97**:729–36.

46. Fracchiolla NS, Luminari S, Baldini L, Lombardi L, Maiolo AT, Neri A. FGFR3 gene mutations associated with human skeletal disorders occur rarely in multiple myeloma. *Blood* 1998; **92**:2987–9.

47. Intini D, Baldini L, Fabris S, Lombardi L, Ciceri G, Maiolo AT, et al. Analysis of FGFR3 gene mutations in multiple myeloma patients with t(4;14). *Br J Haematol* 2001; **17**:362–4.

48. Plowright EE, Li Z, Bergsagel PL, Chesi M, Barber DL, Branch DR, et al. Ectopic expression of fibroblast growth factor receptor 3 promotes myeloma cell proliferation and prevents apoptosis. *Blood* 2000; **95**:992–8.

49. Li Z, Zhu YY, Plowright EE, Bergsagel PL, Chesi M, Patterson B, et al. The myeloma-associated oncogene fibroblast growth factor receptor 3 is transforming in hematopoietic cells. *Blood* 2001; **97**:2413–19.

●50. Stec I, Wright TJ, van Ommen GB, de Boer PAJ, van Haeringen A, Moorman AFM, et al. WHSC1, a 90 kb SET domain-containing gene, expressed in early development and homologous to a Drosophila dysmorphy gene maps in the Wolf–Hirschhorn syndrome critical region and is fused to IgH in t(4;14) multiple myeloma. *Hum Mol Genet* 1998; **7**:1071–82.

51. Cui X, De Vivo I, Slany R, Miyamoto A, Firestein R, Cleary ML. Association of SET domain and myotubularin-related proteins modulates growth control. *Nat Genet* 1998; **18**:331–7.

52. Chesi M, Nardini E, Lim RSC, Smith KD, Kuehl WM, Bergsagel PL. The t(4;14) translocation in myeloma dysregulates both FGFR3 and a novel gene, MMSET, resulting in IgH/MMSET hybrid transcripts. *Blood* 1998; **92**:3025–34.

53. Chesi M, Bergsagel PL, Shonukan OO, Martelli ML, Brents LA, Chen T, et al. Frequent dysregulation of the c-maf proto-oncogene at 16q23 by translocations to an Ig locus in multiple myeloma. *Blood* 1998; **91**:4457–63.

◆54. Bergsagel PL, Kuehl WM. Chromosome translocations in multiple myeloma. *Oncogene* 2001; **20**:5611–22.

55. Kataoka K, Nishizawa M, Kawai S. Structure–function analysis of the maf oncogene product, a member of the b-Zip protein family. *J Virol* 1993; **67**:2133–41.

56. Bednarek AK, Lafflin KJ, Daniel RL, Liao Q, Hawkins KA, Aldaz CM. WWOX, a novel WW domain-containing protein mapping to human chromosome 16q23.3–24.1, a region frequently affected by breast cancer. *Cancer Res* 2000; **60**:2140–5.

57. Iida S, Rao PH, Butler M, Corradini P, Boccadoro M, Klein B, et al. Deregulation of MUM1/IRF4 by chromosomal translocation in multiple myeloma. *Nat Genet* 1997; **17**:226–30.

58. Mittrucker HW, Matsuyama T, Grossman A, Kundig TM, Potter J, Shahinian A, et al. Requirement for the transcription factor LSIRF/IRF4 for mature B and T lymphocyte function. *Science* 1997; **275**:540–3.

59. Yoshida S, Nakazawa N, Iida S, Hayami Y, Sato S, Wakita A, et al. Detection of MUM1/IRF4-IgH fusion in multiple myeloma. *Leukemia* 1999; **13**:1812–16.

60. Shaughnessy J, Gabrea A, Qi Y, Brents L, Zhan F, Tian E, et al. Cyclin D3 at 6p21 is dysregulated by recurrent chromosomal translocations to immunoglobulin loci in multiple myeloma. *Blood* 2001; **98**:217–23.

●61. Avet-Loiseau H, Gerson F, Magrangeas F, Minvielle S, Harousseau JL, Bataille R, et al. Rearrangements of the c-myc oncogene are present in 15% of primary human multiple myeloma tumors. *Blood* 2001; **98**:3082–6.

62. Hatzivassiliou G, Miller I, Takizawa J, Palanisamy N, Rao PH, Iida S, et al. IRTA1 and IRTA2, novel immunoglobulin superfamily receptors expressed in B cells and involved in chromosome 1q21 abnormalities in B cell malignancy. *Immunity* 2001; **14**:277–89.

●63. Nishida K, Tamura A, Nakazawa N, Ueda Y, Abe T, Matsuda F, et al. The Ig heavy chain gene is frequently involved in chromosomal translocations in multiple myeloma and plasma cell leukemia as detected by in situ hybridization. *Blood* 1997; **90**:526–34.

●64. Ho PJ, Brown RD, Pelka G, Basten A, Gibson J, Joshua DE. Illegitimate switch recombinations are present in approximately half of primary myeloma tumors, but do not relate to known prognostic indicators or survival. *Blood* 2001; **97**:490–5.

●65. Avet-Loiseau H, Daviet A, Brigadeau C, Callet-Bauchu E, Terre C, Lafage-Pochitaloff M, et al. Cytogenetic, interphase, and multicolor fluorescence in situ hybridization analyses in primary plasma cell leukaemia: a study of 40 patients at diagnosis, on behalf of the Intergroupe Francophone du Myelome and the Groupe Francais de Cytogenetique Hematologique. *Blood* 2001; **97**:822–5.

66. Zojer N, Konigsberg R, Ackermann J, Fritz E, Dallinger S, Kromer E, et al. Deletion of 13q14 remains an independent adverse prognostic variable in multiple myeloma despite its frequent detection by interphase fluorescence in situ hybridization. *Blood* 2000; **95**:1925–30.

67. Konigsberg R, Zojer N, Ackermann J, Kromer E, Kittler H, Fritz E, et al. Predictive role of interphase cytogenetics for survival of patients with multiple myeloma. *J Clin Oncol* 2000; **18**:804–12.

68. Doughney KB, Williams DM, Penn RL. Multiple myeloma: infectious complications. *South Med J* 1988; **81**:855–85.

69. Joshua DE, Brown G, MacLennan IC. Immune suppression in BALB/c mice bearing the plasmacytoma TEPC-183: evidence for normal lymphocyte but defective macrophage function. *Int J Cancer* 1979; **23**:663–72.

●70. Brown RD, Pope B, Murray A, Esdale W, et al. Dendritic cells from patients with myeloma are numerically normal but functionally defective as they fail to upregulate CD80(B7-1) expression after huCD40LT stimulation because of inhibition by transforming growth factor-beta 1 and interleukin-10. *Blood* 2001; **98**:2992–8.

71. Savage DG, Lindenbaum J, Garret TJ. Biphasic pattern of bacterial infection in multiple myeloma. *Ann Intern Med* 1982; **96**:47–50.

72. Snowdon L, Gibson J, Joshua DE. Frequency of infection in plateau-phase multiple myeloma. *Lancet* 1994; **344**:262.

73. Oken MM, Pomeroy C, Weisdorf D, Bennett JM. Prophylactic antibodies for the prevention of early infection in multiple myeloma. *Am J Med* 1996; **100**:624–8.

74. Raitakari M, Brown RD, Gibson J, Joshua DE. T cells in myeloma. *Haematol Oncol* 2003; **21**:33–42.

75. Mills KHG, Cawley JC. Abnormal monoclonal antibody-defined helper/suppressor T-cell subpopulations in multiple myeloma: relationship to treatment and clinical stage. *Br J Haematol* 1983; **53**:271–5.

76. Serra HM, Mant MJ, Ruether BA, Ledbetter JA, Pilarski LM. Selective loss of CD4$^+$CD45R$^+$ T cells in peripheral blood of multiple myeloma patients. *J Clin Immunol* 1988; **8**:259–65.

77. Massaia M, Bianchi A, Attisano C, Peola S, Redoglia V, Dianzani U, et al. Detection of hyperreactive T cells in multiple myeloma by multivalent cross-linking of the CD3/TCR complex. *Blood* 1991; **78**:1770–80.

78. Reibnegger G, Krainer M, Herold M, Ludwig H, Wachter H, Huber H. Predictive value of interleukin-6 and neopterin in patients with multiple myeloma. *Cancer Res* 1991; **51**:6250–3.

79. Brown RD, Joshua DE, Nelson M, Gibson J, Dunn J, MacLellan ICM. Serum thymidine kinase as a prognostic indicator for patients with multiple myeloma: results from the MRC (UK) V trial. *Br J Haematol* 1993; **84**:238–41.

80. Miguel-Garcia A, Matutes E, Tarin F, Garcia-Talavera J, Miguel-Sosa A, Carbonell F, et al. Circulating Ki67 positive lymphocytes in multiple myeloma and benign monoclonal gammopathy. *J Clin Pathol* 1995; **48**:835–9.

81. Massaia M, Borrione P, Attisano C, Barral P, Beggiato E, Montacchini L, et al. Dysregulated Fas and bcl-2 expression leading to enhanced apoptosis in T cells of multiple myeloma patients. *Blood* 1995; **85**:3679–87.

82. Massaia M, Dianzani U, Bianchi A, Camponi A, Boccadoro M, Pileri A. Defective generation of alloreactive cytotoxic T lymphocytes (CTL) in human monoclonal gammopathies. *Clin Exp Immunol* 1988; **73**:214–18.

83. Massaia M, Bianchi A, Dianzani U, Camponi A, Attisano C, Boccadoro M, et al. Defective interleukin-2 induction of lymphokine-activated killer (LAK) activity in peripheral blood T lymphocytes of patients with monoclonal gammopathies. *Clin Exp Immunol* 1990; **79**:100–4.

84. Ozer H, Han T, Henderson ES, Nussbaum A, Sheedy D. Immunoregulatory T cell function in multiple myeloma. *J Clin Invest* 1981; **67**:779–89.

85. Lahat N, Aghai E, Froom P. T-cells of multiple myeloma patients triggered by the autologous mixed lymphocyte reaction suppress polyclonal immunoglobulin synthesis. *Cancer* 1988; **15**:1124–8.

86. Pilarski LM, Mant MJ, Ruether BA, Carayanniotis G, Otto D, Krowka JF. Abnormal clonogenic potential of T cells from multiple myeloma patients. *Blood* 1985; **66**:1266–71.

87. Wen T, Mellstedt H, Jondal M. Presence of clonal T cell populations in chronic B lymphocytic leukemia and smoldering myeloma. *J Exp Med* 1990; **171**:659–66.

●88. Brown RD, Yuen E, Nelson M, Gibson J, Joshua D. The prognostic significance of T cell receptor beta gene rearrangements and idiotypic-reactive T cell in multiple myeloma. *Leukaemia* 1997; **11**:1312–17.

89. Janson CH, Grunewald J, Osterborg A, DerSimonian H, Brenner MB, Mellstedt H, et al. Predominant T cell receptor V gene usage in patients with abnormal clones of B cells. *Blood* 1991; **77**:1776–80.

●90. Moss P, Gillespie G, Frodsham P, Bell J, Reyburn H. Clonal populations of CD4$^+$ and CD8$^+$ T cells in patients with multiple myeloma and paraproteinemia. *Blood* 1996; **87**:3297–306.

●91. Raitakari M, Brown RD, Sze D, Yuen E, Barrow L, Nelson M, et al. T-cell expansion in patients with multiple myeloma have a phenotype of cytotoxic T cells. *Br J Haematol* 2000; **110L**:203–9.

●92. Halapi E, Werner A, Wahlstrom J, Osterborg A, Jeddi-Tehrani M, Yi Q, et al. T cell repertoire in patients with multiple myeloma and monoclonal gammopathy of undetermined significance: clonal CD8$^+$ T cell expansions are found preferentially in patients with a low tumor burden. *Eur J Immunol* 1997; **27**:2245–52.

●93. Sze DM, Giesajtis G, Brown RD, Raitakari M, Gibson J, Ho J, et al. Clonal cytotoxic T cells are expanded in myeloma and reside in the CD8(+)CD57(+)CD28(−) compartment. *Blood* 2001; **98**:2817–27.

●94. Osterborg A, Masucci M, Bergenbrandt S, Holm G, Lefvert AK, Mellstedt H. Generation of T cell clones binding f(ab')2 fragments of the idiotypic immunoglobulin in patients with monoclonal gammopathy. *Cancer Immunol Immunother* 1991; **34**:157–62.

95. Osterborg A, Yi Q, Bergenbrandt S, Holm G, Lefvert A-K, Mellstedt H. Idiotype-specific T cells in multiple myeloma stage I: an evaluation by four different function tests. *Br J Haematol* 1995; **89**:110–16.

96. Yi Q, Holm G, Lefvert AK. Idiotype-induced T cell stimulation requires antigen presentation in association with HLA-DR molecules. *Clin Exp Immunol* 1996; **104**:359–65.

97. Dembic Z, Schenck K, Bogen B. Dendritic cells purified from myeloma are primed with tumor-specific antigen (idiotype) and activate CD4$^+$ T cells. *Proc Natl Acad Sci USA* 2000; **97**:2697–702.

98. Osterborg A, Janson CH, Bergenbrandt S, Holm G, Lefvert A-K, Wigzell H, et al. Peripheral blood T lymphocytes in patients with monoclonal gammopathies: expanded subsets as depicted by capacity to bind to autologous monoclonal immunoglobulins or reactivity with anti-V gene-restricted antibodies. *Eur J Haematol* 1991; **47**:185–91.

99. Parker KC, Bednarek MA, Coligan JE. Scheme for ranking potential HLA-A2 binding peptides based on independent binding of individual peptide side-chains. *J Immunol* 1994; **152**:163–75.

100. Trojan A, Schulze JL, Witzens M, Vonderheide RH, Ladetto M, Donovan JW, et al. Immunoglobin framework-derived peptides function as cytotoxic T-cell epitopes commonly expressed in B-cell malignancies. *Nat Med* 2000; **6**:667–72.

101. Sze DM-Y, Brown RD, Gibson J, Ho J, Yang S, Pelka G, et al. Multiple myeloma idiotypic peptide-cytotoxic T cell interaction constitutes a minimal anti-tumor response. *Blood* 2001; **98**:154a (abstract).

102. Cook G, Campbell JD, Carr CE, Boyd KS, Franklin IM. Transforming growth factor beta from multiple myeloma cells inhibits proliferation and IL-2 responsiveness in T lymphocytes. *J Leucocyte Biol* 1999; **66**:981–8.

103. Villunger A, Egle A, Marschitz I, Kos M, Bock G, Ludwig H, et al. Constitutive expression of Fas (Apo-1/Cd95) ligand or multiple myeloma cells: a potential mechanism of tumor-induced suppression of immune surveillance. *Blood* 1997; **90**:12–20.

104. Shima Y, Nishimoto N, Ogata A, Fujii Y, Yoshizaki K, Kishimoto T. Myeloma cells express Fas antigen/APO-1 (CD95) but only some are sensitive to anti-Fas antibody resulting in apoptosis. *Blood* 1995; **85**:757–64.

●105. Abbas K, Perry LL, Bach BA, Greene MI. Idiotype-specific T cell immunity. I. Generation of effector and suppressor T lymphocytes reactive with myeloma idiotypic determinants. *J Immunol* 1980; **124**:1160–6.

◆106. Abbas AK. Antigen and T lymphocyte mediated suppression of myeloma cells: model systems for regulation of lymphocyte function. *Immunol Rev* 1979; **48**:245–64.

107. Lynch RG. Immunoglobulin-specific suppressor T cells. *Adv Immunol* 1987; **40**:135–51.

108. Milburn GL, Lynch RG. Anti-idiotypic regulation of IgA expression in myeloma cells. *Mol Immunol* 1983; **20**:931–40.

109. Bogen B, Snodgrass R, Briand JP, Hannestad K. Synthetic peptides and beta-chain gene rearrangements reveal a diversified T cell repertoire for a lambda light chain third hypervariable region. *Eur J Immunol* 1986; **16**:1379–89.

110. Bogen B, Lauritzsen GF, Weiss S. A stimulatory monoclonal antibody detecting T cell receptor diversity among idiotype-specific, major histocompatibility complex-restricted T cell clones. *Eur J Immunol* 1990; **20**:2359–62.

111. Broder S, Humphrey R, Durm M, Blackman M, Meade B, Goldman C, et al. Impaired synthesis of polyclonal (non-paraprotein) immunoglobulins by circulating lymphocytes from patients with multiple myeloma. *N Engl J Med* 1957; **293**:888–92.

112. Bertz H, Burger JA, Kunzmann R, Mertelsmann R, Finke J. Adoptive immunotherapy for relapsed multiple myeloma after allogeneic bone marrow transplantation (BMT): evidence for a graft-versus-myeloma effect. *Leukemia* 1997; **11**:281–3.

113. Cabrera R, Diaz-Espada F, Barrios Y, Briz M, Fores R, Barbolla L, et al. Infusion of lymphocytes obtained from a donor immunised with the paraprotein idiotype as a treatment in a relapsed myeloma. *Bone Marrow Transplant* 2000; **25**:1105–8.

114. Kwak LW, Taub DD, Duffey PL, Bensinger WI, Bryant EM, Reynolds CW, et al. Transfer of myeloma idiotype-specific immunity from an actively immunised marrow donor. *Lancet* 1995; **345**:1016–20.

115. Kroger N, Kruger W, Renges H, Zabelina T, Stute N, Jung R, et al. Donor lymphocyte infusion enhances remission status in patients with persistent disease after allografting for multiple myeloma. *Br J Haematol* 2001; **112**:421–3.

116. Chiriva-Internati M, Du J, Cannon M, Barlogie B, Yi Q. Myeloma-reactive allospecific cytotoxic T lymphocytes lyse target cells via the granule exocytosis pathway. *Br J Haematol* 2001; **112**:410–20.

117. Orsini E, Alyea EP, Schlossman R, Canning C, Soiffer RJ, Chillemi A, et al. Changes in T cell receptor repertoire associated with graft-versus-tumor effect and graft-versus-host disease in patients with relapsed multiple myeloma after donor lymphocyte infusion. *Bone Marrow Transplant* 2000; **25**:623–32.

118. Sawanobori M, Suzuki K, Nakagawa Y, Inoue Y, Utsuyama M, Hirokawa K. Natural killer cell frequency and serum cytokine levels in monoclonal gammopathies: correlation of bone marrow granular lymphocytes to prognosis. *Acta Haematol* 1997; **98**:150–4.

119. Ishiyama T, Watanabe K, Fukuchi K, Yajima K, Koike M, Tomoyasu S, et al. The increase of CD5LOW-NK cells in patients with multiple myeloma and plasmacytoma. *Anticancer Res* 1994; **14**:725–30.

120. Garcia-Sanz R, Gonzalez M, Orfao A, Moro MJ, Hernandez JM, Borrego D, et al. Analysis of natural killer-associated antigens in peripheral blood and bone marrow of multiple myeloma patients and prognostic implications. *Br J Haematol* 1996; **93**:81–8.

121. King MA, Radicchi-Mastroianni MA. Natural killer cells and CD56[+] T cells in the blood of multiple myeloma patients: analysis by 4-colour flow cytometry. *Cytometry* 1996; **26**:121–4.

122. Davies FE, Raje N, Hideshima T, Lentzsch S, Young T, Tai YT, et al. Thalidomide and immunomodulatory derivatives augment natural killer cell cytotoxicity in multiple myeloma. *Blood* 2001; **98**:210–16.

◆123. Joshua DE, Brown RD, Gibson J. Multiple myeloma: why does the disease escape from plateau phase? *Br J Haematol* 1994; **88**:667–71.

124. Das H, Wang L, Kamath A, Bukowski JF. Vgamma2Vdelta2 T-cell receptor-mediated recognition of aminobis-phosphonates. *Blood* 2001; **98**:1616–18.

125. Brown RD, Pope B, Murray A, Sze D, Gibson J, Ho JP, et al. CD80[+] T cells in myeloma: an acquired marker of prior antigen presentation and unresponsiveness. *Blood* 2001; **98**:49276 (abstract).

126. Hawkins RE, Russell SJ, Marcus R, Ashworth LJ, Brissnik J, Zhang J, et al. A pilot study of idiotypic vaccination for follicular B-cell lymphoma using a genetic approach. *Hum Gene Ther* 1997; **8**:1287–99.

127. Van Baren N, Brasseur F, Godelaine D, Hames G, Ferrant A, Lehmann F, et al. Genes encoding tumor-specific antigens are expressed in human myeloma cells. *Blood* 1999; **94**:1156–64.

128. Brossart P, Schneider A, Dill P, Schammann T, Grunebach F, Wirths S, et al. The epithelial tumor antigen MUC1 is expressed in hematological malignancies and is recognized by MUC1-specific cytotoxic T-lymphocytes. *Cancer Res* 2001; **61**:6846–50.

129. Treon SP, Anderson KC. The use of rituximab in the treatment of malignant and nonmalignant plasma cell disorders. *Semin Oncol* 2000; **27**:79–85.

130. Ono K, Ohtomo T, Yoshida K, Yoshimura Y, Kawai S, Koishihara Y, et al. The humanized anti-HM1.24 antibody effectively kills multiple myeloma cells by human effector cell-mediated cytotoxicity. *Mol Immunol* 1999; **36**:387–95.

4

Molecular biology and cytogenetics

JOHANNES DRACH, JUTTA ACKERMANN, SONJA SEIDL AND HANNES KAUFMANN

INTRODUCTION

Chromosomal abnormalities leading to altered expression and dysregulated function of genes, which are critically involved in normal cell growth and differentiation, are a hallmark of cancer cells. The importance of specific cytogenetic aberrations has been particularly evident in acute leukemias, where the identification of chromosomal abnormalities has contributed to the understanding of leukemia cell biology and the establishment of a prognostically as well as a clinically relevant classification of the disease. In recent years, considerable progress has also been made in the cytogenetic and molecular genetic investigation of lymphoproliferative disorders, and most investigators believe that almost every case is characterized by a chromosomally abnormal clone. This is also true for multiple myeloma (MM),[1] although cytogenetic studies of MM cells are often hampered by the low mitotic rate of the myelomatous clone. For this reason, use of molecular cytogenetic techniques, which do not necessarily depend on dividing cells, has greatly enhanced our possibilities to investigate MM and monoclonal gammopathy of undetermined significance (MGUS) at the cytogenetic level and to derive clinically relevant information from these studies.

CYTOGENETIC ABNORMALITIES IN MM

Metaphase cytogenetic studies

The ability to obtain karyotypic information in MM is greatly influenced by the aggressiveness and the proliferative capacity of the malignant clone.[2] Abnormal karyotypes are, therefore, almost never observed in MGUS; in MM, chromosomally abnormal clones can be found in 30–40% of patients with newly diagnosed disease, in up to 60% of patients with relapsed disease, and in up to 80% of patients with plasma cell leukemia.[3–8] Karyotypes in MM typically exhibit a complex set of numerical and structural abnormalities. Frequent karyotypic abnormalities of MM cells are summarized in Table 4.1; it should be noted,

Table 4.1 *Chromosomal abnormalities associated with multiple myeloma*

Abnormality	Comments
Trisomies of chromosomes 3, 5, 7, 9, 11, 15, 19	Characteristically found in hyperdiploid karyotypes
14q32 translocations	Translocation partner frequently unidentified, in karyotypes described as a 14q$^+$ chromosome
t(11;14)(q13;q32)	Results in overexpression of CYCLIN-D1
t(4;14)(p16.3;q32)	Only detectable by molecular cytogenetics
Monosomy 13/deletion of 13q	Found in 15% of MM patients by metaphase cytogenetics, in about 45% by FISH Prognostic implications
Abnormalities of 1p/1q	No apparent locus specificity of translocations, gains and deletions
Deletions of 6q21 and 8p	

however, that a disease-specific aberration has not yet been identified.

Cytogenetic studies performed in large patient populations have reproducibly shown that two main groups of MM patients can be distinguished based on the number of chromosomes in the abnormal metaphases.[3–9] One group is characterized by the presence of a hyperdiploid clone (with mean chromosome numbers between 50 and 53) with frequent occurrence of trisomies of chromosomes 3, 5, 7, 9, 11, 15, and 19. Structural abnormalities may or may not be present along with these numerical gains. The second group is defined by hypodiploid and pseudodiploid karyotypes, which are invariably associated with structural aberrations. This pattern of chromosomal changes obviously represents distinct MM entities, which is also reflected by the different clinical course of these patient populations (see later).

Studies using molecular cytogenetic techniques

Failure to obtain informative metaphases from MM cells can be circumvented by using molecular cytogenetic techniques. One approach is fluorescence *in situ* hybridization (FISH), which utilizes DNA from interphase nuclei and thus targets chromosomal regions of interest in non-dividing cells (Fig. 4.1, Plate 1). The limitation of FISH, however, is the fact that it requires chromosome- or region-specific DNA probes and, therefore, the technique depends on knowledge of candidate regions. By comparative genomic hybridization (CGH), a genomewide analysis for chromosomal gains and losses is performed, but balanced translocations not resulting in changes of the DNA content remain unrecognized by this approach.

It also needs to be pointed out that differences between cytogenetic techniques exist with respect to the ability of detecting small aberrations. Metaphase karyotyping detects gross chromosomal abnormalities in the range of 10–12 megabases; comparative genomic hybridization may be somewhat more sensitive (2–10 megabases). FISH will identify even smaller aberrant regions targeted by the DNA probes (usually 20–50 kilobases) and may, therefore, enable the detection of submicroscopic changes.

The application of molecular cytogenetic techniques has not only redefined the true incidence of specific abnormalities in MM, but these techniques have also contributed to the identification of some previously unidentified chromosomal aberrations.[1,10–13] FISH studies even with a limited number of DNA probes have demonstrated chromosomal aneuploidy in more than 90% of patients with MM. Studies using CGH suggested that the most frequent chromosomal events in MM are gains of chromosome 19p and partial or complete loss of chromosome 13. Other recurrent abnormalities include gains of chromosomes 1q, 9q, 11q, 12q, 15q, 17q, and 22q as well as losses of 6q, 8p, and 16q. Recently, multicolor spectral karyotyping (SKY) has been described to resolve complex chromosomal abnormalities. SKY analysis makes use of multicolor FISH and allows visualization of each chromosome in a different color, but depends on the availability of

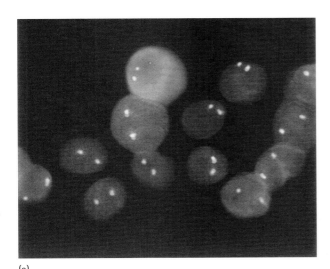
(a)

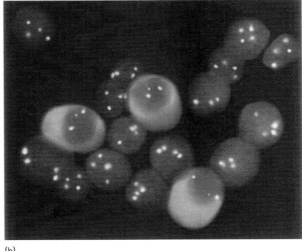
(b)

Figure 4.1 *Interphase fluorescence* in situ *hybridization of myelomatous plasma cells. (a) Detection of a translocation involving the* IgH *locus at 14q32. Two probes flanking the breakpoints are used; thus, presence of a red/green fusion signal indicates a normal pattern, whereas separation of the red and green signals indicates presence of a translocation. The plasma cell is identified after staining for cytoplasmic immunoglobulin light-chain expression and shows evidence for a IgH translocation, whereas a normal pattern of 14q32 is observed in the surrounding bone marrow cells. (b) Detection of a deletion of 13q14. The red signals are derived from a retinoblastoma-1 (rb-1) gene specific probe (13q14) and green signals represent a reference probe hybridizing to the centromeric region of chromosome 11. Note loss of an* rb-1 *signal in all plasma cells.*

metaphase chromosomes. By this approach, new recurrent translocations, t(14;16)(q32;q22–23) and t(9;14)(p13;q32), have been identified.[13]

Since chromosomal aberrations in MM may be detected at different frequencies depending on the cytogenetic technique employed, it will be an important goal to define diagnostic standards, particularly in the context of prognostically relevant chromosomal aberrations.

SPECIFIC CYTOGENETIC ABNORMALITIES IN MM AND THEIR MOLECULAR CONSEQUENCES

Translocations involving the immunoglobulin heavy chain locus (14q32)

14q32 translocations in MM involve the switch region of the immunoglobulin heavy chain (IgH) gene locus. Unlike the physiological process where Ig gene sequences are brought together during switch recombination, 14q32 translocations in MM are characterized by juxtaposition of IgH gene sequences with non-Ig DNA sequences (so-called illegitimate switch rearrangements; see Chapter 3).[14] These translocations are an almost universal event in MM cell lines.[15] By interphase FISH analyses, it was reported that IgH translocations are present in about 50% of patients with MGUS, in 75% of patients with MM, and in more than 80% of patients with plasma cell leukemia.[8,16–18] Translocation partners are quite heterogenous (see Table 4.2), with 11q13, 4p16.3, and 16q23 being most commonly involved in 14q32 translocations in MM. As a consequence of these translocations, genes that may

function as oncogenes, growth factors or transcription factors may be dysregulated.

11q13

A t(11;14)(q13;q32) can be found in 15–20% of patients with MM and may lead to overexpression of *cyclin D1*.[19,20] In contrast to mantle cell lymphoma, breakpoints on 11q13 in MM are not clustered in the major translocation cluster, but are scattered over a relatively large genomic region.[21] Probably as a result of this heterogeneity, a t(11;14) may also result in dysregulation of a second gene (myeloma overexpressed gene, *myeov*), which is located centromeric to *cyclin D1*.[22]

4p16.3

A t(4;14)(p16;q32) is present in about 15% of MM cases[20,23,24] using FISH and other molecular techniques but cannot be detected by conventional cytogenetics owing to the telomeric breakpoint on chromosome 4. This translocation results in dysregulated expression of two genes, *fgfr3* (fibroblast growth factor receptor 3) on the derivative chromosome 14 and *mmset* (multiple myeloma SET domain) on the derivative chromosome 4.[23–26] *fgfr3*, which is not expressed by normal plasma cells, is overexpressed as a consequence of the translocation and, in some cases, activating mutations have also been found on the translocated allele. Observations that expression of *fgfr3* promotes myeloma cell proliferation and prevents apoptosis, and that activation of *fgfr3* is a transforming event in hematopoietic cells further substantiate an oncogenic role for *fgfr3* in MM.[27–29] Thus, FGFR3 could represent a specific therapeutic target in MM cases carrying a t(4;14). In addition, the presence of a t(4;14) could influence the choice of cytotoxic agents, since in the murine myeloma cell line B9, cells overexpressing *fgfr3* were resistant to treatment with dexamethasone, but not to exposure with anthracyclines or alkylating agents.[30]

As with *fgfr3*, *mmset* overexpression only occurs in the presence of a t(4;14). Recent data suggest that presence of a *mmset/IgH* fusion transcript and expression of MMSET protein, but lack of FGFR3 expression, may occur in up to a third of MM cases with a t(4;14).[31] These cases may be characterized by loss of one copy of *fgfr3*. In another study, expression of *fgfr3* transcripts was observed in only 23 of 31 MM cases (74%) carrying the t(4;14).[32] Collectively, these data suggest that activation of *mmset* may be the critical transforming event in at least part of MM cases with a t(4;14), although the role of *mmset* for MM pathogenesis awaits further characterization.

16q23

The t(14;16)(q32;q23), which is present in 5–10% of patients with MM, results in expression of c-*maf* in MM

Table 4.2 *Partner chromosomes frequently involved in 14q32 translocations in multiple myeloma*

Chromosome	Gene	Function/comment
11q13	cyclin-D1/myeov	Overexpession of CYCLIN-D1; proliferation; favorable prognosis
4p16.3	fgfr3/mmset	Transcription factor; unfavorable prognosis
16q23	c-maf	Transcription factor; unfavorable prognosis
6p25	mum/irf4	Transcription factor
8q24	c-myc	Proliferation, differentiation, apoptosis
18q21	bcl-2	Inhibition of apoptosis
20q11	mafB	Probably secondary translocation
12q24	?	? (recently identified by SKY analysis)

cells at a high level.[13,33] c-*maf* has been identified as a transcription factor in lymphoid cells involved in regulation of expression of interleukin-4 (IL-4),[34] but its role in the molecular pathology of MM still needs to be determined.

OTHER TRANSLOCATION PARTNERS

There are several other chromosomal regions that have been reported as partner loci for 14q32 translocations in MM,[35] but each of them appears to occur in fewer than 5% of patients with MM. In some instances, the breakpoints have been cloned and information on dysregulated genes is available. These include t(6;14) (p21;q32) leading to overexpression of *cyclin D3*[36] and t(6;14) (p25;q32) with the *IRF-4/MUM-1* gene being expressed at high levels in the MM cell lines carrying the translocation.[37]

In about half of the patients with MM, in whom FISH analysis demonstrates presence of a 14q32 translocation, the partner chromosome remains unidentified.[18]

Deletion of chromosome 13q

Partial or complete loss of chromosome 13q has been observed as the most frequent chromosomal region that is recurrently deleted in MM karyotypes. This abnormality has gained considerable interest owing to the strong association between the presence of a chromosome 13 deletion and the shorter survival of MM patients. By metaphase cytogenetics, a chromosome 13q abnormality can be found in about 15% of MM patients at diagnosis,[3–9,38] whereas interphase FISH studies have shown a higher frequency of 13q deletions in MM, occurring in 39–54% of newly diagnosed cases.[39–43] By using an extended panel of DNA probes covering 11 regions on 13q, an even higher frequency of deletions has been reported (86% of patients, some of whom were heavily pre-treated).[44]

The molecular consequences of 13q deletions in MM are still poorly characterized. In the majority of cases with a 13q deletion, large proportions of the 13q arm are deleted, indicating loss of the entire chromosome arm or even monosomy 13.[42,45] However, interstitial deletions mainly involving band 13q14,[46] as well as dual loss at 13q14 and 13q34 with an intact intervening region,[47] have recurrently been observed. Recently, it has been suggested that a common deleted region including the *D13S319* locus is located at 13q14 between the *RB-1* and *D13S25* gene loci.[47] This genomic region encompasses an area rich in expressed sequence tagged sites and contains the *DLEU1, DLEU2,* and *RFP2* genes. Direct sequencing of the *RFP2* gene did not reveal any mutations in six patients and four cell lines exhibiting a 13q14 deletion. It has not yet been investigated as to whether *RFP2* may be involved in the pathogenesis

of MM by means of other mechanisms of inactivation, e.g. haploinsufficiency.

A chromosome 13 abnormality may be associated with specific 14q translocations:[18,48] data obtained thus far indicate that there are significant associations between t(4;14) and the presence of a deletion 13q (>80%) as well as t(14;16) and deletion 13q (100% in the few reported cases). In contrast, patients lacking any 14q translocation displayed significantly less frequent abnormalities of chromosome 13q (about 25% of cases). No correlations were found between t(11;14) and deletion 13q; likewise, there is no apparent association between a 14q32 translocation with an unknown partner chromosome and deletion 13q.

Abnormalities of chromosome 1

Abberrations of chromosome 1 belong to the most frequent structural abnormalities, which are recurrent in MM karyotypes. Both the p- and q-arms of chromosome 1 may be involved in these aberrations, although no specific locus appears to be predominantly affected by deletions, gains, or translocations.[3–7,35] Frequent breakpoints were reported to involve 1q12–q21.[49] Partial trisomies of 1q are a recurrent finding and may also occur as so-called jumping translocations, when the 1q segment moves around the karyotype to more than one non-homologous chromosome.[50] Specific translocations include the der(16)t(1;16)(q11;q11)[51] and the t(1;14)(q21;q32), which may be found in 1–2% of patients with advanced MM.[13]

OTHER MOLECULAR EVENTS IN MM

Translocations involving c-*myc*

Chromosomal aberrations of 8q24 (c-*myc* gene locus) have only rarely been reported by classical karyotypic analyses of MM. Similarly, a t(8;14)(q24;q32), as studied by interphase FISH, was present in only three of 140 primary MM tumors.[16] However, multicolor FISH studies of metaphase chromosomes obtained from patients with advanced MM indicated that complex translocations involving c-*myc* occur in about 40% of the 38 cases investigated.[52] In contrast to Burkitt's lymphoma, where c-*myc* is rearranged with Ig gene loci as a primary molecular event, translocations with c-*myc* in MM mostly involve non-Ig gene sequences and represent a late event in the pathogenesis of MM.

Mutations of N- and K-*ras*

Whereas mutations of N- and K-*ras* are absent in MGUS and solitary plasmacytoma, they may be present in about 30% of patients with MM at diagnosis and at even greater frequency in MM at an advanced and terminal stage. Activating mutations of *ras* can contribute to growth factor-independent proliferation of myeloma cells.[53] MM cell lines carrying a t(4;14) without activating mutation of *fgfr3* may have mutations of N- and K-*ras*, providing further evidence for a role of such mutations during progression of MM.[28]

Abnormalities of *p53*

p53 mutations are a rare event in MM at diagnosis, but they may be found with increasing frequency in patients with relapsed disease and plasma cell leukemia.[54] Deletions of 17p13 including the *p53* gene may also be present in MM at diagnosis but, since these abnormalities are often small interstitial deletions, molecular cytogenetic techniques are required for their detection.[55]

Epigenetic abnormalities of cell–cycle regulators and tumor suppressor genes

Epigenetics is the study of modifications in gene expression that do not involve changes in DNA nucleotide sequences.[56] Modifications in gene expression through methylation of DNA and remodeling of chromatin via histone proteins are believed to be the most important epigenetic changes. Current interest in the role of methylation has focused on the potential of aberrant methylation in silencing tumor suppressor genes.

In MM, hypermethylation of genes including *death-associated protein (DAP)-kinase*, *SOCS-1*, and the cell cycle regulators *p15* and *p16* has been established to be associated with gene inactivation. *p15* and *p16* proteins are cell-cycle regulators involved in the inhibition of G1-phase progression. They compete with cyclin D for binding to CDK4/CDK6 and, therefore, inhibit CDK4/6 complex kinase activity, resulting in dephosphorylation of pRb and related G1 growth arrest. Frequencies of *p16* or *p15* gene methylation up to 75% have been reported in MM and in myeloma-derived cell lines,[57,58] and *p16* methylation was associated with an increased proliferative rate of plasma cells and a poor prognosis.[59] Methylation of *p16* and *p15* was also detected in MGUS, suggesting that methylation of these genes is an early event and not associated with transition from MGUS to MM.[60]

Loss of DAP-kinase expression was recognized to be associated with promoter hypermethylation in 67% of MM. *DAP-kinase* is a gene-regulating apoptosis induced by INFγ. Preliminary findings suggest prognostic implications of DAP kinase in MM.[57] The *SOCS-1*-protein has been shown to be involved into the Jak/STAT pathway. It suppresses signaling by a wide variety of cytokines including IL-6, IL-4, leukemia inhibitory factor, oncostatin M, growth hormone, prolactin, thrombopoietin,

and interferons.[61] It has been shown that regulation of cytokine signaling by SOCS-1 is important in normal lymphocyte development and differentiation. *SOCS-1* is inactivated by hypermethylation in almost 63% of MM patient samples.[62]

The frequent demonstration of aberrant gene-promotor methylation in MM and MGUS not only provides new insights into the biology of MM but also suggests that this pathway may be a potential target for novel therapeutic interventions. Hypermethylation-associated gene silencing is a potentially reversible phenomenon,[63] and demethylating agents, such as 5-aza-2′deoxycytidine, have been shown to exert clinical activity in patients with myelodysplastic syndromes.[64]

Genetic events defined by global gene expression profiling of MM

Global gene expression profiling utilizes arrays that contain thousands of oligonucleotide probes packed at extremely high densities. By exploiting the complementary base pairing of nucleic acids, a large number of genes can be monitored in a single experiment.[65] First results obtained with this new technique indicated that MM plasma cells can be differentiated from normal plasma cells by approximately 120 genes, whereas MGUS plasma cells and MM cells are currently indistinguishable by this approach.[66] Among MM plasma cells, genes associated with B-cell differentiation may be highly variable and, based upon the pattern of expression of early and late differentiation antigens, four MM subgroups could be identified.[66] The MM1 subgroup contained samples that were more like normal plasma cells and MGUS plasma cells, whereas the MM4 subgroup contained samples resembling MM cell lines. The most significant gene expression patterns differentiating MM1 and MM4 were cell-cycle control and DNA metabolism genes. Furthermore, the MM4 subgroup was more likely to have abnormal cytogenetics, elevated serum β_2-microglobulin, elevated creatinine, and deletions of chromosome 13, suggesting that the MM4 subgroup may represent a high-risk clinical entity. This system represents the framework for a new molecular classification system of MM and identifies the genetic differences associated with these distinct subgroups.

Thus, knowledge of the molecular genetics of this particular subgroup should provide insight into its biology and possibly provide a rationale for appropriate subtype-specific therapeutic interventions.

CYTOGENETIC ABNORMALITIES IN MGUS

Owing to the low number of clonal bone marrow plasma cells and their low proliferative rate, virtually no informative karyotypes are available from individuals with MGUS. FISH studies, however, have demonstrated that chromosomal aneuploidy is a common finding already present at the level of MGUS: plasma cells from individuals with MGUS may exhibit not only numerical changes (trisomies of chromosomes 3, 7, 9, and 11),[67,68] but also structural aberrations like 14q translocations and deletions of 13q.[16,17,69]

Translocations involving the *IgH* locus have been reported to occur in 46% of patients with MGUS by interphase FISH analysis (36 of 79 patients in the study by Avet-Loiseau *et al.*,[16] 27 of 59 patients in the study by Fonseca *et al.*[17]). A t(11;14)(q13;q32) was found to be the most common translocation in MGUS. The t(4;14) can also be detected in MGUS (either by FISH or by a reverse-transcriptase polymerase chain reaction for the *IgH-MMSET* transcript) but was reported to occur in fewer than 10% of cases.[16,17,24] As in MM, presence of a t(4;14) can result in expression of the FGFR3 protein. Thus, all 14q translocations observed in MM also appear to be present in MGUS, including the t(14;16).[17] So far, no association of a specific translocation with progression of MGUS to MM has been reported.

Several studies also show the presence of a chromosome 13q deletion in the clonal plasma cells of patients with MGUS, with a prevalence ranging between 15% and 50%.[16,17,41,69] With respect to 14q translocations, about 50% of patients with a t(11;14) had a concomitant deletion of 13q, whereas there was a strong association between t(4;14) and deletion 13q (similar to observations in MM).[16,17,48] There is some evidence that a chromosome 13 abnormality may be important for the progression of MGUS to MM,[41,70] but this issue needs to be addressed in larger cohorts of patients.

DEVELOPMENT OF MONOCLONAL GAMMOPATHIES AS A MULTISTEP PROCESS

From cytogenetic and molecular studies in MM and MGUS, one can conclude that critical chromosomal abnormalities leading to karyotypic instability already occur in MGUS plasma cells, and that additional genetic events take place during evolution of MM and further progression to advanced stages of the disease. A model has, therefore, been proposed implicating multiple genetic events in the pathogenesis of monoclonal gammopathies (Fig. 4.2).[71] One of the earliest chromosomal events may be the occurrence of a 14q32 translocation with consecutive activation of an oncogene at one of the various translocation partner regions, which results in immortalization of the plasma cell clone. It is unclear at present whether this event may even precede the development of MGUS, because B cells carrying chromosomal translocations with involvement of *IgH* genes can also be found in normal individuals.[72] Karyotypic instability becomes apparent in MGUS plasma cells and may be even more pronounced as soon as the disease progresses. Acquisition of additional chromosomal changes (including deletion 13q) as well as activation of oncogenes may then lead to transformation and development of MM. Factors produced by MM cells further generate a milieu in the bone marrow that supports proliferation of the malignant clone. During this phase of the disease, MM cells remain growth factor dependent and thus are localized just in the bone marrow. Late-occurring genetic and molecular events (secondary translocations, dysregulation of additional oncogenes) characterize MM cell growth that becomes more and more independent of the supportive role of

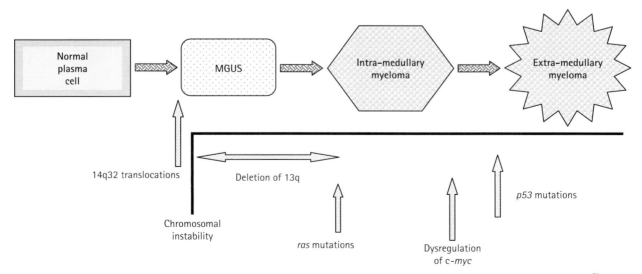

Figure 4.2 *Genetic and molecular events during development and progression of MGUS and MM. (Adapted from Hallek et al.[71])*

bone marrow stroma cells. This phase is clinically characterized by an aggressive course with frequent development of extramedullary manifestations.

CLINICAL AND PROGNOSTIC IMPLICATIONS OF CHROMOSOMAL ABNORMALITIES IN MM

There is now increasing evidence that information about cytogenetic abnormalities in MM provides important prognostic information.

Hypodiploidy as an indicator of poor prognosis

Measurements of total DNA content by flow cytometry have indicated that presence of a hypodiploid DNA stemline is associated with a poor prognosis in patients with MM.[73] This observation has recently been confirmed by large cytogenetic studies, which have demonstrated the association of hypodiploid MM karyotypes with poor outcome (see Fig. 4.3).[9,74,75] Specific monosomies, in particular monosomy 13 or deletion of 13q (see later), may also be important, but the presence of monosomies could also be regarded as surrogate markers of hypodiploid MM. Two study groups have reported that among MM patients with hypodiploid karyotypes, monosomy 13 did not add prognostic significance.[9,75] This is in contrast to data reported from Little Rock showing an independent prognostic value of both hypodiploidy and monosomy 13/deletion of 13q.[76] Some differences may be related to the fact that metaphase cytogenetics underestimates the true incidence of specific chromosomal abnormalities in MM.

Compared with MM patients with a hypodiploid karyotype, the group of patients with hyperdiploid MM is characterized by a rather favorable outcome (Fig. 4.3).[9,75,76]

Chromosome 13q and prognosis

Among specific abnormalities, partial or complete loss of chromosome 13q has been identified as an indicator of poor prognosis. Table 4.3 summarizes studies reporting a significant association of a deletion of 13q with short survival of MM patients not only after standard-dose chemotherapy but also after high-dose melphalan and autologous stem cell transplantation (see also Fig. 4.4). Multivariate analyses have shown that deletion of 13q provides independent prognostic information, and

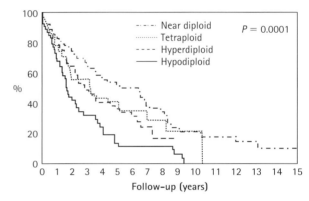

Figure 4.3 *Overall survival of MM patients grouped according to ploidy status after karyotypic analysis. The patient population was treated by standard-dose chemotherapy and the survival time since diagnosis is presented on the x-axis in years. (Adapted from Debes-Marun et al.[75])*

Table 4.3 *Unfavorable prognosis of multiple myeloma with deletion of chromosome 13q*

Study	Therapy	Method	13q	n	OS (months)	P
Tricot et al.[38]	HDT	CG	Normal	127	50+	
			−13/13q−	22	29	0.001
Seong et al.[77]	SDT	CG	−13/13q−	17	10	
Desikan et al.[82]	HDT	CG	Normal	830	44	
			−13/13q−	163	16	<0.0001
Perez-Simon et al.[39]	SDT	FISH	Normal	32	60	
			Deleted	16	14	0.001
Zojer et al.[40]	SDT	FISH	Normal	51	60+	
			Deleted	46	24	<0.005
Fonseca et al.[78]	SDT	FISH	Normal	149	51	
			Deleted	176	35	0.02
Worel et al.[79]	HDT	FISH	Normal	17	72+	
			Deleted	11	24	0.012
Facon et al.[80]	HDT	FISH	Normal	68	65	
			Deleted	42	26	0.0001

CG, metaphase cytogenetics; FISH, fluorescence *in situ* hybridization; HDT, high-dose therapy; n, number of patients; OS, overall survival; SDT, standard-dose chemotherapy.

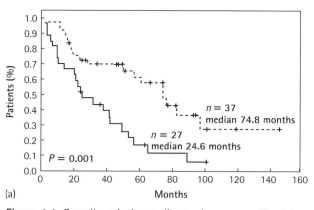
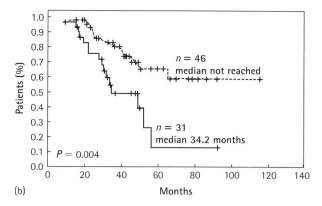

Figure 4.4 *Overall survival according to chromosome 13q status according to fluorescence* in situ *hybridization FISH (dotted line, normal chromosome 13q; solid line, deletion of 13q). Presence of a 13q deletion is associated with significantly shortened survival, both after standard-dose (a) and high-dose (b) chemotherapy.*

Table 4.4 *Prognostic model in multiple myeloma based on chromosome 13q and β_2-microglobulin*

Study	Risk	Features	Median overall survival (months)
Königsberg *et al.*[81]	Low	Normal 13q and B2M < 4 mg/L	102
	Intermediate	Del(13q) or B2M > 4 mg/L	46
	High	Del(13q) and B2M > 4 mg/L	11
Facon *et al.*[80]	Low	Normal 13q and B2M < 2.5 mg/L	111+
	Intermediate	Del(13q) or B2M > 2.5 mg/L	47
	High	Del(13q) and B2M > 2.5 mg/L	25

combinations of chromosome 13 with other powerful prognostic factors can identify patient populations with significantly different outcome. This is particularly true for a prognostic model using chromosome 13q status (FISH analysis) and serum levels of β_2-microglobulin, which allows the identification of MM patients with low-, intermediate-, and high-risk disease (compare with Table 4.4).

There is also evidence that patients with normal chromosome 13 may have long-term disease-free survival after high-dose therapy. Desikan *et al.* identified a favorable prognostic group being characterized by absence of chromosome 13 abnormalities (metaphase cytogenetics), low β_2-microglobulin ($\leq$2.5 mg/L), low C-reactive protein ($\leq$4 mg/L), and short preceding standard-dose therapy ($\leq$12 months). Among 112 MM patients with these disease characteristics and a complete remission after high-dose therapy, 52% have remained in continuous complete remission at 5 years.[82]

Since a deletion of 13q can be detected up to three times more frequently by FISH than by metaphase cytogenetic analysis, it has been a matter of debate as to whether a deletion 13q by FISH carries the same negative prognostic information as chromosome 13 abnormalities identified by metaphase cytogenetics. The direct comparison of both cytogenetic techniques in 231 patients with newly diagnosed MM revealed chromosome 13 abnormalities by metaphase analysis in 14% and a deletion 13q by FISH in

51% of patients.[43] Patients who exhibited a chromosome 13 abnormality, either by metaphase cytogenetics or FISH, experienced significantly shortened event-free survival and overall survival. However, with respect to early treatment failure after an intensive treatment program including tandem autologous transplantation, the 29 patients with a cytogenetic chromosome 13 abnormality had a relapse rate at 3 years of 61% versus 38% in 111 patients with a FISH deletion 13q ($P = 0.02$); the corresponding 3-year mortality rates were 43% and 35% ($P = 0.1$).[43] Thus, both cytogenetic abnormalities of chromosome 13 and FISH deletion 13q provide prognostic information in MM, although the approximately 15% of MM patients with cytogenetically detected chromosome 13 abnormalities appear to be the group of patients with the worst outcome. This could reflect the association of presence of an abnormal karyotype with increased proliferative activity.[2]

14q32 translocations and prognosis

As summarized above, illegitimate rearrangements of IgH-sequences at 14q32 occur in 70–75% of patients with MM. According to recent results, specific 14q32 translocations are of prognostic importance: a t(11;14) was originally reported to be associated with poor outcome. However, two cytogenetic studies were based on small numbers of patients,[19,83] and in the study by Tricot *et al.*,[38] the t(11;14) was part of the patient population summarized as the group with 11q abnormalities.

Two larger studies performed with FISH now suggest that presence of a t(11;14) is rather associated with a favorable outcome. In a retrospective analysis of 336 patients enrolled in a standard-dose chemotherapy protocol, 16% of patients had a t(11;14) by FISH. Patients with a t(11;14) appeared to have higher response rates and longer survival, although this did not reach statistical significance.[84] In a study of MM patients receiving intensive chemotherapy,[18] expected survival at 80 months was 87.5% versus 55.4% for patients without t(11;14) ($P = 0.05$). Most notably, among patients with a t(11;14), chromosome 13 abnormalities did not significantly influence the outcome. Even in the most aggressive form of plasma cell malignancies, i.e. plasma cell leukemia, presence of a t(11;14) was associated with the longest survival.[8]

On the other hand, a t(4;14) predicted for short event-free and overall survival, with an expected survival at 80 months of only 22.8% (as opposed to 66% in the group of patients without t(4;14); $P = 0.002$).[18] Owing to a strong correlation with a chromosome 13 deletion, t(4;14) did not show independent prognostic significance by multivariate analysis. In a second study, the clinical impact of a t(4;14) was confirmed: presence of a t(4;14) was predictive of poor response to first-line chemotherapy and short overall survival, even in patients with lack of expression of FGFR3.[32]

CONCLUSIONS AND FUTURE DIRECTIONS

From a clinical perspective, it has long been recognized that MM is characterized by a heterogeneous group of entities with distinct biological behavior. We are now at the beginning of a molecular classification of MM. At present, it can be concluded that distinct MM entities can be defined by specific chromosomal abnormalities. It appears that a particularly favorable outcome can be predicted for MM patients presenting with a t(11;14) and/or absence of a chromosome 13 deletion. Together with low β_2-microglobulin, these patients appear to benefit most from intensive chemotherapy. In contrast, such treatment is still insufficient for sustained disease control in patients with unfavorable prognostic indicators, in particular deletion 13q and t(4;14). For these patients, innovative therapeutic interventions will be required.

Many important issues remain to be clarified. In the context of 14q32 translocations, it will be important to resolve the question of yet unknown translocation partners, and their contribution to biology and clinical behavior. Likewise, it will be relevant to study molecular events in the 25% of MM patients not exhibiting a 14q32 translocation. Also, candidate genes that are dysregulated by a 13q deletion and other chromosomal losses need to be defined. Finally, molecular events leading to transition from MGUS to MM are still poorly characterized.

It is anticipated that systematic use of novel molecular techniques, in particular global gene expression profiling,[66,85] may lead to new insights into molecular changes of MM. It can also be envisioned that elucidation of fundamental genetic events in monoclonal gammopathies may lead to the definition of specific targets for future, more effective therapeutic interventions, in particular for MM patients with unfavorable cytogenetic features.

KEY POINTS

- Plasma cells from patients with multiple myeloma (MM) are characterized by a high degree of karyotypic instability leading to a complex set of chromosomal abnormalities in almost every patient.
- Molecular data suggest that a series of genetic events is involved in the development and progression of monoclonal gammopathies.
- Translocations of the immunoglobulin heavy chain locus at 14q32, in which many different partner chromosomes may be involved, are among the earliest chromosomal changes in monoclonal gammopathies and occur in about 75% of patients with MM.
- Frequent translocation partners of 14q32 are 11q13 (with overexpression of cyclin-D1) and 4p16.3 (with dysregulation of two genes, *fgfr3* and/or *mmset*).
- The presence of a t(11;14)(q13;q32) is associated with a rather favorable clinical course of MM, whereas a hypodiploid karyotype, a deletion of chromosome 13q, and a t(4;14)(p16.3;q32) are indicators of short survival of MM patients.
- Gene expression profiling, along with standard cytogenetic and molecular techniques, may lead to a molecular classification of MM and to identification of specific targets for future therapeutic interventions.

REFERENCES

● = Key primary paper
◆ = Major review article

1. Zandecki M, Lai JL, Facon T. Multiple myeloma: almost all patients are cytogenetically abnormal. *Br J Haematol* 1996; **94**:217–33.
2. Rajkumar SV, Fonseca R, Dewald GW, Therneau TM, Lacy MQ, Kyle RA, *et al.* Cytogenetic abnormalities correlate with the

plasma cell labeling index and extent of bone marrow involvement in myeloma. *Cancer Genet Cytogenet* 1999; **113**:73–7.

3. Dewald GW, Kyle RA, Hicks GA, Greipp PR. The clinical significance of cytogenetic studies in 100 patients with multiple myeloma, plasma cell leukemia, or amyloidosis. *Blood* 1985; **66**:380–90.

4. Weh HJ, Gutensohn K, Selbach J, Kruse R, Wacker-Backhaus G, Seeger D, *et al*. Karyotype in multiple myeloma and plasma cell leukemia. *Eur J Cancer* 1993; **29A**:1269–73.

5. Sawyer JR, Waldron JA, Jagannath S, Barlogie B. Cytogenetic findings in 200 patients with multiple myeloma. *Cancer Genet Cytogenet* 1995; **82**:41–9.

6. Lai JL, Zandecki M, Mary JY, Bernardi F, Izydorczyk V, Flactif M, *et al*. Improved cytogenetics in multiple myeloma: a study of 151 patients including 117 patients at diagnosis. *Blood* 1995; **85**:2490–7.

7. Calasanz MJ, Cigudosa JC, Odero MD, Ferreira C, Ardanaz MT, Fraile A, *et al*. Cytogenetic analysis of 280 patients with multiple myeloma and related disorders: primary breakpoints and clinical correlations. *Genes Chromosomes Cancer* 1997; **18**:84–93.

8. Avet-Loiseau H, Daviet A, Brigaudeau C, Callet-Bauchu E, Terre C, Lafage-Pochitaloff M, *et al*. Cytogenetic, interphase, and multicolor fluorescence in situ hybridization analyses in primary plasma cell leukemia: a study of 40 cases, on behalf of the Intergroupe Fancophone du Myelome and the Groupe Francais de Cytogenetique Hematologique. *Blood* 2001; **97**:822–5.

9. Smadja NV, Bastard C, Brigaudeau C, Leroux D, Fruchart C, on behalf of the Groupe Francais de Cytogenetique Hematologique. Hypodiploidy is a major prognostic factor in multiple myeloma. *Blood* 2001; **98**:2229–38.

●10. Drach J, Schuster J, Nowotny H, Angerler J, Rosenthal F, Fiegl M, *et al*. Multiple myeloma: high incidence of chromosomal aneuploidy as detected by interphase fluorescence *in situ* hybridization. *Cancer Res* 1995; **55**:3854–9.

11. Cigudosa JC, Rao PH, Calasanz MJ, Odero MD, Michaeli J, Jhanwar SC, *et al*. Characterization of non-random chromosomal gains and losses in multiple myeloma by comparative genomic hybridization. *Blood* 1998; **91**:3007–13.

12. Rao PH, Cigudosa JC, Ning Y, Calasanz MJ, Iida S, Tagawa S, *et al*. Multicolor spectral karyotyping identifies recurring breakpoints and translocations in multiple myeloma. *Blood* 1998; **92**:1742–8.

●13. Sawyer JR, Lukacs JL, Munshi N, Desikan KR, Singhal S, Mehta J, *et al*. Identification of new nonrandom translocations in multiple myeloma with multicolor spectral karyotyping. *Blood* 1998; **92**:4269–76.

◆14. Willis TG, Dyer MJS. The role of immunoglobulin translocations in the pathogenesis of B-cell malignancies. *Blood* 2000; **96**:808–22.

●15. Bergsagel PL, Chesi MC, Nardini E, Brents LA, Kirby SL, Kuehl WH. Promiscuous translocations into IgH switch regions in multiple myeloma. *Proc Natl Acad Sci USA* 1996; **93**:13931–6.

16. Avet-Loiseau H, Facon T, Daviet A, Godon C, Rapp MJ, Harrousseau JL, *et al*. 14q32 translocations and monosomy 13 observed in monoclonal gammopathy of undetermined significance delineate a multistep process for the oncogenesis of multiple myeloma. *Cancer Res* 1999; **59**:4546–50.

17. Fonseca R, Bailey RJ, Ahmann GJ, Rajkumar SV, Hoyer JD, Lust JA, *et al*. Genomic abnormalities in monoclonal gammopathy of undetermined significance. *Blood* 2002; **100**:1417–24.

●18. Moreau P, Facon T, Leleu X, Morineau N, Huyghe P, Harousseau JL, *et al*. Recurrent 14q32 translocations determine the prognosis of multiple myeloma, especially in patients receiving intensive chemotherapy. *Blood* 2002; **100**:1579–83.

19. Fonseca R, Witzig TE, Gertz MA, Kyle RA, Hoyer JD, Jalal SM, *et al*. Multiple myeloma and the translocation t(11;14) (q13;q32): a report on 13 cases. *Br J Haematol* 1998; **101**:296–301.

20. Avet-Loiseau H, Li JY, Facon T, Brigaudeau C, Morineau N, Maloisel F, *et al*. High incidence of translocations t(11;14)(q13;q32) and t(4;14)(p16;q32) in patients with plasma cell malignancies. *Cancer Res* 1998; **58**: 5640–5.

21. Ronchetti D, Finelli P, Richeldi R, Baldini L, Rocci M, Viggiano L, *et al*. Molecular analysis of 11q13 breakpoints in multiple myeloma. *Blood* 1999; **93**:1330–7.

22. Janssen JW, Vaandrager JW, Heuser T, Jauch A, Kluin PM, Geelene E, *et al*. Concurrent activation of a novel putative transforming gene, myeov, and cyclin D1 in a subset of multiple myeloma cell lines with t(11;14)(q13;q32). *Blood* 2000; **95**:2691–8.

●23. Chesi M, Nardini E, Brents LA, Schrock E, Ried T, Kuehl WM, *et al*. Frequent translocation t(4;14)(p16.3;q32.3) in multiple myeloma is associated with increased expression and activating mutations of fibroblast growth factor receptor 3. *Nat Genet* 1997; **16**:260–5.

24. Sibley K, Fenton JAL, Dring AM, Ashcroft AJ, Rawstron AC, Morgan GJ. A molecular study of the t(4;14) in multiple myeloma. *Br J Haematol* 2002; **118**:514–20.

25. Finelli P, Fabis S, Zagano S, Baldini L, Intini D, Nobili L, *et al*. Detection of t(4;14)(p16.3;q32) chromosomal translocation in multiple myeloma by double color fluorescence in situ hybridization. *Blood* 1999; **94**:724–32.

26. Richelda R, Ronchetti D, Baldini L, Cro L, Viggiano L, Marzella R, *et al*. A novel chromosomal translocation t(4;14) (p16.3;q32) in multiple myeloma involves the fibroblast growth factor receptor 3 gene. *Blood* 1997; **90**:4062–9.

27. Plowright EE, Li Z, Bergsagel PL, Chesi M, Barber DL, Branch DR, *et al*. Ectopic expression of fibroblast growth factor receptor 3 promotes myeloma cell proliferation and prevents apoptosis. *Blood* 2000; **95**:992–8.

28. Chesi M, Brents LA, Ely SA, Bais C, Robbiani DF, Mesri EA, *et al*. Activated fibroblast growth factor receptor 3 is an oncogene that contributes to tumor progression in multiple myeloma. *Blood* 2001; **97**:729–36.

29. Li Z, Zhu YX, Plowright EE, Bergsagel PL, Chesi M, Patterson B, *et al*. The myeloma-associated fibroblast growth factor receptor 3 is transforming in hematopoietic cells. *Blood* 2001; **97**:2413–9.

30. Pollett BP, Trudel S, Stern D, Li Z, Stewart AK. Overexpression of the myeloma-associated oncogene fibroblast growth factor receptor 3 (FGFR3) confers dexamthasone resistance. *Blood* 2002; **100**:3819–21.

31. Santra M, Zhan F, Tian E, Barlogie B, Shaughnessy J. A subset of multiple myeloma harboring the t(4;14)(p16;q32) translocation lack FGFR3 expression but maintain an *IGH/MMSET* fusion transcript. *Blood* 2003; **101**:2374–6.

32. Keats JJ, Reiman T, Maxwell CA, Taylor BJ, Mant MJ, Belch AR, *et al.* In multiple myeloma t(4;14)(p16;q32) is an adverse prognostic factor irrespective of FGFR3 expression. *Blood* 2003; **101**:1520–9.

33. Chesi M, Bergsagel PL, Shonukan OO, Martelli ML, Brents LA, Chen T, *et al.* Frequent dysregulation of the c-maf proto-oncogene at 16q23 by translocation to an Ig locus in multiple myeloma. *Blood* 1998; **91**:4457–63.

34. Ho IC, Hodge MR, Rooney JW, Glimcher LH. The proto-oncogene c-maf is responsible for tissue-specific expression of interleukin-4. *Cell* 1996; **85**:973–83.

35. Taniwaki M, Nishida K, Takashima T, Nakagawa H, Fujii H, Tarnaki T, *et al.* Nonrandom chromosomal rearrangements of 14q32.3 and 19p13.3 and preferential deletion of 1p in 21 patients with multiple myeloma and plasma cell leukemia. *Blood* 1994; **84**:2283–90.

36. Shaughnessy J, Gabrea A, Qi Y, Brents L, Zhan F, Tian E, *et al.* Cyclin D3 at 6p21 is dysregulated by recurrent chromosomal translocations to immunoglobulin loci in multiple myeloma. *Blood* 2001; **98**:217–23.

37. Iida S, Rao PH, Butler M, Corradini P, Boccadoro M, Klein B, *et al.* Deregulation of MUM1/IRF4 by chromosomal translocation in multiple myeloma. *Nat Genet* 1997; **17**:226–30.

●38. Tricot G, Barlogie B, Jagannath S, Bracy D, Mattox S, Vesole DH, *et al.* Poor prognosis in multiple myeloma is associated only with partial or complete deletions of chromosome 13 or abnormalities involving 11q and not with other karyotype abnormalities. *Blood* 1995; **86**:4250–6.

39. Perez-Simon JA, Garcia-Sanz R, Tabernero MD, Almeida J, Gonzales M, Fernandez-Calvo J, *et al.* Prognostic value of numerical chromosome aberrations in multiple myeloma: a FISH analysis of 15 different chromosomes. *Blood* 1998; **91**:3366–71.

40. Zojer N, Königsberg R, Ackermann J, Fritz E, Dallinger S, Krömer E, *et al.* In multiple myeloma, deletion of 13q14 remains an independent adverse prognostic parameter despite its frequent detection by interphase FISH. *Blood* 2000; **95**:1925–30.

41. Avet-Loiseau H, Li JY, Morineau N, Facon T, Brigaudeau C, Harrousseau JL, *et al.* Monosomy 13 is associated with the transition of monoclonal gammopathy of undetermined significance to multiple myeloma. *Blood* 1999; **94**: 2583–9.

42. Fonseca R, Oken MM, Harrington D, Bailey RJ, Van Wier SA, Henderson KJ, *et al.* Deletions of chromosome 13 in multiple myeloma identified by interphase FISH usually denote large deletions of the q arm or monosomy. *Leukemia* 2001; **15**:981–6.

43. Shaughnessy J, Tian E, Sawyer J, McCoy J, Tricot G, Jacobson J, *et al.* Prognostic impact of cytogenetic and interphase fluorescence in situ hybridization-defined chromosome 13 deletion in multiple myeloma: early results of total therapy II. *Br J Haematol* 2003; **120**:44–51.

44. Shaughnessy J, Tian E, Sawyer J, Bumm K, Landes R, Badros A, *et al.* High incidence of chromosome 13 deletion in

45. multiple myeloma detected by multiprobe interphase FISH. *Blood* 2001; **96**:1505–11.

45. Avet-Loiseau H, Daviet A, Saunier S, Bataille R. Chromosome 13 abnormalities in multiple myeloma are mostly monosomy 13. *Br J Haematol* 2000; **111**:1116–17.

46. Nomdedeu JF, Lasa A, Ubeda J, Saglio G, Bellido M, Casas S, *et al.* Interstitial deletions at the long arm of chromosome 13 may be as common as monosomies in multiple myeloma. A genotypic study. *Haematologica* 2002; **87**:828–35.

47. Elnenaei MO, Hamoudi RA, Swansbury J, Gruszka-Westwood AM, Brito-Babapulle V, Matutes E, *et al.* Delineation of the minimal region of loss at 13q14 in multiple myeloma. *Genes Chromosom Cancer* 2003; **36**:99–106.

48. Fonseca R, Oken MM, Greipp PR. The t(4;14)(p16.3;q32) is strongly associated with chromosome 13 abnormalities in both multiple myeloma and monoclonal gammopathy of undetermined significance. *Blood* 2001; **98**:1271–2.

49. Le Baccon P, Leroux D, Dascalescu C, Duley S, Marais D, Esmenjaud E, *et al.* Novel evidence of a role for chromosome 1 pericentric heterocromatin in the pathogenesis of B-cell lymphoma and multiple myeloma. *Genes Chromosomes Cancer* 2001; **32**:250–64.

50. Sawyer JR, Tricot G, Mattox S, Jagannath S, Barlogie B. Jumping translocations of chromosome 1q in multiple myeloma: evidence for a mechanism involving decondensation of pericentromeric heterochromatin. *Blood* 1998; **91**:1732–41.

51. Mugneret F, Sidaner I, Favre B, Manone L, Maynadie M, Caillot D, *et al.* Der(16)t(1;16)(q10;p10) in multiple myeloma: a new non-random abnormality that is frequently associated with Burkitt's type translocations. *Leukemia* 1995; **9**:277–81.

52. Shou Y, Martelli ML, Gabrea A, Qi Y, Brents LA, Roschke A, *et al.* Diverse karyotypic abnormalities of the c-myc locus associated with c-myc dysregulation and tumor progression in multiple myeloma. *Proc Natl Acad Sci USA* 2000; **97**:228–33.

53. Billadeau D, Jelinek DF, Shah N, Le Bien TW, Van Ness B. Introduction of an activated N-ras oncogene alters the growth characteristics of the interleukin-6 dependent myeloma cell line ANBL6. *Cancer Res* 1995; **55**:3640–6.

54. Neri A, Baldini L, Trecca D, Cro L, Polli E, Maiolo AT. p53 gene mutations in multiple myeloma are associated with advanced forms of malignancy. *Blood* 1993; **81**:128–33.

55. Drach J, Ackermann J, Fritz E, Krömer E, Schuster R, Gisslinger H, *et al.* Presence of a p53 gene deletion in patients with multiple myeloma predicts for short survival after conventional-dose chemotherapy. *Blood* 1998; **92**:802–7.

56. Jones PA, Baylin SB. The fundamental role of epigenetic events in cancer. *Nature Rev Genet* 2002; **3**:415–28.

57. Ng MH, To KW, Lo KW, Chan S, Tsang KS, Cheng SH, *et al.* Frequent death-associated protein kinase promoter hypermethylation in multiple myeloma. *Clin Cancer Res* 2001; **7**:1724–9.

58. Gonzalez M, Mateos MV, Garcia-Sanz R, Balanzategui A, Lopez-Perez R, Chillon MC, *et al.* De novo methylation of tumor suppressor gene p16/INK4a is a frequent finding in multiple myeloma patients at diagnosis. *Leukemia* 2000; **14**:183–7.

59. Mateos MV, Garcia-Sanz R, Lopez-Perez R, Moro MJ, Ocio E, Hernandez J, et al. Methylation is an inactivating mechanism of the p16 gene in multiple myeloma associated with high plasma cell proliferation and short survival. Br J Haematol 2002; **118**:1034–40.

●60. Guillerm G, Gyan E, Wolowiec D, Facon T, Avet-Loiseau H, Kuliczkowski K, et al. p16(INK4a) and p15(INK4b) gene methylations in plasma cells from monoclonal gammopathy of undetermined significance. Blood 2001; **98**:244–6.

61. Greenhalgh CJ, Hilton DJ. Negative regulation of cytokine signaling. J Leukocyte Biol 2001; **70**:348–56.

62. Galm O, Yoshikawa H, Esteller M, Osieka R, Herman JG. SOCS-1, a negative regulator of cytokine signaling, is frequently silenced by methylation in multiple myeloma. Blood 2003; **101**:2784–8.

63. Cameron EE, Bachman KE, Myohanen S, Herman JG, Baylin SB. Synergy of demethylation and histone deacetylase inhibition in the re-expression of genes silenced in cancer. Nat Genet 1999; **21**:103′–7.

64. Wijermans P, Lubbert M, Verhoef G, Bosly A, Ravoet C, Andre M, et al. Low-dose 5-aza-2′-deoxycytidine, a DNA hypomethylating agent, for the treatment of high-risk myelodysplastic syndrome: a multicenter phase II study in elderly patients. J Clin Oncol 2000; **18**:956–62.

65. DeRisi J, Penland L, Brown PO, Bittner ML, Meltzer PS, Ray M, et al. Use of a cDNA microarray to analyse gene expression patterns in human cancer. Nat Genet 1996; **14**:457–60.

●66. Zhan F, Hardin J, Kordsmeier B, Bumm K, Zheng M, Tian E, et al. Global gene expression profiling of multiple myeloma, monoclonal gammopathy of undetermined significance, and normal bone marrow plasma cells. Blood 2002; **99**:1745–57.

●67. Drach J, Angerler J, Schuster J, Rothermund C, Thalhammer R, Haas OA, et al. Interphase fluorescence in situ hybridization identifies chromosomal abnormalities in plasma cells from patients with monoclonal gammopathy of undetermined significance. Blood 1995; **86**:3915–21.

68. Zandecki M, Obein V, Bernardi F, Soenen V, Flactif M, Lai JL, et al. Monoclonal gammopathy of undetermined significance: chromosomal changes are a common finding within bone marrow plasma cells. Br J Haematol 1995; **90**:693–6.

69. Königsberg R, Ackermann J, Kaufmann H, Zojer N, Urbauer E, Krömer E, et al. Deletions of chromosome 13q in monoclonal gammopathy of undetermined significance. Leukemia 2000; **14**:1975–9.

70. Kaufmann H, Ackermann J, Nösslinger T, Gisslinger H, Krömer E, Ludwig H, et al. Deletion of chromosome 13q is a frequent abnormality in multiple myeloma evolving from a preexisting monoclonal gammopathy of undetermined significance. Blood 2002; **100**:103a.

◆71. Hallek M, Bergsagel PL, Anderson KC. Multiple myeloma: increasing evidence for a multistep transformation process. Blood 1998; **91**:3–21.

72. Kuppers R, Dalla-Favera R. Mechanisms of chromosomal translocations in B-cell lymphomas. Oncogene 2001; **20**:5580–94.

73. Barlogie B, Alexanian R, Dixon D, Smith L, Smallwood L, Delasalle K. Prognostic implications of tumor cell DNA and RNA content in multiple myeloma. Blood 1985; **66**:338–41.

74. Calasanz MJ, Cigudosa JC, Odero MD, Garcia-Foncillas J, Marin J, Ardana MT, et al. Hypodiploidy and 22q11 rearrangements at diagnosis are associated with poor prognosis in patients with multiple myeloma. Br J Haematol 1997; **98**:418–25.

75. Debes-Marun CS, Dewald GW, Bryant S, Picken E, Santana-Davila R, Gonzalez-Paz N, et al. Chromosome abnormalities clustering and its implications for pathogenesis and prognosis in myeloma. Leukemia 2003; **17**:427–36.

76. Fassas A, Spencer J, Sawyer J, Zangari M, Choon-Kee, Anaissie E, et al. Both hypodiploidy and deletion of chromosome 13 independently confer poor prognosis in multiple myeloma. Br J Haematol 2002; **118**:1041–7.

77. Seong C, Delasalle K, Hayes K, Weber D, Dimopoulos M, Swantkowski J, et al. Prognostic value of cytogenetics in multiple myeloma. Br J Haematol 1998; **101**:189–94.

78. Fonseca R, Harrington D, Oken MM, et al. Biological and prognostic significance of interphae fluorescence in situ hybridization detection of chromosome 13 abnormalities (Δ13) in multiple myeloma. Cancer Res 2002; **62**:715–20.

79. Worel N, Greinix H, Ackermann J, Kaufmann H, Urbauer E, Höcker P, et al. Deletion of chromosome 13q14 detected by FISH has prognostic impact on survival after high-dose therapy in patients with multiple myeloma. Ann Hematol 2001; **80**:345–8.

●80. Facon T, Avet-Loiseau H, Guillerm G, et al. Chromosome 13 abnormalities identified by FISH analysis and serum (2-microglobulin produce a powerful myeloma staging system for patients receiving high-dose therapy. Blood 2001; **97**:1566–71.

81. Königsberg R, Zojer N, Ackermann J, Krömer E, Kittler H, Fritz E, et al. Predictive role of interphase cytogenetics for survival of patients with multiple myeloma. J Clin Oncol 2000; **18**:804–12.

●82. Desikan R, Barlogie B, Sawyer J, Ayers D, Tricot G, Bardos A, et al. Results of high-dose therapy for 1000 patients with multiple myeloma: durable complete remissions and superior survival in the absence of chromosome 13 abnormalities. Blood 2000; **95**:4008–10.

83. Lai JL, Michaux L, Dastugue N, Vasseur F, Dau Dignon A, Facon T, et al. Cytogenetics in multiple myeloma: a multicenter study of 24 patients with t(11;14)(q13;q32) or its variant. Cancer Genet Cytogenet 1998; **104**:133–8.

84. Fonseca R, Blood EA, Oken MM, Kyle RA, Dewald GW, Bailey RJ, et al. Myeloma and the t(11;14)(q13;q32): evidence for a biologically defined unique subset of patients. Blood 2002; **99**:3735–41.

85. Claudio JO, Masih-Khan E, Tang H, Goncalves J, Voralia M, Li ZH, et al. A molecular compendium of genes expressed in multiple myeloma. Blood 2002; **100**:2175–86.

5

Biology of the malignant plasma cell

FEDERICO CALIGARIS-CAPPIO

INTRODUCTION

Multiple myeloma (MM) is characterized by the uncontrolled proliferation and accumulation of monoclonal plasmablasts and plasma cells (PCs) in the bone marrow (BM).[1,2] Normal PCs are the effector arm of the humoral immune response and are the mainstay of the immune defence against foreign invaders. Although morphologically homogeneous, PCs are a functionally heterogeneous compartment of terminally differentiated B-cell populations. They all develop from mature B cells upon antigen (Ag) stimulation but, when arising in different environmental scenarios, become endowed with different biological properties. Until recently, little has been known about the biology of normal PCs and, while advances have been made in some areas, such as the molecular events that are necessary for a B-lineage cell to become a PC, other aspects of normal PC biology, such as the life span of PCs, remain incompletely defined.

A number of features of malignant PCs that are central to the clinical presentation and evolution of MM are not clearly related to the biology of normal PCs. In contrast to the distribution of normal PCs, MM PCs localize uniquely within the BM, and MM cells are widespread throughout the BM from the early stages of the disease, even though an overt invasion of the peripheral blood by malignant B-lineage cells is not apparent. This suggests that human MM cells need to reach the proper microenvironment (i.e. the BM microenvironment) in order to exploit their potential fully and it is, therefore, crucial to identify the links between MM cells and the BM microenvironment that confer a growth advantage and an extended cell survival to the malignant clone. The interactions between BM stromal cells and malignant PCs induce stromal cells to produce a variety of cytokines and angiogenetic factors that build up the milieu most favorable to the malignant PC growth and accumulation, and the development of osteolytic lesions. Differences in the microenvironment may explain why MM and monoclonal gammopathy of undetermined significance (MGUS) have such a different behavior.

WHAT IS NEEDED TO BECOME A PLASMA CELL?

The fundamental task of PCs is to synthesize and secrete immunoglobulins of predetermined specificity. This requires abundant amounts of immunoglobulin (Ig) heavy and light chain (and, when needed, also of J chain) mRNA and a change to secreted versus membrane mRNA forms. The process of differentiation from B cells to PCs is also marked by important modifications of the spectrum of B-cell surface molecules.[2] Most B-specific and B-associated surface molecules are lost during the transition to the PC stage and conventional B-cell surface markers are almost absent in PCs. Numerous cell membrane molecules that are necessary for the B-cell response to antigen, including CD19, CD21, CD22, and, above all, MHC class II, are downregulated.[3] This is necessary to avoid further Ag presentation and to allow PCs to follow their program undisturbed. MHC class II is absent because of the lack of class II transactivator (CIITA), a coactivator necessary for the transcription of MHC class II invariant chain, and HLA-DR.

Surface molecules that control interactions with other cells are also significantly modified: a very large array of adhesion structures are acquired and the expression of chemokine receptors is reshaped. The adhesion molecules syndecan-1 (CD138) and very late antigen-4 (VLA-4) are upregulated in PCs, while the chemokine receptors CXCR5 and CCR7 are downregulated.[3] The implication is that PCs retain the properties of cell-matrix binding and cell–cell adhesion but have lost the capacity to respond to the B- and T-cell zone chemokines CXCL13, CCL19, and CCL21, and thus have become unresponsive to the microenvironmental signals that might distract them from the production of Ig.[4] PCs retain the expression of CXCR4, which may mediate their adequate location in the proper microenvironments by recognizing the chemokine CXCL12.[4]

Development into a PC entails cell-cycle arrest and the loss of the B-cell capacity to undergo activation and response. These events are regulated by lineage-restricted transcription factors.[5] Three factors play a major role: the transcriptional repressor Bcl-6, the B-lymphocyte-induced maturation protein 1 (Blimp-1) – which is a target of Bcl-6 repressor activity – and the X-box-binding protein 1 (XBP1). XBP1 and Blimp-1 independently act as master genes that regulate PC differentiation. So far, XBP1 is the only transcription factor that loss-of-function studies have shown to be essential for the terminal differentiation of B lymphocytes.[6] Furthermore, the generation of high-affinity antibody-producing PCs from the progeny of germinal center (GC) B cells is associated with the downregulation of Bcl-6. This leads to the emergence of the previously repressed Bcl-6-target gene Blimp-1[7] and, in turn, the Blimp-1 gene product indirectly represses several genes involved either in B-cell proliferation (e.g. c-myc) or in B-cell function (e.g. CIITA).[3,7]

THE HETEROGENEITY OF NORMAL PCs AND THEIR RELATIONSHIP TO MM CELLS

Antigen stimulation triggers normal B cells to proliferate and differentiate into memory B cells and Ig-producing PCs. Depending on the nature of the Ag, the type of T cell response – T-cell-dependent (TD) vs. T-cell-independent (TI) response – and the number of Ag exposures (primary

vs. secondary response), there are quantitative and qualitative differences in the immune responses generated.[8–12] In TD responses, protein Ag that cannot directly evoke an antibody response are processed by Ag-presenting cells (APCs) and presented by MHC Class II molecules to T-helper cells, which then trigger the Ag-specific B-cell response. TI responses are directly elicited by Ag presented in an immunogenic form as multimeric Ag that efficiently cross-links B-cell receptors, stimulating B-cell proliferation and differentiation.

The different B-cell responses to Ag occur in different specialized microenviroments (Fig. 5.1),[8–12] which include:

1. macrophage-rich areas, such as the red pulp of the spleen, where TI responses take place;
2. areas of extrafollicular lymphoid tissues rich in T lymphocytes and interdigitating cells;
3. GC of secondary lymphoid follicles where follicular dendritic cells (FDC) and T lymphocytes gather in a specific fashion.

It follows that normal PC populations are heterogeneous in terms of Ig isotype, anatomical distribution, and life span. PCs generated in macrophage-rich areas after TI Ag stimulation secrete IgM and are short-lived. PCs generated in the extrafollicular areas after primary TD Ag challenge are IgM-secreting, are short-lived, and remain in the lymph node extramedullary regions. Secondary TD antibody (Ab) responses that lead to the production of IgG- or IgA-secreting PCs with a life span of at least a few weeks occur in the specialized microenvironments of the dark and light zone of GC in peripheral lymphoid follicles.[13] The dark zone is packed with proliferating centroblasts that undergo somatic hypermutations of Ig genes and differentiate into centrocytes.[14] The light zone is occupied mainly by non-dividing centrocytes, which

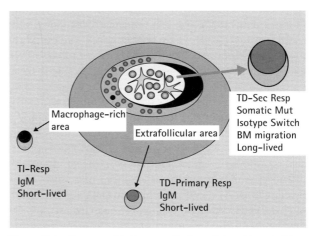

Figure 5.1 *Plasma cell heterogeneity in peripheral lymphoid tissues. Somatic Mut, somatic mutations; TD-Primary Resp, T-dependent primary response; TD-Sec-Resp, T-dependent secondary response; TI-Resp, T-independent response.*

are in close contact with the intertwining processes of FDCs that facilitate a long-standing stimulation of Ag-specific B cells and switch their Ig isotype under the control of cytokines.[14] Only the centrocytes able to express Ig with a high affinity for the FDC-presented Ag are selected to give rise to memory B cells and to plasmablasts. Memory B cells are very efficient in presenting Ag to T cells. The renewed Ag encounter evokes a very rapid anamnestic response that can take place without further hypermutation outside the GC, or can entail a new round of GC mutation and selection processes that expands and optimizes the B-cell response and the generation of plasmablasts.

GC-derived plasmablasts are characterized by a switched isotype, somatic hypermutations, and specific traffic commitments.[9,11,14] Plasmablasts generated in the follicles of the spleen or peripheral lymph nodes migrate to the BM a few days after the antigenic challenge, while those derived from the follicles of Peyer's patches or mesenteric lymph nodes migrate to the lamina propria of the gut.[15] Even if the steps of Ag processing and presentation that lead to the generation of IgG and IgA PCs occur only in secondary lymphoid follicles, the BM is a major site where immunoglobulins are produced in TD secondary immune responses.[16,17] Conceivably BM-seeking PC precursors receive a differentiation signal when they come into physical contact with inductive BM stromal microenvironment.

THE ANATOMICAL DISTRIBUTION AND LIFE SPAN OF PLASMA CELLS

Plasma cells have a widespread anatomical distribution: at least 70% of them are present in the gut where they secrete IgA.[15,18] This observation raises the interesting issue that, although the intestine's lamina propria contains more Ig-producing cells than all other tissues in the body, it is never a site where MM develops, not even IgA-producing MM. Likewise, the involvement of the spleen and/or lymph nodes, which is typical of Waldenström's macroglobulinemia, is very unusual in MM.

MM paraproteins may be directed against a wide variety of infectious agents, suggesting that the development of MM may be causally related to some sort of chronic Ag stimulation.[19–21] The Ig isotype of MM PCs is generally IgG or IgA, demonstrating that the predominant phenotype of MM tumor cells is that of a post-switch B cell. Clonal MM cells also have somatically hypermutated Ig genes.[22,23] These observations suggest that the development and evolution of MM is an Ag-triggered process, although the specific causal Ag is generally unknown. An interesting difference observed between MM and MGUS is that ongoing somatic mutations are present in MGUS, but not in MM, suggesting that MM is an Ag-selected, while MGUS is an Ag-driven process.[24] All the data so far discussed lead to the conclusion that the most likely candidate for the physiological equivalent of MM PC precursor is either an activated B memory cell or a plasmablast generated in peripheral lymphoid organs during secondary TD Ab response, which is programmed to home to the BM and committed to differentiate in close association with the local microenvironment.

The result is that MM is a BM-restricted malignancy even if the clonal founder cell may originate from the periphery. However, it remains unclear whether the BM is merely the site where progenitors migrating from peripheral lymphoid organs find the optimal soil to develop into fully fledged plasma cells, or whether PCs can differentiate *in situ* from *in situ*-generated or *in situ*-located progenitors. An answer to this problem will become possible once we are able to answer the fundamental and unresolved question of what makes long-lived PCs capable of a long life, in which environment(s), and dependent on which factors. Most data would suggest that PCs may have an unlimited survival provided they are lodged in the proper niches and are rescued by specific factors.[25] In rodents different subsets of Ag-experienced PC precursors have been identified in the BM.[26] These precursors arise several days after immunization, persist for several months, and can give rise to either short-lived or long-lived PCs. The precise origin, roles, and features of these different precursors in humans need to be thoroughly explored.

MM AND THE BM: A TENTATIVE MODEL

Even if we accept that the clonal founder cells of MM and MGUS have developed within peripheral lymphoid organs, it is evident that their progeny have a predilection for the BM microenvironment, which supports their extended survival. Other chronic B-cell malignancies like follicular lymphoma (FL) and chronic lymphocytic leukemia (CLL) are also characterized by clonal founder cells originating in the periphery and a striking propensity to invade the BM. However, the pattern of BM invasion is different in FL and CLL, and in MM.[27] BM involvement in FL is essentially characterized by malignant nodules whose architecture recapitulates the basic structure of neoplastic follicles in peripheral lymphoid organs with abundant FDC and CD4[+] T cells.[13] A similar pattern of BM invasion is observed in the early stages of CLL, whose progressive evolution from a nodular to a diffuse pattern remains characterized by the presence of numerous and frequently activated CD4[+] T cells in proliferation centers.[28] In contrast, no FDC are observed in MM BM and CD4[+] T cells are sparse, if present at all.[27] The most prominent aspect of the MM BM microenvironment is the impressive amount of BM-derived endogenous stromal cells,[29] which are highly activated.[30] In patients with MM, BM stromal cells cultured *in vitro*[29,31] form a confluent meshwork of intertwining elements that may be used as a feeder layer for autologous peripheral blood mononuclear cells and allow the development of a monoclonal B-lineage cell population.[29] Four major populations can be identified in MM BM stromal cell cultures: fibroblasts, myofibroblasts, macrophages, and osteoclasts, all fully equipped with adhesion molecules.[32] The same populations are observed in MGUS, but in MGUS the BM stromal cells are definitely less active.[30] The stromal

cells growing *in vitro* from MGUS BM are low in number, do not support the growth of autologous B cells, and produce very low amounts of interleukin-6 (IL-6) in the culture supernatants.[29]

Taken together, these observations may be assembled into a model (Fig. 5.2),[27] the 'importing vs. instructing model.' In FL and CLL patients, BM appears to 'import' from the periphery the cellular components that are necessary to create a microenvironment favorable to the dissemination and progression of the malignant clone. Conversely, MM plasma cells appear to 'instruct' the local components of BM environment to help the expansion

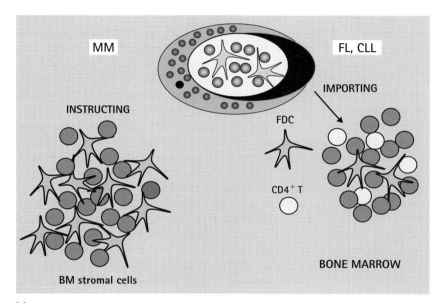

(a)

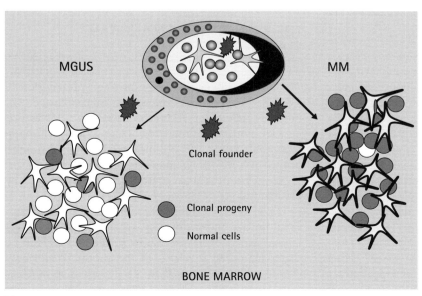

(b)

Figure 5.2 *(a) A model tentatively explaining the different pattern of bone marrow (BM) invasion in follicular lymphoma (FL) and chronic lymphocytic leukemia (CLL) as compared with multiple myeloma (MM). (b) A model tentatively explaining the bone marrow differences between multiple myeloma and monoclonal gammopathy of undetermined significance (MGUS). The clonal founder cells of MM and MGUS appear to originate in the periphery and to invade the BM. The most prominent aspect of the MM BM microenvironment is the impressive amount of BM-derived endogenous stromal cells, which are highly activated. The overall picture of the BM microenvironment is essentially identical in MGUS with a major difference: MGUS BM stromal cells are definitely less active. MM plasma cells appear to 'instruct' the local components of the BM environment to help the expansion of the malignant clone. The acquisition of the capacity to activate endogenous stromal cells may mark the evolution from MGUS to MM. FDC, follicular dendritic cell.*

of the malignant clone. The 'importing vs. instructing' model may allow some predictions. The frequent presence of activated CD4[+] T cells in both FL and CLL lesions suggests that CD4[+] T cells may have a driving role in the natural history of these diseases. In contrast, despite the fact that the clonal founder cell of MM must have been involved in a TD antigenic response, the evolution of the MM malignant clone appears to be T-cell independent but strongly dependent on the stimulating and nourishing activity of BM stromal cells, explaining why MM is confined within the BM. It may be asked why these stromal cells, which would normally be quiescent, especially in the age range of MM patients, are activated in the BM of MM. As normal, BM stromal cells produce IL-6 after activation by inflammatory cytokines like IL-1,[33] the activated state of stromal cells in MM may be a direct consequence of the influence of accessory cell-activating cytokines produced by the expanding monoclonal B-cell population. In MGUS patients, the clonal population is below the theshold size that may produce enough cytokines to initiate the activation of BM stromal cells. Once the threshold size is reached, BM stromal cells become activated and trigger a self-perpetuating mechanism of mutual help and recruitment between malignant PCs and BM stromal cells that favors the progressive expansion of the B-cell clone. In conclusion, it is not unreasonable to postulate that the acquisition by PCs of the capacity to activate endogenous stromal cells is the real turning point in the natural history of MGUS, giving a decisive impulse to growth of the malignant clone and marking the progression of MGUS into overt MM (Fig. 5.2).

PLASMA CELL PRECURSORS IN MM

The long-standing observation that MM cells are widespread troughout the BM even when very few PCs are seen in the peripheral blood has suggested that the malignancy may be disseminated by circulating clonogenic cells distinct from the MM PC compartment.[34] Such a possibility is reinforced by the observation that a similar situation is operating in the mouse model.[35] Polymerase chain reaction (PCR) studies based on amplification of the complementarity-determining region (CDR)3 of the clone-specific IgH gene have shown that circulating monoclonal tumor-related cells are present in myeloma patients, independent of both tumor burden and stage of disease,[36] and may easily be detected even after successful autologous BM transplantation.[37,38] The precise phenotypic and functional definition of these circulating cells is still unclear, despite several experimental approaches, a multitude of papers, and frequent controversies. More specifically, it is unclear whether circulating PC precursors

in MM are plasmablasts or mature B cells. Precursors might conceivably circulate in disguise as small mature-looking lymphocytes or they might be plasmablasts capable of acquiring different morphological and phenotypic features.

The proportion of circulating clonal MM cells within the lymphocyte population is debated[39,40] and the possibility that the putative PC precursors might be mature lymphocytes has been challenged by the observation that tumor-specific aneuploidy is not detected in CD19 positive B lymphoid cells.[41] Pre-switch B cells clonally related to malignant plasma cells have been detected in the BM of MM patients by means of the CDR3 amplification of rearranged H chain alleles.[42,43] This population is numerically very small, shows somatic hypermutations, and is not seen in PB where only post-switch B cells have been observed. The precise place of BM pre-switch cells in the evolution of MM clone is unknown but their existence is not unique to MM. A similar population has been detected in the rare cases of IgG-positive CLL, where mRNA transcripts coding for patient-specific H-chain variable region have been found to be linked to $C\mu$ and $C\alpha$ H-chain genes.[44] These data suggest that either BM pre-switch cells represent clonal B memory cells, which have not yet completed their full differentiation into switched cells, or that they are a sort of 'blind alley' in the natural history of the malignant clone.

In conclusion, it is reasonable to believe that circulating clonal precursors exist but their precise nature is unclear. The relationship of the cells that belong to the circulating vs. the tissue compartments is not known. Circulating precursor cells may spill over from the BM environment into the blood or they may be travelling to the BM from peripheral lymphoid organs.

THE PHENOTYPE OF MALIGNANT PLASMA CELLS

The use of microarray gene expression profiling of PC (MM, MGUS, normal), although still in its infancy,[45] will probably make observations about phenotypic differences between normal and malignant PCs outdated within the foreseeable future,[46-48] but meanwhile the immunophenotype of MM PCs remains a useful clinical tool.[49]

At present, the most useful surface markers of MM plasma cells are CD38 and CD138 (Fig. 5.3; see Plate 2). CD38 is an elusive molecule, which is not restricted to the B lineage and is not stage-specific within the B-cell lineage, as it is expressed also by B blasts proliferating in the GC.[50] CD38 is related to the enzyme ADP-ribosyl cyclase, which is involved in a pathway of intracellular Ca^{2+} mobilization distinct from the inositol 1,4,5-triphosphate pathway, but its functional role in PCs is

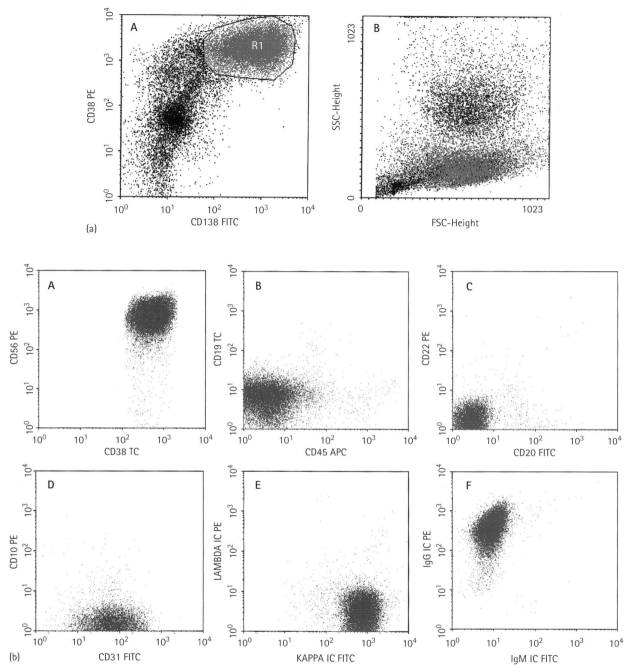

Figure 5.3 *(a) Typical co-expression of CD38 at high fluorescence intensity and CD138 in multiple myeloma plasma cells (A) and their physical distribution compared to lymphocytes (B) in a bone marrow sample. (b) Immunophenotype of multiple myeloma plasma cells. Usually CD56 is expressed at high density (A); CD19 CD45 (B), CD20 and CD22 (C) are negative; CD31 is expressed on the majority of cases; CD10, usually negative on myeloma, can be positive on plasma cell leukemias (D), monoclonal immunoglobulin light and heavy chains are detectable in the cytoplasm (E and F).*

unknown.[51,52] Malignant PCs tend to co-express CD38 and its natural ligand CD31, a member of the Ig gene superfamily characterized by a unique adhesive ability, which is mediated by homophilic and heterophilic mechanisms.[53]

CD138 (syndecan 1) is an adhesion molecule that promotes MM cell adhesion and spreading on extracellular matrix (ECM) proteins and also favors homotypic aggregation.[54] An interesting observation whose implications still have to be fully explored is that CD138 co-localizes with growth factors in the MM PC uropods.[55] For example, hepatocyte growth factor (HGF) upon binding to CD138 promotes the HGF-mediated signaling and results in enhanced activation of its receptor, the tyrosine kinase proto-oncogene c-*met*.[56,57]

In a proportion of MM patients, both BM PCs and some monoclonal B cells are CD10+,[34,58] and PCR analysis has shown that a small population of CD10+ clonal cells exists in most patients with MM.[59] As CD10 is expressed not only by early B-lineage committed cells in the BM[34] but also by GC B blasts and activated B lymphocytes,[58] this CD10 expression by MM PCs is consistent with the possible peripheral B-cell nature of MM PC precursors.

Another interesting molecule that may be expressed by MM PCs is CD28, a T-cell associated molecule that is absent on the surface of normal B cells and PCs, but becomes expressed by MM cell lines and by PCs of several fresh samples.[60] The expression of CD28 appears to correlate with the advanced state of MM. The stimulation of CD28 mediates NF-κB activation possibly via the serine/threonine kinase Akt and has been shown to upregulate numerous MM genes, including IL-8, a chemokine with angiogenesis-promoting properties.

Besides CD138, MM PCs express on the membrane other adhesion molecules, such as H-cellular adhesion molecule (H-CAM; CD44), intercellular adhesion molecule-1 (ICAM-1; CD54), N-cellular adhesion molecule (N-CAM; CD56), leukocyte function antigen-3 (LFA-3; CD58), a receptor for hyaluronan-mediated motility, and frequently also CD11/CD18.[61–67] It is conceivable that MM surface adhesion structures, by interacting with their homologous ligands in the BM microenvironment, may allow malignant B cells to be entrapped within the BM stromal cell web and favor their exposure to the locally produced cytokines. The integrin VLA-4 plays a crucial role in binding malignant PCs to stromal cells in the BM microenvironment. Recently, it has been reported that VLA-4-mediated adhesion may be modulated by the chemokine stromal-cell-derived factor-1α (SDF-1α), and so the production of SDF-1α could contribute to the trafficking and BM compartmentalization of MM PCs.[68]

It has also been reported that CD44 expression may favor the spread of malignant cells[69] and that the expression of different CD44 splicing patterns defines different prognostic subgroups.[67] MM PCs are almost invariably CD56+,[62,65] and a correlation has been observed between expression of CD56 and the presence of lytic bone lesions.[70] CD56 binds specifically to heparan sulfate, a member of the ECM protein family and it might thus be involved in tumor cell–ECM protein interactions.[71] It has also been implicated in the homotypic adhesions of tumor cells, which lead to the formation of MM PC nodules and clusters.[62,71] Consistent with this possibility, the loss of CD56 has been reported to be associated with a more aggressive clinical course and a tendency to the development of PC leukemia.[62]

CYTOKINES AND MM PLASMA CELLS

Multiple myeloma plasma cells are not simply secreting monoclonal Ig. They also secrete a number of cytokines that are capable of influencing the different cell populations of the BM microenvironment involved in MM pathophysiology. MM PCs are also responsive to several cytokines and growth factors, while other cytokines appear to exert an inhibitory effect.[72]

The cytokines produced by MM PCs include IL-1β, tumor necrosis factor β (TNFβ), and a functionally active truncated version of monocyte–macrophage colony stimulating factor (M-CSF).[73–76] All these cytokines activate stromal and accessory cells and may also influence osteoclast activity.

Interleukin–15

Interleukin-15 induces proliferation and promotes cell survival of human T and B lymphocytes, natural killer cells, and neutrophils. Both MM cell lines and fresh MM samples constitutively express a functional IL-15 receptor (IL-15R) and frequently also have detectable expression of IL-15 transcript and protein,[77] suggesting the possible existence of an autocrine IL-15 loop and pointing to the potential paracrine stimulation of myeloma cells by IL-15 released from the cellular microenvironment. It has been shown that blocking autocrine IL-15 production increases the rate of spontaneous apoptosis in cell lines and that adding IL-15 to short-term cultures of primary myeloma cells reduces the percentage of tumor cells spontaneously undergoing apoptosis.[77]

Interleukin–6

A minority of human MM cell lines autonomously produce small amounts of IL-6, while it is debated whether, and to what extent, fresh MM PCs may also produce IL-6.[78–80] *In vitro*, the growth of human MM cell lines can be improved by IL-6 or is dependent on IL-6 producing feeder cells.[79,81,82] IL-6 is the most relevant known growth factor not only for human MM cell lines, but also for fresh MM samples.[79–84] High levels of IL-6 are observed in the sera of patients with aggressive or progressive MM,[85] and tumor responses have been observed following the infusion of anti-IL-6 Ab in patients with plasma cell leukemia or refractory to MM.[86] IL-6, besides promoting B-cell proliferation and differentiation, has also been shown to have an important osteoclast activating factor role.[87]

Whatever the source of IL-6, the crucial point is that malignant MM PCs express IL-6 receptor (IL-6R).[80,88] The IL-6R is a complex of two molecules, CD126 (IL-6Ra) and gp130 (CD130). CD126 contains the ligand-binding site, which allows the binding – albeit at a low affinity – to IL-6. It is relevant that CD126 expression is restricted to malignant PCs, both from MM and from MGUS, while it is absent in normal PCs.[89] The binding of IL-6 to CD126 triggers the association of CD130 that allows high-affinity binding and signal transduction. CD130 is a transducer common to several distantly related cytokines,[88] including IL-6, oncostatin M (OM), leukemia inhibiting factor (LIF), ciliary neurotrophic factor (CNTF), IL-11, and cardiotrophin-1 (CT-1). Accordingly, a number of cytokines that use gp130 as common signal transducer pathway, like CNTF, LIF, and OM, act *in vitro* as MM growth factors.[80,88,90]

Interleukin–10

Another potentially important cytokine for the expansion of MM clones is IL-10, which has been shown to support the growth of MM cell lines and to enhance the proliferative activity of fresh MM tumor samples.[91] The precise effect of IL-10 has not been fully elucidated, but it may modulate the expression of other cytokines and cytokine receptors.

Other stimulating factors

Other growth factors produced in the BM milieu are potentially involved in the proliferation of MM, including granulocyte – macrophage colony-stimulating factor (GM-CSF), stem cell factor (SCF), IL-3, TNFα, insulin-like growth factors 1 and 2 (IGF-1, IGF-2), and HGF.[2,91–93] Both HGF and its ligand c-met have been detected in MM PCs and elevated serum concentrations of HGF have been found in patients with poor prognosis.[94]

Inhibitory factors

Numerous factors have been found to inhibit the growth of MM cells, including interferon γ (IFNγ) and IFNα, although the data so far obtained have not been useful to clinical practice.[2] More relevant appears to be the role of the Fas antigen (CD95), a member of the TNF receptor (R) superfamily, which is expressed on virtually all MM cell lines and fresh samples. The cellular effects of CD95 stimulation have been shown to be antagonized by IL-6 activation.[2]

It is extremely difficult to establish appropriate *in vitro* experimental systems that prevent the redundant and frequently synergistic and/or antagonistic effects of cytokines and allow the clarification of the functional relevance of individual cytokines. It is difficult to obtain *in vitro* preparations of BM MM samples totally devoid of microenvironmental components but, on the other hand, results obtained using MM cell lines may not reflect the situation in MM patients. The results obtained using material from different patients and in different phases of the disease are highly variable, as opposed to the straightforward and consistent results provided by MM cell lines. Finally, it is useful to remember that the biologically active concentrations of IL-6 operating *in vitro* (and found *in vivo*) are 500–5000-fold higher than the concentrations of other MM growth factors.[95] With all these caveats in mind, the following conclusions can be safely drawn:

- the balance between stimulatory and inhibitory cytokines is tilted toward stimulation and has important implications for the growth and survival of MM PCs in the BM microenvironment;
- IL-6 appears to be the most important stimulatory cytokine. It is essentially provided by the microenvironment, and there is thus a paracrine circuit of stimulation between the MM cells and the microenvironment;
- the cytokines produced by MM PCs are able to 'activate' BM stromal cells.

These conclusions lead to the view that the increasing tumor mass provides increasing amounts of activating cytokines to the microenvironment, which in turn becomes able to produce large amounts of the MM-stimulating-cytokine IL-6. This close relationship between PCs and the microenvironment is lost when the development of new genetic abnormalities allows the stroma-independent growth of the malignant clone.[2]

APOPTOSIS AND MM PLASMA CELLS

Multiple myeloma plasma cells have an extended life span owing to defective apoptosis. Both external stimuli and intrinsic genetic defects may contribute to the ability of MM PCs to avoid apoptosis.[2] In the initial phases of the disease, when the malignant clone growth is highly dependent upon the supportive role of the BM stromal microenvironment, the stroma itself may be involved in the production of anti-apoptotic factors. The survival of MM PCs is accounted for at least partly by the direct cell–cell contacts with BM stromal cells that increase IL-6 production. IL-6 is able to support the MM clonal expansion not only by inducing proliferation but also by preventing apoptosis induced by different conditions, including exposure to dexamethasone or anti-Fas antibodies.[80,88] Other factors like IGF-1 are also capable of favoring not only the growth but also the extended survival of MM cells.[92] Conversely, IL-6R antagonists, which block the effects of IL-6 stimulation, act as pro-apoptotic factors for MM PCs.[96]

Investigations of this resistance to apoptosis have focused the attention on the *Bcl-2* gene family. The *Bcl-2* gene product, which is the prototype antiapoptotic factor, is consistently overexpressed in MM PCs, although the mechanisms that regulate the overexpression have not yet been clarified.[97] *Bcl-2* overexpression contributes to the resistance of MM PCs to the apoptosis that might occur in a number of different situations, including dexamethasone treatment or IL-6 deprivation. Another antiapoptotic member of the *Bcl-2* gene family – Bcl-XL has been observed more frequently in cells from patients in relapse and has been associated with resistance to chemotherapy.[98] Recently, an important role has been ascribed to a third antiapoptotic member of the family, myeloid cell factor-1 (*Mcl-1*). It has been shown that knocking out Mcl-1 induced PC apoptosis, while increasing its levels with transfection induced even greater resistance to cell death.[99] The mechanisms that control the expresssion of *Mcl-1* in MM PCs are yet undefined and it is not clear whether it is dependent on extrinsic factors or whether there is constitutive *Mcl-1* expression. In support of the 'extrinsic' hypothesis, it has been reported that IL-6 may significantly upregulate *Mcl-1* expression.[100] On the other hand, it is intriguing that *Mcl-1* transgenic mice develop lymphomas,[101] suggesting that the constitutive overexpression of *Mcl-1* may favor the development of lymphoid malignancies. Another interesting intrinsic mechanism that might contribute to the defective apoptosis (coupled to increased proliferation) of MM PCs is related to the ectopic expression of fibroblast growth factor receptor 3 (FGFR3) in patients with the t(4;14) translocation.[102]

The defective apoptosis observed in MM PCs raises the possibility of a therapeutic intervention. There is current interest in the effects of TNF-related apoptosis-inducing ligand (TRAIL), a member of the superfamily of cell-death ligands that include TNFα and Fas ligand (FasL). TRAIL induces apoptosis of a variety of cancer cells, while sparing normal cells, and has been shown to induce apoptosis of MM cell lines and of fresh cells *in vitro*.[103] TRAIL is highly expressed by PCs of patients with aggressive disease together with FasL, and it has been reported that FasL+/TRAIL+ highly malignant PCs exert a negative regulation on erythroblast maturation and may thereby contribute to the development of anemia in MM.[104]

In conclusion, numerous combinations of antiapoptotic mechanims of both intrinsic and extrinsic origin are operating in MM, and their individual contribution may vary in different phases (early vs. late, smoldering vs. aggressive) of the disease to ensure the survival of the malignant clone. The multiplicity of mechanisms underlines the complexity of a therapeutic approach based upon interfering with the mechanisms that prevent MM PC apoptosis.

CELL SIGNALING PATHWAYS IN MM PLASMA CELLS

As the expansion of MM clone results from both enhanced proliferation and defective apoptosis, the signal transduction pathways involved are the subject of intense investigation, with the aim of developing drugs that can selectively inhibit or interrupt specific molecular targets.[105]

IL-6 is of central importance in the pathophysiology of MM. It induces intracellular signaling through multiple pathways that affect proliferation and survival. Binding of IL-6 to CD126 results in the formation of a hexameric receptor complex, which is formed by two IL-6, two CD126, and two CD130 molecules, the CD130 molecules representing the signal-transducing elements.[2,88] Tyrosine kinases, including members of the Janus kinase (JAK) and Src family, that are constitutively bound to CD130 become activated and phosphorylated. This results in the recruitment and phosphorylation of members of the signal transducer and activator of transcription (STAT) family that dimerize, move to the nucleus, and regulate the target gene expression.[105] An interesting outcome of this pathway is the overexpression of Bcl-XL and the inhibition of Fas-mediated apoptosis.[106] Further, studies in MM cell lines have recently suggested that MM cell proliferation in response to IL-6 also requires the IL-6-independent activation of Src family kinase activity associated with CD45 expression.[107]

Another important signaling pathway that appears to influence MM PC proliferation is mediated by the Ras-MAPK (mitogen-activated protein-kinase) cascade.[105] The term Ras or p21^{ras} defines a complex of three proteins encoded by the three human ras genes (H-*ras*, K-*ras*, N-*ras*) that are membrane-associated guanosine triphospatases (GTPases) and mediate many biological responses stimulated by tyrosine kinases. Activation of Ras leads to the activation of a number of important kinases that include MAPK (alternatively termed extracellular signal regulated kinases, ERKs).[108] IL-6 activates Ras-MAPK and its substrates, which in turn may activate the endogenous production of IL-6. This brings in the important point that Ras mutations are relatively common in MM patients and increase with disease progression, suggesting the possibility that MM growth may be sustained by an altered Ras-MAPK signal transduction pathway.[109]

A third pathway through which IL-6 may influence survival of MM PCs is via the activation of protein tyrosine phosphatase (SHP2), which blocks the activation of related adhesion focal tyrosine kinase (RAFTK) in response to dexamethasone and prevents dexamethasone-induced apoptosis.[110]

Finally, both IL-6 and IGF-1 may activate the phosphatidylinositol 3-kinase (PI3-K)/AKT kinase pathway in MM cell lines.[111,112] This observation supports an independent role for the PI3-K/AKT pathway in cytokine-dependent responses in myeloma cells and suggests that PI3-K/Akt signaling mediates growth, survival and cell-cycle regulatory effects of IL-6 and IGF-1. Interestingly, immunohistochemical studies have shown that AKT kinase is activated in fresh human MM samples but not in MGUS samples.[113] The interruption of AKT activity in cultures of primary MM cells resulted in inhibition of MM cell growth *in vitro*.[113]

ANGIOGENESIS

Angiogenesis, the process of new vessel formation, is essential for the growth and metastasis of most solid tumors. Four main pieces of evidence support the concept that angiogenesis may be important also in MM (Fig. 5.4; see Plate 3):[114–118]

- microvascular density is definitely more prominent in smouldering, newly diagnosed, and relapsing

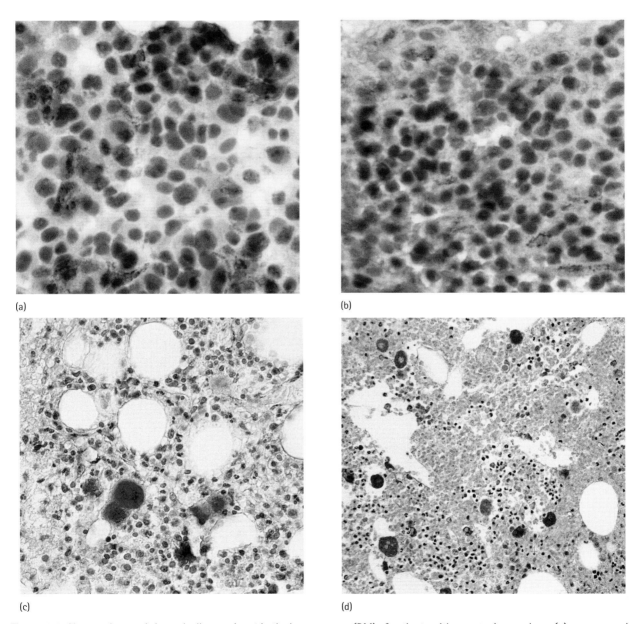

(a)

(b)

(c)

(d)

Figure 5.4 *Neo-angiogenesis is markedly prominent in the bone marrow (BM) of patients with progressive myeloma (a) as compared with the BM of patients who undergo disease remission (b) and patients with monoclonal gammopathy of undetermined significance (MGUS) (c). Anti-factor VIII immunostaining (d) (megakaryocyte positivity provides the internal positive control). (Courtesy of Professor A. Vacca, University of Bari, Italy.)*

MM than in controls, including MGUS and primary amyloidosis;

- a high correlation has been observed between the extent of BM angiogenesis, evaluated as microvessel area, and the PC labeling index;
- patients' survival has been shown to be inversely related to the entity of angiogensis;
- clinical responses have been obtained with thalidomide, which has well-known antiangiogenic properties.[119]

All these observations make a strong case for the role of angiogenesis in MM, and further underline the close interactions between the microenvironment and the malignant clone. As usual, a note of caution is needed, as most of the observed newly formed vessels are microvessels detected by factor VIII-related antigen, are frequently distorted and telangiectatic, and may represent an epiphenomenon owing to the production of angiogenetic factors by malignant PCs. PCs produce a number of angiogenetic factors, notably vascular endothelial growth factor (VEGF) – a potent angiogenic peptide with numerous biologic effects – whose receptors are expressed by BM stromal cells.[116] A number of observations link VEGF and IL-6, i.e. PCs and the microenvironment, and are of considerable therapeutic interest. VEGF secretion by MM PCs is upregulated by their interaction with BM stromal cells and exposure of stromal cells to VEGF induces a significant increase in the stromal cell production of IL-6, which in turn stimulates VEGF expression and secretion by PCs.[120,121] It is also important to point out that VEGF can replace M-CSF in promoting early osteoclast development.[122] This finding adds bone loss to the list of activities mediated by VEGF and triggered by the interactions of PCs with the microenvironment.

THE OVERALL CONCLUDING PICTURE: INTERACTIONS BETWEEN MALIGNANT PLASMA CELLS AND BM MICROENVIRONMENT

Normal BM microenvironment regulates normal B lymphopoiesis. B-cell generation occurs in intimate contact with an array of inductive stromal cells, and is mediated by multiple molecular contacts mediated by adhesion molecules and ECM proteins.[123–126] Cell–cell contacts switch on a specialized and selective program of gene expression that initiates B-cell commitment and leads to the stromal cell secretion of cytokines and chemokines. Growth factors are functionally active when bound to ECM proteins like proteoglycans and laminin. A strict interplay exists between cytokines and adhesion molecules: cytokines may regulate cell adhesion, which, in return, may modify the cellular response to cytokines.[125,126] It is also of interest that B-lymphoid lineage cells may affect the pathophysiology of bone by regulating osteoclastogenesis.[127,128] BM B-lineage cells are a source of receptor activator of NF-κB ligand (RANKL) and support osteoclast differentiation *in vitro*.[129] Further, osteoprotegerin (OPG), an important regulator of bone metabolism, also regulates B-cell maturation and development of efficient Ab responses.[130]

MM provides one of the best examples to illustrate the concept that host–tumor interactions contribute to cancer cell proliferation, survival, and progression, and to show that both the 'seed' and the 'soil' are important (Fig. 5.5).[105,131–133] It also outlines, although in a perverted way, the dynamic relationhips between the immune system and bone. BM microenvironmental stromal cells play an essential role in the growth of plasma cell tumors both

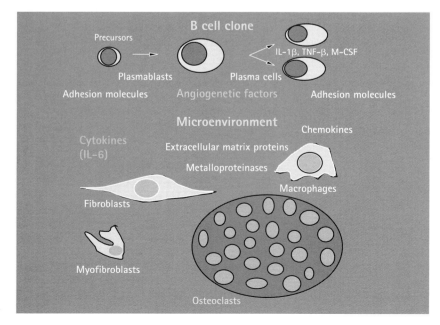

Figure 5.5 *Multiple interactions between the malignant cell clone and bone marrow microenvironment allow the progression of the disease.*

in mice[35] and in humans.[29] MM BM stromal cells are well equipped with a large series of adhesion molecules and ECM proteins that mediate homotypic and heterotypic interactions and provide anchorage sites to cells selectively exposed to locally released growth factors.[132,133] MM BM stromal cells also produce cytokines, such as IL-6, that play a crucial role in the evolution of the disease.[29,79] In turn, MM malignant plasma cells produce a number of cytokines and angiogenetic factors. Thus, the whole BM environment in MM contributes to the development of myeloma bone disease (see Chapter 6).

A multitude of experimental findings, linked to clinical observations, have led to the plausible hypothesis that a self-maintaining series of mutually interacting paracrine loops may occur between the malignant B-cell clone and the BM microenvironment and, through the production of ever-increasing amounts of cytokines, favor the progression of MM (Fig. 5.5). Dissecting the multiple molecular mechanisms that underlie these interactions is a formidable task but may lead to effective new therapeutic interventions.

KEY POINTS

- The transcriptional repressor Bcl-6, B-lymphocyte maturation protein 1 (Blimp-1), and X-box-binding protein 1 (XBP1) are the most important genes for plasma cell differentiation.
- The most likely candidate for the physiological equivalent of the multiple myeloma plasma cell (MM PC) precursor is either an activated B memory cell or a plasmablast generated in peripheral lymphoid organs during secondary T-dependent antibody response.
- Multiple myeloma is a bone marrow (BM)-restricted malignancy, even though the clonal founder cell may originate from the periphery.
- Circulating clonal precursors of MM PCs probably exist but their precise nature is unclear.
- MM PCs express several adhesion molecules. The best surface markers of MM plasma cells are CD38 and CD138.
- MM PCs secrete a number of cytokines able to influence the BM microenvironment and are also responsive to various cytokines. Interleukin-6 (IL-6) is the most relevant known growth factor for MM PCs.
- IL-6 affects proliferation and survival of MM PCs by intracellular signaling through multiple pathways: the JAK/STAT pathway, the Ras-MAPK

cascade, and the activation of SHP2 that blocks the activation of RAFTK.
- MM PCs have an extended life span owing to defective apoptosis. Both external stimuli and intrinsic genetic defects influence the ability of MM PCs to avoid apoptosis.
- Angiogenesis is more pronounced in MM than in monoclonal gammopathy of undetermined significance (MGUS). Patients' survival appears to be inversely related to the entity of angiogensis.
- MM plasma cells appear to 'instruct' the BM environment to help the expansion of the malignant clone. The capacity to activate endogenous stromal cells marks the evolution from MGUS to MM.
- A self-maintaining series of mutually interacting paracrine loops occurs between the malignant B-cell clone and the BM microenvironment, and favors the progression of MM.

ACKNOWLEDGMENTS

The author's work is supported by Associazione Italiana per la Ricerca sul Cancro (AIRC), Milan, Italy and by MURST.

REFERENCES

◆ = Key primary paper
● = Major review article

◆1. Bataille R, Harousseau JL. Multiple myeloma. *N Engl J Med* 1997; **336**:1657–64.
◆2. Hallek M, Bergsagel PL, Anderson KC. Multiple myeloma: increasing evidence for a multistep transformation process. *Blood* 1998; **91**:3–21.
◆3. Calame KL. Plasma cells: finding new light at the end of B cell development. *Nature Immunology* 2001; **2**:1103–108.
4. Cyster JG. Chemokines and cell migration in secondary lymphoid organs. *Science* 1999; **286**:2098–102.
5. Schebesta M, Heavey B, Busslinger M. Transcriptional control of B-cell development. *Curr Opin Immunol* 2002; **14**:216–23.
◆6. Reimold AM, Iwakoshi NN, Manis J, Vallabhajosyula P, Szomolanyi-Tsuda E, Gravallese EM, *et al.* Plasma cell differentiation requires the transcription factor XBP-1. *Nature* 2001; **412**:300–7.
●7. Shaffer AL, Yu X, He Y, Boldrick J, Chan EP, Staudt LM. BCL-6 represses genes that function in lymphocyte differentiation, inflammation, and cell cycle control. *Immunity* 2000; **13**:199–212.
◆8. MacLennan ICM, Gray D. Antigen-driven selection of virgin and memory B cells. *Immunol Rev* 1986; **91**:61–85.
9. MacLennan ICM, Chan EYT. The origin of bone marrow plasma cells. In: Obrams GI, Potter M (eds) *Epidemiology and*

biology of multiple myeloma. Berlin: Springer-Verlag, 1991:129–35.

10. Liu YJ, Johnson GD, Gordon J, MacLennan ICM. Germinal centres in T-cell dependent antibody responses. *Immunol Today* 1992; **13**:17–21.

11. McHeyzer-Williams MG, Ahmed R. B cell memory and the long-lived plasma cell. *Curr Opin Immunol* 1999; **11**:172–9.

12. Rolink A, Melchers F. Generation and regeneration of cells of the B-lymphocyte lineage. *Curr Opin Immunol* 1993; **5**:207–17.

13. Stein H, Gerdes J, Mason DY. The normal and malignant germinal centre. *Clin Haematol* 1982; **11**:531–59.

14. Kelsoe G. Life and death in germinal centers (Redux). *Immunity* 1996; **4**:107–11.

15. Brandtzaeg P, Farstad IN, Johansen FE, Morton HC, Norderhaug IN, Yamanaka T. The B-cell system of human mucosae and exocrine glands. *Immunol Rev* 1999; **171**:45–87.

16. Benner R, Hijmans W, Haaijman JJ. The bone marrow: the major source of serum immunoglobulins, but still a neglected site of antibody formation. *Clin Exp Immunol* 1981; **46**:1–8.

17. DiLosa RM, Maeda K, Masuda A, Szakal AK, Tew JG. Germinal center B cells and antibody production in the bone marrow. *J Immunol* 1991; **146**:4071–7.

18. Brandtzaeg P, Farstad IN, Haraldsen G. Regional specialization in the mucosal immune system: primed cells do not always home along the same track. *Immunol Today* 1999; **20**:267–77.

●19. Potter M. Myeloma proteins (M-components) with antibody-like activity. *N Engl J Med* 1971; **284**:831–8.

20. Seligmann M, Brouet JC. Antibody activity of human myeloma globulins. *Semin Hematol* 1973; **10**:163–77.

21. Konrad RJ, Kricka LJ, Goodman DBP, Goldman J, Silberstein LE. Myeloma-associated paraprotein directed against the HIV-1 p24 antigen in an HIV-1-seropositive patient. *N Engl J Med* 1993; **328**:1817–19.

●22. Bakkus MHC, Heirman C, Van Riet I, Van Camp B, Thielemans K. Evidence that multiple myeloma Ig heavy chain VDJ genes contain somatic mutations but show no intraclonal variation. *Blood* 1992; **80**:2326–35.

23. Vescio R, Cao J, Hong CH, Lee JC, Wu CH, Der-Danielian M, et al. Myeloma Ig heavy chain V region sequences reveal prior antigenic selection and marked somatic mutation but no intraclonal diversity. *J Immunol* 1995; **155**:2487–97.

24. Sahota SS, Leo R, Hamblin TJ, Stevenson FK. Ig VH gene mutational pattern indicate different tumor cell status in human myeloma and monoclonal gammopathy of undetermined significance. *Blood* 1996; **87**:746–55.

25. Manz RA, Radbruch A. Plasma cells for a lifetime? *Eur J Immunol* 2002; **32**:923–7.

●26. O'Connor BP, Cascalho M, Noelle RJ. Short-lived and long-lived bone marrow plasma cells are derived from a novel precursor population. *J Exp Med* 2002; **195**:737–45.

27. Ghia P, Granziero L, Chilosi M, Caligaris-Cappio F. Chronic B cell malignancies and bone marrow microenvironment. *Semin Cancer Biol* 2001; **12**:149–55.

28. Ghia P, Strola G, Granziero L, Geuna M, Guida G, Sallusto F, et al. Chronic lymphocytic leukemia B cells are endowed with the capacity to attract CD4+, CD40L+ T cells by producing CCL22. *Eur J Immunol* 2002; **32**:1403–13.

●29. Caligaris-Cappio F, Bergui L, Gregoretti MG, Gaidano G, Gaboli M, Schena M, et al. Role of bone marrow stromal cells in the growth of human multiple myeloma. *Blood* 1991; **77**:2688–93.

30. Merico F, Bergui L, Gregoretti MG, Ghia P, Aimo G, Lindley IJD, et al. Cytokines involved in the progression of multiple myeloma. *Clin Exp Immunol* 1993; **92**:27–31.

31. Bernerman ZN, Chen ZZ, Ramael M, Van Hoof V, Peetermans ME. Human long-term bone marrow cultures (HLTBMCs) in myelomatous disorders. *Leukemia* 1989; **3**:151–4.

32. Gregoretti MG, Gottardi D, Ghia P, Bergui L, Merico F, Marchisio PC, et al. Characterization of bone marrow stromal cells from multiple myeloma. *Leuk Res* 1994; **18**:675–8.

33. Nemunaitis J, Andrews F, Mochizuki D, Lilly MB, Singer JW. Human marrow stromal cells: response to interleukin-6 (IL-6) and control of Il-6 expression. *Blood* 1989; **74**:1929–36.

34. Caligaris-Cappio F, Bergui L, Tesio L, Pizzolo G, Malavasi F, Chilosi M, et al. Identification of malignant plasma cell precursors in the bone marrow of multiple myeloma. *J Clin Invest* 1985; **76**:1243–51.

●35. Degrassi A, Hilbert DM, Rudikoff S, Anderson AO, Potter M, Coon HG. In vitro culture of primary plasmacytomas requires stromal cell feeder layers. *Proc Natl Acad Sci USA* 1993; **90**:2060–4.

36. Billadeau D, Quam L, Thomas W, Kay N, Greipp P, Kyle R, et al. Detection and quantitation of malignant cells in the peripheral blood of multiple myeloma patients. *Blood* 1992; **80**:1818–24.

37. Corradini P, Voena C, Astolfi M, Ladetto M, Tarella C, Boccadoro M, et al. High-dose sequential chemoradiotherapy in multiple myeloma: residual tumor cells are detectable in bone marrow and peripheral blood harvests and after autografting. *Blood* 1995; **85**:1596–602.

38. Lemoli RM, Fortuna A, Motta MR, Rizzi S, Giudice V, Nannetti A, et al. Concomitant mobilization of plasma cells and hematopoietic progenitors into peripheral blood of multiple myeloma patients: positive selection and transplantation of enriched CD34+ cells to remove circulating tumor cells. *Blood* 1996; **87**:1625–34.

39. Szczepek AJ, Seeberger K, Wizniak J, Mant MJ, Belch AR, Pilarski LM. A high frequency of circulating B cells share clonotypic Ig heavy-chain VDJ rearrangements with autologous bone marrow plasma cells in multiple myeloma, as measured by single-cell and in situ reverse transcriptase-polymerase chain reaction. *Blood* 1998; **92**:2844–55.

40. Chen BJ, Epstein J. Circulating clonal lymphocytes in myeloma constitute a minor subpopulation of B cells. *Blood* 1996; **87**:1972–6.

41. McSweeney PA, Wells DA, Shults KE, Nash RA, Bensinger WI, Duckner CD, et al. Tumor-specific aneuploidy not detected in CD19+ B-Lymphoid cells from myeloma patients in a multidimensional flow cytometric analysis. *Blood* 1996; **88**:622–32.

42. Billadeau D, Ahmann G, Greipp P, Van Ness B. The bone marrow of multiple myeloma patients contains B cell populations at different stages of differentiation that are clonally related to the malignant plasma cell. *J Exp Med* 1993; **178**:1023–31.

43. Corradini P, Boccadoro M, Voena C, Pileri A. Evidence for a bone marrow B cell transcribing malignant plasma cell VDJ joined to Cm sequence in IgG and IgA secreting multiple myelomas. *J Exp Med* 1993; **178**:1091–6.

44. Dono M, Hashimoto S, Fais F, Trejo V, Allen SL, Lichtman SM, *et al.* Evidence for progenitors of chronic lymphocytic leukemia B cells that undergo intraclonal differentiation and differentiation. *Blood* 1996; **87**:1586–94.

●45. Zhan F, Hardin J, Kordsmeier B, Bumm K, Zheng M, Tian E, Sanderson R, *et al.* Global gene expression profiling of multiple myeloma, monoclonal gammopathy of undetermined significance, and normal bone marrow plasma cells. *Blood* 2002; **99**:1745–57.

46. Kawano MM, Huang N, Harada H, Harada Y, Sakai A, Tanaka H, *et al.* Identification of immature and mature myeloma cells in the bone marrow of human myelomas. *Blood* 1993; **82**:564–70.

●47. Harada H, Kawano MM, Huang N, Harada Y, Iwato K, Tanabe O, *et al.* Phenotypic difference of normal plasma cells from mature myeloma cells. *Blood* 1993; **81**:2658–63.

48. Medina F, Segundo C, Campos-Caro A, Gonzalez-Garcia I, Brieva JA. The heterogeneity shown by human plasma cells from tonsil, blood, and bone marrow reveals graded stages of increasing maturity, but local profiles of adhesion molecule expression. *Blood* 2002; **99**:2154–61.

49. San Miguel JF, Almeida J, Mateo G, Blade J, Lopez-Berges C, Caballero D, *et al.* Immunophenotypic evaluation of the plasma cell compartment in multiple myeloma: a tool for comparing the efficacy of different treatment strategies and predicting outcome. *Blood* 2002; **99**:1853–6.

50. Malavasi F, Caligaris-Cappio F, Milanese C, Dellabona P, Richiardi P, Carbonara AO. Characterization of a murine monoclonal antibody specific for human early lymphohemopoietic cells. *Hum Immunol* 1984; **9**:9–20.

51. States DJ, Walseth TF, Lee HC. Similarities in amino acid sequences of aplysia ADP-ribosyl cyclase and human lymphocyte antigen CD38. *Trends Biochem Sci* 1992; **17**:495–9.

52. Galione A. Cyclic ADP-ribose: a new way to control calcium. *Science* 1993; **259**:325–6.

53. Vallario A, Chilosi M, Adami F, Montagna L, Deaglio S, Malavasi F, *et al.* Human myeloma cells express the CD38 ligand CD31. *Br J Haematol* 1999; **105**:441–4.

●54. Ridley RC, Xiao H, Hata H, Woodliff J, Epstein J, Sanderson RD. Expression of syndecan regulates human myeloma plasma cell adhesion to type I collagen. *Blood* 1993; **81**:767–74.

55. Borset M, Hjertner O, Yaccoby S, Epstein J, Sanderson RD. Syndecan-1 is targeted to the uropods of polarized myeloma cells where it promotes adhesion and sequesters heparin-binding proteins. *Blood* 2000; **96**:2528–36.

56. Seidel C, Borset M, Hjertner O, Cao D, Abildgaard N, Hjorth-Hansen H, *et al.* High levels of soluble syndecan-1 in myeloma-derived bone marrow: modulation of hepatocyte growth factor activity. *Blood* 2000; **96**:3139–46.

57. Derksen PWB, Keehnen RMJ, Evers LM, van Oers MHJ, Spaargaren M, Pals ST. Cell surface proteoglycan syndecan-1 mediates hepatocyte growth factor binding and promotes Met signaling in multiple myeloma. *Blood* 2002; **99**:1405–10.

58. Warburton, Joshua DE, Gibson J, Brown RD. CD10-(CALLA)-positive lymphocytes in myeloma:evidence that they are a malignant precursor population and are of germinal centre origin. *Leuk Lymph* 1989; **1**:11–20.

59. Cao J, Vescio RA, Rettig MB, Hong CH, Kim A, Lichtenstein AK, *et al.* A CD10-positive subset of malignant cells is identified in multiple myeloma using PCR with patient-specific immunoglobulin gene primers. *Leukemia* 1995; **9**:1948–53.

60. Shapiro VS, Mollenauer MN, Weiss A. Endogenous CD28 expressed on myeloma cells up-regulates interleukin-8 production: implications for multiple myeloma progression. *Blood* 2001; **98**:187–93.

61. Uchiyama H, Barut BA, Chauhan D, Cannistra SA, Anderson KC. Characterization of adhesion molecules on human myeloma cell lines. *Blood* 1990; **80**:2306–14.

●62. Van Camp B, Durie BGM, Spier C, DeWaele M, Van Riet I, Vela, Frutiger Y, *et al.* Plasma cells in multiple myeloma express a natural killer cell-associated antigen: CD56 (NKH-1; Leu-19). *Blood* 1990; **76**:377–82.

63. Turley EA, Belch AJ, Poppema S, Pilarski L. Expression and function of a receptor for hyaluronan-mediated motility on normal and malignant B lymphocytes. *Blood* 1993; **81**:446–53.

64. Van Riet I, Van Camp B. The involvement of adhesion molecules in the biology of multiple myeloma. *Leuk Lymphoma* 1993; **9**:441–52.

65. Drach J, Gattringer C, Huber H. Expression of the neural cell adhesion molecule (CD56) by human myeloma cells. *Clin Exp Immunol* 1991; **83**:418–22.

66. Ashmann EJM, Lokhorst HM, Dekker AW, Bloem AC. Lymphocyte function-associated antigen-1 expression on plasma cells correlates with tumor growth in multiple myeloma. *Blood* 1992; **79**:2068–75.

67. Stauder R, Van Driel M, Schwarzler C, Thaler J, Lokhorst HM, Kreuser ED, *et al.* Different CD44 splicing patterns define prognostic subgroups in multiple myeloma. *Blood* 1996; **88**:3101–8.

68. Sanz-Rodriguez F, Hidalgo A, TeixidòJ. Chemokine stromal cell-derived factor-1α modulates VLA-4 integrin-mediated multiple myeloma cell adhesion to CS-1/fibronectin and VCAM-1. *Blood* 2001; **97**:346–51.

69. Masellis-Smith A, Belch AR, Mant MJ, Turley EA, Pilarski LM. Hyaluronan-dependent mobility of B cells and leukemic plasma cells in blood, but not of bone marrow plasma cells, in multiple myeloma: alternate use of receptor for hyaluronan-mediated motility (RHAMM) and CD44. *Blood* 1996; **87**:1891–9.

70. Ely SA, Knowles DM. Expression of CD56/neural cell adhesion molecule correlates with the presence of lytic bone lesions in multiple myeloma and distinguishes myeloma from monoclonal gammopathy of undetermined significance and lymphomas with plasmacytoid differentiation. *Am J Pathol* 2002; **160**:1293–9.

71. Barker HF, Hamilton MS, Ball J, Drew M, Franklin IM. Expression of adhesion molecules LFA-3 and N-CAM on normal and malignant human plasma cells. *Br J Haematol* 1992; **81**:331–5.

72. Anderson KC, Jones RM, Morimoto C, Leavitt P, Barut A. Response patterns of purified myeloma cells to hematopoietic growth factors. *Blood* 1989; **73**:1915–24.

73. Cozzolino F, Torcia M, Aldinucci D, Rubartelli A, Miliani A, Shaw AR, *et al.* Production of Interleuchin-1 by bone marrow myeloma cells. *Blood* 1989; **74**:380–7.

●74. Mundy GR, Raisz LG, Cooper RA, Schechter GP, Salmon SE. Evidence for the secretion of an osteoclast stimulating factor in myeloma. *N Engl J Med* 1974; **291**:1041–6.

75. Ross Garrett I, Durie BGM, Nedwin GE, Gillespie A, Bringman T, Sabatini M, *et al.* Production of lymphotoxin, a bone-resorbing cytokine, by cultured human myeloma cells. *N Engl J Med* 1987; **317**:526–32.

76. Nakamura M, Merchav S, Carter A, Ernst TJ, Demetri GD, Furukawa Y, *et al.* Expression of a novel 3.5-kb macrophage colony-stimulating factor transcript in human myeloma cells. *J Immunol* 1989; **143**:3543–7.

77. Tinhofer I, Marschitz I, Henn T, Egle A, Greil R. Expression of functional interleukin-15 receptor and autocrine production of interleukin-15 as mechanisms of tumor propagation in multiple myeloma. *Blood* 2000; **95**:610–18.

●78. Kawano M, Hirano T, Matsuda T, Taga T, Horii Y, Iwato K, *et al.* Autocrine generation and requirement of BSF-2/IL-6 for human multiple myeloma. *Nature* 1988; **332**:83–6.

●79. Klein B, Zhang XG, Jourdan M, Content J, Houssiau F, Aarden L, *et al.* Paracrine rather than autocrine regulation of myeloma-cell growth and differentiation by interleukin-6. *Blood* 1989; **73**:517–26.

◆80. Klein B, Zhang XG, Lu ZY, Bataille R. Interleukin-6 in human multiple myeloma. *Blood* 1995; **85**:863–72.

81. Nilsson K, Jernberg H, Pettersson M. IL-6 as a growth factor for human multiple myeloma cells – a short overview. *Curr Top Microbiol Immunol* 1990; **166**:3–8.

82. Jernberg H, Pettersson M, Kishimoto T, Nilsson K. Heterogeneity in response to Interleukin 6 (IL-6), expression of IL-6 and IL-6 receptor mRNA in a panel of established human multiple myeloma cell lines. *Leukemia* 1991; **5**:255–65.

83. Lokhorst HM, Lamme T, deSmet M, Klein S, de Weger RA, van Oers R, *et al.* Primary tumor cells of myeloma patients induce interleukin-6 secretion in long-term bone marrow cultures. *Blood* 1994; **84**:2269–74.

84. Chauhan D, Uchiyama H, Akbarali Y, Urashima M, Yamamoto KI, Libermann TA, *et al.* Multiple myeloma cell adhesion-induced interleukin-6 expression in bone marrow stromal cells involves activation of NF-kB. *Blood* 1996; **87**:1104–12.

85. Bataille R, Jourdan M, Zhang XG, Klein B. Serum levels of interleukin-6, a potent myeloma cell growth factor, as a reflection of disease severity in plasma cell dyscrasias. *J Clin Invest* 1989; **84**:2008–11.

86. Klein B, Wijdenes J, Zhang XG, Jourdan M, Boiron JM, Brochier J, *et al.* Murine anti-Interleuchin-6 monoclonal antibody therapy for a patient with plasma cell leukemia. *Blood* 1991; **78**:1198–204.

87. Udagawa N, Takahashi N, Katagiri T, Tamura T, Wada S, Findlay DM, *et al.* Interleukin (IL)-6 induction of osteoclast differentiation depends on IL-6 receptors expressed on osteoblastic cells but not on osteoclast progenitors. *J Exp Med* 1995; **182**:1461–8.

◆88. Kishimoto T, Akira S, Narazaki M, Taga T. Interleukin-6 family of cytokines and gp130. *Blood* 1995; **86**:1243–54.

89. Rawstron C, Fenton JAL, Ashcroft J, English A, Jones RA, Richards SJ, *et al.* The interleukin-6 receptor alpha-chain (CD126) is expressed by neoplastic but not normal plasma cells. *Blood* 2000; **96**:3880–6.

90. Chauhan D, Kharbanda SM, Ogata A, Urashima M, Frank D, Malik N, *et al.* Oncostatin M induces association of Grb2 with janus kinase JAK2 in multiple myeloma cells. *J Exp Med* 1995; **182**:1801–6.

91. Lu ZY, Zhang XG, Rodriguez C, Wijdenes J, Gu ZJ, Morel-Fournier B, *et al.* Interleukin-10 is a proliferation factor but not a differentiation factor for human myeloma cells. *Blood* 1995; **85**:2521–7.

92. Georgii-Hemming P, Jernberg-Wiklund H, Ljunggren O, Nilsson K. IGF-I is a growth and survival factor in human myeloma cell lines. *Blood* 1996; **88**:2250–8.

93. Borset M, Hjorth-Hansen H, Seidel C, Sundan A, Waage A. Hepatocyte growth factor and its receptor c-met in multiple myeloma. *Blood* 1996; **88**:3998–4004.

94. Seidel C, Borset M, Turesson I, Abildgaard N, Sundan A, Waage A. Elevated serum concentrations of hepatocyte growth factor in patients with multiple myeloma. The nordic myeloma study group. *Blood* 1998; **91**:806–12.

95. Jourdan M, De Vos J, Mechti N, Klein B. Regulation of Bcl-2-family proteins in myeloma cells by three myeloma survival factors: interleukin-6, interferon-alpha and insulin-like growth factor 1. *Cell Death Differ* 2000; **7**:1244–52.

96. Demartis A, Bernassola F, Savino R, Melino G, Ciliberto G. Interleukin-6 receptor superantagonists are potent inducers of human multiple myeloma cell death. *Cancer Res* 1996; **56**:4213–18.

97. Schwarze MM, Hawley RG. Prevention of myeloma cell apoptosis by ectopic bcl-2 expression or interleukin 6-mediated up-regulation of bcl-xL. *Cancer Res* 1995; **55**:2262–5.

98. Gauthier ER, Piche L, Lemieux G, Lemieux R. Role of bcl-X(L) in the control of apoptosis in murine myeloma cells. *Cancer Res* 1996; **56**:1451–6.

99. Zhang B, Gojo I, Fenton RG. Myeloid cell factor-1 is a critical survival factor for multiple myeloma. *Blood* 2002; **99**:1885–93.

100. Puthier D, Derenne S, Barille S, Moreau P, Harousseau JL, Bataille R, *et al.* Mcl-1 and Bcl-xL are co-regulated by IL-6 in human myeloma cells. *Br J Haematol* 1999; **107**:392–5.

101. Zhou P, Levy NB, Xie H, Qian L, Lee CY, Gascoyne RD, *et al.* MCL1 transgenic mice exhibit a high incidence of B-cell lymphoma manifested as a spectrum of histologic subtypes. *Blood* 2001; **97**:3902–9.

102. Plowright EE, Li Z, Bergsagel PL, Chesi M, Barber DL, Branch DR, *et al.* Ectopic expression of fibroblast growth factor receptor 3 promotes myeloma cell proliferation and prevents apoptosis. *Blood* 2000; **95**:992–8.

103. Mitsiades N, Mitsiades CS, Poulaki V, Anderson KC, Treon SP. Intracellular regulation of tumor necrosis factor-related apoptosis-inducing ligand-induced apoptosis in human multiple myeloma cells. *Blood* 2002; **99**:2162–71.

104. Silvestris F, Cafforio P, Tucci M, Dammacco F. Negative regulation of erythroblast maturation by Fas-L[+]/TRAIL[+] highly malignat plasma cells: a major pathogenetic mechanism of anemia in multiple myeloma. *Blood* 2002; **99**:1305–13.

105. Dalton WS, Bergsagel PL, Kuehl WM, Anderson KC, Harousseau JL. Multiple myeloma. *Hematology* 2001:157–77.

106. Catlett-Falcone R, Landowski TH, Oshiro MM, Turkson J, Levitzki A, Savino R, *et al.* Constitutive activation of Stat3

signaling confers resistance to apoptosis in human U266 myeloma cells. *Immunity* 1999; **10**:105–15.

107. Ishikawa H, Tsuyama N, Abroun S, Liu S, Li FJ, Taniguchi O, *et al*. Requirements of src family kinase activity associated with CD45 for myeloma cell proliferation by interleukin-6. *Blood* 2002; **99**:2172–8.

108. Ogata A, Chauhan D, Teoh G, Treon SP, Urashima M, Schlossman RL, *et al*. IL-6 triggers cell growth via the Ras-dependent mitogen-activated protein kinase cascade. *J Immunol* 1997; **159**:2212–21.

109. Neri A, Murphy JP, Cro L, Ferrero D, Tarella C, Baldini L, *et al*. Ras oncogene mutation in multiple myeloma. *J Exp Med* 1989; **170**:1715–25.

110. Hideshima T, Nakamura N, Chauhan D, Anderson KC. Biologic sequelae of interleukin-6 induced PI3-K/Akt signaling in multiple myeloma. *Oncogene* 2001; **20**:5991–6000.

111. Tu Y, Gardner A, Lichtenstein A. The phosphatidylinositol 3-kinase/AKT kinase pathway in multiple myeloma plasma cells: roles in cytokine-dependent survival and proliferative responses. *Cancer Res* 2000; **60**:6763–70.

112. Hyun T, Yam A, Pece S, Xie X, Zhang J, Miki T, *et al*. Loss of PTEN expression leading to high Akt activation in human multiple myelomas. *Blood* 2000; **96**:3560–8.

113. Hsu JH, Shi Y, Krajewski S, Renner S, Fisher M, Reed JC, *et al*. The AKT kinase is activated in multiple myeloma tumor cells. *Blood* 2001; **98**:2853–5.

●114. Vacca A, Ribatti D, Roncali L, Ranieri G, Serio G, Silvestris F, *et al*. Bone marrow angiogenesis and progression in multiple myeloma. *Br J Haematol* 1994; **87**:503–8.

115. Vacca A, Ribatti D, Presta M, Minischetti M, Iurlaro M, Ria R, *et al*. Bone marrow neovascularization, plasma cell angiogenic potential, and matrix metalloproteinase-2 secretion parallel progression of human multiple myeloma. *Blood* 1999; **93**:3064–73.

116. Bellamy WT, Richter L, Frutiger Y, Grogan TM. Expression of vascular endothelial growth factor and its receptors in hematopoietic malignancies. *Cancer Res* 1999; **59**:728–33.

117. Bellamy WT. Expression of vascular endothelial growth factor and its receptors in multiple myeloma and other hematopoietic malignancies. *Semin Oncol* 2001; **28**:551–9.

118. Rajkumar SV, Kyle RA. Angiogenesis in multiple myeloma. *Semin Oncol* 2001; **28**:560–4.

119. Singhal S, Mehta J, Desikan R, Ayers D, Roberson P, Eddlemon P, *et al*. Antitumor activity of thalidomide in refractory multiple myeloma. *N Engl J Med* 1999; **341**:1565–71.

120. Dankbar B, Padrò T, Leo R, Feldmann B, Kropff M, Masters RM, *et al*. Vascular endothelial growth factor and interleukin-6 in paracrine tumor-stromal cell interactions in multiple myeloma. *Blood* 2000; **95**:2630–6.

121. Gupta D, Treon SP, Shima Y, Hideshima T, Podar K, Tai YT, *et al*. Adherence of multiple myeloma cells to bone marrow stromal cells upregulates vascular endothelial growth factor secretion: therapeutic applications. *Leukemia* 2001; **15**:1950–61.

122. Niida S, Kaku M, Amano H, Yoshida H, Kataoka H, Nishikawa S, *et al*. Vascular endothelial growth factor can substitute for macrophage colony-stimulating factor in the support of osteoclastic bone resorption. *J Exp Med* 1999; **190**:293–8.

123. Thiery JP, Boyer B. The junction between cytokines and cell adhesion. *Curr Opin Cell Biol* 1992; **4**:782–92.

124. Hynes RO. Integrins: versatility, modulation and signalling in cell adhesion. *Cell* 1992; **69**:11–25.

125. Juliano RL, Haskill S. Signal transduction from the extracellular matrix. *J Cell Biol* 1993; **120**:577–85.

126. Giancotti FG, Ruoslahti E. Integrin signaling. *Science* 1999; **285**:1028–32.

●127. Choi SJ, Cruz JC, Craig F, Chung H, Devlin RD, Roodman GD, *et al*. Macrophage inflammatory protein 1-alpha is a potential osteoclast stimulatory factor in multiple myeloma. *Blood* 2000; **96**:671–5.

128. Kong YY, Yoshida H, Sarosi I, Tan HL, Timms E, Capparelli C, *et al*. OPGL is a key regulator of osteoclastogenesis, lymphocyte development and lymph-node organogenensis. *Nature* 1999; **397**:315–23.

129. Manabe N, Kawaguchi H, Chikuda H, Miyaura C, Inada M, Nagai R, *et al*. Connection between B lymphocyte and osteoclst differentiation pathways. *J Immunol* 2001; **167**:2625–31.

130. Yun TJ, Tallquist MD, Aicher A, Raffarty KL, Marshall AJ, Moon JJ, *et al*. Osteoprotegerin, a crucial regulator of bone metabolism, also regulates B cell development and function. *J Immunol* 2001; **166**:1482–91.

131. Tricot G. New insights into role of microenvironment in multiple myeloma. *Lancet* 2000; **355**:248–9.

132. Caligaris-Cappio F, Gregoretti MG, Ghia P, Bergui L. In vitro growth of human multiple myeloma: implications for biology and therapy. *Hematol Oncol Clin North Am* 1992; **6**:257–71.

133. Shain KH, Landowski TH, Dalton WS. The tumor microenvironment as a determinant of cancer cell survival: a possible mechanism for de novo drug resistance. *Curr Opin Oncol* 2000; **12**:557–63.

6

Pathophysiology of myeloma bone disease

BABATUNDE O. OYAJOBI AND GREGORY R. MUNDY

INTRODUCTION

Multiple myeloma is characterized by a unique form of destructive bone disease, which occurs in the majority of patients. The bone destruction, which is progressive, is responsible for the most prominent and distressing clinical features of this disease, namely intractable bone pain, fractures occurring either spontaneously or following trivial injury, and hypercalcemia with its attendant symptoms and signs. Although myeloma is a disease with protean features resulting from the effects of the disease on multiple organ systems, perhaps its most important clinical manifestation, and certainly the one that most often heralds the onset of the disease, is its effects on the skeleton. This chapter will focus on the pathophysiology of the bone lesions in myeloma.

NATURE OF THE BONE DISEASE

The bone lesions in myeloma, which typically appear on radiographs as radiolucent areas, occur in several patterns. Occasionally, patients develop single osteolytic lesions that are associated with solitary plasmacytomas. Some patients have diffuse bone loss (osteopenia), which mimics the appearance of osteoporosis, owing to the

dissemination of the myeloma cells throughout the axial skeleton. However, in most patients, there are multiple, discrete, lytic bone lesions occurring at the site of deposits or nests of myeloma cells. Rarely, patients with myeloma have an increase in the formation of new bone around myeloma cells rather than lytic lesions or bone loss, a rare condition known as osteosclerotic myeloma. The extent of the bone disease is an important factor in the prognosis of a patient with myeloma.

Bone remodeling is profoundly impaired in almost all patients with myeloma. Although some patients with other hematopoietic malignancies, such as B-cell lymphoma and adult T-cell leukemia, occasionally have skeletal manifestations, they are rarely as severe and certainly not as common as in myeloma. There is evidence that excessive bone resorption is an early tumor-induced event in myeloma and is often associated with progression from quiescent monoclonal gammopathy of undetermined significance (MGUS) or smoldering myeloma to active myeloma.[1] Bone pain is a major cause of morbidity in myeloma, and 75–80% of patients present with bone pain as a predominant symptom.[1,2] The bone pain is often unremitting but occasionally fluctuates in intensity for reasons that are unknown. Patients with myeloma bone disease are susceptible to fractures occurring either spontaneously or following trivial injury. These pathological fractures mainly involve the vertebrae, ribs, and long bones (most commonly), but occasionally occur at other sites, such as the sternum and pelvis. Hypercalcemia, which occurs in about a third of patients with advanced disease, mainly as a consequence of osteolysis, is accompanied by its characteristic attendant symptoms and signs. Occasionally hypercalcemia is exacerbated by concomitant renal failure, which frequently complicates the course of the disease.

PATHOPHYSIOLOGY OF BONE LESIONS IN MYELOMA

Although the precise molecular mechanisms mediating myeloma bone disease remain unclear, observations over the past 30 years have revealed the following:

1 Osteolysis in myeloma is due to an increase in the number and activity of osteoclasts, the only cells known to have the capacity to resorb mineralized bone. This is the only cellular mechanism for bone destruction, which is clearly evident in myeloma.

2 Excessive osteoclast activity in myeloma almost always occurs adjacent to foci of myeloma tumor cells.[3] In some patients, lytic lesions occur adjacent to nests of myeloma cells, resulting in a discrete osteolytic lesion. As mentioned earlier, only rarely are the myeloma cells spread more diffusely throughout the marrow, resulting in osteopenia. Thus, it appears that the predominant mechanism by which osteoclasts are stimulated in myeloma is a local one, whereby myeloma cells (or host cells) produce local factors (cytokines) responsible for increasing osteoclast formation and activation in an autocrine, paracrine, or juxtacrine fashion.

3 It has been known for several years that cultures of human myeloma cells *in vitro* express and secrete several osteoclast-activating factors (OAFs) into conditioned media. Earlier work had identified a number of soluble mediators with bone-resorptive activity, including lymphotoxin (tumor necrosis factor β), tumor necrosis factor α, interleukin-1α and β, and interleukin-6, capable of acting locally. Most of these putative mediators were identified in conditioned media from myeloma cells cultured independently. However, these *in vitro* studies have not clarified the nature of the critical mediator *in vivo*, and our understanding of how and to what extent these soluble mediators influence bone resorption in myeloma remains limited. More recent information suggests that other putative factor(s) with substantial bone-resorbing activity are produced only when myeloma cells are in contact with marrow stromal cells (see later).

4 Hypercalcemia occurs in many patients with myeloma at some time during the course of the disease. Hypercalcemia is almost always associated with markedly increased bone resorption and frequently with impaired renal function that is fixed and due to direct effects of the disease on renal function. Glomerular filtration may be further compromised by concurrent volume depletion and hypercalcemia.

5 The increase in osteoclastic bone resorption in myeloma is usually associated with impaired osteoblast function and the rate of new bone formation is often markedly reduced.[4] In contrast to other types of osteolytic bone disease, such as breast cancer, serum alkaline phosphatase activity is decreased or within the normal range, and radionuclide scans do not always show evidence of increased uptake.

6 Recent evidence suggests that the frequency of osteolytic bone disease may be correlated with the pattern of infiltration of the marrow by myeloma cells, the highest frequency of lytic lesions being seen in patients with nodular or diffuse, rather than interstitial, involvement.[5,6]

7 Occasionally, patients with myeloma show a predominant increase in new bone formation with subsequent osteosclerosis. This is often associated with polyneuropathy, organomegaly, endocrinopathy, monoclonal gammopathy, and skin changes (POEMS) syndrome.

FACTORS IMPLICATED IN MYELOMA-ASSOCIATED BONE DESTRUCTION

It has been recognized for over a quarter of a century that bone lesions in myeloma are caused by increased production of locally acting osteoclastogenic and/or resorptive factors, which are overexpressed in the bone marrow microenvironment of patients with myeloma. Nonetheless, it has proven very difficult to identify these factors.[7,8] It is now becoming apparent that the reason may be that, in patients with myeloma, there are complex interactions between myeloma cells and the marrow microenvironment such that tumor cells and bone cells or marrow stromal cells that exist in their immediate vicinity together form a complex neoplastic unit, which actively produces bone-resorbing factors. This may explain why it has been hitherto so difficult to elucidate the mechanism of bone destruction in myeloma.

As mentioned above, earlier work had implicated a number of powerful bone-resorbing cytokines in the pathogenesis of myeloma bone disease. These include lymphotoxin, interleukin-1 (IL-1), IL-6, and parathyroid hormone-related protein (PTH-rP). More recently, other putative cell-surface-bound cytokines, such as receptor activator of nuclear factor κ B (RANK) ligand (RANKL), and soluble mediators, such as macrophage inflammatory protein 1α (MIP-1α), have also been identified as playing

Table 6.1 *Factors implicated in development and progression of osteolysis in myeloma* in vivo

Cytokine	Cell of origin	Osteoclast formation	Osteoclast activation	Induces RANKL	Role in MBD *in vivo*	References
TNFα/lymphotoxin (TNFβ)	MM	+	+	+	??	12
IL-1β	MM	+	+	+	??	18–22
IL-6/sIL-6R	MM, BMSC, Obl, Ocl	+	±	+	??	24–26
PTH–rP	MM, BMSC, Obl	+	−	+	??	41–47
RANKL	MM, BMSC, Obl	+	+	N/A	Yes	69, 71, 72, 74, 78, 79
MIP-1α	MM, BMSC, Obl	+	+	+	Yes	88–90, 97, 98, 100, 101

BMSC, bone marrow stromal cells; IL, interleukin; MBD, myeloma bone disease; MIP-1α, macrophage inflammatory protein 1α; MM, myeloma cells; Obl, osteoblasts; Ocl, osteoclasts; PTH–rP, parathyroid hormone-related protein; RANKL, receptor activator of nuclear factor κ B ligand; TNFα/β, tumor necrosis factor α/β.

critical roles in the development and progression of bone lesions in myeloma (see Table 6.1).

Lymphotoxin

Lymphotoxin (tumor necrosis factor β; TNFβ) is a normal activated lymphocyte product that is also produced by lymphoid cell lines in culture, and in particular by B-lymphoblastoid cell lines. Lymphotoxin enhances bone resorption[9] and stimulates the formation of osteoclasts from precursors in marrow cell cultures.[10] Moreover, lymphotoxin activates mature isolated osteoclasts to form resorption pits on bone slices.[11] Lymphotoxin has identical effects to those of TNFα, IL-1α, and IL-1β on bone resorption and repeated injections of recombinant human lymphotoxin induce severe hypercalcemia in normal mice.[12] The tumor cells from a number of myeloma cell lines express lymphotoxin messenger RNA and the conditioned media contains biologic activity ascribable to lymphotoxin,[12] including bone resorbing activity, which is partially neutralized by lymphotoxin antibodies.

Interleukin-1α and β

Interleukin-1α and β are powerful stimulators of osteoclastic bone resorption *in vitro*[13–15] and cause severe hypercalcemia in mice *in vivo* through this mechanism.[16,17] They have also been implicated in myeloma bone disease, although this remains controversial. Freshly isolated whole-marrow harvests from patients with myeloma, which contain both myeloma cells and stromal cells, have been shown to express and produce IL-1α in the conditioned media.[18–20] The bone-resorbing activity produced by these cells in cultures can be neutralized by antibodies to IL-1α.[19] In contrast, cell lines from patients with myeloma, which represent relatively homogeneous populations of tumor cells, do not express IL-α.[12] The reason for these discrepancies probably relates to the nature and

composition of the cells that were studied and artifacts could readily occur in both model systems. Established cell lines could have 'differentiated' in culture to secrete factors not produced by parent cells *in situ* and vice versa. Alternatively, freshly isolated myeloma tumor cells (which contain dead and dying elements) likely release factors that are not released *in situ* (as has been shown previously for prostaglandins). Furthermore, there is controversy as to the contribution of IL-1 produced by myeloma cells to the development and progression of bone lesions, since an IL-1 receptor antagonist, the natural receptor antagonist of IL-1β, inhibits OAF activity produced by cultures of myeloma cells,[21] but has no effect on either development or progression of myeloma bone disease in an *in vivo* model of myeloma bone disease.[22]

Interleukin-6

Interleukin-6 is a multifunctional cytokine that is thought to play an important role in the pathophysiology of myeloma, although its significance in myeloma bone disease is also controversial.[23] Early evidence had suggested that it may be an important growth factor in myeloma and that neutralizing antibodies to IL-6 may have important effects on the course of the disease.[24–26] However, others have reported that serum IL-6 has neither discriminatory nor prognostic role in multiple myeloma.[27] Nevertheless, these two observations are not necessarily contradictory as IL-6 presumably works locally. Notably, the effects of IL-6 on bone resorption *in vitro* and calcium homeostasis *in vivo* are different from those of IL-1 and the TNFs.[28] Like IL-1 and the TNFs, IL-6 promotes formation of osteoclast-like cells from hematopoietic precursors *in vitro*, albeit in the presence of its soluble receptor protein.[29] However, whether IL-6 can activate mature osteoclasts to resorb bone *in vivo* remains equivocal because positive effects have been demonstrated in some, but not other, *in vitro* systems.[30–32]

Elevated circulating levels of IL-6 also causes hypercalcemia *in vivo*, as observed in mice carrying tumors with transfected CHO cells expressing IL-6,[28] although the increase in blood calcium induced by IL-6 is much less than that caused by IL-1 or lymphotoxin.

IL-6 may also have effects in the bone marrow microenvironment in myeloma that are different from those of the other bone-resorbing cytokines. Although bone cells isolated from trabecular bone surfaces (bone lining cells) express cytokines, such as IL-1, TNFα, macrophage colony-stimulating factor (M-CSF), and IL-6, it is only in the case of IL-6 that these bone cells produce more of a cytokine when exposed to osteotropic factors, such as parathyroid hormone, IL-1, and TNFα.[33] The majority of myeloma cells freshly isolated from patients do not produce appreciable amounts of IL-6. However, myeloma cells induce normal human osteoblasts and bone marrow stromal cells to secrete IL-6.[34–38] It has also been speculated that vascular endothelial cell growth factor (VEGF) produced by myeloma cells in response to cell–cell interactions between myeloma tumor cells and bone marrow stromal cells, in turn, induces IL-6 production by the stromal cells.[39]

Parathyroid hormone–related protein (PTH–rP)

As in breast cancer-associated skeletal metastases, where PTH-rP has been shown to be the major mediator of osteolysis, it has been suggested that PTH-rP may also play a role in the destructive bone lesions associated with myeloma.[40–42] PTH-rP, which induces osteoclast formation primarily by stimulating RANKL expression in osteoblasts and bone marrow stromal cells, has been identified by immunohistochemistry and by *in situ* hybridization in the bone marrow biopsies from patients with myeloma, and elevated serum levels have also been demonstrated in some myeloma patients.[42–48] A specific role of PTH-rP relative to other cytokines that are likely important in myeloma has yet to be clarified but an increase in serum IL-6 levels has been noted in a subset of patients with elevated serum PTH-rP levels.[48] This may be important because PTH-rP does have synergistic effects with IL-6 on osteoclastic bone resorption and inducing hypercalcemia.[49] Unlike classic humoral hypercalcemia of malignancy, which is primarily mediated by PTH-rP, it is unclear what role, if any, PTH-rP plays in the pathogenesis of hypercalcemia in myeloma, as some patients with hypercalcemia have normal serum PTH-rP levels, while others remain mormocalcemic despite markedly elevated serum PTH-rP levels.[43]

The importance of the aforementioned soluble cytokine mediators in the pathophysiology of the bone lesions associated with myeloma thus remains unclear. It is possible that a combination of these factors work in concert to enhance bone resorption in myeloma and it is also possible that other factors may be involved. These factors have been difficult to identify by traditional identification methods (purification) from myeloma cell cultures, possibly because important cell–cell interactions in the bone microenvironment are involved (see later).

MYELOMA, CELL–CELL INTERACTIONS, AND THE BONE MICROENVIRONMENT

There have been major advances recently in our understanding of the molecular mechanisms by which tumor cells stimulate osteoclastogenesis and osteoclast activity with various studies highlighting the critical role of complex adhesion molecule-mediated interactions between tumor cells and neighboring marrow stromal cells.[50] Earlier studies to determine which cytokines are most important in causing osteolysis in patients with myeloma did not take into consideration the importance of these complex interactions (cell–cell and cell–matrix) between the myeloma tumor cells and its microenvironment in the regulation of putative mediators. These interactions between myeloma cells and resident bone cells are almost certainly more complicated than simple excess production of a particular osteoclastotrophic factor by myeloma cells. For example, there are data suggesting that products elaborated as a consequence of osteoclastic bone resorption may influence the avidity with which myeloma cells grow in bone compared with other hematologic malignancies that situate in bone and this is exemplified by IL-6 factor for myeloma cells.[34] There is increasing evidence that production of IL-6 in the bone microenvironment may be related to direct cellular interactions between myeloma cells and other resident cells, such as stromal cells, osteoblasts, and even osteoclasts.[34,35,37] In this paradigm, a vicious cycle exists whereby myeloma cells stimulate excessive formation of osteoclasts and also activate these osteoclasts to resorb bone aggressively by inducing the production of osteotropic cytokines including, but not limited to, IL-6. Osteoclasts produce prodigious amounts of IL-6, considerably more than other cell types and certainly more than other types of bone cells.[51] It is, therefore, likely that, as a consequence of the myeloma-induced increase in osteoclast activity, large amounts of IL-6 are secreted by cells involved in the resorption process, and this serves to further enhance the growth and survival of myeloma cells in bone. This vicious cycle could mean that the greater the bone destruction, the more aggressive the behavior of myeloma cells, which then may cause even greater bone destruction. Thus, bone may not be simply a passive bystander in this disease but rather may act indirectly to amplify the growth of myeloma cells in bone.[37]

Data from recent studies provide further evidence that interactions between vascular cell adhesion molecule 1 (VCAM-1) expressed on the surface of bone marrow stromal cells and its cognate receptor, the very late antigen 4 (VLA-4; α4β1) integrin receptor, expressed on myeloma tumor cells may be responsible for the osteolytic bone destruction.[52] Such important cell–cell interactions in myeloma have also been described by others.[39,53,54] Myeloma cells bind avidly to bone marrow stromal cells, in part through these VLA-4/VCAM-1 interactions.[52,55] A soluble recombinant form of VCAM-1 stimulated myeloma cells to produce a bone-resorbing activity, and this activity produced by myeloma cells was abrogated in the presence of neutralizing antibodies to either VCAM-1 or to the α4 integrin subunit.[52] Importantly, the increasing recognition of the critical role of these interactions has led to the recent identification of other cytokines such as RANKL and MIP-1α that appear to play a pivotal role in pathogenesis of the bone lesions in myeloma (see later).

EXPERIMENTAL ANIMAL MODELS OF HUMAN MYELOMA BONE DISEASE: OPPORTUNITY TO STUDY MYELOMA CELLS IN THEIR NORMAL MICROENVIRONMENT

Until a decade ago, a major drawback to studying the mechanisms responsible for myeloma bone disease has been the lack of suitable animal models of the human disease. Human myeloma cells do not home to the bone marrow in naive nude mice even when injected systemically. This has meant that it has been difficult to establish an acceptable animal model of the human disease not only to study the pathogenetic mechanisms but also to determine the efficacy of various novel therapies. The importance of cell–cell interactions between myeloma cells and resident cells in the bone microenvironment not only in facilitating growth and survival of the tumor cells, but also in promoting osteolysis, spurred a number of groups to develop experimental animal models of human myeloma bone disease that are useful for studying the mechanisms involved. These include models in which human myeloma cells are xenografted in irradiated or non-irradiated athymic (T-cell-deficient) or SCID mice (B- and T-cell deficient).[36,56–60] In addition to being immunodeficient, most of these models are further compromised by the requirement for irradiation to ensure tumor engraftment in medullary cavities, a procedure that almost certainly affects the bone microenvironment. To date, the only myeloma model utilizing immunocompetent, non-irradiated hosts is a murine syngeneic model originally characterized by Radl et al. in 1988, who described a myeloma bone disease, which occurs spontaneously in

aging mice of the C57BL/KaLwRij strain.[61,62] These series of myelomas, designated 5T myelomas, developed at the rate of approximately one in every 200 aged mice and caused a monoclonal gammopathy with features reminiscent of the human disease, including infiltration of the bone marrow by the myeloma cells and, most importantly, characteristic myelomatous skeletal lesions. Osteolytic lesions were found in most tumor-bearing mice and, as in humans, very infrequently some mice developed osteosclerotic lesions. Either freshly dispersed 5T myeloma cells from the bone marrow or involved spleens of myeloma-bearing mice can be serially transplanted by tail-vein or intraperitoneal injections into fresh naive recipients of the same strain, or by direct bone marrow inoculation with the disease being faithfully transmitted from mouse to mouse.[26,63–65] In order to develop a more convenient animal model of the human myeloma bone disease, we[26,63] and others[66] have developed cell lines from one of these myelomas, the 5T33 myeloma, which can be studied both in vitro and in vivo. The cell line that we established, designated 5TGM1, which also reproducibly causes characteristic osteolytic bone lesions in young C57BL/KaLwRij mice when injected via the tail vein, produces the monoclonal IgG2bκ paraprotein and IL-6 but grows independent of exogenous IL-6 in vitro. Identical results are obtained when 5TGM1 cells are inoculated into immunodeficient (bg/nu/xid) mice. Some but not all mice carrying these myelomas become mildly hypercalcemic, again reminiscent of the human myeloma bone disease. Importantly, histomorphometric analysis shows that the osteolytic bone lesions in tumor-bearing mice are associated with an increase in osteoclast numbers and activity confirming the validity of this model for studies of pathogenetic mechanisms in myeloma and for pre-clinical evaluation of novel antitumor and antiosteolytic strategies.

RANKL/osteoprotegerin system

RANKL together with its cognate receptor (RANK) and its soluble decoy receptor osteoprotegerin (OPG) are members of the TNF ligand and receptor superfamilies, respectively, that regulate osteoclastogenesis and bone resorption in vivo (Fig. 6.1). RANK mediates signals that are indispensable for osteoclast formation, activation and survival. OPG, which is naturally secreted, acts solely as a decoy receptor.[67,68] Once it was established that RANKL and OPG are central to the regulation of normal bone resorption, we postulated that dysregulation of their expression in the bone microenvironment plays a major role in the excessive osteoclastic resorption in myeloma. We also hypothesized that direct cell–cell interactions between myeloma cells and neighboring bone marrow stromal cells are critical for this to happen, and this would

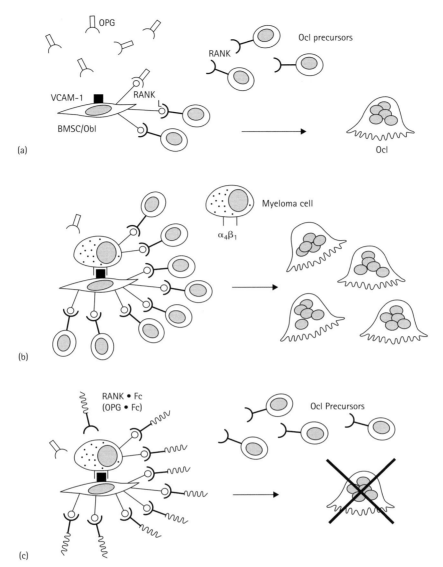

Figure 6.1 *Expression of the receptor activator of the nuclear factor kappa B ligand (RANKL) and osteoprotegenin (OPG) in the bone microenvironment: dysregulated expression in myeloma and the effect of RANK.Fc and OPG.Fc. (a) Expression of RANKL and OPG in the bone microenvironment. Bone marrow stromal cells (BMSC) and osteoblasts (Obl) express RANKL on their cell surface in vitro and in vivo. RANKL expression in BMSC is largely inducible, whereas Obl express the cytokine constitutively. Interaction of RANKL with its cognate receptor RANK, expressed on osteoclast (Ocl) precursors, promotes osteoclast differentiation and the interaction of the ligand with RANK on mature Ocl results in their activation and prolonged survival. The OPG present in the bone microenvironment is secreted primarily by BMSC/Obl and in this milieu (and in conditioned media harvested from BMSC and Obl cultures), there is an excess of OPG. In vivo, OPG blocks the interaction of RANKL with its cognate receptor RANK on Ocl precursors as well as on mature Ocl, thus acting as a physiological regulator of bone resorption. (b) Overexpression of RANKL and downregulation of OPG in myeloma. BMSC/Obl cells bind avidly to myeloma cells, via vascular cell adhesion molecule 1 (VCAM-1) and its cognate receptor ($\alpha 4\beta 1$) on myeloma cells. This interaction results in overexpression of RANKL in the bone microenvironment (increased expression in both BMSC/Obl and in myeloma cells, which also do not express RANKL constitutively), and downregulation of OPG production by BMSC/Obl. The consequent increase in RANKL/OPG ratio is responsible for the exaggerated Ocl formation, enhanced Ocl activation, and prolonged Ocl survival that characterize myeloma bone disease. (c) Effect of RANK.Fc and OPG.Fc in myeloma in vivo. The chimeric synthetic antagonists, RANK.Fc and OPG.Fc, act as decoys in a similar fashion to naturally occurring OPG. RANK.Fc, and OPG.Fc, bind to RANKL expressed on both myeloma cells and BMSC/Obl cells, thus blocking the interaction of the ligand with RANK on Ocl precursors and mature Ocl. As a consequence, there is less 'free' RANKL available to interact with RANK resulting overall in decreased Ocl numbers, reduced resorptive activity, and increased osteoclast apoptosis. Total blockade of RANKL binding to RANK can be achieved with saturating quantities of the synthetic antagonists, resulting in complete stoppage of Ocl formation.*

explain why myeloma cells that aggressively destroy bone *in vivo* produce low or undetectable levels of bone-resorbing cytokines when cultured alone.

Indeed, it was observed that co-culture of myeloma cells and bone-marrow-derived stromal cells led to marked induction of RANKL expression by both cell types, even though neither cell type expressed the cytokine at an appreciable level constitutively. Furthermore, there was concomitant downregulation of OPG expression by the bone marrow stromal cells.[69] It appears that these changes are mediated by adhesion of myeloma cells to stromal cells. Both RANKL induction and downregulation of OPG in the myeloma cell-stromal cell co-cultures was abrogated in the presence of a neutralizing antibody to the α4 integrin receptor subunit, while treatment of myeloma cells with a recombinant soluble form of VCAM-1 was sufficient to induce RANKL expression.[69] These data suggested that cell–cell interactions, mediated by stromal cell-expressed VCAM-1 binding to VLA-4 on myeloma cells, are necessary for the tumor cells to express RANKL.

Data from a number of studies have now shown that neutralizing the biological effects of this overexpressed RANKL *in vivo* will reduce bone destruction and have a beneficial effect in murine models of multiple myeloma, e.g. using a genetically engineered soluble form of RANK (RANK.Fc; Immunex), which acts as a decoy receptor by binding to RANKL, thus preventing it from interacting with its native receptor on hematopoietic precursors and osteoclasts. This chimeric protein, constructed by fusing the extracellular domain of murine RANK to the Fc region of human IgG1, inhibits normal and pathological osteoclastic bone resorption in a mouse model of tumor-induced hypercalcemia.[70] The inhibitory effect of RANK.Fc was evaluated in the Radl 5TGM1 myeloma model that, as described earlier, has features similar to those of human multiple myeloma.[26,63] RANK.Fc was administered by daily subcutaneous injection, as with other established cytokine receptor–human IgG fusion proteins, such as p75 TNFR.Fc, the molecule was minimally antigenic in mice and the daily injections were well tolerated with no observable indications of toxicity in either tumor-bearing mice or non-tumor-bearing mice. Administration of RANK.Fc to tumor-bearing mice resulted in a profound inhibition of resorptive activity with markedly increased bone trabeculae in the metaphyseal regions (Fig. 6.2).

Unexpectedly, however, we also observed reductions in tumor growth rate in bone and overall tumor burden, as assessed by skeletal tumor volume and serum monoclonal IgG2bκ levels, raising the intriguing possibility that RANKL/RANK interactions facilitate myeloma growth.[71]

Consistent with these data, other investigators have reported that RANK.Fc ameliorates myeloma tumor burden in bone and lowers serum paraprotein levels in the SCID-hu mouse model of myeloma.[72,73] Interestingly, OPG.Fc had a similar inhibitory effect on development of osteolytic lesions with reductions in serum IgG levels when administered to mice bearing 5T33 and 5T2 mouse myeloma tumors.[74,75] Importantly, neutralizing monoclonal antibodies raised against the mouse α4 integrin subunit also decreased osteolysis as well as overall tumor load in the 5TGM1 myeloma model,[76] consistent with our data that RANKL levels are modulated by stromal cell-expressed VCAM-1 binding to VLA-4 (α4β1) on myeloma cells.[52,69] Taken together, the available data strongly suggest that RANKL is the final common mediator of osteoclast activation and that aberrant expression of RANKL within the myeloma bone microenvironment is likely to be pivotal in initiating and maintaining the characteristic bone destruction.

Unlike most of the other mediators previously implicated in myeloma bone disease, RANKL is expressed in various cell types as a transmembrane protein rather than being secreted, although it can be cleaved in activated T cells to yield a soluble form that remains biologically active.[68] Murine 5TGM1 and 5T2 myeloma cells freshly sorted by flow cytometry from diseased marrow of tumor-bearing mice express RANKL.[69,74] However, there has been controversy over whether human myeloma cells freshly harvested from patients, which have also just been in contact with bone microenvironment, actually express RANKL protein on their cell-surface; some groups have reported unequivocal expression,[77,78] whereas others have not been able to detect any cell-surface expression by flow cytometry or immunocytochemically.[72,79,80] The reason for this discrepancy is presently unclear but it may relate to technical differences.[78] Nevertheless, whether or not the predominant source of RANKL in the myeloma bone microenvironment is the tumor cells, the marrow stromal cells, or both, the consequent exaggerated osteoclast formation and activation is likely to be exacerbated by a concomitant decrease in locally available OPG. The reduced levels of OPG in bone marrow of patients with myeloma is likely to be further exacerbated by the tumor cells binding, internalizing and degrading OPG.[81] Consistent with this, serum OPG levels in myeloma patients are significantly reduced compared with in healthy controls.[82]

Collectively, the available data demonstrate the potential utility of RANK.Fc (and OPG.Fc) to inhibit RANKL action *in vivo* and suggest that therapeutic interventions targeted at blockade of RANKL/RANK interactions and/or disruption of signaling cascades downstream of RANK would have disease-modifying effect on myeloma-associated bone destruction, and possibly myeloma itself. Moreover, targeting this ligand–receptor interaction is particularly attractive, since almost all of the soluble cytokines implicated in myeloma to date stimulate

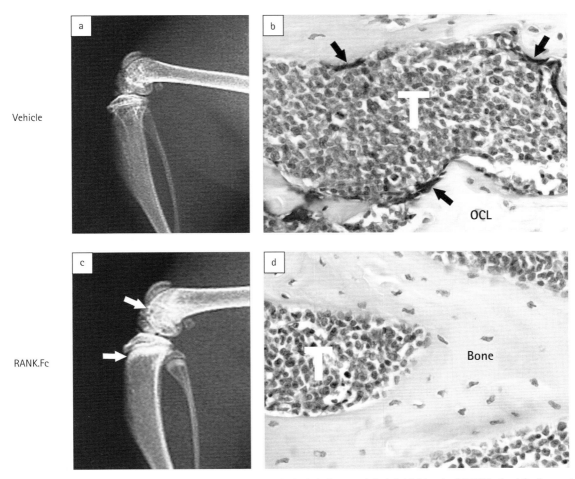

Figure 6.2 *Radl 5TGM1 myeloma model: radiographs showing the lytic lesions and their inhibition by RANK.Fc. (a,c) Radiographs from 5TGM1 myeloma-bearing mice. (b,d) Photomicrograph of section through long bone of 5TGM1 myeloma-bearing mice stained for TRAP activity to reveal osteoclasts (OCL). RANK.Fc inhibits osteolytic lesion induced by 5TGM1 myeloma cells in distal femoral and proximal tibial metaphyses in syngeneic mice. Note the increased radiodensity in RANK.Fc-treated mice (white arrows) and complete absence of osteoclasts in RANK.Fc-treated bone even in presence of myeloma tumor (T).*

osteoclast differentiation and activation, in part, by enhancing RANKL expression.[67]

It is worth noting that OPG and OPG.Fc, unlike RANK.Fc, which is specific for RANKL, also bind and inhibit TRAIL,[83] a ubiquitous TNF-related ligand that is selectively cytotoxic to myeloma cells,[84] and is under development for its antitumor properties.[85] Thus, in contrast to OPG, RANK.Fc is unlikely to abrogate any potential beneficial effect of TRAIL in myeloma and may well be a better molecule for further pre-clinical development.

MACROPHAGE INFLAMMATORY PROTEIN

Macrophage inflammatory protein 1α is a chemokine that has been implicated in various malignancy-associated processes.[86] There is now an accumulating body of evidence also implicating MIP-1α as an important mediator in the bone disease associated with myeloma. MIP-1α is produced excessively by human and murine myeloma cell lines, by freshly isolated plasma cells from myeloma patients, and is present in the bone marrow and marrow supernatants of patients with myeloma bone disease at much higher levels in comparison to patients with other hematological malignancies and normal controls.[87–90] MIP-1α, which is a chemoattractant for cells of the monocyte–macrophage lineage, including granulocyte–macrophage colony-forming units (CFU-GM) osteoclast precursors,[91,92] stimulates osteoclastic differentiation and resorption *in vitro*,[93–96] and there is now convincing evidence that MIP-1α also stimulates osteoclast differentiation and bone resorption *in vivo* when expressed adjacent to bone surfaces,[97] consistent with the notion that it plays an important role in the pathogenesis of myeloma-associated osteolysis *in vivo*. Interestingly, MIP-1α is also produced by osteoblast-like cells in response to stimulation by IL-1 and TNFα.[96] As mentioned earlier, both cytokines are secreted by myeloma cells.[98] This would serve to further amplify the concentrations of the chemokine locally in the bone microenvironment.[88]

MIP-1α signaling receptors (CCR-1 and CCR-5) have been reported to be expressed by human myeloma cell lines[99] and we have also found that murine 5TGM1 myeloma cells, which secrete MIP-1α also express mouse CCR-1 mRNA, raising the possibility that MIP-1α may also have previously unidentified autocrine effects on myeloma cell growth/survival. In accord with this notion, recent studies have shown that MIP-1α triggers migration of and signaling cascades in myeloma cells.[100] Based on these observations, we evaluated the effect of neutralizing MIP-1α bioactivity on the development and/or progression of myeloma lesions *in vivo*. Systemic (intraperitoneal) administration of neutralizing antibodies to MIP-1α ameliorated myeloma-induced osteolysis and limited disease progression in the murine 5TGM1 myeloma model assessed by radiography and histomorphometry.[97] Treatment of tumor-bearing mice anti-MIP-1α antibodies resulted in a significant reduction in serum monoclonal paraprotein IgG2bκ levels and the titers also correlated directly with splenic wet weights. Histomorphometric analyses of long bones and vertebrae revealed that blockade of MIP-1α function resulted in not only a reduction in tumor volume within the medullary spaces, but also a reduction in the number and intensity of tartrate-resistant acid phosphatase (TRAP) staining of osteoclasts lining bone surfaces. These data strongly implicate MIP-1α in the pathogenesis of myeloma-associated bone destruction and possibly myeloma itself. Interestingly, others have recently reported that inhibiting MIP-1α production using an anti-sense approach also impaired osteolysis in irradiated SCID mice bearing ARH-77 B-lymphoblastoid cells.[101] Taken together, these data provide a basis for further pre-clinical studies to determine efficacy of orally bioavailable small molecule synthetic antagonists of the receptors that mediate the effects of MIP-1α (CCR-1 and CCR-5) as adjuncts to current standard anti-osteolytic, and possibly antitumor, therapeutic approaches in myeloma. Although it is presently unclear which of the MIP-1α signaling receptors mediates its osteoclastogenic activity, both CCR-1 and CCR-5 antagonists are currently under development for other disease conditions.[102–104]

In contrast to a previous report that the osteoclastogenic effect of MIP-1α *in vitro* is RANKL-independent,[105] recent studies using wild-type and RANK-null mutant mice (from Immunex) found that an intact RANK signaling pathway is indispensable for the osteoclastogenic effect of MIP-1α *in vivo*,[97] lending further support to the notion that RANKL is, indeed, the final common mediator of the excessive osteoclast number and activity in myeloma. The knowledge that novel antagonists of RANKL bioactivity, such as RANK.Fc and OPG.Fc, show antiosteolytic efficacy in pre-clinical models of multiple myeloma provides a rationale for development of therapeutic approaches that target these cytokines.

HYPERCALCEMIA IN MYELOMA BONE DISEASE

Hypercalcemia in myeloma is due primarily to increased osteoclastic bone resorption, which leads to efflux of calcium into the extracellular fluid. This overwhelms the patient's capacity to maintain normal calcium homeostasis, resulting in elevated serum calcium levels. However, the pathogenesis of hypercalcemia in myeloma is probably more complex than this. Firstly, not all patients with significant myeloma bone disease develop hypercalcemia.[106] Approximately one-third of patients develop hypercalcemia, although usually late in the course of the disease, and this frequency may be decreasing in recent years with the advent of bisphosphonates as standard therapy for cancer-induced osteolysis. Nevertheless, hypercalcemia is most common in patients who have the largest tumor volume, irrespective of serum PTH-rP status. The reasons for this are unclear but may be related to the amount of bone-resorbing activity produced by the myeloma cells, as well as glomerular filtration status. Measurements of total body myeloma cell burden together with production of bone-resorbing activity by cultured bone marrow myeloma cells *in vitro* do not correlate closely with hypercalcemia, although they do correlate somewhat with extent of osteolytic bone lesions.[107] Thus, there are clearly other factors that are involved in the pathogenesis of hypercalcemia in addition to those that promote osteoclast formation and induce osteoclast activation. Probably the most important of these is the impairment of renal function, which occurs frequently and complicates the course of the disease in patients with myeloma. In addition to impaired glomerular filtration, increased renal tubular calcium reabsorption may also be a contributing factor to the pathophysiology of hypercalcemia[108] and elevated serum PTH-rP levels may play a role in this regard in a subset of patients.[43–45] It is unclear why myeloma patients present with this increase in renal tubular calcium reabsorption. There are other differences between the hypercalcemia that occurs in myeloma and humoral hypercalcemia in patients with solid tumors. For example, in patients with hypercalcemia due to myeloma, there is almost always impaired renal function and an increase in serum phosphate owing to the decreased glomerular filtration rate. Markers of bone formation, such as serum alkaline phosphatase, are usually not increased in patients with myeloma, since bone formation is often not increased and, in fact, may be suppressed, for reasons that are not entirely clear (see later). Patients with hypercalcemia due to myeloma usually respond very rapidly to treatment with corticosteroids, unlike patients with humoral hypercalcemia due to solid tumors,[109] although the efficacy of steroids in this setting is mainly due to their rapid suppression of myeloma tumor growth.

BONE MARKERS AND BONE MINERAL DENSITY FOR MONITORING MYELOMA BONE DISEASE

Bone markers (Table 6.2) may eventually be useful for non-invasive monitoring of the response of cancer-induced osteolytic bone disease to therapy. The current most accurate and precise marker for osteoclastic bone resorption is the measurement of deoxypyridinoline (Dpyr) crosslinks of collagen,[110] although the usefulness of this and other markers in assessing and monitoring patients with myeloma remains to be unequivocally established.[111] Dpyr cross-links can be readily measured in the urine (u-Dpyr) by chemical assays or by enzyme-linked immunosorbant assay (ELISA), and sensitive as well as specific serum-based assays are becoming increasingly available. Dpyr measurement is much improved over previous markers, such as urinary hydroxyproline, urinary pyridinoline, or fasting urine calcium. Moreover, a number of studies have suggested that u-Dpyr is more sensitive in distinguishing between treated and untreated patients, and not only may help in differentiating between multiple myeloma and MGUS, but may also serve as a marker of the underlying osteolytic bone disease activity.[112–114] Other breakdown products of type I collagen that can be measured are the carboxy-terminal telopeptide (CTX or ICTP) and the amino-terminal telopeptide (NTX). A number of studies have suggested that serum levels of ICTP may be a sensitive prognostic marker of bone disease in myeloma.[115–118] Clearly, further studies are needed to show correlation between the levels of these markers, alone or in combination, and evidence of changes in the markers that correlate with bone disease progression in myeloma patients treated with or without bisphosphonates. It remains to be determined whether these markers could facilitate determination of the efficacy of dose, determination of optimal mode of administration, as well as facilitate follow-up of bone turnover in patients with myeloma bone disease, especially after specialized treatments, such as autologous transplantation.[119]

Parameters of bone formation, such as serum alkaline phosphatase, are often decreased in patients with myeloma, unless the patient has an active fracture undergoing repair. In myeloma patients, measurements of osteocalcin (bone GLA protein), a marker of bone formation show a large scatter. Serum osteocalcin is usually decreased in myeloma patients with advanced disease and more extensive bone lesions consistent with the impaired bone formation. By contrast, serum osteocalcin levels may be normal or even increased earlier in the disease, and in patients who have less aggressive or no obvious bone disease.[4,116,117,120] More recently, bone mineral density (BMD) has been shown to increase in myeloma patients in sustained remission after chemotherapy who have never been on bisphosphonates.[121]

MANAGEMENT OF MYELOMA BONE DISEASE: BISPHOSPHONATES AND OTHER POTENTIAL THERAPEUTIC APPROACHES

The major symptoms and the high morbidity and mortality rates associated with myeloma are due largely to the progressive bone destruction. Since patients may survive for a number of years post-diagnosis, clinicians have attempted to devise therapeutic approaches in myeloma that would relieve disabling symptoms, especially bone pains, thereby improving quality of life. An early approach was the use of fluoride, and later calcium and fluoride, although this combination was ineffective and, in fact, probably detrimental because of associated side effects. More recently, bisphosphonates, which inhibit osteoclastic bone resorption mainly by inducing osteoclast apoptosis, have become the standard antiosteolytic therapy for myeloma-induced bone disease. Several groups have shown that the more potent second-generation (pamidronate; Aredia) and third-generation (zoledronic acid; Zometa) bisphosphonates relieve bone pain, and produce a rapid, sustained, and significant decrease in the urinary excretion of calcium and hydroxyproline, indicating decreased bone turnover.[122,123] The use of bisphosphonates is discussed in detail in Chapter 21.

RANK.Fc and OPG.Fc also inhibit osteoclast activation, but they may be more effective antiosteolytic agents in myeloma because they also effectively prevent osteoclast formation. Importantly, emerging independent data

Table 6.2 *Biochemical markers of bone turnover*

Bone destruction	Bone formation
Pyridinoline	Bone-specific alkaline phosphatase (BSALP)
Deoxypyridinoline	Osteocalcin (bone Gla-protein)
Carboxy-terminal telopeptide of type I collagen (CTX/ICTP[a])	Carboxy-terminal propeptide of type I collagen (PICP)
N-terminal telopeptide of type I collagen (NTX)	N-terminal telopeptide of type I collagen (PINP)

[a] Assays for different epitopes.

from our group and others suggest that the two novel molecules have additional effects in myeloma *in vivo*, beyond those on inhibiting osteolysis, notably a modest but significant reduction in tumor burden, assessed histomorphometrically and by monoclonal paraprotein titers, in different pre-clinical models of human bone myeloma disease.[70–74] Although the mechanistic basis of this unanticipated reduction in myeloma tumor load remains to be elucidated, these findings potentially constitute a major advance, as bisphosphonates have not been shown to date to exert an antitumor effect either in pre-clinical models[63,73,124,125] or in myeloma patients.[126–129] Although reduction in tumor load as a primary endpoint is not being examined, in ongoing phase I studies, a single subcutaneous dose of OPG.Fc has been shown to be as effective as an intravenously administered bolus of pamidronate.[130,131] It remains to be determined whether antitumor efficacy can be demonstrated with these novel molecules in phase II and III clinical trials in myeloma patients.

KEY POINTS

- In the myeloma bone microenvironment, receptor activator of NF-κ B ligand (RANKL) is expressed by tumor cells and overexpressed by osteoblasts and bone marrow stromal cells. Concomitantly, the production of its naturally occurring decoy receptor, osteoprotegerin (OPG), by bone marrow stromal cells is markedly downregulated.
- The change in RANKL/OPG in favor of RANKL is responsible for the exaggerated osteoclast formation and activity seen in patients.
- RANK.Fc and OPG.Fc, synthetic chimeric antagonists of RANKL/RANK interactions, block osteolytic lesions in pre-clinical mouse models of multiple myeloma.
- Macrophage inflammatory protein 1α (MIP-1α) is overexpressed in bone marrow of myeloma patients compared with other hematological neoplasms, and has been implicated in myeloma-induced osteolysis.
- Neutralizing anti-MIP-1α antibodies and MIP-1α antisense block osteolytic lesions and myeloma tumor progression in pre-clinical mouse models of multiple myeloma.
- RANKL and MIP-1α represent novel therapeutic targets in myeloma.
- Bone markers and bone mineral density measurements may be useful for non-invasive monitoring of the response to antitumor and/or antiosteolytic therapy in myeloma patients.

ACKNOWLEDGMENTS

The authors' studies were supported by NIH/NCI Program Project Grant PO1 CA 40035 (GRM), NIH/NCI Minority Investigator Research Supplement (for BOO), the International Myeloma Foundation, and the Multiple Myeloma Research Foundation.

REFERENCES

● = Key primary paper
♦ = Major review article

1. Bataille R, Chappard D, Basle M. Quantifiable excess of bone resorption in monoclonal gammopathy is an early sign of malignancy: a prospective study of 87 bone biopsies. *Blood* 1996; **87**:4762–9.
2. Bataille R, Harrousseau J-L. Multiple myeloma. *N Engl J Med* 1997; **336**:1657–64.
3. Bataille R, Chappard D, Basle M. Excessive bone resorption in human plasmacytomas: direct induction by tumor cells *in vivo*. *Br J Haematol* 1995; **90**:721–4.
4. Bataille R, Delmas PD, Chappard D, Sany J. Abnormal serum bone GLA protein levels in multiple myeloma: crucial role of bone formation and prognostic implications. *Cancer* 1990; **66**:67–72.
5. Goasguen JE, Zandecki M, Mathiot C, Scheiff JM, Bizet M, Ly-Sunnaram B, et al. Mature plasma cells as indicator of better prognosis in multiple myeloma. New methodology for the assessment of plasma cell morphology. *Leuk Res* 1999; **23**:1133–40.
6. Bartl R, Frisch B, Burkhardt R, Fateh-Moghadam A, Mahl G, Gierster P, et al. Bone marrow histology in myeloma: its importance in diagnosis, prognosis, classification and staging. *Br J Haematol* 1982; **51**:361–75.
7. Mundy GR, Raisz LG, Cooper RA, Schechter GP, Salmon SE. Evidence for the secretion of an osteoclast stimulating factor in myeloma. *N Engl J Med* 1974; **291**:1041–6.
8. Mundy GR. Myeloma bone disease. *Eur J Cancer* 1998; **34**:246–251.
9. Bertolini DR, Nedwin GE, Bringman TS, Smith DD, Mundy GR. Stimulation of bone resorption and inhibition of bone formation in vitro by human tumour necrosis factors. *Nature* 1986; **319**:516–18.
10. Pfeilschifter J, Chenu C, Bird A, Mundy GR, Roodman GD. Interleukin-1 and tumor necrosis factor stimulate the formation of human osteoclast-like cells *in vitro*. *J Bone Miner Res* 1989; **4**:113–18.
11. Thomson BM, Mundy GR, Chambers TJ. Tumor necrosis factors alpha and beta induce osteoblastic cells to stimulate osteoclastic bone resorption. *J Immunol* 1987; **138**:775–9.
12. Garrett IR, Durie BGM, Nedwin GE, Gillespie A, Bringman T, Sabatini M, et al. Production of the bone resorbing cytokine lymphotoxin by cultured human myeloma cells. *N Engl J Med* 1987; **317**:526–32.
13. Gowen M, Meikle MC, Reynolds JJ. Stimulation of bone resorption in vitro by a non-prostanoid factor released by

human monocytes in culture. *Biochem Biophys Acta* 1983; **762**:471–4.

14. Gowen M, Wood DD, Ihrie EJ, McGuire MK, Russell RG. An interleukin 1-like factor stimulates bone resorption *in vitro*. *Nature* 1983; **306**:378–80.

15. Gowen M, Nedwin G, Mundy GR. Preferential inhibition of cytokine stimulated bone resorption by recombinant interferon gamma. *J Bone Miner Res* 1986; **1**:469–74.

16. Sabatini M, Boyce B, Aufdemorte T, Bonewald L, Mundy GR. Infusions of recombinant human interleukin-1α and β cause hypercalcemia in normal mice. *Proc Natl Acad Sci USA* 1988; **85**:5235–9.

17. Boyce BF, Aufdemorte TB, Garrett IR, Yates AJP, Mundy GR. Effects of interleukin-1 on bone turnover in normal mice. *Endocrinology* 1989; **125**:1142–50.

18. Cozzolino F, Torcia M, Aldinucci D, Rubartelli A, Miliani A, Shaw AR, *et al.* Production of interleukin-1 by bone marrow myeloma cells. *Blood* 1989; **74**:380–7.

19. Kawano M, Tanaka H, Ishikawa H, *et al.* Interleukin-1 accelerates autocrine growth of myeloma cells through interleukin-6 in human myeloma. *Blood* 1989; **73**:2145–8.

20. Sati HI, Greaves M, Apperley JF, Russell RG, Croucher PI. Expression of interleukin-1 beta and tumor necrosis factor-alpha in plasma cells from patients with multiple myeloma. *Br J Haematol* 1999; **104**:350–7.

21. Torcia M, Lucibello M, Vannier E, Fabiani S, Miliani A, Guidi G, *et al.* Modulation of osteoclast-activating factor activity of multiple myeloma bone marrow cells by different interleukin-1 inhibitors. *Exp Hematol* 1996; **24**:868–74.

22. Ferguson VL, Simke SJ, Ayers RA, Bateman TA, Wang HT, Bendele A, *et al.* Effect of MPC-11 myeloma and MPC-11 + IL-1 receptor antagonist treatment on mouse bone properties. *Bone* 2002; **30**:109–16.

23. Lauta VM. Interleukin-6 and the network of several cytokines in multiple myeloma: an overview of clinical and experimental data. *Cytokine* 2001; **16**:79–86.

24. Klein B, Zhang XG, Jourdan M, *et al.* Cytokines involved in human multiple myeloma. *Monoclonal Gammopathies II* 1989; **12**:55–9.

25. Bataille R, Jourdan M, Zhang XG, Klein B. Serum levels of interleukin-6, a potent myeloma cell growth factor, as a reflection of dyscrasias. *J Clin Invest* 1989; **84**:2008–11.

26. Garrett IR, Dallas S, Radl J, Mundy GR. A murine model of myeloma bone disease. *Bone* 1997; **20**:515–20.

27. Schaar CG, Kaiser U, Snijder S, Ong F, Hermans J, Franck PFH, *et al.* Serum interleukin-6 has no discriminatory role in paraproteinaemia nor a prognostic role in multiple myeloma. *Br J Haematol* 1999; **107**:132–8.

28. Black K, Garrett IR, Mundy GR. Chinese hamster ovarian cells transfected with the murine interleukin-6 gene cause hypercalcemia as well as cachexia, leukocytosis and thrombocytosis in tumor-bearing nude mice. *Endocrinology* 1991; **128**:2657–9.

29. Tamura T, Udagawa N, Takahashi N, Miyaura C, Tanaka S, Yamada Y, *et al.* Soluble interleukin-6 receptor triggers osteoclast formation by interleukin 6. *Proc Natl Acad Sci USA* 1993; **90**:11924–8.

30. Lowik CWGM, Van der pluijm G, Bloys H, Hoekman K, Bijvoet OL, Aarden LA, *et al.* Parathyroid hormone (PTH) and PTH-like protein (Plp) stimulate interleukin-6 production by osteogenic cells: a possible role of interleukin-6 in osteoclastogenesis. *Biochem Biophys Res Commun* 1989; **162**:1546–52.

31. Ishimi Y, Miyaura C, Jin CH, Akatsu T, Abe E, Nakamura Y, *et al.* IL-6 is produced by osteoblasts and induces bone resorption. *J Immunol* 1990; **145**:3297–303.

32. Al-Humidan A, Ralston SH, Hughes DE, Chapman K, Aarden L, Russell RG, *et al.* Interleukin-6 does not stimulate bone resorption in neonatal mouse calvariae. *J Bone Miner Res* 1991; **6**:3–8.

33. Feyen JHM, Elford P, DiPadova FE, Trschel U. Interleukin-6 is produced by bone and modulated by parathyroid hormone. *J Bone Miner Res* 1989; **4**:633–8.

34. Uchiyama H, Barut BA, Mohrbacher AF, Chauhan D, Anderson KC. Adhesion of human myeloma-derived cell lines to bone marrow stromal cells stimulates interleukin-6. *Blood* 1993; **82**:3712–20.

35. Lokhorst HM, Lamme T, de Smet M, Klein S, de Weger RA, van Oers R, *et al.* Primary tumor cells of myeloma patients induce interleukin-6 secretion in long-term bone marrow cultures. *Blood* 1994; **84**:2269–77.

36. Urashima M, Chen BP, Chen S, Pinkus GS, Bronson RT, Dedera DA, *et al.* The development of a model for the homing of multiple myeloma cells to human bone marrow. *Blood* 1997; **90**:754–65.

37. Bloem AC, Lamme T, De Smet M, Kok H, Vooijs W, Wijdenes J, *et al.* Long-term bone marrow cultured stromal cells regulate myeloma tumor growth *in vitro*: studies with primary tumor cells and LTBMC-dependent cell lines. *Br J Haematol* 1998; **100**:166–75.

38. Karadag A, Oyajobi BO, Apperley JF, Russell RGG, Croucher PI. Human myeloma cells promote the production of interleukin-6 by primary human osteoblasts. *Br J Haematol* 2000; **108**:383–90.

39. Dankbar B, Padro T, Leo R, Feldman B, Kropff M, Mesters RM, *et al.* Vascular endothelial growth factor and interleukin-6 in paracrine tumor–stromal cell interactions in multiple myeloma. *Blood* 2000; **95**:2630–6.

40. Budayr AA, Nissenson RA, Klein RF, Pun KK, Clark OH, Diep D, *et al.* Increased serum levels of a parathyroid hormone-like protein in malignancy-associated hypercalcemia. *Ann Intern Med* 1989; **11**:807–12.

41. Suzuki A, Takahashi T, Okuno Y, Tsuyuoka R, Sasaki Y, *et al.* Production of parathyroid hormone-related protein by cultured human myeloma cells. *Am J Hematol* 1994; **45**:88–90.

42. Firkin F, Seymour JF, Watson AM, Grill V, Martin TJ. Parathyroid hormone-related protein in hypercalcemia associated with haematological malignancy. *Br J Haematol* 1996; **94**:486–92.

43. Horiuchi T, Miyachi T, Nakamura T, Mori M, Ito H. Raised plasma concentrations of parathyroid hormone-related peptide in hypercalcemic multiple myeloma. *Horm Metab Res* 1996; **29**:4690–71.

44. Tsujimura H, Nagamura F, Iseki T, Kanazawa S, Saisho H. Significance of parathyroid hormone-related protein as a factor stimulating bone resorption and causing hypercalcemia in myeloma. *Am J Hematol* 1998; **59**:168–70.

45. Ohmori M, Nagai M, Fujita M, Dobashi H, Tasaka T, Yamaoka G, *et al.* A novel mature B-cell line (DOBIL-6) producing both parathyroid hormone-related protein and interleukin-6 from a myeloma patient presenting with hypercalcaemia. *Br J Haematol* 1998; **101**:688–93.

46. Schneider HG, Kartsogiannis V, Zhou H, Chou ST, Martin TJ, Grill V. Parathyroid hormone-related protein mRNA and protein expression in multiple myeloma: a case report. *J Bone Miner Res* 1998; **13**:1640–3.

47. Zeimer H, Firkin F, Grill V, Slavin J, Zhou H, Martin TJ. Assessment of cellular expression of parathyroid hormone-related protein mRNA and protein in multiple myeloma. *J Pathol* 2000; **192**:336–41.

48. Kitazawa R, Kitazawa S, Kajimoto K, Sowa H, Sugimoto T, Matsui T, *et al.* Expression of parathyroid hormone-related protein (PTHrP) in multiple myeloma. *Pathol Int* 2002; **52**:63–8.

49. De La Mata J, Uy H, Guise TA, Story B, Boyce BF, Mundy GR, *et al.* IL-6 enhances hypercalcemia and bone resorption mediated by PTH-rP *in vivo*. *J Clin Invest* 1995; **95**:2846–52.

50. Roodman GD. Role of the bone marrow microenvironment in multiple myeloma. *J Bone Miner Res* 2002; **17**:1921–5.

51. Roodman GD. Cell biology of the osteoclast. *Exp Hematol* 1999; **27**:1229–41.

52. Michigami T, Shimizu N, Williams PJ, Niewolna M, Dallas SL, Mundy GR, *et al.* Cell-cell contact between marrow stromal cells and myeloma cells via VCAM-1 and α4β1-integrin enhances production of osteoclast-stimulating activity. *Blood* 2000; **96**:1953–60.

53. Barille S, Collette M, Bataille R, Amiot M. Myeloma cells upregulate interleukin-6 secretion in osteoblastic cells through cell-to-cell contact but down-regulate osteocalcin. *Blood* 1995; **86**:3151–9.

54. Teoh G, Anderson KC. Interaction of tumor and host cells with adhesion and extracellular matrix molecules in the development of multiple myeloma. *Hematol Oncol Clin North Am* 1997; **11**:27–42.

55. Sanz-Rodriguez F, Teixido J. VLA-4 dependent myeloma cell adhesion. *Leuk Lymphoma* 2001; **41**:239–45.

56. Yaccoby S, Barlogie B, Epstein J. Primary myeloma cells growing in SCID-hu mice: a model for studying the biology and treatment of myeloma and its manifestations. *Blood* 1998; **92**:2908–13.

57. Yaccoby S, Epstein J. The proliferative potential of myeloma plasma cells manifest in the SCID-hu host. *Blood* 1999; **94**:3576–82.

58. Hjorth-Hansen H, Seifert MF, Borset M, Aarset H, Ostlie A, Sundan A, *et al.* Marked osteoblastopenia and reduced bone formation in a model of multiple myeloma bone disease in severe combined immunodeficiency mice. *J Bone Miner Res* 1999; **14**:256–63.

59. Barton BE, Cullison J, Jackson J, Murphy T. A model that reproduces syndromes associated with human multiple myeloma in nonirradiated SCID mice. *Proc Soc Exp Biol Med* 2000; **223**:190–7.

60. Pilarski LM, Hipperson G, Seeberger K, Pruski E, Coupland RW, Belch AR. Myeloma progenitors in the blood of patients with aggressive or minimal disease: engraftment and self-renewal of primary human myeloma in the bone marrow of NOD SCID mice. *Blood* 2000; **95**:1056–65.

61. Radl J, Croese JW, Zurcher C, van den Enden-Vieveen MM, de Leeuw AM. Animal model of human disease: multiple myeloma. *Am J Pathol* 1988; **132**:593–7.

62. Asosingh K, Radl J, Van Riet I, Van Camp B, Vanderkerken K. The 5TMM series: a useful in vivo mouse model of human multiple myeloma. *Hematol J* 2000; **1**:351–6.

63. Dallas SL, Garrett IR, Oyajobi BO, Dallas MR, Boyce BF, Bauss F, *et al.* Ibandronate reduces osteolytic lesions but not tumor burden in a murine model of myeloma bone disease. *Blood* 1999; **93**:1697–706.

64. Vanderkerken K, Goes E, De Raeve H, Radl J, Van Camp B. Follow-up of bone lesions in an experimental multiple myeloma mouse model: description of an in vivo technique using radiography dedicated for mammography. *Br J Cancer* 1996; **73**:1463–5.

65. Vanderkerken K, De Raeve H, Goes E, Van Meirvenne S, Radl J, Van Riet I, *et al.* Organ involvement and phenotypic adhesion profile of 5T2 and 5T33 myeloma cells in the C57BL/KaLwRij mouse. *Br J Cancer* 1997; **76**:451–60.

66. Manning LS, Berger JD, O'Donoghue HL, Sheridan GN, Claringbold PG, Turner JH. A model of multiple myeloma: culture of 5T33 murine myeloma cells and evaluation of tumorigenicity in the C57BL/KalwRij mouse. *Br J Cancer* 1992; **66**:1088–93.

67. Hofbauer LC, Neubauer A, Heufelder AE. Receptor activator of nuclear factor-kappaB ligand and osteoprotegerin: potential implications for the pathogenesis and treatment of malignant bone diseases. *Cancer* 2001; **92**:460–70.

♦68. Theill LE, Boyle WJ, Penninger JM. RANK-L AND RANK: T Cells, bone loss, and mammalian evolution. *Annu Rev Immunol* 2002; **20**:795–823.

69. Oyajobi BO, Traianedes K, Harris MA, Harris SE, Yoneda T, Mundy GR. RANK ligand expression in a model of myeloma bone disease: dependence on tumor cell-marrow stromal cell interactions. *J Clin Invest* (submitted).

●70. Oyajobi BO, Anderson DM, Traianedes K, Williams PJ, Yoneda T, Mundy GR. Therapeutic efficacy of a soluble receptor activator of nuclear factor kappaB-IgG Fc fusion protein in suppressing bone resorption and hypercalcemia in a model of humoral hypercalcemia of malignancy. *Cancer Res* 2001; **61**:2572–8.

71. Oyajobi B, Garrett IR, Williams PJ, Yoneda T, Anderson DM, Mundy GR. A soluble murine Receptor Activator of NF-κB-human immunoglobulin fusion protein (RANK.Fc) inhibits bone resorption in a murine model of human multiple myeloma bone disease [abstract]. *J Bone Miner Res* 2001; **15**(Suppl):S176.

●72. Pearse RN, Sordillo EM, Yaccoby S, Wong BR, Liau DF, Colman N, *et al.* Multiple myeloma disrupts the TRANCE/osteoprotegerin cytokine axis to trigger bone destruction and promote tumor progression. *Proc Natl Acad Sci USA* 2001; **98**:11581–6.

73. Yaccoby S, Pearse RN, Johnson CL, Barlogie B, Choi Y, Epstein J. Myeloma interacts with the bone marrow microenvironment to induce osteoclastogenesis and is dependent on osteoclast activity. *Br J Haematol* 2002; **116**:278–90.

●74. Croucher PI, Shipman CM, Lippitt J, Perry M, Asosingh K, Hijzen A, *et al.* Osteoprotegerin inhibits the development of osteolytic bone disease in multiple myeloma. *Blood* 2001; **98**:3534–40.

75. Vanderkerken K, Asosingh K, Van Camp B, Croucher PI. Anti-tumor effect of recombinant osteoprotegerin in the murine 5T33 model [abstract]. *Blood* 2001; **98**(Suppl):637a.

76. Mori Y, Michigami T, Dallas M, Niewolna M, Story B, Lobb R, *et al.* Anti-α4 integrin antibody suppresses the bone

disease of myeloma and disrupts myeloma-marow stromal cell interactions [abstract]. *J Bone Miner Res* 1999; **14**(Suppl):S173.

77. Sezer O, Heider U, Jakob C, Zavrski I, Eucker J, Possinger K, et al. Immunocytochemistry reveals RANKL expression of myeloma cells [letter]. *Blood* 2002; **99**:4646–7.

78. Sezer O, Heider U, Jakob C, Eucker J, Possinger K. Human bone marrow myeloma cells express RANKL [letter]. *J Clin Oncol* 2002; **20**:353–4.

●79. Giuliani N, Bataille R, Mancini C, Lazzaretti M, Barille S. Myeloma cells induce imbalance in the osteoprotegerin/ osteoprotegerin ligand system in the human bone microenvironment. *Blood* 2001; **98**:3527–33.

80. Roux S, Meignin V, Quillard J, Meduri G, Guiochon-Mantel A, Fermand J-P, et al. RANK (receptor activator of nuclear factor-κB) and RANKL expression in multiple myeloma. *Br J Haematol* 2002; **117**:86–92.

●81. Seidel C, Hjertner O, Abildgaard N, Heickendorf L, Hjorth M, Westin J, et al. Serum osteoprotegerin levels are reduced in patients with multiple myeloma with lytic bone disease. *Blood* 2001; **98**:2269–71.

82. Emery JG, McDonnell P, Burke MB, Deen KC, Lyn S, Silverman C, et al. Osteoprotegerin is a receptor for the cytotoxic ligand TRAIL. *J Biol Chem* 1998; **273**:14363–7.

83. Mariani SM, Matib M, Armandola EA, Kramer PH. Interleukin-1β-converting enzyme related protease/ caspases are involved in TRAIL-induced apoptosis of myeloma and leukemia cells. *J Exp Med* 1995; **137**:221–9.

84. French LE, Tschopp J. The TRAIL to selective tumor death. *Nat Med* 1999; **5**:146–8.

85. Standal T, Seidel C, Hjertner O, Plesner T, Sanderson RD, Waage A, et al. Osteoprotegerin is bound, internalized and degraded by multiple myeloma cells. *Blood* 2002; **100**:3002–7.

86. Gerard C, Rollins BJ. Chemokines and disease. *Nat Immunol* 2001; **2**:108–15.

87. Chauhan D, Auclair D, Robinson EK, Hideshima T, Li G, Podar K, et al. Identification of genes regulated by dexamethasone in multiple myeloma cells using oligonucleotide arrays. *Oncogene* 2002; **21**:1346–58.

●88. Choi S, Cruz JC, Craig J, Anderson J, Roodman GD, Alsina M. Macrophage inflammatory protein (MIP)-1α is a potential osteoclast stimulatory factor in myeloma. *Blood* 2000; **96**:671–5.

●89. Abe M, Hiura K, Wilde J, Moriyama K, Hashimoto T, Ozaki S, et al. Role for macrophage inflammatory protein (MIP)-1α and MIP-1β in the development of osteolytic lesions in multiple myeloma. *Blood* 2002; **100**:2195–202.

90. Uneda S, Hata H, Matsuno F, Harada N, Mitsuya Y, Kawano F, et al. Macrophage inflammatory protein-1alpha is produced by human multiple myeloma (MM) cells and its expression correlates with bone lesions in patients with MM. *Br J Haematol* 2003; **120**:53–5.

91. Fuller K, Owens JM, Chambers TJ. Macrophage inflammatory protein-1α and IL-8 stimulate the motility but suppress the resorption of isolated rat osteoclasts. *J Immunol* 1995; **154**:6065–72.

92. Broxmeyer HE, Cooper S, Hangoc G, Gao J-L, Murphy PM. Dominant myelopoietic effector functions mediated by chemokine receptor CCR1. *J Exp Med* 1999; **189**:1987–92.

93. Kukita T, Nomiyama H, Ohmoto Y, Kukita A, Shuto T, Hotokebuchi T, et al. Macrophage inflammatory protein-1α (LD78) expressed in human bone marrow: its role in regulation of hematopioesis and osteoclast recruitment. *Lab Invest* 1997; **76**:399–406.

94. Kukita T, Nakao J, Hamada F, Kukita A, Inai T, Kurisu K, Nomiyama H. Recombinant LD78 protein, a member of the small cytokine family, enhances osteoclast differentiation in rat bone marrow culture system. *Bone Miner* 1992; **19**:215–23.

95. Scheven BAA, Milne JS, Hunter I, Robins SP. Macrophage inflammatory protein-1α regulates preosteoclast differentiation *in vitro*. *Biochem Biophys Res Commun* 1999; **254**:773–8.

96. Votta BJ, White JR, Dodds RA, James IE, Connor JR, Lee-Rykaczewski E, et al. CKα-8 (CCL23), a novel CC chemokine, is chemotactic for human osteoblast precursors and is expressed in bone tissues. *J Cell Physiol* 2000; **183**:196–207.

●97. Oyajobi BO, Franchin G, Williams PJ, Pulkrabek D, Gupta A, Munoz S, et al. Dual effects of macrophage inflammatory protein-1α on osteolysis and tumor burden in the murine 5TGM1 model of myeloma bone disease. *Blood* 2003; **102**:311–19.

98. Taichman RS, Reilly MJ, Matthew LS. Human osteoblast-like cells and osteosarcoma cell lines synthesize macrophage inhibitory protein 1α in response to interleukin 1β and tumour necrosis factor-β stimulation *in vitro*. *Br J Haematol* 2000; **108**:275–83.

99. Arendt BK, Miller AL, Arora T, Tschumper RC, Jelinek DF. Evidence for functional chemokine receptors on myeloma cells [abstract]. Blood 1998; **92**(Suppl):100a.

100. Lentzch S, Gies M, Janz M, Bargou R, Dorken B, Mapara MY. Macrophage inflammatory protein 1 alpha (MIP-1α) triggers migration and signaling cascades mediating survival and proliferation in multiple myeloma (MM) cells. *Blood* 2003; **101**:3568–73.

●101. Choi SJ, Oba Y, Gazitt Y, Alsina M, Cruz J, Anderson J, et al. Antisense inhibition of macrophage inflammatory protein 1a blocks bone destruction in a model of myeloma bone disease. *J Clin Invest* 2001; **108**:1833–41.

102. Liang M, Mallari C, Rosser M, Ng HP, May K, Monahan S, et al. Identification and characterization of a potent, selective and orally active antagonist of the CC chemokine receptor-1. *J Biol Chem* 2000; **275**:19000–8.

103. Proudfoot AE. Chemokine receptors: multi-faceted therapeutic targets. *Nat Rev Immunol* 2002; **2**:106–15.

104. Proudfoot AEI, Power CA, Wells TNC. The strategy of blocking the chemokine system to combat disease. *Immunol Rev* 2000; **177**:246–56.

●105. Han JH, Choi SJ, Kurihara N, Koide M, Oba Y, Roodman GD. Macrophage inflammatory protein-1 alpha is an osteoclastogenic factor in myeloma that is independent of receptor activator of nuclear factor kappa B ligand. *Blood* 2001; **97**:3349–53.

106. Snnaper I, Kahn A. *Myelomatosis*. Basel: Karger, 1971.

107. Durie BGM, Salmon SE, Mundy GR. Relation of osteoclast activating factor production to the extent of bone disease in multiple myeloma. *Br J Haematol* 1981; **47**:21–30.

108. Tuttle KR, Kunau RT, Loveridge N, Mundy GR. Altered renal calcium handling in hypercalcemia of malignancy. *J Am Soc Nephrol* 1991; **2**:191–9.

109. Binstock ML, Mundy GR. Effects of calcitonin and glucocorticoids in combination in hypercalcemia of malignancy. *Ann Intern Med* 1980; **193**:269–72.

110. Watts NB. Clinical utility of biochemical markers of bone remodeling. *Clin Chem* 1999; **5**:1359–68.

♦111. Fontana A, Delmas PD. Markers of bone turnover in bone metastases. *Cancer* 2000; **88**(Suppl):2952–60.

112. Nawawi H, Samson D, Apperley J, Girgis S. Biochemical bone markers in patients with multiple myeloma. *Clin Chim Acta* 1996; **253**:61–77.

113. Diamond T, Levy S, Smith A, Day P, Manoharan A. Non-invasive markers of bone turnover and plasma cytokines differ in osteoporotic patients with multiple myeloma and monoclonal gammopathies of undetermined significance. *Intern Med J* 2001; **31**:272–8.

114. Alexandrakis MG, Passam FH, Malliaraki N, Katachanakis C, Kyriakou DS, Margioris AN. Evaluation of bone disease in multiple myeloma: a correlation between biochemical markers of bone metabolism and other clinical parameters in untreated multiple myeloma patients. *Clin Chim Acta* 2002; **325**:51–7.

115. Abildgaard N, Bentzen SM, Nielsen JL, Heickendorff L. Serum markers of bone metabolism in multiple myeloma: prognostic value of the carboxyterminal propeptide of type I collagen (ICTP). *Br J Haematol* 1997; **96**:103–10.

116. Abildgaard N, Glerup H, Rungby, Bendix-Hansen K, Kassem M, Brixen K, et al. Biochemical markers of bone metabolism reflect osteoclastic and osteoblastic activity in multiple myeloma. *Eur J Haematol* 2000; **64**:121–9.

117. Fonseca R, Trendle MC, Leong T, Kyle RA, Oken MM, Kay NE, et al. Prognostic value of serum markers of bone metabolism in untreated multiple myeloma patients. *Br J Haematol* 2000; **109**:24–9.

118. Carlson K, Larsson A, Simonsson B, Turesson I, Westin J, Ljunghall S. Evaluation of bone disease in multiple myeloma: a comparison between the resorption markers urinary deoxypyridinoline/creatinine (DPD) and serum ICTP, and an evaluation of the DPD/osteocalcin and ICTP/osteocalcin ratios. *Eur J Haematol* 1999; **62**:300–6.

119. Clark RE, Fraser WD. Bone turnover following autologous transplantation in multiple myeloma. *Leuk Lymphoma* 2002; **43**:511–16.

120. Woitge HW, Horn E, Keck AV, Auler B, Seibel MJ, Pecherstorfer M. Biochemical markers of bone formation in patients with plasma cell dyscrasias and benign osteoporosis. *Clin Chem* 2001; **47**:686–93.

121. Roux S, Bergot C, Fermand JP, Frija J, Brouet JC, Mariette X. Evaluation of bone mineral density and fat-lean distribution in patients with multiple myeloma in sustained remisssions. *J Bone Miner Res* 2003; **18**:231–6.

122. Van Breukelen FJM, Bijvoet OLM, Van Oosterom AT. Inhibition of osteolytic bone lesions by (3-amino-1-hydroxypropylidene)-1, 1-bisphosphonate (APD). *Lancet* 1979; **i**:803–5.

123. Siris ES, Sherman WH, Baquiran DC, Schlatterer JP, Osserman EF, Canfield RE. Effects of dichloromethylene diphosphonate on skeletal mobilization of calcium in multiple myeloma. *N Engl J Med* 1980; **302**:310–15.

124. Cruz JC, Alsina M, Craig F, Yoneda T, Anderson JL, Dallas M, et al. Ibandronate decreases bone disease development and osteoclast stimulatory activity in an *in vivo* model of human myeloma. *Exp Hematol* 2001; **29**:441–7.

125. Shipman CM, Vanderkerken K, Rogers MJ, Lippitt JM, Asosingh K, Hughes DE, et al. The potent bisphosphonate ibandronate does not induce myeloma cell apoptosis in a murine model of established multiple myeloma. *Br J Haematol* 2000; **111**:283–6.

●126. Berenson JR, Rosen LS, Howell A, Porter L, Coleman RE, Morley W, et al. Zoledronic acid reduces skeletal-related events in patients with osteolytic metastases. *Cancer* 2001; **91**:1191–200.

127. Martin A, Garcia-Sanz R, Hernandez J, Blade J, Suquia B, Fernandez-Calvo J, et al. Pamidronate induces bone formation in patients with smouldering or indolent myeloma, with no significant anti-tumour effect. *Br J Haematol* 2002; **118**:239–42.

128. Menssen HD, Sakalova A, Fontana A, Herrmann Z, Boewer C, Facon T, et al. Effects of long-term intravenous ibandronate therapy on skeletal-related events, survival, and bone resorption markers in patients with advanced multiple myeloma. *J Clin Oncol* 2002; **20**:2353–9.

●129. Rosen LS, Gordon D, Antonio BS, Kaminski M, Howell A, Belch A, et al. Zoledronic acid versus pamidronate in the treatment of skeletal metastases in patients with breast cancer or osteolytic lesions of multiple myeloma: a phase III, double-blind, comparative trial. *Cancer J* 2001; **7**:377–87.

130. Greipp P, Facon T, Williams CD, Lipton A, Mariette X, Fermand J-P, et al. A single subcutaneous dose of an osteoprotegerin (OPG) construct (AMGN-0007) causes a profound and sustained decrease of bone resorption comparable to standard intravenous bisphosphonate in patients with multiple myeloma [abstract]. *Blood* 2001; **98**(Suppl):775a.

●131. Body JJ, Greipp P, Coleman RE, Facon T, Geurs F, Fermand JP, et al. A Phase I study of AMGN-0007, a recombinant osteoprotegerin construct, in patients with multiple myeloma or breast carcinoma related bone metastases. *Cancer* 2003; **97**(3 Suppl):887–92.

PART 3

Clinical features, diagnosis, and investigation

7

Clinical features

DIETRICH PEEST

INTRODUCTION

Multiple myeloma (MM) is characterized by malignant plasma cells infiltrating the bone marrow and, in some patients, other organs and extramedullary tissues. In most cases, monoclonal immunoglobulin molecules or immunoglobulin light chains can be measured in the serum or urine and used as a specific marker for diagnosis and follow up (Table 7.1). Presenting symptoms depend on tumor burden and individual complications induced by each myeloma plasma cell clone. The clone may produce and secrete monoclonal immunoglobulin, different cytokines, and less defined biological and physically active factors, which interfere with bone metabolism, renal function, hematopoiesis, immune mechanisms, and other organ systems. Different patterns of such complications contribute to the heterogeneity of MM patients in terms of symptoms, treatment strategy, and prognosis. This chapter will present an overview of the clinical features of myeloma. Particular complications are dicussed in more detail in subsequent chapters.

Roughly 40–70% of MM patients present with bone pain, 20–60% with weakness, 10–20% with infections, 10–20% with hypercalcemia, and 15% with weight loss at diagnosis (Table 7.2). Other symptoms, such as tumors, hepatosplenomegaly, lymphadenopathy, clinical signs of renal involvement, hemorrhage, and others are less frequent.[1–3] Some patients are asymptomatic and the diagnosis is made by chance as a result of electrophoresis

Table 7.1 *Monoclonal immunoglobulins (% of patients studied)*[6,113]

Serum	
IgG	59–61
IgA	23
IgD	0–1
IgE	0–2
IgM	<1
Negative for heavy chain	14–17
Bence Jones protein in the urine	
Kappa	35–47
Lambda	23–33
Negative	20–42

Table 7.2 *Symptoms at presentation*

Bone pain	40–70%
Weakness	20–60%
Infections	10–20%
Hypercalcemia	10–20%
Weight loss	10–15%
Tumors	6%
Clinical signs of renal involvement	3%
Hemorrhage	2%
Hepatosplenomegaly	2–4%
Lymphadenopathy	1–4%

performed for unrelated reasons or to explain an elevated erythrocyte sedimentation rate. In one study, three series of MM patients collected during three consecutive decades (years 1960–1986) were compared.[2] The proportion of symptomatic patients fell from 90 to 66% over this time period, suggesting an earlier diagnosis of MM than in the past, i.e. an increase in the number of patients diagnosed by chance.

Clinical features of patients change throughout the course of MM. Many patients in remission, particularly after high-dose chemotherapy, are asymptomatic with a good quality of life. In advanced disease, high tumor burden, chemotherapy resistance and dedifferentiation of tumor cells, bone marrow dysfunction induced by prior chemotherapy and radiation, impairment of organ performance by deposition of monoclonal immunoglobulins, and other complications are increasingly prominent. In a study of 52 MM patients consecutively autopsied at one single institution, 64% of the patients had distant extraosseous growth of tumor cells, mainly in the kidney, spleen and liver.[4] Sixty percent were proven to have infection. Hemorrhage, infection, and renal failure accounted for death in approximately 70% of the patients.

MM is a disease of older age groups. An overview of 6633 MM patients described 11% aged <50 years, 44% aged 50–64 years, 33% aged 65–74 years, and 10% aged >75 years at presentation.[5] Only 2% of patients are younger than 40 years.[6] The presenting features of younger patients are not substantially different as compared with older patients.[3,7] There is, however, evidence that overall survival is longer in younger than in elderly MM patients.[3] This has been supported by a larger series of patients with a 5-year survival of 31% for MM patients >50 years vs. 27%, 21%, and 12% for patients 50–64 years, 65–74 years, and >75 years, respectively.[5] It has been suggested that malignant clones in older patients might be more aggressive. However, overall survival in older patients is increasingly influenced by co-morbidity and the natural mortality rate becomes more important. It is, therefore, not certain whether there is a real difference in tumor-related survival between younger and older patients.[8]

ASYMPTOMATIC MULTIPLE MYELOMA

Approximately 10–40% of MM are asymptomatic at diagnosis.[2,9,10] These patients feel healthy without any treatment until they develop progressive disease. In some patients this might occur early, but in others after a long time of observation. Such patients are designated as smoldering or asymptomatic myeloma, and are defined by the following criteria (see also Chapter 12): more than 30 g/L monoclonal serum protein and/or more than 10% bone marrow plasma cells without any clinical and laboratory evidence of overt symptomatic MM.[11] Asymptomatic patients with less than 30 g/L monoclonal serum protein, less than 10% bone marrow plasma cells, and an absence of lytic bone lesions, anemia, hypercalcemia, and renal insufficiency related to monoclonal protein are defined as patients with monoclonal gammopathy of undetermined significance (MGUS).[12] The risk of progression of MGUS to MM or related disorders is about 1% per year (see Chapter 24).[13] Discrimination between smoldering myeloma and MGUS on the one hand and an early stage of progressing multiple myeloma on the other is sometimes difficult. In these cases, determinations of plasma cell labeling index and morphologic criteria are helpful (see Chapter 8), and close follow-up is mandatory.

Using the Durie/Salmon classification,[14] the German Myeloma Treatment Group observed that 95% of stage I and up to 40% of stage II MM patients have stable disease without significant symptoms at diagnosis.[10] These patients were observed without treatment; 60% of untreated stage I patients remained progression-free at 4 years, and 50% of the stage II patients were progression-free after 1 year. In other studies of asymptomatic MM patients, the median time to progression was between 12 and 48 months.[9,15–18] A high level of monoclonal serum protein, the presence of a Bence Jones protein, a low serum hemoglobin, a high degree of bone marrow plasmocytosis, the presence of lytic bone lesions using conventional X-rays, and an abnormal bone marrow pattern on magnetic resonance imaging (MRI) have been been described as adverse prognostic parameters for time to progression (see also Chapters 12 and 13).[9,15,17,18]

HYPERCALCEMIA AND BONE DESTRUCTION

Active bone destruction in MM (Table 7.3) is caused by excessive stimulation of normal osteoclasts[19] associated with an impaired osteoblast function in patients with high tumor burden,[20] thus resulting in an uncoupling of the normal bone remodeling sequence, which requires a precise balance of osteoclast and osteoblast activity.[21] In vitro or in animal models, several osteoclast-activating factors produced by the malignant myeloma tumor cells themselves or by other cells of the bone marrow environment have been identified, including tumor necrosis factor β (TNFβ), interleukin-1β (IL-1β), receptor activator

Table 7.3 Bone destruction as identified by conventional roentgenographics (% of patients studied)[1,6,113]

Osteoporosis only	6–16%
Lytic lesions only	10–13%
Combined (osteoporosis, lytic lesions, fractures)	57–78%
Negative	6–21%

of nuclear factor kappa B (RANK) ligand, and IL-6 (see Chapter 6).[21]

In 20–30% of MM patients hypercalcemia may occur as a result of the osteoclast activity and increased release of calcium from the skeleton. Hypercalcemia leads to impaired tubular concentrating ability owing to decreased sodium reabsorption in the loop of Henlé and to interference with antidiuretic hormone (ADH) action, leading to increased natriuresis and loss of water. Calcium hyperfiltration causes further inhibition of sodium reabsorption leading to a progressive decrease of the extracellular fluid volume (ECV). This, in turn, stimulates the renin–aldosterone circuit, which leads to hypokalemia because of the increased sodium level in the distal nephron. Glomerular filtration is further impaired by hypercalcemia-induced constriction of afferent glomerular arterioles. Furthermore, hypercalcemia causes transiently increased hydrogen ion secretion, e.g. in the stomach, thus producing alkalemia. Histologically, tubular injury resulting from hypecalcemia is first seen in the distal loop of Henlé and in the collecting ducts; progressive tubular necrosis and scarring finally leads to renal tubular acidosis and renal failure. In the presence of renal failure and dehydration, impaired calcium excretion and enhanced calcium reabsorption in the proximal tubuli constitute additional mechanisms leading to hypercalcemia.[22]

Clinically, mild hypercalcemia (>2.6–<3.5 mmol/L) can be distinguished from the severe or toxic form (>3.5 mmol/L) requiring more intensive treatment. Symptoms of mild hypercalcemia are polyuria, polydipsia, constipation, nausea, malaise, and neuromuscular weakness, while patients with toxic hypercalcemia may suffer from polyuria followed by dehydration, oliguria, anuria, and acute renal failure, cardiac ventricular arrhythmia, shortening of QT interval, and somnolence followed by coma. In patients with hypercalcemia, adequate early chemotherapy, intravenous bisphosphonates, and intravenous fluid replacement are the most important treatment measures.

Persistent high osteoclast activity will induce bone destruction, such as osteopenia, lytic lesions, and pathological fractures of vertebrae and other bones with the consequence of often severe incapacitating bone pain. Forty to seventy percent of MM patients have bone pain at presentation and there are still patients with a history of several months of unsuccessful symptomatic treatment before the diagnosis of MM was established.

Local radiation therapy in combination with effective chemotherapy are the basis for treating myeloma bone disease,[23] although in some patients chemotherapy may have little or no effect on the progression of bone destruction. Merlini et al. were first to show that prolonged intermittent intravenous/intramuscular administration of bisphosphonates, in addition to the usual care of MM patients, significantly reduced bone pain, the appearance of new osteolytic lesions, and the incidence of pathological fractures.[24] A placebo-controlled study using oral clodronate reported similarly favorable results with decreased progression of osteolytic bone lesions and disappearance of bone pain.[25] New-generation bisphosphonates for intravenous application are more potent, i.e. these drugs are active at very low doses. Pamidronate was tested in a randomized double-blind study and a significant decrease of skeletal events was observed, with less bone pain and a better quality of life.[26] Zoledronic acid seems to be of similar effectiveness with the advantage of a shorter infusion time (see Chapter 21).[27]

INFECTIONS

Many MM patients suffer from frequent bacterial infections[28] and death rates due to infections in the range of 15–60% of all MM cases have been observed.[4,8,29] Tumor-induced immunosuppression aggravated by chemotherapy and/or irradiation forms the basis for a complex immunodeficiency syndrome in these patients. In addition to impaired cellular defence due to neutropenia, reduced T-lymphocyte functions,[30] and natural killer cell activity,[31] the most prominent defect concerns the production of polyclonal immunoglobulins.[28] Nearly all MM patients show reduced concentrations of polyclonal serum immunoglobulins and impaired antibody responses to vaccination with different antigens have been demonstrated.[32–36] Pre-B- and B-lymphocyte compartments are reduced in MM.[37] Furthermore, monocytes from MM patients inhibit in vitro mitogen-induced polyclonal immunoglobulin production when tested in cocultures with normal or MM B-lymphocytes.[38,39] Soluble suppressor activity could be measured in supernatants of cultured mononuclear cells isolated from the bone marrow of MM patients.[40,41] Such supernatants inhibit the proliferation of normal polyclonal B lymphocytes, while the differentiation of the lymphoblastoid B-cell line CESS into immunoglobulin (Ig)-secreting cells remains undisturbed. These observations in humans are compatible with studies in mice showing that plasmacytoma cells produce a soluble factor (PC factor), which stimulates macrophages to produce a second factor (PIMS), capable of inhibiting the primary antibody response of splenic B lymphocytes.[42]

The most common infections are those of the respiratory tract, i.e. bronchitis and pneumonia; infections of the urinary tract, septicemia, and skin infections are less common.[28,34,35] Patients in stable plateau phase have significantly fewer infections as compared with patients with active MM.[35] In non-neutropenic MM patients, the infections most frequently reported are due to *Streptococcus pneumoniae* or *Haemophilus influenzae* as seen in other groups of patients with humoral immunodeficiency. However, during periods of neutropenia following intensive chemotherapy and in advanced disease, infections due to *Staphylococcus aureus* and Gram-negative bacteria predominate.

MM patients presenting with bacterial infection should be managed in the same way as other immunodeficient patients. Early complete diagnosis (e.g. bacterial cultures from blood and other specimens, chest X-rays, bronchoscopy with bronchoalveolar lavage) followed by intensive bactericidal antibiotic therapy to cover the predominant spectrum of bacteria in these patients is mandatory.

Immunoglobulin preparations for intravenous application have been tested in controlled trials for the prevention of infections in multiple myeloma,[34,43] where doses between 10 g every 3–4 weeks and 0.4 g/kg bodyweight monthly have been administered. A significant reduction of both frequency and severity of infections as compared with control groups could be observed, although there was no survival benefit. Patients not responding to vaccination with pneumococcal vaccine, i.e. those with a pronounced immunodeficiency, have profited most from intravenous immunoglobulin treatment.[34] This corresponds to the observation that patients with low or negative antibody titers against lipid A have significantly more infections than those with titers within the normal range.[44]

Viral and fungal infections are important in association with intensive treatment and transplantation (covered in Chapter 17), but do not seem to be a major problem in untreated or conventionally treated patients.

RENAL DYSFUNCTION

Approximately 20–35% of all MM patients present with impairment of kidney function at diagnosis.[45–47] These patients have a significantly worse prognosis than those without.[45] The main cause of renal failure in myeloma is deposition of Bence Jones protein in the renal tubules, but many other factors may be involved in damaging the kidneys.[47] Hypercalcemia, dehydration, excess of uric acid, infections, and nephrotoxic drugs (including nonsteroidal anti-inflammatory drugs and antibiotics) are non-specifically harmful. Amyloid light chain, light-chain deposition disease, and light- and heavy-chain deposition disease are characteristic complications of monoclonal gammopathies, such as MM. Radiographic contrast agents may induce acute renal failure, particularly in dehydrated MM patients.

The morphology of myeloma kidney is characterized by eosinophilic or polychromatophilic, sometimes laminated, casts in the distal and collecting tubules.[48] The distal tubules are often dilated and present an atrophic flattened epithelium. Multinucleated syncytial epithelial cells and fibrotic changes of the interstitium may be found. The casts contain immunoglobulin light chains, complete immunoglobulin molecules, or albumin.[49,50] Glomeruli are usually affected only if amyloidosis is present. In nephrocalcinosis, calcium is deposited in the epithelial cells of the tubules.[48]

Renal failure in MM is highly associated with the presence of Bence Jones proteinuria, indicating a central role of immunoglobulin light chains in kidney injury. Healthy persons produce an excess of free polyclonal immunoglobulin light chains, which has been calculated to be filtered through the glomeruli in the order of 5 mg/kg body weight/day.[51] Only a small fraction (0.04 mg/kg body weight/day) will be excreted in the urine, as most of the immunoglobulin light chains will be reabsorbed in the proximal tubules and catabolized by the epithelial cells. In monoclonal gammopathies with pronounced production of free monoclonal immunoglobulin light chains, the normal capacity of reabsorption and catabolism is often not sufficient to eliminate the protein. Consequently, Bence Jones proteinuria will develop, and casts of monoclonal protein and toxic catabolism products may accumulate in the epithelial cells, resulting in tubular damage.[52] Although the mechanisms are not fully understood, individual physicochemical properties of the monoclonal immunoglobulin light chains are thought to explain the various degrees of renal involvement. Using an animal model, it is possible to test the individual potential of a given human Bence Jones proteins to induce deposits and renal damage.[50]

Early clinical signs of myeloma kidney are impairment of renal tubular functions, such as capability to concentrate and to acidify the urine. An adult Fanconi syndrome with specific reabsorption defects of glucose, amino acids, phosphate, and electrolytes can be observed in some patients.[53] Later stages are characterized by the loss of nephrons with the consequence of progressive reduction of glomerular filtration rates. A non-selective proteinuria is suggestive of amyloidosis, particularly if associated with nephrotic syndrome.

Hydration and administration of adequate chemotherapy is essential for MM patients with renal failure (Chapter 22). In a prospective trial, it has been shown that fluid intake of at least 3 L/day can improve or even reverse renal failure in many patients.[54] Furthermore, there are patients with oliguric renal failure whose renal function improves after an intermittent period of dialysis and appropriate chemotherapy reducing the tumor clone and thus decreasing Bence Jones protein production. Studies with small numbers of patients suggest that plasmapheresis combined with dialysis and chemotherapy may improve the likelihood of renal recovery compared with dialyis and chemotherapy alone.[55,56] It is well worthwhile to offer chronic hemodialysis to MM patients with terminal renal failure provided that chemotherapy successfully controlling the tumor is available.[57,58]

LIGHT-CHAIN AMYLOIDOSIS, LIGHT-CHAIN DEPOSITION DISEASE, AND LIGHT- AND HEAVY-CHAIN DEPOSITION DISEASE

Light-chain amyloidosis (AL) (Chapter 27), light-chain deposition disease (LCDD), and light- and heavy-chain deposition disease (LHCDD) (Chapter 28) are pathologically similar complications associated with monoclonal gammopathies such as MM, and may be summarized under the term monoclonal immunoglobulin deposition diseases (MIDD).[59,60] Differences among MIDD can be defined only by histochemical or immunohistochemical methods. In AL, monoclonal immunoglobulin light chains or light-chain fragments are linked together forming amyloid fibrils with β-pleated sheet formation, which can be stained with Congo red. Additionally, an amyloid P-component is present. These characteristics are missing from the amorphous deposits of LCDD and LHCDD.

The amyloidogenic capacity of an individual monoclonal immunoglobulin light chain is determined by physicochemical properties of the molecule. Sequence analyses have failed to identify a distinct chemical structure responsible for amyloid formation. Almost all of the known light chain V-region subgroups have been found in AL. Proteolysis of light chains may be involved[61] because proteolytic cleavage of certain Bence Jones proteins resulted in the formation of amyloid fibrils in vitro. Tissue-specific proteolytic enzymes may then determine the pattern of organ involvement in individual patients.

The deposits that develop in less than 10% of MM patients can affect nearly all organs (e.g. kidney, heart, liver, nervous system, gut, skin, vessels, etc.).[62] Clinical signs include weakness, weight loss, edema, dyspnea, paresthesias, carpal tunnel syndrome, macroglossia, liver enlargement, and slight splenomegaly. Skin bleeding may occur owing to fragile vessels and a deficiency of clotting factor X, as a result of factor X binding to amyloid (see 'Coagulation defects' later).

Examination of biopsies of clinically affected organs will allow the diagnosis in most cases.[59] In addition to standard staining procedures (Congo red staining, polarization microscopy), immunohistochemical analyses must be applied. Rectal biopsies, which have to include submucosal tissue, have a sensitivity of about 80%, while bone marrow or gingival biopsies are less valuable (sensitivity <50%). The sensitivity of subcutaneous fat aspiration was found to be 50–70% provided suitable techniques were used.[63–65]

BONE MARROW DYSFUNCTION

Hematopoiesis is frequently impaired in MM. Twenty-five percent of stage II and 62% of stage III patients (classification according to tumor cell mass[66]) present with an anemia of <10 g hemoglobin/dL at diagnosis (unpublished results of GMTG trial MM02),[10] indicating a correlation between degree of anemia and tumor cell load. The mechanisms inducing anemia in MM are unknown, although it is clearly not due to marrow replacement, as significant neutropenia and thrombocytopenia are unusal at presentation. Renal failure and damage of hematopoietic precursors by radiation or numerous chemotherapy cycles in advanced stage patients may aggravate anemia. In newly diagnosed MM patients, anemia will rapidly improve after several cycles of chemotherapy successfully reducing the tumor load. However, red blood cell transfusions are frequently needed in advanced MM patients to achieve a better quality of life. A hemoglobin level >10 g/dL should be maintained, particularly in elderly patients and those with cardiovascular diseases. In some MM patients, including those without renal failure, anemia can be sufficiently corrected by the application of recombinant erythropoietin in a dose of 150–200 IU/kg body weight thrice weekly.[67,68]

A mild reduction of granulocyte and platelet counts is often found in MM patients at diagnosis; severe reductions are rare. Patients with platelet counts ⩾150 000 μL have a significantly better prognosis than those with less thrombocytes.[43,69]

An increased incidence of acute leukemias of non-lymphocytic type has been reported in MM patients.[70] Such leukemias often develop after a period of myelodysplasia with pancytopenia in the peripheral blood. In a Canadian MM trial, the risk of converting into leukemia has been determined as 17% at 50 months' treatment with alkylating agents, more than 200 times higher than in the normal population.[71] While measuring a lower incidence (3% after 5 years), another group demonstrated a significant correlation to duration of melphalan treatment.[72] This association was not found in the control group treated with cyclophosphamide. Since occurrence of leukemias has been reported also in untreated patients with monoclonal gammopathies, it has been postulated that the development of leukemia may be a variant of the natural course of MM and might be explained by a defect of early hematopoietic stem cells in MM.[73,74] Chemotherapy and radiation probably escalate this intrinsic risk. The prognosis of MM patients developing secondary leukemias is poor. Induction of remissions with standard regimens for leukemia should be attempted, although elevated toxicity and complication rates have to be expected, owing to pre-treatment-induced reduction of stem-cell reserve, age of the patients, and myeloma-related impairment of different organ functions.

NEUROLOGIC COMPLICATIONS

Radicular pain, typically aggravated by coughing, is an early sign of spinal cord or nerve root compression by fractured vertebrae or extramedullary extension of myeoma deposits. Sensory or motor defects, paraplegia, and loss of sphincter control are late symptoms (Chapter 23). Early diagnostis is needed to prevent permanent damage. Magnetic resonance imaging is presently the most suitable method because it can detect paravertebral tumors and osteolytic destructions before conventional X-rays are positive.[75] Usually MRI can replace a myelogram, which may only be needed in a few exceptional cases for diagnosing imminent spinal cord compression.

Since MM tumors are very sensitive to X-rays, radiation with a local dose of 40 Gy is the therapy of choice, which should be applied even before symptoms occur, if diagnostic methods indicate a risk of neurologic complications. High doses of steroids, e.g. 16 mg dexamethasone/day orally, should be given as a supplement in patients with a spinal cord compression syndrome. If the diagnosis of local MM growth is certain, decompression laminectomy is rarely necessary.

Meningeal and cerebral involvement is uncommon in MM, and only a few cases are described in the literature.[76,77] Most of these patients are in the late stages of disease with a high myeloma cell burden, but it may also be a presenting feature of MM. Symptoms include changes in mental state, headache, cranial nerve palsies, disturbances of gait and speech, leg weakness, and other neurological defects. MRI is often unspecific or negative in myelomatous meningitis, and therefore cytological analysis of the cerebrospinal fluid is essential. Treatment includes systemic steroids, intrathecal chemotherapy, and craniospinal irradiation. However, the prognosis of these patients is very poor. Median survival calculated from cases or small series reported in the literature is 1.5 months from time of diagnosis.[77]

Non-chemotherapy-induced polyneuropathy is a rare complication in MM.[78–80] It may be induced by amyloidosis or hyperviscosity. Polyneuropathy is also part of an incompletely understood MM-associated syndrome characterized by polyneuropathy, organomegaly, endocrinopathy, monoclonal gammopathy, and skin changes (POEMS syndrome).[81] Furthermore, individual monoclonal proteins may have an affinity to neural constituents, although most of them belong to the IgM class.[82–84] Specific therapy is lacking. Improvement of polyneuropathic symptoms has been observed after response to chemotherapy in many patients. However, therapy remains disappointing in others.

HYPERVISCOSITY

A hyperviscosity syndrome is a rare complication of MM, occurring more often in immunocytoma (Waldenström's macroglobulinemia), owing to the tendency of monoclonal IgM to form polymers (Chapter 29).[85–87] IgA and IgG3 myeloma proteins may also polymerize, and thus cause clinical symptoms associated with pathologically increased blood viscosity. Symptoms are slowly developing vertigo, lethargy, fatigue, blurred vision, fundus paraproteinemicus, angina pectoris, intestinal angina, bleeding tendency (platelet 'coatover' effect), somnolence, and coma. However, no straightforward relationship between plasma, or whole blood viscosity, serum protein concentration, and clinical symptoms has been established for monoclonal gammopathies,[88] so that individual factors, such as age, presence of atherosclerotic blood vessel and/or organ lesions, cardiac performance, and anemia may all contribute. Blood being a non-Newtonian fluid, its dynamic viscosity depends to a large extent on the shearing velocity, which increases with decreasing blood vessel diameter and reaches its highest value within capillaries. Here, single red blood cells suspended in blood plasma travel through the vessel lumen, so that increased plasma viscosity may impair local oxygen supply. Different methods are being used to measure plasma viscosity, precluding the comparison of results from one laboratory to the next. Hence the term 'hyperviscosity syndrome' remains a comparatively ill-defined clinical entity and other causes of the observed symptoms must be excluded in every case. Specific treatment measures are not at hand; adequate chemotherapy will result in decreased M-protein levels and thus alleviate symptoms. In severe cases, plasmapheresis is indicated[89] but will only bring about short-lived relief unless accompanied by effective chemotherapy.

CRYOGLOBULINEMIA

Cryoglobulinemia is a rare complication in MM and commonly induces acrocyanosis, Raynaud's phenomenon, and purpura.[90,91] The M-components of these patients bind other immunoglobulin molecules upon cooling, resulting in reversible protein precipitation, gelification, increase of serum viscosity, or complement activation by immune complexes. Cryoglobulinemia type I (containing only the M-component in the precipitate) and type II (containing the M-component and polyclonal immunoglobulins) are associated with monoclonalgammopathies, while type III (containing polyclonal components) is not.

COAGULATION DEFECTS

Bleeding due to acquired coagulation defects is a rare but serious complication in MM and other monoclonal gammopathies. There are reports describing patients with inhibition of fibrin monomer polymerization by myeloma immunoglobulin,[92,93] circulating heparin-like anticoagulants,[94] and a monoclonal thrombin inhibitor.[95] Acquired von Willebrand disease is often associated with lymphoproliferative disorders, such as MM or MGUS.[96,97] In some of these cases, myeloma proteins specific for von Willebrand factor were idendified.[98–100] A factor X deficiency can be found in patients with AL amyloidosis, where the coagulation factor is prematurely cleared by the amyloid deposits.[101] Lupus-like anticoagulants have also been reported in myeloma patients.[102,103]

OTHER MANIFESTATIONS

High cardiac output failure

A syndrome of high cardiac output failure has been reported in MM.[104] In that study, eight of 34 MM patients had a cardiac index $\geq 4.0\,L/min/m^2$. Neither known causes of high output states (hyperthyroidism, large arteriovenous malformation, Paget's disease, etc.) nor severe anemia were identified. Four patients developed high output congestive heart failure; two of them died. Although an association with extensive bone disease could be demonstrated, the reason for high cardiac output states in MM is still unknown.

Sweet's syndrome

Sweet's syndrome is rare and was first described as a benign disease of unknown etiology. The features are fever, neutrophil polymorphonuclear leukocytosis, and painful erythematous plaques affecting the limbs, face, and neck. Histologically dense infiltration with neutrophils can be demonstrated in the dermal plaques. The syndrome may be idiopathic or may occur after infections, as a side effect after drug medication, and as a paraneoplatic condition.[105] In a review of the literature, 54 cases with malignancies associated with Sweet's syndrome were collected.[106] Most patients (21 out of 54) had acute myelogenous leukemia, while only three of 54 had MM. Usually the symptoms respond well to systemic steroid treatment.

Necrobiotic xanthogranuloma

Necrobiotic xanthogranuloma is also rare. A few cases have been described in association with MM or paraproteinemia.[107,108] It is a histiocytic skin disease of non-caseating granuloma and areas of fat necrosis. Clinically, it manifests as non-pruritic nodules or plaques involving the periorbital area, trunk, and extremities. The lesions are usually painless; they tend to ulcerate and heal with scar formation.

IgM, IgD, AND IgE MYELOMAS

IgM MM

IgM MM can be distinguished from Waldenström's macroglobulinemia (WM) by histomorphology. While in WM a lymphoplasmacytoid proliferation will be found in the bone marrow, IgM MM is characterized by mainly mature, sometimes less differentiated plasma cells. Only a few cases have been reported in the literature; it has been suggested that IgM MM may account for approximately 0.5% of MM.[109] Clinical features of IgM MM usually are not different from MM of other types, although in some cases symptoms found in WM, such as hyperviscosity, lymphadenopathy, and hepatosplenomegaly, may occur.

IgD MM

IgD MM will be found in larger studies of MM in up to 1% of cases (Table 7.1). A study of a single institution described 53 IgD MM patients (1.8%) out of 2952 MM patients seen,[110] while 133 cases were collected in a review of the condition.[111] IgD MM patients usually present with a small or no visible monoclonal spike in electrophoresis (see Chapter 9) and it cannot be excluded that some patients with IgD MM are falsely diagnosed as non-secretors. Clinical features are similar to those of other MM patients, although Bence Jones proteinuria, extramedullary involvement, and amyloidosis seem to be more frequent, and IgD MM patients appear to be of younger age (median 50–60 years).

IgE MM

Only a few patients with IgE MM have been repored in the literature. In a review, one case from the authors' institution and ten others described in the literature were summarized.[112] The clinical feature of these patients and MM patients of other types are similar.

KEY POINTS

- Symptoms and signs presented by MM patients result from complications induced by the plasma cell clone.
- Approximately 10–40% of MM patients are asymptomatic at diagnosis. These patients feel healthy without any treatment until they develop progressive disease.
- Active bone destruction in MM is a result of excessive stimulation of normal osteoclasts by the tumor clone. More than 70% of MM patients develop bone destruction and 20–30% experience periods of hypercalcemia during the course of the disease.
- Many MM patients suffer from frequent bacterial infections due to a complex immunodeficiency syndrome. An important cause is the impaired production of normal polyclonal immunoglobulins.
- Up to 50% of all MM patients develop renal impairment at some stage of their disease.
- Monoclonal immunoglobulin deposition diseases (including amyloidosis) may affect various organs. In most of these cases, monoclonal immunoglobulin light chains are contained in the deposits.
- Hematopoiesis is frequently impaired in MM. An increased incidence of acute leukemias of non-lymphocytic type has been reported.
- Sensoric or motoric defects due to nerve root or spinal cord compression occur not infrequently in MM patients; however, non-chemotherapy-induced polyneuropathy is a rare complication.
- A hyperviscosity syndrome, cryoglobulins, and acquired coagulation defects can rarely be observed in MM patients.

REFERENCES

● = Key primary paper
♦ = Major review article

♦1. Ludwig H. Die Klinik des multiplen Myeloms. *Onkologie* 1986; **9**:202–8.

●2. Riccardi A, Gobbi PG, Ucci G, Bertoloni D, Luoni R, Rutigliano L, et al. Changing clinical presentation of multiple myeloma. *Eur J Cancer* 1991; **27**:1401–5.

●3. Blade J, Kyle RA, Greipp PR. Presenting features and prognosis in 72 patients with multiple myeloma who were younger than 40 years. *Br J Haematol* 1996; **93**:345–51.

●4. Oshima K, Kanda Y, Nannya Y, Kaneko M, Hamaki T, Suguro M, et al. Clinical and pathologic findings in 52 consecutively autopsied cases with multiple myeloma. *Am J Hematol* 2001; **67**:1–5.

●♦5. Combination chemotherapy versus melphalan plus prednisone as treatment for multiple myeloma: an overview of 6633 patients from 27 randomized trials. Myeloma Trialists' Collaborative Group. *J Clin Oncol* 1998; **16**:3832–42.

●6. Kyle RA. Multiple myeloma: review of 869 cases. *Mayo Clin Proc* 1975; **50**:29–40.

●7. Rodon P, Linassier C, Gauvain JB, Benboubker L, Goupille P, Maigre M, et al. Multiple myeloma in elderly patients: presenting features and outcome. *Eur J Haematol* 2001; **66**:11–17.

●8. Peest D, Coldewey R, Deicher H. Overall vs. tumour-related survival in multiple myeloma. *Eur J Cancer* 1991; **27**:672–2.

●9. Wisloff F, Andersen P, Andersson TR, Brandt E, Eika C, Fjaestad K, et al. Incidence and follow-up of asymptomatic multiple myeloma. The myeloma project of health region I in Norway. II. *Eur J Haematol* 1991; **47**:338–41.

●10. Peest D, Deicher H, Coldewey R, Leo R, Bartl R, Bartels H, et al. A comparison of polychemotherapy and melphalan/prednisone for primary remission induction, and interferon-alpha for maintenance treatment, in multiple myeloma. A prospective trial of the German Myeloma Treatment Group. *Eur J Cancer* 1995; **31A**:146–51.

●11. International Myeloma Working Group. Criteria for the classification of monoclonal gammopathies, multiple myeloma and related diorders: a report of the International myeloma Working Group. *Br J Haematol* 2003; **121**:749–57.

♦12. Kyle RA, London U. Monoclonal gammopathy of undetermined significance (MGUS): a review. In: Salmon SE (ed.) *Clinics in haematology*, Vol. 11, No. 1, *Myeloma and related disorders*. London: WB Saunders, 1982:123–50.

●13. Kyle RA, Therneau TM, Rajkumar SV, Offord JR, Larson DR, Plevak MF, et al. A long-term study of prognosis in monoclonal gammopathy of undetermined significance. *N Engl J Med* 2002; **346**:564–9.

●14. Durie BGM, Salmon SE. A clinical staging system for multiple myeloma. *Cancer* 1975; **36**:842–54.

●15. Dimopoulos MA, Moulopoulos A, Smith T, Delasalle KB, Alexanian R. Risk of disease progression in asymptomatic multiple myeloma. *Am J Med* 1993; **94**:57–61.

●16. Hjorth M, Hellquist L, Holmberg E, Magnusson B, Rödjer S, Westin J. Initial versus deferred melphalan-prednisone therapy for asymptomatic multiple myeloma stage I – a randomized study. Myeloma Group of Western Sweden. *Eur J Haematol* 1993; **50**:95–102.

●17. Facon T, Menard JF, Michaux JL, Euller-Ziegler L, Bernard JF, Grosbois B, et al. Prognostic factors in low tumour mass asymptomatic multiple myeloma: a report on 91 patients. Groupe d'Etudes et de Recherche sur le Myelome (GERM). *Am J Hematol* 1995; **48**:71–5.

●18. Weber DM, Dimopoulos MA, Moulopoulos LA, Delasalle KB, Smith T, Alexanian R. Prognostic features of asymptomatic multiple myeloma. *Br J Haematol* 1997; **97**:810–14.

♦19. Mundy GR. Hypercalcemia of malignancy revisited. *J Clin Invest* 1988; **82**:1–6.

●20. Taube T, Beneton MN, McCloskey EV, Rogers S, Greaves M, Kanis JA. Abnormal bone remode' in patients with myelomatosis and normal biochemical indices of bone resorption. *Eur J Haematol* 1992; **49**:192–8.

♦21. Callander NS, Roodman GD. Myeloma bone disease. *Semin Hematol* 2001; **38**:276–85.

♦22. Hosking DJ. Assessment of renal and skeletal components of hypercalcemia. *Calcif Tissue Int* 1990; **46**(Suppl):S11–S19.

●23. Adamietz IA, Schöber C, Schulte RW, Peest D, Renner K. Palliative radiotherapy in plasma cell myeloma. *Radiother Oncol* 1991; **20**:111–16.

●24. Merlini G, Parrinello GA, Piccinini L, Crema F, Fiorentini ML, Riccardi A, et al. Long-term effects of parenteral dichloromethylene bisphosphonate (CL2MBP) on bone disease of myeloma patients treated with chemotherapy. *Hematol Oncol* 1990; **8**:23–30.

●25. Lahtinen R, Laakso M, Palva I, Virkkunen P, Elomaa I. Randomised, placebo-controlled multicentre trial of clodronate in multiple myeloma. Finnish Leukaemia Group. *Lancet* 1992; **340**:1049–52.

●26. Berenson JR, Lichtenstein A, Porter L, Dimopoulos MA, Bordoni R, George S, et al. Efficacy of pamidronate in reducing skeletal events in patients with advanced multiple myeloma. Myeloma Aredia Study Group. *N Engl J Med* 1996; **334**:488–93.

●27. Berenson JR, Rosen LS, Howell A, Porter L, Coleman RE, Morley W, et al. Zoledronic acid reduces skeletal-related events in patients with osteolytic metastases. *Cancer* 2001; **91**:1191–200.

♦28. Jacobson DR, Zolla-Pazner S. Immunosuppression and infection in multiple myeloma. *Semin Oncol* 1986; **13**:282–90.

●29. Twomey JJ, Houston MB. Infections complicating multiple myeloma and chronic lymphocytic leukemia. *Arch Intern Med* 1973; **132**:562–5.

●30. Massaia M, Dianzani U, Bianchi A, Camponi A, Boccadoro M, Pileri A. Defective generation of alloreactive cytotoxic T lymphocytes (CTL) in human monoclonal gammopathies. *Clin Exp Immunol* 1988; **73**:214–18.

●31. Österborg A, Nilsson B, Björkholm M, Holm G, Mellstedt H. Natural killer cell activity in monoclonal gammopathies: relation to disease activity. *Eur J Haematol* 1990; **45**:153–7.

●32. Fahey JL, Scoggins R, Utz JP, Szwed CF. Infection, antibody response and gamma globulin components in multiple myeloma and macroglobulinemia. *Am J Med* 1963; **35**:698–707.

●33. Krull P, Deicher H. Primäre Antikörperbildung bei Patienten mit malignen lymphoretikulären Systemerkrankungen und metastasierenden Tumoren. *Z Immunitats forsch Exp Klin Immunol* 1973; **145**:70–7.

●34. Chapel HM, Lee M, Hargreaves R, Pamphilon DH, Prentice AG. Randomised trial of intravenous immunoglobulin as prophylaxis against infection in plateau-phase multiple myeloma. The UK Group for Immunoglobulin Replacement Therapy in Multiple Myeloma. *Lancet* 1994; **343**:1059–63.

●35. Hargreaves RM, Lea JR, Griffiths H, Faux JA, Holt JM, Reid C, et al. Immunological factors and risk of infection in plateau phase myeloma. *J Clin Pathol* 1995; **48**:260–6.

●36. Robertson JD, Nagesh K, Jowitt SN, Dougal M, Anderson H, Mutton K, et al. Immunogenicity of vaccination against influenza, Streptococcus pneumoniae and Haemophilus influenzae type B in patients with multiple myeloma. *Br J Cancer* 2000; **82**:1261–5.

●37. Duperray C, Bataille R, Boiron JM, Haagen IA, Cantaloube JF, Zhang XG, et al. No expansion of the pre-B and B-cell compartments in the bone marrow of patients with multiple myeloma. *Cancer Res* 1991; **51**:3224–28.

●38. Broder S, Humphrey R, Durm M, Blackman M, Meade B, Goldman C, et al. Impaired synthesis of polyclonal (non-paraprotein) immunoglobulins by circulating lymphocytes from patients with multiple myeloma. *N Engl J Med* 1975; **293**:887–92.

●39. Peest D, Brunkhorst U, Schedel I, Deicher H. In vitro immunoglobulin production by peripheral blood mononuclear cells from multiple myeloma patients and patients with benign monoclonal gammopathy. Regulation by cell subsets. *Scand J Immunol* 1984; **19**:149–57.

●40. Peest D, Hölscher R, Weber R, Leo R, Deicher H. Suppression of polyclonal B cell proliferation mediated by supernatants from human myeloma bone marrow cell cultures. *Clin Exp Immunol* 1989; **75**:252–7.

●41. Quesada S, Leo R, Deicher H, Peest D. Functional and biochemical characteristics of a soluble B lymphocyte proliferation-inhibiting activity produced by bone marrow cells from multiple myeloma patients. *Cell Immunol* 1995; **162**:275–81.

●42. Berman JE, Zolla-Pazner S. Control of B cell proliferation: inhibition of responses to B cell mitogens induced by plasma cell tumors. *J Immunol* 1985; **134**:2872–8.

●43. Schedel I. Application of immunoglobulin preparations in multiple myeloma. In: Nydegger UE, Morell A (eds) *Clinical use of intravenous immunoglobulins*. London: Academic Press, 1986:123–32.

●44. Stoll C, Schedel I, Peest D. Serum antibodies against common antigens of bacterial lipopolysaccharides in healthy adults and in patients with multiple myeloma. *Infection* 1985; **13**:115–19.

●45. Peest D, Coldewey R, Deicher H, Sailer M, Vykoupil C, Leo R, et al. Prognostic value of clinical, laboratory, and histological characteristics in multiple myeloma: improved definition of risk groups. *Eur J Cancer* 1993; **29A**:978–83.

♦46. Durie BGM. Staging and kinetics of multiple myeloma. In: Salmon SE (ed.) *Clinics in haematology* Vol. 11, No. 1. London: WB Saunders, 1982:3–18.

♦47. Clark AD, Shetty A, Soutar R. Renal failure and multiple myeloma: pathogenesis and treatment of renal failure and management of underlying myeloma. *Blood Rev* 1999; **13**:79–90.

●48. Zlotnick A, Rosenmann E. Renal pathologic findings associated with monoclonal gammopathies. *Arch Intern Med* 1975; **135**:40–5.

●49. Levi DF, Williams RC Jr, Lindstrom FD. Immunofluorescent studies of the myeloma kidney with special reference to light chain disease. *Am J Med* 1968; **44**:922–33.

●50. Solomon A, Weiss DT, Kattine AA. Nephrotoxic potential of Bence Jones proteins. *N Engl J Med* 1991; **324**:1845–51.

●51. Waldmann TA, Strober W, Mogielnicki RP. The renal handling of low molecular weight proteins. II. Disorder of serum protein catabolism with tubular proteinuria, the nephrotic syndrom, or uremia. *J Clin Invest* 1972; **51**:2162–74.

♦52. Clyne DH, Pollak VE. Renal handling and pathophysiology of Bence Jones proteins. *Contrib Nephrol* 1981; **24**:78–87.

♦53. Maldonado JE, Velosa JA, Kyle RA, Wagoner RD, Holley KE, Salassa RM. Fanconi syndrome in adults: a manifestation of a latent form of myeloma. *Am J Med* 1975; **58**:354–64.

●54. Analysis and management of renal failure in fourth MRC myelomatosis trial. MRC working party on leukaemia in adults. *Br Med J* 1984; **288**:1411–16.

●55. Feest TG, Burge PS, Cohen SL. Successful treatment of myeloma kidney by diuresis and plasmaphoresis. *Br Med J* 1976; **1**:503–4.

●56. Pasquali S, Cagnoli L, Rovinetti C, Rigotti A, Zucchelli P. Plasma exchange therapy in rapidly progressive renal failure due to multiple myeloma. *Int J Artif Organs* 1985; **8**(Suppl 2): 27–30.

●57. Coward RA, Mallick NP, Delamore IW. Should patients with renal failure associated with myeloma be dialysed? *Br Med J* 1983; **287**:1575–8.

●58. Johnson WJ, Kyle RA, Pineda AA, O'Brien PC, Holley KE. Treatment of renal failure associated with multiple myeloma. Plasmapheresis, hemodialysis, and chemotherapy. *Arch Intern Med* 1990; **150**:863–9.

♦59. Buxbaum J. Mechanisms of disease: monoclonal immunoglobulin deposition. Amyloidosis, light chain deposition disease, and light and heavy chain deposition disease. *Hematol Oncol Clin North Am* 1992; **6**:323–46.

♦60. Buxbaum J, Gallo G. Nonamyloidotic monoclonal immunoglobulin deposition disease. Light-chain, heavy-chain, and light- and heavy-chain deposition diseases. *Hematol Oncol Clin North Am* 1999; **13**:1235–48.

●61. Linke RP, Zucker-Franklin D, Franklin EC. Morphologic, chemical, and immunologic studies of amyloid-like fibrils formed from Bence Jones proteins by proteolysis. *J Immunol* 1973; **111**:10–23.

♦62. Kyle RA. Amyloidosis. In: Salmon SE (ed.) *Clinics in hematology*, Vol. 11, No. 1, *Myeloma and related disorders*. London: WB Saunders, 1982:151–80.

●63. Gertz MA, Li CY, Shirahama T, Kyle RA. Utility of subcutaneous fat aspiration for the diagnosis of systemic amyloidosis (immunoglobulin light chain). *Arch Intern Med* 1988; **148**:929–33.

●64. Breedveld FC, Markusse HM, MacFarlane JD. Subcutaneous fat biopsy in the diagnosis of amyloidosis secondary to chronic arthritis. *Clin Exp Rheumatol* 1989; **7**:407–10.

●65. Duston MA, Skinner M, Meenan RF, Cohen AS. Sensitivity, specificity, and predictive value of abdominal fat aspiration for the diagnosis of amyloidosis. *Arth Rheum* 1989; **32**:82–5.

●66. Salmon SE, Wampler SE. Multiple myeloma: quantitative staging and assessment of response with a programmable pocket calculator. *Blood* 1977; **49**:379–89.

●67. Ludwig H, Fritz E, Kotzmann H, Höcker P, Gisslinger H, Barnas U. Erythropoietin treatment of anemia associated with multiple myeloma. *N Engl J Med* 1990; **322**:1693–9.

●68. Österborg A, Boogaerts MA, Cimino R, Essers U, Holowiecki J, Juliusson G, *et al.* Recombinant human erythropoietin in transfusion-dependent anemic patients with multiple myeloma and non-Hodgkin's lymphoma – a randomized multicenter study. *Blood* 1996; **87**:2675–82.

●69. Cavo M, Galieni P, Zuffa E, Baccarani M, Gobbi M, Tura S. Prognostic variables and clinical staging in multiple myeloma. *Blood* 1989; **74**:1774–80.

●70. Gonzalez F, Trujillo JM, Alexanian R. Acute leukemia in multiple myeloma. *Ann Intern Med* 1977; **86**:440–3.

♦71. Bergsagel DE, Bailey AJ, Langley GR, MacDonald RN, White DF, Miller AB. The chemotherapy of plasma-cell myeloma and the incidence of acute leukemia. *N Engl J Med* 1979; **301**:743–8.

●72. Cuzick J, Erskine S, Edelman D, Galton DA. A comparison of the incidence of the myelodysplastic syndrome and acute myeloid leukaemia following melphalan and cyclophos- phamide treatment for myelomatosis. A report to the Medical Research Council's working party on leukaemia in adults. *Br J Cancer* 1987; **55**:523–9.

♦73. Bergsagel DE. Chemotherapy of myeloma: drug combinations versus single agents, an overview, and comments on acute leukemia in myeloma. *Hematol Oncol* 1988; **6**:159–66.

●74. Economopoulos T, Pappa V, Panani A, Stathakis N, Dervenoulas J, Papageorgiou E, *et al.* Myelopathies during the course of multiple myeloma. *Haematologica* 1991; **76**:289–92.

●75. Ludwig H, Frühwald F, Tscholakoff D, Rasoul S, Neuhold A, Fritz E. Magnetic resonance imaging of the spine in multiple myeloma. *Lancet* 1987; **II**:364–6.

●76. Patriarca F, Zaja F, Silvestri F, Sperotto A, Scalise A, Gigli G, *et al.* Meningeal and cerebral involvement in multiple myeloma patients. *Ann Hematol* 2001; **80**:758–62.

●♦77. Petersen SL, Wagner A, Gimsing P. Cerebral and meningeal multiple myeloma after autologous stem cell transplantation. A case report and review of the literature. *Am J Hematol* 1999; **62**:228–33.

●78. Kelly JJ, Kyle RA, Miles JM, O'Brien PC, Dyck PJ. The spectrum of peripheral neuropathy in myeloma. *Neurology* 1981; **31**:24–31.

●79. Read DJ, Vanhegan RI, Matthews WB. Peripheral neuropathy and benign IgG paraproteinaemia. *J Neurol Neurosurg Psychiatry* 1978; **41**:215–19.

●80. Delauche MC, Clauvel JP, Seligmann M. Peripheral neuropathy and plasma cell neoplasias: a report of 10 cases. *Br J Haematol* 1981; **48**:383–92.

●81. Resnick D, Greenway GD, Bardwick PA, Zvaifler NJ, Gill GN, Newman DR. Plasma-cell dyscrasia with polyneuropathy, organomegaly, endocrinopathy, M-protein, and skin changes: the POEMS syndrome. *Radiology* 1981; **140**:17–22.

●82. Dellagi K, Dupouney P, Brouet JC, Billecocq A, Gomez D, Clauvel JP, *et al.* Waldenström's macroglobulinemia and peripheral neuropathy: a clinical and immunological study of 25 patients. *Blood* 1983; **62**:280–5.

●83. Wehmeier U, Rilke H, Patzold U, Schedel I, Deicher H. Crossreacting idiotypes of kappa-monoclonal immunoglobulins M in sera of patients with Waldenström's macroglobulinemia. *Immunobiology* 1987; **176**:144–53.

●84. Hoppe U, Dräger HS, Patzold U, Stark E, Wurster U, Deicher H. Polyneuropathy in Waldenström's macroglobulinaemia. Passive transfer from man to mouse. *Acta Neurol Scand* 1987; **75**:112–16.

●85. Fahey JL, Barth WF, Solomon A. Serum hyperviscosity syndrome. *J Am Med Assoc* 1965; **192**:464–7.

●86. McGrath MA, Penny R. Paraproteinemia: blood hyperviscosity and clinical manifestations. *J Clin Invest* 1976; **58**:1155–62.

●87. Preston FE, Cooke KB, Foster ME, Winfield DA, Lee D. Myelomatosis and the hyperviscosity syndrome. *Br J Haematol* 1978; **38**:517–30.

●88. Crawford J, Cox EB, Cohen HJ. Evaluation of hyperviscosity in monoclonal gammopathies. *Am J Med* 1985; **79**:13–22.

●89. Isbister JP, Biggs JC, Penny R. Experience with large volume plasmapheresis in malignant paraproteinemia and immune disorders. *Aust N Z J Med* 1978; **8**:154–64.

●90. Osterland CK, Espinoza LR. Biological properties of myeloma proteins. *Arch Intern Med* 1975; **135**:32–6.

●91. Brouet JC, Clauvel JP, Danon F, Klein M, Seligmann M. Biologic and clinical significance of cryoglobulins. A report of 86 cases. *Am J Med* 1974; **57**:775–88.

●92. Lackner H, Hunt V, Zucker MB, Pearson J. Abnormal fibrin ultrastructure, polymerization, and clot retraction in multiple myeloma. *Br J Haematol* 1970; **18**:625–36.

●93. O'Kane MJ, Wisdom GB, Desai ZR, Archbold GP. Inhibition of fibrin monomer polymerisation by myeloma immunoglobulin. *J Clin Pathol* 1994; **47**:266–8.

●◆94. Tefferi A, Nichols WL, Bowie EJ. Circulating heparin-like anticoagulants: report of five consecutive cases and a review. *Am J Med* 1990; **88**:184–8.

●95. Colwell NS, Tollefsen DM, Blinder MA. Identification of a monoclonal thrombin inhibitor associated with multiple myeloma and a severe bleeding disorder. *Br J Haematol* 1997; **97**:219–26.

◆96. Tefferi A, Nichols WL. Acquired von Willebrand disease: concise review of occurrence, diagnosis, pathogenesis, and treatment. *Am J Med* 1997; **103**:536–40.

●◆97. Nitu-Whalley IC, Lee CA. Acquired von Willebrand syndrome – report of 10 cases and review of the literature. *Haemophilia* 1999; **5**:318–26.

●98. Bovill EG, Ershler WB, Golden EA, Tindle BH, Edson JR. A human myeloma-produced monoclonal protein directed against the active subpopulation of von Willebrand factor. *Am J Clin Pathol* 1986; **85**:115–23.

●99. Mohri H, Noguchi T, Kodama F, Itoh A, Ohkubo T. Acquired von Willebrand disease due to inhibitor of human myeloma protein specific for von Willebrand factor. *Am J Clin Pathol* 1987; **87**:663–8.

●100. Mohri H, Tanabe J, Ohtsuka M, Yoshida M, Motomura S, Nishida S, et al. Acquired von Willebrand disease associated with multiple myeloma; characterization of an inhibitor to von Willebrand factor. *Blood Coagul Fibrinolysis* 1995; **6**:561–6.

●101. Furie B, Voo L, McAdam KP, Furie BC. Mechanism of factor X deficiency in systemic amyloidosis. *N Engl J Med* 1981; **304**:827–30.

●102. Dührsen U, Paar D, Kolbel C, Boekstegers A, Metz-Kurschel U, Wagner R, et al. Lupus anticoagulant associated syndrome in benign and malignant systemic disease – analysis of ten observations. *Klin Wochenschr* 1987; **65**:852–9.

●103. Bellotti V, Gamba G, Merlini G, Montani N, Bucciarelli E, Stoppini M, et al. Study of three patients with monoclonal gammopathies and 'lupus-like' anticoagulants. *Br J Haematol* 1989; **73**:221–7.

●104. McBride W, Jackman J-DJ, Grayburn PA. Prevalence and clinical characteristics of a high cardiac output state in patients with multiple myeloma. *Am J Med* 1990; **89**:21–4.

●105. Breier F, Hobisch G, Groz S. Sweet-Syndrom. Akute neutrophile Dermatose bei multiplem Myelom. *Hautarzt* 1993; **44**:229–31.

●◆106. Berth-Jones J, Hutchinson PE. Sweet's syndrome and malignancy: a case associated with multiple myeloma and review of the literature. *Br J Dermatol* 1989; **121**:123–7.

●◆107. Valentine EA, Friedman HD, Zamkoff KW, Streeten BW. Necrobiotic xanthogranuloma with IgA multiple myeloma: a case report and literature review. *Am J Hematol* 1990; **35**:283–5.

●108. Hafner O, Witte T, Schmidt RE, Vakilzadeh F. Nekrobiotisches Xanthogranulom bei IgG-kappa-Plasmozytom und Quincke-Odem. *Hautarzt* 1994; **45**:339–43.

109. Dierlamm T, Laack E, Dierlamm J, Fiedler W, Hossfeld DK. IgM myeloma: a report of four cases. *Ann Hematol* 2002; **81**:136–9.

●110. Blade J, Lust JA, Kyle RA. Immunoglobulin D multiple myeloma: presenting features, response to therapy, and survival in a series of 53 cases. *J Clin Oncol* 1994; **12**:2398–404.

◆111. Jancelewicz Z, Takatsuki K, Sugai S, Pruzanski W. IgD multiple myeloma. Review of 133 cases. *Arch Intern Med* 1975; **135**:87–93.

●◆112. Endo T, Okumura H, Kikuchi K, Munakata J, Otake M, Nomura T, et al. Immunoglobulin E (IgE) multiple myeloma: a case report and review of the literature. *Am J Med* 1981; **70**:1127–32.

●113. Peest D, Deicher H, Coldewey R, Schmoll HJ, Schedel I. Induction and maintenance therapy in multiple myeloma: a multicenter trial of MP versus VCMP. *Eur J Cancer Clin Oncol* 1988; **24**:1061–7.

8

Hematologic investigations: morphologic and phenotypic features of myeloma marrow diagnosis

THOMAS M. GROGAN, DEBORAH GELBSPAN AND LISA RIMSZA

INTRODUCTION

This chapter emphasizes both the morphologic and phenotypic features of the bone marrow in plasma cell myeloma. It details the morphologic features of both trephine biopsies and marrow aspirations. It emphasizes the salient phenotypic features of marrow myeloma cells, in contrast with normal plasma cells. The myeloma cell phenotype is discussed from the perspective of both tissue section immunohistochemistry (IHC) and flow cytometry (FACS analysis). The specific criteria for myeloma diagnosis are discussed and illustrated in Figs 8.1–8.21. Finally, the differential diagnosis of myeloma is discussed emphasizing the key morphologic and phenotypic diagnostic criteria of each entity.

MARROW MORPHOLOGY

The diagnosis of myeloma is an integrated activity combining radiographic findings of osteolytic lesions, serologic or urologic evidence of a monoclonal gammophathy, and morphologic evidence of an atypical marrow plasmacytosis. This section emphasizes that, ultimately, the diagnosis of multiple myeloma requires the morphologic identification of abnormal sheets or clusters of plasma cells (Figs 8.1–8.4).[1] The finding of plasma cells in sheets or aggregates producing a 'mass' effect indicates displacement of normal tissue through plasma cell infiltration – evidencing the uncontrolled growth of a malignant clone (Figs 8.1 and 8.2).[1–4] This pathologic microanatomic property contrasts with the usual randomly dispersed, non-aggregated plasma cells in a benign reactive plasmacytosis. Beyond a 'mass' effect, additional cytologic properties favor a neoplastic process. Specifically, these include the findings of multinucleated plasma cells and plasma cell immaturity or anaplasia (Figs 8.1, 8.3, and 8.4, p. 104).[5,6] Since 1–5% of reactive-plasma cells may be binucleate or, rarely, trinucleate, it is the finding of bizarre multinucleate (greater than trinucleate) forms that is considered pathologic (Fig. 8.5).[7,8] The findings of immaturity include dispersed nuclear chromatin, high nuclear/cytoplasmic ratio and prominent nucleoli, giving a 'blastic' appearance indicative of plasmablasts (Figs 8.6 and 8.7).[6] Since nuclear–cytoplasmic asynchrony and immaturity rarely occur in reactive circumstances, they are reliable indicators of 'atypical' or pleomorphic plasmacytosis greatly favoring

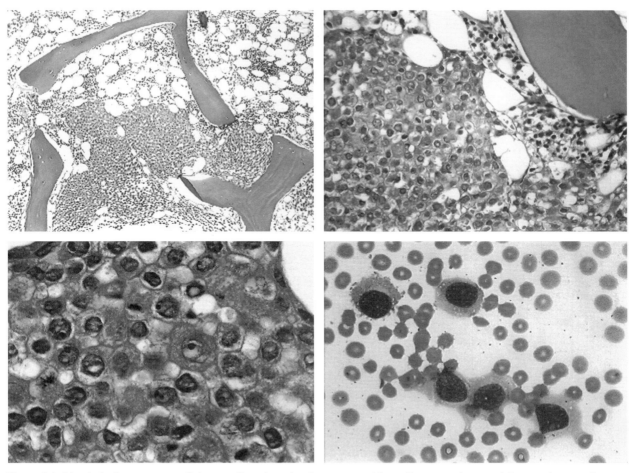

Figure 8.1 *Morphologic appearance of plasma cell myeloma in a bone marrow biopsy. Upper panels: several discrete plasma cell masses displace normal marrow fat cells and hematopoietic elements. This 'displacing' mass contrasts with the normal fat cell pattern. Lower panels: left, monomorphosis sheet of plasma cells; right, neoplastic plasma cells from marrow aspirated (40×, 150×, 100×, 100×).*

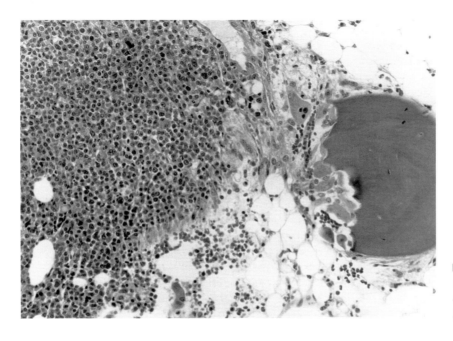

Figure 8.2 *Plasma cell myeloma mass with prominent osteoclastic activity eroding associated trabecular bone (250×).*

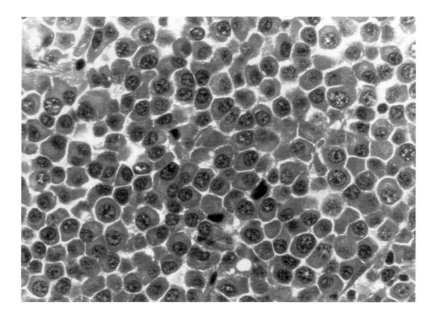

Figure 8.3 *Monomorphosis 'mass' of plasma cell myeloma cells (H&E, 400×).*

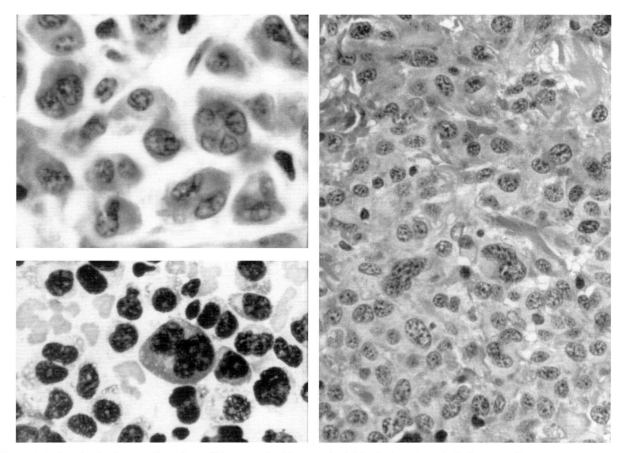

Figure 8.4 *Anaplastic plasma cell myeloma. This composite illustrates both histologic and cytologic features of immature, pleomorphic, polylobated, and multinucleate 'anaplastic' plasma cell myeloma. A combination of vestigial 'clock-face' chromatin; the presence of eccentric nuclei, low N/C ratio, abundant cytoplasm with occasional Golgi combined with an immunoperoxidase demonstration of cytoplasmic Ig, without pan-B antigens, leads to the diagnosis of plasma cell malignancy even in the face of substantial morphologic 'immaturity'.*

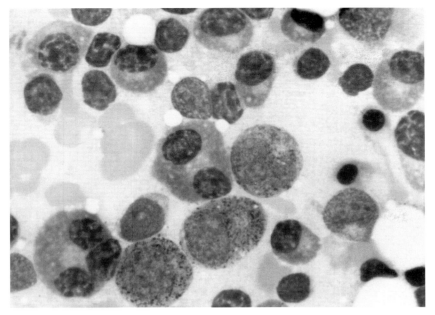

Figure 8.5 *Reactive marrow plasmacytosis, marrow aspirate. This striking plasmacytosis (>50% plasma cells) occurred in the recovery phase of marrow agranulocytosis related to drug therapy. Note the mature, 'block', 'clock-face' chromatin and inapparent nuclei heralding a 'typical' plasmacytosis. Also note binucleate and a trinucleate plasma cell in a 'benign' circumstance. The prominent promyelocytes reflect the 'recovery' from agranulocytosis. On the basis of this and other extreme reactive cases, the numeric plasma cell count alone obviously does not establish a diagnosis of myeloma (630×).*

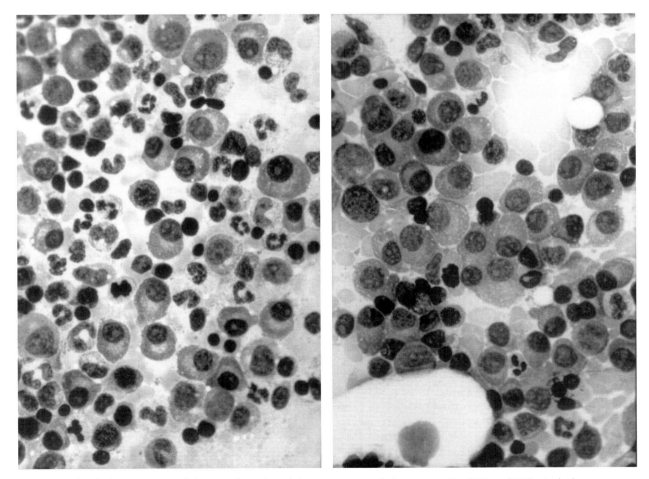

Figure 8.6 *Cytologic appearance of plasma cell myeloma in bone marrow aspirates representing 20% and 65% atypical plasmacytosis, respectively. The designation 'atypical' stems from the nuclear immaturity evidenced by prominent nucleoli and fine chromatin patterning (Wright-Giemsa stain, 400×).*

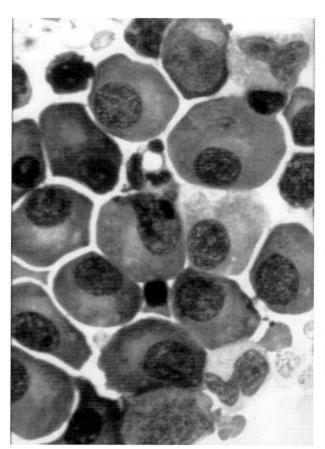 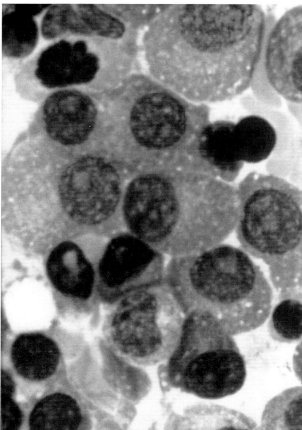

Figure 8.7 *Morphologic variants of plasma cell myeloma based on cell maturity. Left,* mature *myeloma cells with clumped nuclear chromatin, abundant cytoplasm and low nuclear-cytoplasmic ratio compared with* intermediate *maturity myeloma cells, on the right, with more prominent nucleoli, loose reticular chromatin, and moderate nuclear-cytoplasmic ratio (630×).*

a diagnosis of neoplasia.[2] Even given this atypicality, it is said that no single morphologic feature distinguishes between normal and malignant plasma cells.[2] Nevertheless, a constellation of findings including cytologic pleomorphism and tissue evidence of a displacing mass or abnormal aggregates strongly favors neoplasia. Beyond diagnosis, plasma cell immaturity, in the form of variants resembling lymphoid precursors and plasmablasts, has been highly associated with an adverse prognosis (Fig. 8.8).[6]

In contrast with the frequent telltale nuclear changes, the cytoplasmic features of neoplastic plasma cells typically simulate normalcy. The round or egg-shaped plasma cell with eccentrically placed nucleus contains abundant basophilic cytoplasm with a paranuclear clear zone (Figs 8.1, 8.6, and 8.7). Electron microscopy reveals highly developed endoplasmic reticulum specialized for immunoglobulin (Ig) synthesis.[2] The blue of Romanowsky-type stains reflects high RNA content, while the paranuclear clear zone reflects the Golgi where Ig is processed and glycosylated for secretion.[9] A great variety of cytoplasmic appearances may be found, including multiple

pale bluish-white grape-like accumulations (Mott cells, Morula cells) (Fig. 8.9), cherry-red round bodies (Russell bodies) (Fig. 8.9), vermilion-staining patterns ('flame cells'), cells 'overstuffed' with 'silky fibrils' (Gaucher-like cells, thesaurocytes), cells with 'hairy-cell'-like appearance and crystalline rods.[10–13] These inclusions all represent either aggregated, altered, retained, phagocytosed, condensed, or crystallized cytoplasmic Ig or glycoproteins.[10,11] While morphologically remarkable, these cytoplasmic changes are not pathognomonic of myeloma or plasma cell neoplasia, since they may also be seen in reactive plasma cells, particularly in inflammatory disorders of chronicity.[2] These disorders include syphilis, rheumatoid arthritis, tuberculosis, and secondary amyloidosis, in particular.[14]

The morphologic diagnosis of multiple myeloma almost invariably is made by bone marrow aspiration or biopsy. The scattered, focal bony disease may pose sampling difficulties such that failure to demonstrate marrow plasmacytosis does not rule out multiple myeloma. Rather, other sites should be aspirated especially at specific sites of bony tenderness or radiologic evidence of

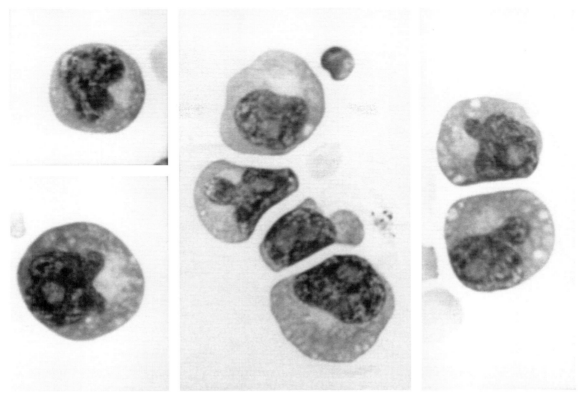

Figure 8.8 *Immature plasmablasts from a plasmablastic myeloma with prominent nucleoli, reticular chromatin, and high nuclear-cytoplasmic ratios. (Wright-Giemsa stain, 630×).*

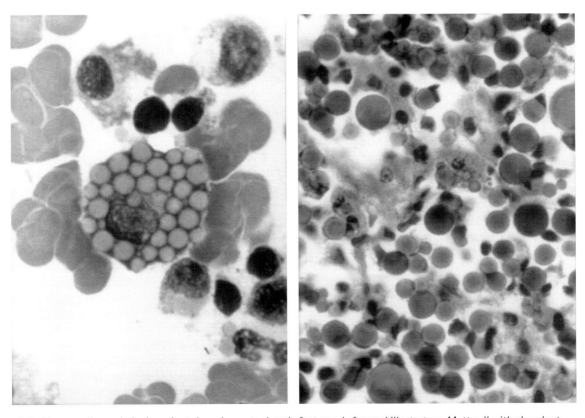

Figure 8.9 *Plasma cell morphologic variants based on cytoplasmic features. Left panel illustrates a Mott cell with abundant 'grape-like' cytoplasmic inclusions of immunoglobulin (630×), and right panel the presence of Russell bodies representing both cytoplasmic and extracellular inclusions seen in bone marrow biopsy (250×).*

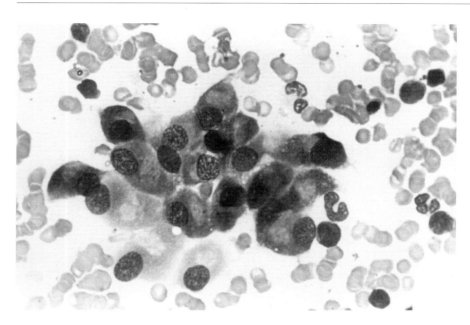

Figure 8.10 *A clump of osteoblasts in a bone marrow aspirate. The prominent Golgi, eccentric nuclei, abundant cytoplasm, and 'clumped' appearance may falsely suggest plasma cell myeloma (400×).*

osteolysis.[15] Involved marrow usually contains greater than 10% plasma cells (normal marrow <5% plasma cells) with 20% and 30%, respectively, meeting minor and major diagnostic criteria (see later).[16–18] Core biopsy reveals an excess of plasma cells occurring in foci, nodules, or sheets (Figs 8.1 and 8.2). In contrast to normal marrow, where the reactive plasma cells usually occur in small clusters of five or six cells around branching arterioles, the myelomatous plasma cells infiltrate the medullary adipocytes and islands of hematocytopoiesis.[4] Characteristically, in myeloma there is displacement of normal hematopoietic cells with adjacent areas of bony erosion or resorption due to osteoclastic activity (Fig. 8.1). Clumped osteoblasts found in children with active bone growth should not be confused with clumped plasma cells (Fig. 8.10).

The degree of marrow plasma cell infiltration has prognostic value. Specifically, three stages (stage I <20%, stage II 20–50%, stage III >50% plasma cells) predict progressively poorer prognoses.[3] When the latter staging is coupled with cytologic features (plasmacytic versus plasmablastic), there is strong predictive power of good-, moderate-, and poor-risk groups representing median survivals of 72, 23, and 6 months, respectively.[5] The main constraint of this strict morphologic predictive system is the common observation that the percentage of plasma cells in the marrow varies greatly with the sample and is not always a reliable measure of the total amount of disease present.[15] The recent finding that the highest plasma cell count from combined counts of marrow core biopsy, aspirate, and clot has the greatest clinical predictive value suggests added sampling to find the highest plasma cell count is a methodologic improvement.[19] Another suggested refinement entails using marrow core biopsy

immunophenotypic assay for CD138 as a more demonstrative method of plasma cell identification and counting.[20]

IMMUNOPHENOTYPIC PROPERTIES OF MYELOMA CELLS

Multiple myeloma as a malignancy of plasma cells, the most mature cell in the B-cell series, expectedly manifests expression of monotypic cytoplasmic immunoglobulin and plasma cell-associated antigens (CD38, Vs38c, CD138) with the unexpected absence of most pan-B-cell antigens except for the Ig-associated pan-B antigen (CD79a) (Figs 8.11 and 8.12).[21–23] In contrast with normal plasma cells, which express CD19 and lack the adhesion molecules CD56 and CD58, malignant plasma cells lack CD19 and express CD56 and CD58.[24,25] The latter adhesion molecules are thought relevant to bone marrow localization. Besides CD56 and CD58, the collagen-1 binding proteoglycan, syndecan-1 (CD138) found on myeloma and normal plasma cells, is also relevant to plasma cell marrow anchoring (Fig. 8.11).[26,27]

The interleukin-6 receptor α chain (CD126) is expressed by neoplastic and not normal plasma cells.[28] Plasma cells also typically strongly express transcription factors from the interferon regulatory factor (IRP) family. In particular, the product of the MUMI/IRF4 gene is detected in the nuclei and cytoplasm of plasma cells.[29]

The typical combined phenotype of neoplastic plasma cells is as follows: cIg+CD19−20−38+43+45−56+58+126+138+ (Figs 8.11–8.14). Normal plasma cells in contrast express CD19+ and lack CD56−58− and 126−.[30] The characteristic loss of CD19

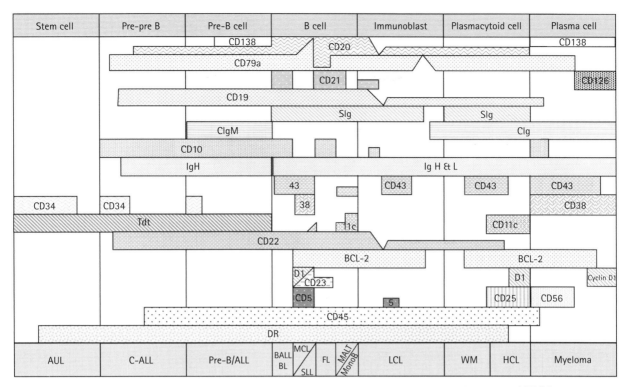

Figure 8.11 *Myeloma cell phenotype in the context of normal B-cell development. Illustrated are the expected CD (cluster designations) expected for plasma cell myeloma. AUL, acute undifferentiated leukemia; B-ALL, B-cell ALL; BL, Burkitt lymphoma; C-ALL, common (ALL) acute lymphocytic leukemia; FL, follicular lymphoma; HCL, hairy cell leukemia; LCL, large cell lymphoma; MALT, mucosa-associated lymphoma; MCL, mantle cell lymphoma; MONOB, monocytoid B-cell lymphoma; SLL, small lymphocytic lymphoma; WM, Waldenström's macroglobulinemia.*

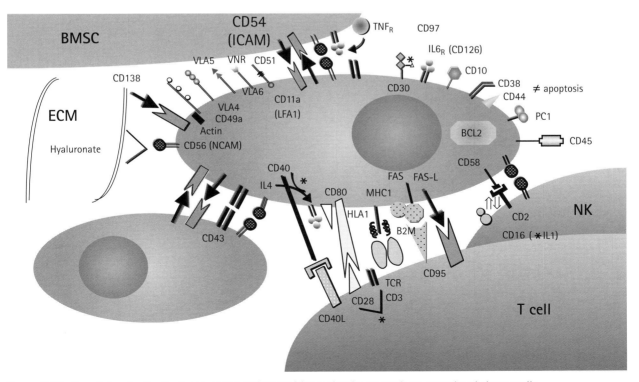

Figure 8.12 *Repertoire of cell adhesion signaling and recognition molecules on myeloma-associated plasma cells.*

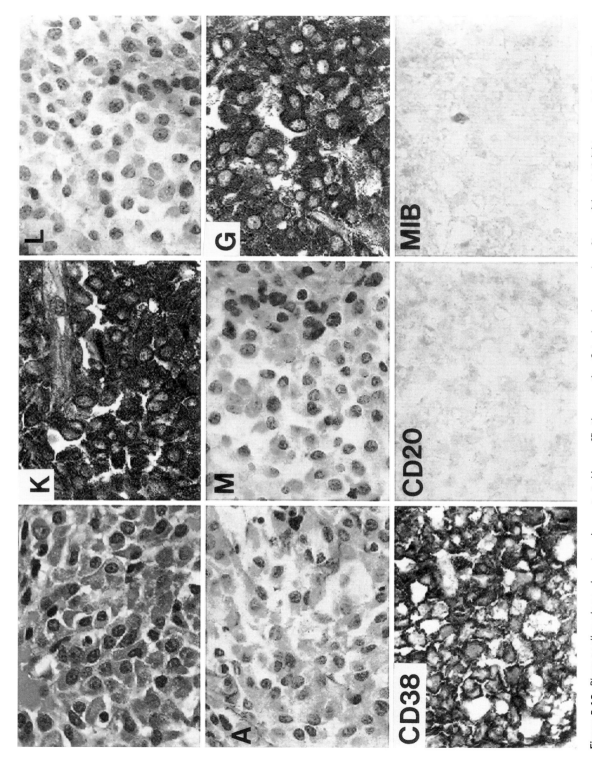

Figure 8.13 *Plasma cell myeloma phenotype demonstrated in paraffin tissue section. Cytoplasmic expression of kappa (K) and IgG (D) immunoglobulins with absence of lambda (L) light chain and IgM (M) and IgA (A) heavy chains is shown. Also characteristic is the prominent expression of CD38 and absent CD20 (400×).*

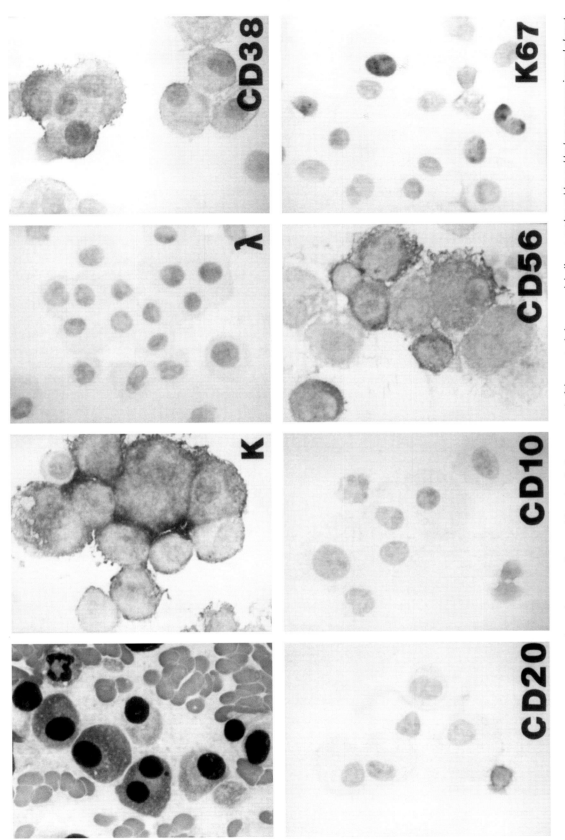

Figure 8.14 Typical plasma cell myeloma aspirate phenotype. Immunohistochemical assay reveals: (1) monotypic immunoglobulin expression evidenced by kappa expression and absent lambda; (2) plasma cell antigen expression (CD38); (3) absent mature (CD20) and immature (CD10) B-cell antigens; (4) cell adhesion molecule (CAM) expression – N-CAM (neuronal-CAM, CD56); (5) nuclear proliferation antigen as detected by Ki67 (K67) (immunoperoxidase studies, 400×).

expression reflects altered expression of the *pax-5* gene on chromosome 9.[31]

Besides the marrow plasma cells, the neoplastic clone includes circulating monoclonal idiotype-identical B lymphocytes, which might represent the myeloma stem cell.[32,33] These circulating B cells express the same idiotype and isotype as the paraprotein secreted by the malignant plasma cells. Occasionally, both components, lymphoid and plasma cell, may manifest immature B-cell antigen expression, e.g. common acute lymphoblastic leukemia antigen (CALLA) CD10 (Fig. 8.15).[34–36] This has been referred to as CALLA+ myeloma, representing a clinically significant finding portending a poor prognosis.[35] Some CALLA+ myeloma cells have a pre-B-cell phenotype[37–39] with cytoplasmic mu chain and nuclear terminal deoxynucleotidyl transferase (TdT) expression (Fig. 8.15). These highly proliferative myeloma pre-B cells could represent a significant component of the self-renewal or stem cell population of myeloma.[21] The view that myeloma may begin with normal precursor pre-B cells is questioned by the novel nature of the myeloma pre-B cells that co-express both immature B-cell and plasma cell antigens (Fig. 8.15). They may simply represent myeloma cells with aberrant or disorganized gene expression that produce novel phenotypes.[37,38] Malignant myeloma cells may not express antigens in the normal one-way progressive, sequential fashion found in normal B-cell differentiation (Fig. 8.15).[38] Clinically, CALLA+ myeloma survival appears favorably altered by therapy directed at the immature acute lymphoblastic leukemia-like component.[37]

MYELOID AND T-CELL ANTIGENS

Occasionally (13%), myeloma may present with aberrant co-expression of myelomonocytic antigens preceding overt leukemia (Fig. 8.16).[40,41] Since many myelomonocytic myelomas express IgA, a possible receptor for granulocyte–macrophage colony-stimulating factor (GM-CSF), the potential role of cytokine modulation is envisioned.[40] These myeloid 'lineage infidelities' or phenotypic 'platypuses' question the true cell of origin in certain cases. Myelomonocytic myeloma, as an obvious contradiction in terms, suggests that myeloma clonal origin may entail the concept of sequential lineage commitment during hematopoiesis rather than a stochastic model of development.[42] The very rare occurrence of T-cell antigen co-expression in myeloma adds fuel to this speculative model.[43] The more recent demonstration by multiparameter flow cytometry studies of erythroid or

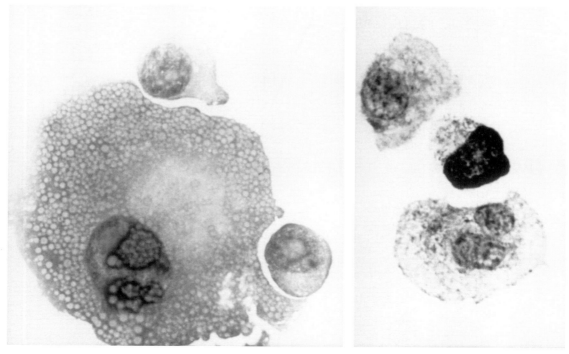

Figure 8.15 *Pre-B-cell lymphoid component associated with plasma cell myeloma. Left, note a large plasma cell with cytoplasmic inclusions (Mott cell) and nuclear inclusions (Dutcher body). Adjacent are two small lymphoblasts with an immature pre-B-cell phenotype: cytoplasmic mu+, light chain−, CD10+, nuclear Tdt+ (as shown on the right panel) (Wright-Giemsa and immunoperoxidase, 1000×).*

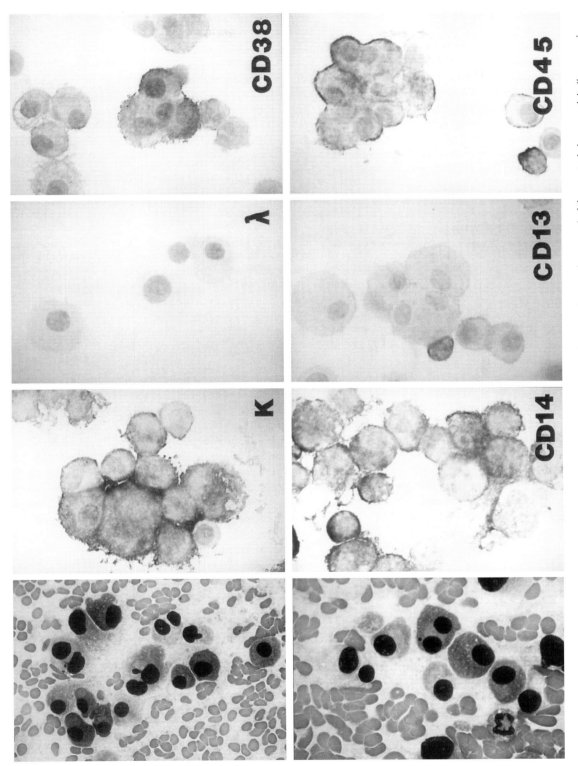

Figure 8.16 *Myelomonocytic myeloma aspirate phenotype. Immunocytochemical assay of this myeloma variant reveals: (1) monotypic immunoglobulin expression (kappa+, lambda−); (2) plasma cell antigen expression (CD38+); (3) myeloid antigen expression (CD14+, CD13+); (4) leukocyte common antigen expression (CD45+) (immunoperoxidase, 400×).*

megakaryocytic antigens on myeloma cells further favors the presence of a myeloma stem cell early in hematopoietic development as in chronic myelogenous leukemia (CML).[41,44] The analogy to CML may also have clinical relevance as CML-like myeloma has a long initial stable period followed by a terminal blastic phase.[44]

These aberrantly acquired, mutated lineage infidelities may directly herald myeloma progression. A case in point is the emergence of CD28+ myeloma cells.[45] This T-cell antigen initially lacking in myeloma presentation is commonly expressed in myeloma relapse and extramedullary spread. CD28 doubly adds to myeloma aggressiveness by facilitating both myeloma cell survival (via overexpression of *Bcl-x*) and proliferation (via increased labeling index).[45]

DRUG RESISTANCE PROTEIN

Resistance to cytotoxic chemotherapy is a major problem in the treatment of patients with multiple myeloma. This phenomenon of multidrug resistance is associated with a variety of molecular mechanisms including P-glycoprotein,[46–52] the lung resistance protein (LRP-56).[53,54] P-glycoprotein is a surface efflux pump, which removes toxic substances from plasma cells protecting them from chemotherapy (Fig. 8.17).[46,47] P-glycoprotein overexpression is induced specifically by known doses of Adriamycin (>300 mg) and of vincristine (>20 mg), resulting in clinical resistance to the vincristine–Adriamycin–dexamethasone (VAD) regimen.[48] While P-glycoprotein-mediated drug resistance could be favorably modulated by chemomodifiers,[49] the clinical benefit to patients was limited as other drug resistance mechanisms emerged (e.g. LRP56).[50,53] The multifactorial nature of multidrug resistant glycoproteins is a factor explaining the current incurability of myeloma.[50–52]

PROLIFERATION ANTIGENS

Tritiated thymidine labeling, DNA 'S'-phase assay and bromodeoxyuridine (BDUR) immunofluorescence are all measures of cell kinetics that have previously proven valuable predictors of myeloma outcome.[55–57] While most myeloma patients at presentation typically show low proliferative activity, more symptomatic, progressive myeloma patients demonstrate higher plasma cell labeling indices associated with shorter survival (Fig. 8.18).[8,57] The utility of these proliferative assays recently has been greatly facilitated by monoclonal antibodies to nuclear proliferation antigens (Ki67, PCNA).[58,59] A Ki67 index predicts poor prognosis, as illustrated in Fig. 8.1.[4] Ki67 has also demonstrated high proliferative activity in myeloma

pre-B cells, adding to the impression that the pre-B cell may be the stem cell accounting for myeloma self-renewal.[38] In 25% of myeloma cases, a higher proliferation rate is associated with nuclear overexpression of cyclin D1 owing to the translocation (t(11:14)) of the *bcl-1* gene. Cyclin D1 plays a key role in driving cells in cycle from G1 to S phase. Thus, cyclin D1 overexpression is thought to give myeloma cells a growth advantage.[60–62]

APOPTOSIS–RELATED ANTIGENS

Myeloma cell immortalization may be, firstly, a consequence of unending proliferation or, secondly, due to prolonged survival through a failure of cell death or apoptosis.[63–65] In myeloma, the latter factor (cell death avoidance) is likely a more important factor, since myeloma is characterized by a latent accumulation of 'resting' plasma cells, which are not in cycle and typically display a very low proliferative activity (<1% Ki67 in 90% of myeloma patients). Thus, in the pathogenesis of myeloma, the key event is not loss of growth control, but rather enhanced myeloma cell survival through inhibition of apoptosis. Myeloma cell death (apoptosis) is determined by a complex balance of survival versus contravailing death-specific factors. Survival factors (e.g. Bcl-2, NF-κB) confer long-term cell survival by blocking programmed cell death. Dexamethasone-induced cytotoxicity in myeloma cells is thought to be the consequence of decreased *bcl-2* expression.[63]

Regarding pro-apoptotic death factors, the CD95 (FAS) antigen through its ligand (FAS-L) or anti-Fas antibodies triggers the cascade of signals for apoptosis in myeloma cells.[64] As myeloma progresses, suppression of FAS (CD95) antigen expression on tumor cells renders them resistant to the FAS-L on tumor-infiltrating T-cells averting any antitumor immunosurveillance.[64] Remarkably, the recent finding of constitutive expression FAS-L on myeloma cells presents another potential mechanism of tumor-induced suppression of immunosurveillance.[65,66] The FAS-L+ myeloma cells foil immunosurveillance by triggering secretion of caspases, granzyme, and perforin, resulting in FAS+ cytotoxic T-cell death.[65,66]

INFILTRATING ACCESSORY CELLS

Contrary to the view that myeloma, as a malignancy, is an entirely autonomous growth, recent findings suggest that the host accessory cell response (T-lymphocytes, monocytes, natural killer cells, etc.) can modulate the disease.[67–70] Specifically, study of the tumor-infiltrating T-lymphocytes (T-TIL) suggests that immunosurveillance is a major factor in myeloma containment. Methodologies like

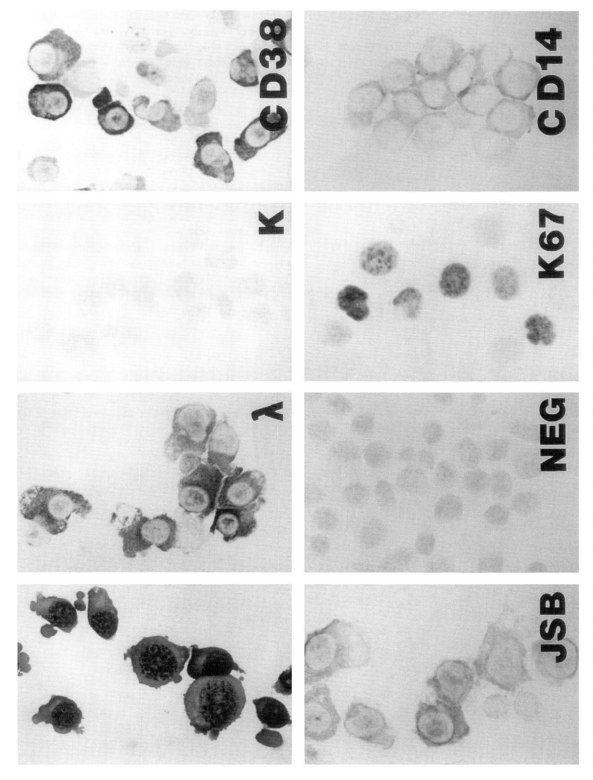

Figure 8.17 Plasma cell leukemia with expression of drug resistance protein (P-glycoprotein). Immunocytochemical assay reveals monotypic Ig, plasma cell antigens, P-glycoprotein (as measured by JSB1), a high proliferative rate (Ki67), and co-expressed myeloid antigen (CD14). Collectively, this suggests combined phenotypic escape, including myeloid and P-glycoprotein escape.

immunohistochemistry, which preserve tumor–host immunoarchitectural relationships, have proven pivotal in delineating these relationships (Fig. 8.19).[71] T suppressor/cytotoxic (s/c) (CD8+) cells within the myeloma tumor have been associated with immunosurveillance.[67–70] *In vitro* culture studies have demonstrated enhanced growth of myeloma cells with removal of Ts/c lymphocytes prior to plating.[71] It is known that myeloma protein stimulates idiotypic specific T-suppressor cell activity relevant to tumor containment.[67–70] T-TIL in myeloma is likely subject to cytokine modulation (e.g. T-TIL adaptive immunotherapy). Knowing that myeloma is a malignancy

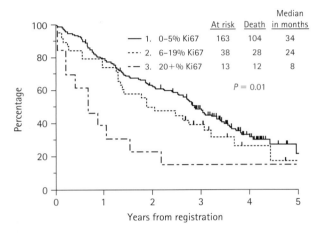

Figure 8.18 *Survival of plasma cell myeloma related to proliferative rate as measured by Ki67 (see Grogan and Spier[4]).*

of immunoregulatory cells rightly leads to consideration of immunoregulatory mechanisms of containment.

Malignant plasma cells may escape myeloma infiltrating T-cell immunosurveillance by a variety of mechanisms. Firstly, as mentioned above, myeloma cells can upregulate their FAS-ligand, which reacts with the FAS+ receptor on activated infiltrating T cells. This FAS-L/FAS interaction induces sequential activation of caspases, resulting in apoptotic death of myeloma T-TIL cells committed to immunosurveillance.[66] Furthermore, the FAS-L+ myeloma cells are thought to cause anemia by destruction of FAS+ erythroblasts and to facilitate osetolysis by destruction of FAS+ osteoblasts.[66] Secondly, myeloma cells may destroy host T cells by direct secretion of granzyme B and perforin.[72] It is hypothesized that myeloma cells may attract host T cells through their antigen-presenting antigens (e.g. HLA-1, CD80, CD86) and then proceed to kill the T cells by secretion of myeloma cell-derived granzyme B and perforin.

Besides T-cell cytolysis caused by myeloma cell, there are other features of immunosuppression. In particular, myeloma-associated CD8+ T cells may have a non-functional CD94 receptor resulting in a form of impaired T-cell response or immunoparesis.[73]

CELL ADHESION MOLECULES

Adhesion cell molecules are important in plasma cell homing and anchoring in the bone marrow (Fig. 8.12).

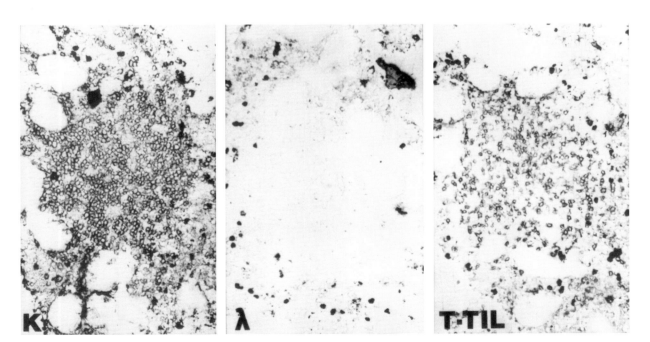

Figure 8.19 *Immunotopography of marrow myeloma. Snap-frozen sections reveal a discrete monotypic immunoglobulin-bearing tumor with striking tumor-infiltrating lymphocytes of T-cell type (T-TIL) representing idiotype specific T-suppressor/cytotoxic cells (immunoperoxidase, 100×).*

Normal plasma cells utilize a repertoire of adhesion molecules including (1) ICAM-1 (CD54), (2) the homing receptor (CD44), (3) fibronectin receptors (VLA-4, VLA-5), and (4) the collagen binding proteoglycan, syndecan-1 (CD138).[26,27,33] Malignant plasma cells have a similar repertoire (Figs 8.11 and 8.12) except for: (1) overexpression of CD44v variant isoforms (e.g. CD44v9),[74] (2) overexpression of LFA-3 (CD58),[25] and (3) overexpression of CD56, the neuronal cell adhesion molecule N-CAM (Figs 8.11, 8.12, and 8.14).[75,76] Because CD56, in particular, is uniquely myeloma-associated, serum levels of N-CAM are especially useful in distinguishing myeloma from benign paraproteinemias (e.g. MGUS).[77] While CD44, CD56, and CD58 are initial landmarks of beginning myeloma relevant to initial myeloma localization, later in the disease there is downregulation of CD56 and CD58, resulting in lost marrow stromal anchoring, enhanced extravasation, and extramedullary dissemination to become plasma cell leukemia.[75,78] Tumor progression in myeloma is also associated with overexpression of CD44v9 variant isoforms known to facilitate tumor metastasis in other tumor types.[79]

ANGIOGENESIS

Angiogenesis is well established as an obligatory factor in the growth, invasion, and metastasis of solid tumors.[80] Recently, angiogenesis has also been associated with progression of myeloma.[81–83] Specific vascular growth factor receptors (e.g. VEGF, AQP1) have been isolated in myeloma cells.[84–86] It has also been demonstrated that VEGF induces interleukin-6 (IL-6) secretion in bone marrow stromal cells.[87] This paracrine cooperation between VEGF and IL-6 may be part of a complex regulatory mechanism sustaining tumor growth and protecting myeloma cells from treatment-induced myeloma.[84–87]

TUMOR CELLS IN THE PERIPHERAL BLOOD

In both a reactive plasmacytosis and malignant myeloma, circulating mature plasma cells are not generally found in the peripheral blood. Rather, circulating tumor cells take the form of lymphoid B-cell precursors, frequently of B-cell and pre-B-cell phenotype. This fact is evidenced by findings of (1) circulating DNA-aneuploid lymphoid cells,[88] (2) concordant Ig gene rearrangement between blood and marrow lymphoid and plasma cells,[89] (3) plasma cell antigens on peripheral B cells,[32,38,90] and (4) idiotype-identical, isotype-concordant surface Ig on both circulating lymphoid and marrow-bound plasma cells.[32,38,91,92] Several of these peripheral blood phenotypic alterations

have been associated with poor survival, including (1) increased peripheral blood lymphocytes (PBL) expressing plasma cell antigen (CD38+),[90] (2) increased T suppressor to T-helper cell ratio,[90] (3) increased CD10 (CALLA)+ lymphoid cells,[34,37,38] and (4) loss of light-chain isotype concordant lymphoid suppression.[93] The increased CD38+ and CD10+ and isotype-specific cells reflect increased neoplastic precursor activity,[90] while the increased T-suppressor cells are thought to represent suppression of tumor clone expression.[68,69] Additionally, as reflected by electrophoresis, decreased non-neoplastic gammaglobulins indicates a reduction of normal peripheral blood B cells. This immunodeficiency and consequent hypogammopathy are concomitants of the monoclonal gammopathy and account for frequent recurrent bacterial infections common among myeloma patients. Suppression of normal B cells in myeloma is thought to occur by a combination of T-suppressor cell effect[68,69] and an Ig-binding factor similar to Ig-FMC receptor shed by T cells.[94] Furthermore, myeloma precursor lymphoid cells are thought to simply displace other B-cell precursors.[32]

PHENOTYPIC ESCAPE

Analogous to chronic myeloid leukemia, terminal myeloma progression is characterized by tumor-cell phenotypic transformation. In some cases this takes the form of a lymphoma-like transition with a high lactic dehydrogenase (LDH) level and lymphoid features with disease in lymph nodes, liver, blood, and brain. This phenomenon is sometimes accompanied by loss of the myeloma M-component and has been referred to as 'phenotypic escape.' Analogous to CML, myeloma in this instance has escaped into a lymphoma-like phenotype. Besides lymphoma-like escape, other modes of escape include (1) acute lymphoid leukemia escape (pre-B and CD10+ phenotypes), (2) transition to acute myelomonocytic leukemia (20% of cases at 5 years), (3) drug-resistant escape (P-glycoprotein found in 75% of drug refractory myeloma in VAD-resistant cases), (4) proliferative escape (high Ki67 or labeling indices characterize many terminal myeloma states), and (5) immunosurveillance escape related to loss of effective immunoregulation. This suggests multiple modes, whereby a myeloma tumor escapes and results in therapeutic failure. Any effective therapeutic strategy necessarily must overcome this multifactorial problem.

In the end, the value of phenotyping myeloma is twofold: (1) in selecting poor prognosis patients as potential candidates for newly proposed aggressive chemotherapy regimens or alternative therapies, such as allogeneic bone marrow transplantation, and (2) in identifying new cellular targets for therapy (e.g. P-glycoprotein, VEGF, cyclin D1).

PHENOTYPING METHODS

Most of the markers discussed above are available for analysis by either intact tissue section methods, e.g. IHC or *in situ* hybridization (ISH) or by cell suspension flow cytometry. Each technique has particular advantages. Flow cytometry can easily demonstrate and exploit differences in antigen intensities and access multiple antigens on single cells. So, for example, by four-color flow cytometry, individual neoplastic plasma cells (CD19−38+56+126+) can be demonstrated to have multiple phenotypic differences compared with individual normal plasma cells (CD19+ 38+56−126−).[95] Also multiparameter flow allows simultaneous DNA-quantification S-phase determin-ation and phenotyping to delineate the active neoplastic component.[96] Flow cytometry is also very sensitive for minimal residual disease detection, such that small populations (<5%) of monoclonal plasma cells can be detected in marrow specimens. Pitfalls include the need for fresh unfixed samples and the well-known loss of plasma cells during preparation and staining so that plasma cell percentages may be underestimated. In contrast, immunohistochemistry can be performed on paraffin-embedded tissues so that tissue architecture and plasma cell populations remain intact. For example, the relationship of host immune response cells (Fas+ T cells) to tumor cell (Fas-L+) phenotype may then be revealed in context.[65,66] The interpretation of monoclonal versus polyclonal plasma cell population in tissue section can be difficult due to the often high background immunoglobulin staining. This issue can be circumvented with tissue ISH (Fig. 8.20) to detect Ig mRNA.

MYELOMA DIAGNOSIS

Plasma cell proliferative disease ranges from asymptomatic patients with an incidental monoclonal gammopathy,

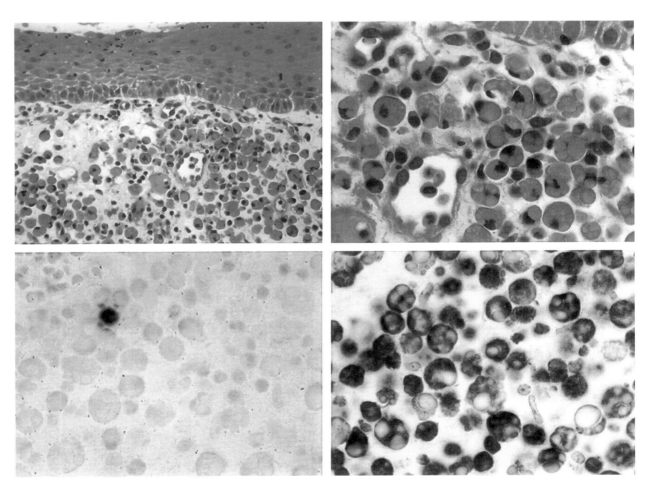

Figure 8.20 *Plasmacytoma of skin with abundant Russel body formation (upper panels), which can produce non-specific staining by immunohistochemistry. In this instance, monoclonality is demonstrated by non-radioactive* in situ *hybridization showing absence of kappa (lower left) and presence of lambda (lower right) mRNA transcripts (100×, 400 × 3).*

known as MGUS, to highly symptomatic myeloma patients with generalized multifocal destructive bone lesions throughout the skeletal system. Between these extremes are a variety of clinical phases representing a spectrum of diseases including indolent myeloma, smoldering myeloma, and solitary plasmacytoma of bone or soft tissue.[97–99] In the case of MGUS with only monoclonal protein in the serum and/or urine, the major diagnostic focus has been on distinction of MGUS from early multiple myeloma. A total of 20–30% of MGUS patients develop myeloma over 10 years, indicating that MGUS is in fact a 'pre-myelomatous' condition.[100,101] The puzzle remains as to which patients will convert.

With overt generalized myeloma, the patients commonly present with bone pain, anemia, and infection (e.g. pneumococcal). Some may also manifest hypercalcemia, renal failure, and/or spinal cord compression.[102] In all of the aforementioned conditions, diagnosis is based on finding an increase in plasma cells. Furthermore, a serum or urinary M-component is found in 99% of patients.[102] In the case of multiple myeloma, skeletal X-ray films reveal multiple 'punched-out' osteolytic bony lesions. Radiographically, the lesions appear as 1–4 cm

punched-out defects without sclerosis. The most common sites of involvement are in areas of active hematocytopoiesis including, in order of frequency, vertebrae, ribs, skull, pelvis, femur, clavicle, and scapula. The bony defects on gross examination are filled with a soft gelatinous, fish-flesh, hemorrhagic tissue.[103] A combination of findings leads to the diagnosis of multiple myeloma, including a marrow plasmacytosis of >10%, osteolytic lesions, and a plasma and/or urinary monoclonal protein.[102] Given the difficulty of sampling spotty disease, a mixture of criteria has been established to diagnose myeloma and its various phases.[102] These criteria are discussed in detail in Chapter 12.[16,97,98,102] In the case of diagnostic uncertainty, the ultimate diagnosis of plasma cell myeloma rests on finding evidence of uncontrolled plasma cell growth, as evidenced by plasma cell sheets, osteolytic lesions, or a progressive increase in the concentration of monoclonal protein.[104]

Marrow plasmacytosis of striking proportions may occur in a number of inflammatory conditions, chronic infections, autoimmune diseases, and hypersensitivity states (Figs 8.5 and 8.21). Specifically, marrow plasmacytosis may be associated with liver cirrhosis, syphilis, agranulocytosis, rheumatoid arthritis, Hodgkin's disease,

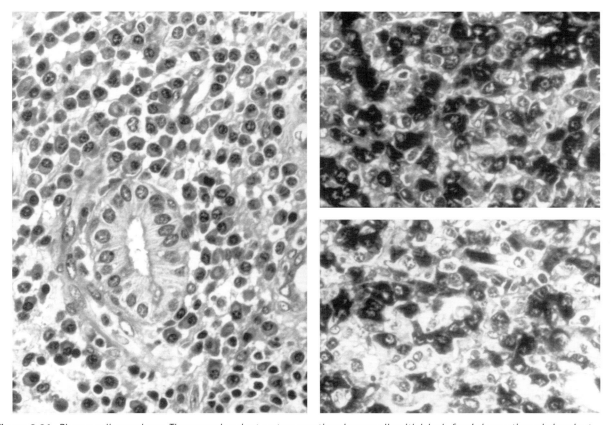

Figure 8.21 *Plasma cell granuloma. There are abundant mature reactive plasma cells with 'clock-face' chromatin and abundant cytoplasm, producing a 'mass effect' simulating a neoplasma. Immunoperoxidase indicates a polyclonal cytoplasmic proliferation with plasma cells containing both kappa (above) and lambda immunoglobulin (400×).*

and aplastic or hypoplastic anemia.[105–107] As mentioned above (morphology section), these reactive plasmacytoses, while sometimes striking (e.g. >50% plasma cells in recovery from agranulocytosis; Fig. 8.5), are generally comprised of scattered, not aggregated, plasma cells and, while binucleate or rare trinucleate plasma cells may be seen, pleomorphism, anaplastic, dysynchronous plasma cells with prominent nucleoli are usually not found in reactive states (Figs 8.4, 8.6–8.8). In these reactive plasmacytoses, electrophoresis generally reveals a broad-based polyclonal hypergammaglobulinemia.[105–107] While scattered, not sheet-like, plasma cells are the general rule in reactive plasmacytoses, a few exceptional circumstances are worthy of note. Both Hashimoto's thyroiditis and plasma cell granuloma are examples of benign conditions that may produce a displacing mass or tumor suggesting neoplasia.[108] In the case of plasma cell granuloma (Fig. 8.21), a primary plasmacytoma is suggested clinically.[108] In this circumstance, of a non-neoplastic tumorous reactive plasmacytosis, there are three important differential properties: (1) lack of plasma cell pleomorphism, dysynchrony, or anaplasia; (2) lack of a monoclonal gammopathy; and (3) direct phenotypic evidence of cytoplasmic plasma cell polyclonal immunoglobulin via immunohistochemistry (Fig. 8.21). These three specific criteria are highly applicable in the head and neck or nasopharyngeal region where the majority of extramedullary plasmacytomas occur, yet there is also a high incidence of chronic mucosal-associated plasmacytosis related to hypersensitivity or allergic states (Fig. 8.21).[109] Comparable confusion may occur in Felty's syndrome, whereby the splenomegaly associated with rheumatoid arthritis is largely the consequence of splenic plasmacytosis. The sheer extent of the latter may suggest neoplasia, but the above-mentioned morphologic and phenotypic criteria, coupled with knowledge of the clinical circumstance, make diagnosis unambiguous.

APPROACH TO DIAGNOSIS

The diagnosis of multiple myeloma requires the correlation of several radiographic and laboratory factors. As described in Chapter 12, the unique triad of osteolytic lesions, atypical marrow plasmacytosis (>10%), and a monoclonal gammopathy generally makes the diagnosis of myeloma straight forward.

The laboratory studies used to diagnose myeloma are listed in Table 8.1. As listed, these studies entail a combination of hematologic, serologic, urologic, and radiographic assessments. The hematologic assessment includes a complete blood count and bone marrow examination. A normochronic, normocytic anemia is present in most myeloma patients. Leukopenia and thrombocytopenia may

Table 8.1 *Laboratory analyses relevant to myeloma diagnosis*

Complete blood cell count (CBCC)
Blood smear examination
Bone marrow aspirate, clot, and core examination
Serum protein electrophoresis
Serum immunofixation
Urine protein electrophoresis
Urine immunofixation (24-hour urine)
Quantitative serum immunoglobulin levels
Serum chemistries, including calcium, blood urea nitrogen, creatinine, and lactic dehydrogenase
Serum b_2-microglobulin
Radiographic skeletal survey
Magnetic resonance imaging or computed tomography scan
Phenotypic analyses:
    Immunohistochemistry
    Flow cytometry
Immunoglobulin mRNA assay by *in situ* hybridization

be concomitant. The blood smear often shows 'stacked-like-coins' red cells known as rouleaux formation – a characteristic myeloma-associated change related to gammopathy. The marrow reveals increased plasma cells (>10%) with atypical cytologic features, as detailed above. A monoclonal gammopathy is established by serum protein electrophoresis (SPEP) and urine protein electrophoresis. A monoclonal spike should then be identified by immunofixation (see Fig. 8.2). Since up to 10% of myelomas may lack a heavy chain (Bence Jones myeloma), the light chain may pass entirely into the urine. Accordingly, electrophoresis must be performed on both serum and urine if myeloma is suspected. Additional useful assays include assessment of normal serum globulin fraction with the frequent of decreased normal immunoglobulin fraction found in myeloma. Additionally, the patients often display azotemia with increased BUN and creatine due to renal impairment. The same impairment results in an elevated B_2-microglobulin, which is further elevated due to secretion by myeloma cells.

Finally, phenotypic analysis, as detailed above, by either immunohistochemistry in intact biopsies or on the aspirate by flow cytometry, will further articulate on aberrant plasma cell phenotype (e.g. Ig-restricted, CD19−20−38+45−56+79a+126+138+).

KEY POINTS

- The diagnosis of multiple myeloma requires the morphological identification of abnormal sheets or clusters of plasma cells in the bone marrow.
- The morphological diagnosis should be made by bone marrow aspiration and/or biopsy. More than one site may have to be investigated.

- Involved marrow usually contains more than 10% plasma cells.
- A marrow core biopsy immunophenotypic assay for CD138 may help in plasma cell identification and counting.
- Immunocytochemistry on bone marrow aspirate by flow cytometry identifying the phenotype CD19−, 20+, 38+, 45−, 56+, 79a+, 126+, 138+ is helpful in identifying the monoclonal plasma cells.

REFERENCES

- = Key primary paper
◆ = Major review article

1. Buss DH, Prichard RW, Hartz JW, Cooper MR, Feigin GA. Initial bone marrow findings in multiple myeloma. Significance of plasma cell nodules. *Arch Pathol Lab Med* 1986; **110**:30–3.
2. Zucker-Franklin D. The pathology of multiple myeloma and related disorders. In Wiernik P, Cannellos, Kyle R, Schiffer C (eds) *Neoplastic diseases of the blood*. New York: Churchill Livingstone, 1985:462.
●3. Bartl R, Frisch B, Burkhardt R, Fateh-Moghadam A, Mahl G, Gierster P, *et al*. Bone marrow histology in myeloma: its importance in diagnosis, prognosis, classification and staging: *Br J Haematol* 1982; **51**:361–75.
◆4. Grogan TM, Spier CM. The B cell immunoproliferative disorders including multiple myeloma and amyloidosis. In Knowles DM (ed.) *Neoplastic hematopathology*, 2nd edn. Philadelphia: Lippincott, Williams and Wilkins, 2001:1235–66.
5. Fritz E, Ludwig H, Kundi M. Prognostic relevance of cellular morphology in multiple myeloma. *Blood* 1984; **63**:1072–9.
●6. Greipp R, Raymond NM, Kyle RA, O'Fallon WM. Multiple myeloma: significance of plasmablastic subtype in morphological classification. *Blood* 1985; **65**:305–10.
◆7. Azar HA. Pathology of multiple myeloma. In Azar HA, Potter M (eds) *Multiple myeloma and related disorders*, Vol. 1. New York: Harper and Row, 1973:5.
●8. Greipp PR, Kyle RA. Clinical morphological and cell kinetic differences among multiple myeloma, monoclonal gammopathy of undetermined significance and smoldering multiple myeloma. *Blood* 1983; **62**:166–71.
9. Farquhar MG, Palade GE. The golgi apparatus (1954–1981) from artifact to center stage. *J Cell Biol* 1981; **91**(Suppl):77–103.
10. Maldonado JE, Brown AL Jr, Bayrd ED, Pease GL. Cytoplasmic and intranuclear electron-dense bodies in the myeloma cell. *Arch Pathol* 1966; **81**:484–500.
11. Pavelta M, Ludwig H. Ultrastructural studies of myeloma cells: observations concerning the golgi apparatus and intermediate-size filaments. *Am J Hematol* 1983; **15**:237–51.
12. Blom J, Mansa B, Wiik A. A study of Russell bodies in human monoclonal plasma cells by means of immunofluorescence and electron microscopy. *Acta Pathol Microbiol Scand* 1976; **84A**:335–49.

13. Maldonado JE, Bayrd ED, Brown AL Jr. The flaming cell in multiple myeloma. A light and electron microscopy study. *Am J Clin Pathol* 1965; **44**:605–12.
14. Jandl J. Multiple myeloma and other differentiated B cell malignancies. In *Blood: textbook of hematology*. Boston: Little Brown & Co, 1987:831.
15. Bergsagel DE. Plasma cell myeloma. In Williams WJ, Beutler E, Erslev AJ, Lichtman MA (eds) *Hematology*, 3rd edn. New York: McGraw-Hill, 1983:831.
◆16. Durie BGM, Salmon SE. Multiple myeloma, macroglobulinemia and monoclonal gammopathies. In Hoffbrand AV, Brian MC, Hirsh J (eds) *Recent advances in hematology*. Edinburgh: Churchill Livingstone, 1977:243.
◆17. Durie BGM. Staging and kinetics of multiple myeloma. *Semin Oncol* 1986; **13**:300–9.
◆18. Salmon SE, Cassady JR: Plasma cell neoplasms. In DeVita VT, Hellman S, Rosenberg S (eds) *Cancer, principles and practice of oncology*. Philadelphia: J.B. Lippincott, 1988:1864.
19. Rajkumar SV, Fonseca R, Dispenzieri A, Lacy MQ, Lust JA, Witzig TE, *et al*. Methods for estimation of bone marrow plasma cell involvement in myeloma: predictive value for response and survival in patients undergoing autologous stem cell transplantation. *Am J Hematol* 2001; **68**:269–75.
20. Costes V, Magen V, Legouffe E, Durand L, Baldet P, Rossi JF, *et al*. The Mi15 monoclonal antibody (anti-syndecan-1) is a reliable marker for quantifying plasma cells in paraffin-embedded bone marrow biopsy specimens. *Hum Pathol* 1999; **30**:1405–11.
21. Anderson KC, Bates MP, Slaughenhoupt B, Schlossman SF, Nadler LM. A monoclonal antibody with reactivity restricted to normal and neoplastic plasma cells. *J Immunol* 1984; **132**:3172–9.
22. Bayer-Garner IB, Sanderson RD, Dhodapkar MV, Owens RB, Wilson CS. Syndecan-1 (CD138) immunoreactivity in bone marrow biopsies of multiple myeloma: shed syndecan-1 accumulates in fibrotic regions. *Mod Pathol* 2001; **4**:1052–8.
23. Ling NR, MacLennan ICM, Mason DY. B-cell and plasma cell antigens: new and previously defined clusters. In McMichael AJ, Beverley PCL, Cobbold S, Crumpton MJ, Gilka W. (eds) *Leukocyte typing III: white cell differentiation antigens*. Oxford: Oxford University Press, 1987:302–35.
24. San Miguel JF, Caballero MD, Gonzalez M, Zola H, Lopez Borrasca A. Immunological phenotype of neoplasms involving the B cell in the last step of differentiation. *Br J Haematol* 1986; **62**:75–83.
25. Harada H, Kawano M, Huang N, *et al*. A Phenotypic difference of normal plasma cells from mature myeloma cells. *Blood* 1993; **81**:2658–63.
26. Barker H, Hamilton M, Ball J, Drew M, Franklin IM. Expression of adhesion molecules LFA-3 and N-CAM on normal and malignant human plasma cells. *Br J Haematol* 1992; **81**:331–5.
27. Ridley R, Xiao H, Hata H, Woodliff J, Epstein J, Sanderson RD. Expression of syndecan regulates human myeloma plasma cell adhesion to type 1 collagen. *Blood* 1993; **81**:767–74.
28. Rawstron AC, Fenton JA, Ashcroft J, English A, Jones RA, Richards SJ, *et al*. The interleukin-6 receptor alpha-chain (CD126) is expressed by neoplastic but not normal plasma cells. *Blood* 2000; **96**:3880–6.
29. Falini B, Fizzotti M, Pucciarini A, Bigerna B, Marafioti T, Gambacorta M, *et al*. A monoclonal antibody (MUM1p)

detects expression of the MUM1/IRF4 protein in a subset of germinal center B cells, plasma cells, and activated T cells. *Blood* 2000; **95**:2084–92.

30. Lima M, Teixeira MA, Fonseca S, Goncalves C, Guerra M, Queiros ML, et al. Immunophenotypic aberrations, DNA content and cell cycle analysis of plasma cells in patients with myeloma and monoclonal gammopathies. *Blood Cells Mol Dis* 2000; **26**:634–45.

●31. Mahmoud MS, Huang N, Nobuyoshi M, Lisukou IA, Tanaka H, Kawana MM. Altered expression of PaX-5 gene in human myeloma cells. *Blood* 1996; **87**:4311–15.

●32. Kubagawa J, Vogler LB, Capra JD, et al. Studies on the clonal origin of multiple myeloma. Use of individually specific (idiotype) antibodies to trace the oncogenic event to its earliest point of expression in B-cell differentiation. *J Exp Med* 1979; **150**:792–807.

33. Van Riet I, Vanderkerken K, De Greef C, Van Camp. Homing behaviour of the malignant cell clone in multiple myeloma. *Med Oncol* 1998; **15**:1554–64.

34. Ruiz-Arüelles GJ, Katzmann JA, Greipp PR, Gouchoroff NJ, Garton JP, Kyle RA. Multiple myeloma: circulating lymphocytes that express plasma cell antigens. *Blood* 1984; **64**:352–6.

35. Durie BGM, Grogan TM. CALLA-positive myeloma: an aggressive subtype with poor survival. *Blood* 1985; **66**:229–32.

36. Caligaris-Cappio F, Berui L, Tesio L, et al. Identification of malignant plasma cell precursors in the bone marrow of multiple myeloma. *J Clin Invest* 1985; **76**:1243–51.

37. Epstein J, Barlogie B, Katzmann J, Alexanian R. Phenotypic heterogeneity in aneuploid multiple myeloma indicates pre-B cell involvement. *Blood* 1988; 71:861–5.

●38. Grogan TM, Durie BGM, Lomen C, Spier C, Wirt DP, Nagle R, et al. Delineation of a novel pre-B cell component in plasma cell myeloma: immunochemical, immunophenotypic, genotypic, cytologic, cell culture and kinetic features. *Blood* 1987; **70**:932–42.

39. Pilarski LM, Mant MJ, Reuther BA. Pre-B cells in peripheral blood of multiple myeloma patients. *Blood* 1985; **66**:416–22.

●40. Grogan TM, Durie BGM, Spier CM, Richter L, Vela E. Myelomonocytic antigen positive multiple myeloma. *Blood* 1989; **73**:763–9.

●41. Epstein J, Xiao H, He X-Y. Markers of multiple hematopoietic cell lineages in multiple myeloma. *N Engl J Med* 1990; **322**:664–8.

42. Brown G, Bunce CM, Howie AJ, Lord JM. Stochastic or ordered lineage commitment during hemopoiesis, editorial. *Leukemia* 1987; **2**:150–3.

43. Spier CS, Grogan TM, Durie BGM, et al. T cell antigen-positive multiple myeloma. *Mod Pathol* 1990; **3**:302–7.

44. Buchsbaum RJ, Schwartz RS. Cellular origins of hematologic neoplasms. *N Engl J Med* 1990; **322**:694–6.

45. Robillard N, Jego G, Pellat-Deceunynck C, Pineau D, Puthier D, Mellerin MP, et al. CD28, a marker associated with tumoral expansion in multiple myeloma. *Clin Cancer Res* 1998; **4**:1521–6.

●46. Dalton WS, Grogan T, Rybski J, Scheper RJ, Richter L, Kailey J, et al. Immunohistochemical detection and quantitation of P-glycoprotein in multiple drug-resistant human myeloma cells: association with level of drug resistance and drug accumulation. *Blood* 1989; **73**:747–52.

47. Grogan T, Dalton W, Rybski J, Spier C, Meltzer P, Richter L, et al. Optimization of immunocytochemical P-glycoprotein assessment in multidrug-resistant plasma cell myeloma using 3 antibodies. *Lab Invest* 1990; **63**:815–24.

48. Grogan T, Spier C, Salmon S, Matzner M, Rybski J, Weinstein RS, et al. P-Glycoprotein expression in human plasma cell myeloma: correlation with prior chemotherapy. *Blood* 1993; **81**:490–5.

49. Durie BGM, Dalton WS. Reversal of drug-resistance in multiple myeloma with verapamil. *Br J Haematol* 1988; **68**:203–6.

50. Wyler B, Shao Y, Schneider E, Cianfriglia M, Scheper RJ, Frey BM, et al. Intermittent exposure to doxorubicin in vitro selects for multifactorial non-P-glycoprotein-associated multidrug resistance in RPMI 8226 human myeloma cells. *Br J Haematol* 1997; **97**:65–75.

51. Dalton WS, Grogan TM, Meltzer PS, Scheper RJ, Durie BG, Taylor CW, et al. Drug-resistance in multiple myeloma and non-Hodgkin's lymphoma: detection of P-glycoprotein and potential circumvention by addition of verapamil to chemotherapy. *J Clin Oncol* 1990; **7**:415–24.

52. Miller TP, Grogan TM, Dalton WS, Spier CS, Scheper RJ, Salmon SE. P-glycoprotein expression in malignant lymphoma and reversal of clinical drug resistance with chemotherapy plus high-dose verapamil. *J Clin Oncol* 1991; **9**:17–24.

53. Rimsza L, Dalton W, Campbell K, Salmon S, Grogan T. In multiple myeloma the non-P-glycoprotein multidrug resistance protein LRP is frequently expressed and an increased proliferative rate (Ki67 > 5%) is associated with a significantly shorter survival. *Leuk Lymphoma* 1999; **10**:123–6.

54. Filipits M, Drach J, Pohl G, Schuster J, Stranzl T, Ackermann J, et al. Expression of the lung resistance protein predicts poor outcome in patients with multiple myeloma. *Clin Cancer Res* 1999; **5**:2426–30.

55. Gratzner H. Monoclonal antibody to 5-bromo- and 5-iododeoxyuridine: a new reagent for detection of DNA replication. *Science* 1982; **218**:474–5.

56. Dolbeare F, Gratzner H, Pallavicini M, Gray JW. Flow cytometric measurement of total DNA content and incorporated bromodeoxyuridine. *Proc Natl Acad Sci USA* 1983; **80**:5573–7.

◆57. Durie BGM, Salmon SE. Staging, kinetics and flow cytometry of multiple myeloma. In Wiernik P, Cannellos G, Kyle R, Schiffer C (eds) *Neoplastic diseases of the blood.* New York: Churchill Livingstone, 1985:513.

58. Gerdes J, Dallenbach F, Lennert K. Growth fractions in malignant non-Hodgkin's lymphomas (NHL) as determined in situ with the monoclonal antibody Ki67. *Hematol Oncol* 1984; **2**:365–71.

59. Grogan TM, Lippman SM, Spier CM, Slymen DJ, Rybski J, Rangel CS, et al. Independent prognostic significance of a nuclear proliferative antigen in diffuse large cell lymphomas as determined by the monoclonal antibody Ki67. *Blood* 1988; **71**:1157–60.

60. Pruneri G, Fabris S, Baldini L, Carboni N, Zagano S, Colombi MA, et al. Immunohistochemical analysis of ayclin D1 shows deregulated expression in multiple myeloma with the t(11;14). *Am J Pathol* 2000; **156**:1505–13.

61. Wilson CS, Butch AW, Lai R, Medeiros LJ, Sawyer JR, Barlogie B, McCourty A, et al. Cyclin D1 and E2F-1 immunoreactivity

in bone marrow biopsy specimens of multiple myeloma: relationship to proliferative activity, cytogenetic abnormalities and DNA ploidy. *Br J Haematol* 2001; **112**:776–82.

62. Hoyer JD, Hanson CA, Foneseca R, Greipp PR, Dewald GW, Kurtin PJ. The (11;14)(q13;q32) translocation in multiple myeloma. A morphologic and immunohistochemical study. Hematopathology t(11:14)(q13:q32) in multiple myeloma. *Am J Clin Pathol* 2000; **113**:831–7.

63. Tosi P, Pellacani A, Visani G, Ottaviani E, Ronconi S, Zamagri E, *et al*. In vitro treatment with retinoids decreases bcl-2 protein expression and enhances dexamethasone-induced cytotoxicity and apoptosis in multiple myeloma cells. *Eur J Haematol* 1999; **62**:143–8.

64. Landowski T, Gleason-Guzman M, Dalton W. Selection for drug resistance to fas-mediated apoptosis. *Blood* 1997; **89**:1854–61.

●65. Villunger A, Egle A, Marschitz I, Kos M, Bock G, Ludwig H, *et al*. Constitutive expression of Fas (Apo-1/CD95) ligand on multiple myeloma cells: a potential mechanism of tumor-induced suppression of immune surveillance. *Blood* 1997; **90**:12–20.

66. Silvestris F, Tucci M, Cafforio P, Dammacco F. Fas-L up-regulation by highly malignant myeloma plasma cells: role in the pathogenesis of anemia and disease progression. *Blood* 2001; **97**:1155–64.

67. Lynch RG, Rohrer JM, Odermatt B, Gebel M, Autry JR, Hoover RG. Immunoregulation of murine myeloma cell growth and differentiation: a monoclonal model of B cell differentiation. *Immunol Rev* 1979; **48**:45–80.

68. Broder S, Humphrey R, Durm M, Blackman M, Meade B, Goldman C, *et al*. Impaired synthesis of polyclonal (non-paraprotein) immunoglobulin by circulating lymphocytes from patients with multiple myeloma: role of suppressor cells. *N Engl J Med* 1975; **293**:887–92.

69. Dianzani U, Pileri A, Boccadoro M, Palumbo S, Massaia M. Activated idiotype-reactive cells in suppressor/cytotoxic subpopulations of monoclonal gammopathies: correlation with diagnosis and disease status. *Blood* 1988; **72**:1064–8.

70. Rai Takari M, Brown RD, Sze D, Yuen E, Barrow L, Nelson M, *et al*. T-cell expansions in patients with multiple myeloma have a phenotype of cytotoxic T-cells. *Br J Haematol* 2000; **110**:203–9.

71. Kronland R, Grogan T, Spier C, Wirt D, Rangel C, Richter L, *et al*. Immunotopographic assessment of lymphoid and plasma cell malignancies in the bone marrow. *Hum Pathol* 1985; **16**:1247–54.

72. Xagoraris I, Paterakis G, Zolota B, Zikos P, Maniatis A, Mouzaki A. Expression of granzyme B and d perforin in multiple myeloma. *Acta Hematol* 2001; **105**:125–9.

73. Besostri B, Beggiato E, Bianchi A, Mariani S, Coscia M, Peola S, *et al*. Increased expression of non-functional killer inhibitory receptor CD94 in CD8+ cells of myeloma patients. *Br J Haematol* 2000; **109**:46–53.

74. Stauder R, Van Driel M, Schwarzler C, Thaler J, Lokhorst HM, Kreuser ED, *et al*. Different CD44 splicing patterns define prognostic subgroups in multiple myeloma. *Blood* 1996; **88**:3101–8.

●75. Van Camp B, Durie BGM, Spier C, De Wacle M, Van Riet I, Vela E, *et al*. Plasma cells in multiple myeloma express a natural killer cell-associated antigen: CD56 (NKH-1; Leu 19). *Blood* 1990; **76**:377–82.

76. Drach J, Gattringer C, Huber H. Expression of the neural cell adhesion molecule (CD56) by human myeloma cells. *Clin Exp Immunol* 1991; **83**:418–22.

77. Ong F, Kaiser U, Seelen P, Hermans J, Wijermans P, Kieviet W, *et al*. Serum neural cell adhesion molecule differentiates multiple myeloma from paraproteinemias due to other causes. *Blood* 1996; **87**:712–16.

78. Pellat-Deceunynck C, Barille S, Jego G, Puthier D, Robillard M, Pineau D, *et al*. The absence of CD56 (NCAM) on malignant plasma cells is a hallmark of plasma cell leukemia and of a special subset of multiple myeloma. *Leukemia* 1998; **12**:1977–82.

79. Van Driel M, Gunthert U, Stauder R, Joling P, Lokhorst H, Bloem A. CD44 isoforms distringuish between bone marrow plasma cells from normal individuals and patients with multiple myeloma at different stages of disease. *Leukemia* 1998; **12**:1821–8.

80. Folkman J. Clinical applications of research on angiogenesis. *N Engl J Med* 1995; **333**:1757–63.

81. Ribatti D, Vacca A, Nico B, Quondamatteo F, Ria R, Minischetti M, *et al*. Bone marrow angiogenesis and mast cell density increase simultaneously with progression of human multiple myeloma. *Br J Cancer* 1999; **79**:451–5.

82. Rajkumar SV, Leong T, Roche PC, Fonseca R, Dispenzieri A, Lacy MQ, *et al*. Prognostic value of bone marrow angiogenesis in multiple myeloma. *Clin Cancer Res* 2000; **6**:3111–16.

83. Vacca A, Ribatti D, Roccaro AM, Frigeri A, Dammacco F. Bone marrow angiogenesis in patients with active multiple myeloma. *Semin Oncol* 2001; **28**:543–50.

84. Bellamy WT. Expression of vascular endothelial growth factor and its receptors in multiple myeloma and other hematopoietic malignancies. *Semin Oncol* 2001; **28**:551–9.

85. Dankbar B, Padro T, Leo R, Feldmann B, Kropff M, Mesters RM, *et al*. Vascular endothelial growth factor and interleukin-6 in paracrine tumor-stromal cell interactions in multiple myeloma. *Blood* 2000; **95**:2630–6.

86. Vacca A, Frigeri A, Ribatti D, Nicchia GP, Nico B, Ria R, *et al*. Miccrovessel overexpression of aquaporin 1 parallels bone marrow angiogenesis in patients with active multiple myeloma. *Br J Haematol* 2001; **113**:415–21.

●87. Bellamy W, Richter L, Frutiger Y, Grogan T. Expression of vascular endothelial growth factor and its receptors in hematopoietic malignancies. *Cancer Res* 1999; **59**:728–33.

◆88. Barlogie B, Latreille J, Swartzenchuber D, *et al*. Quantitative cytology in myeloma research. In Salmon SE (ed.) *Clinics in hematology*. London: Saunders, 1982:19.

89. Berenson J, Wong R, Kim K, Brown N, Lichtenstein A. Evidence for peripheral blood B lymphocyte but not T lymphocyte involvement in multiple myeloma. *Blood* 1987; **70**:1550–3.

90. Omede P, Boccadoro M, Gallone G, Frieri R, Battaglio S, Redoglia V, *et al*. Multiple myeloma: increased circulating lymphocytes carrying plasma cell-associated antigens as an indicator of poor survival. *Blood* 1990; **76**:1375–9.

91. Mellstedt H, Hammarström S, Holm G. Monoclonal lymphocyte population in human plasma cell myeloma. *Clin Exp Immunol* 1974; **17**:371–84.

92. Bast E, Van Camp B, Reynaert P, Wiringa G, Ballieux R. Idiotypic peripheral blood lymphocytes in monoclonal gammopathy. *Clin Exp Immunol* 1982; **47**:677–82.

93. Ruiz-Arüelles GJ, Katzmann JA, Greipp PR, Gouchoroff NJ, Garton JP, Kyle RA. Multiple myeloma: circulating lymphocytes that express plasma cell antigens. *Blood* 1984; **64**:352–6.

94. Ullrich S, Zolla-Pazner S. Immunoregulatory circuits in myeloma. In Hoffbrand AV, Lasch HG, Nathan DG, Salmon SE (eds) *Clinics in haematology*, Vol. 11. Eastbourne: WB Saunders, 1982:87–111.

95. Rawstron AC, Barrans SL, Blythe D, English A, Richards SJ, Fenton JAL, *et al.* In multiple myeloma, only a single stage of neoplastic plasma cell differentiation can be identified by VLA-5 and CD45 expression. *Br J Haematol* 2001; **113**:794–802.

96. Delschlaegel U, Freund D, Range U, Ehninger G, Nowak R. Flow cytometric DNA-quantification of three-color immunophenotyped cells for subpopulation specific determination of aneoploidy and proliferation. *J Immunol Meth* 2001; **253**:145–52.

●97. Alexanian R. Localized and indolent myeloma. *Blood* 1980; **56**:521–5.

●98. Kyle RA, Greipp R. Smouldering multiple myeloma. *N Engl J Med* 1980; **302**:1347–9.

99. Knowling MA, Harwood AR, Bergsagel DE. Comparison of extramedullary plasmacytomas with solitary and multiple plasma cell tumors of the bone. *J Clin Oncol* 1983; **1**:255–62.

◆100. Kyle RA. Monoclonal gammopathy of undetermined significance (MGUS): a review. In Hoffbrand AV, Lasch HG, Nathan DG, Salmon SE (eds) *Clinics in haematology*, Vol. 11. Eastbourne: WB Saunders, 1982:123–50.

●101. Kyle RA. Monoclonal gammopathy of undetermined significance: natural history in 241 cases. *Am J Med* 1978; **64**:814–26.

◆102. Salmon S, Cassady JR. Plasma cell neoplasms. In DeVita VT, Hellman S, Rosenberg S (eds) *Cancer, principles and practice of oncology*. Philadelphia: J.B. Lippincott, 1988:1862.

◆103. Azar HA. Pathology of multiple myeloma. In Azar HA, Potter M (eds) *Multiple myeloma and related disorders*, Vol. 1. New York: Harper and Row, 1973:8.

◆104. Bergsagel DE. Plasma cell myeloma. In Williams WJ, Beutler E, Erslev AJ, Lichtman MA (eds) *Hematology*, 3rd edn. New York: McGraw-Hill, 1983:1090.

105. Bergsagel DE. Plasma cell myeloma. In Williams WJ, Beutler E, Erslev AJ, Lichtman MA (eds) *Hematology*, 3rd edn. New York: McGraw-Hill, 1983:1089.

106. Isobe T, Osserman EF. Pathologic conditions associated with plasma cell dyscrasias: a study of 806 cases. *Ann NY Acad Sci* 1972; **190**:507–18.

107. Williams RC, Bailly RC, Howe RB. Studies of 'benign' serum M-components. *Am J Med Sci* 1969; **257**:275–93.

108. Azar HA. Pathology of multiple myeloma. In Azar HA, Potter M (eds) *Multiple myeloma and related disorders*, Vol. 1. New York, Harper and Row, 1973:10.

109. Kapadia S, Desai U, Cheng U. Extramedullary plasmacytoma of the head and neck: a clinicopathologic study of 20 cases. *Medicine* 1982; **61**:317–29.

9

Biochemical and immunological investigations

JOANNA M. SHELDON AND PAMELA G. RICHES

INTRODUCTION

There are a number of diseases, including myeloma, that are associated with clonal proliferation of B lymphocytes. Biochemical investigations play an important role in their diagnosis, prognosis, and monitoring. The monoclonal immunoglobulin resulting from the clonal proliferation of the B cells is an important tumor marker and reliable detection, typing, and quantification of the monoclonal protein (M-protein or paraprotein) is vital. Measurement of proteins related to B-cell function or turnover, e.g. the polyclonal background immunoglobulins or β_2-microglobulin, can give indications of tumor burden and prognosis. Additionally, in the investigation of patients with B-cell dyscrasias, a wide range of biochemical markers are useful to monitor renal function, bone and calcium metabolism, infection, and the effects of treatments. Where possible, laboratories offering any of the investigations discussed in this chapter should participate in appropriate external quality assurance (EQA) schemes (a list of EQA providers is shown in Appendix A).

Monoclonal proteins may be present at very high concentrations and often show manifestations not seen with normal polyclonal immunoglobulins, such as hyperviscosity, protein precipitation, or interference in analytical systems, where their presence can influence a variety of analytes and methods. Where a monoclonal immunoglobulin directly interferes with an assay, this will be discussed in following sections; however, it is important to

remember that monoclonal components are not 'normal' constituents of blood and may indirectly influence assays. They can influence the serum viscosity, reactions of the serum with other fluids, bind non-specifically to themselves or to other proteins, and precipitate non-specifically. There should be a low index of suspicion when samples containing monoclonal components show unexpected or markedly aberrant results.

Immunoglobulin structure

Immunoglobulins produced by cells of the B-lymphocyte lineage are proteins that show antibody activity. The basic monomeric immunoglobulin unit consists of two identical heavy chains and two identical light chains arranged in a Y-shape (Fig. 9.1). In humans, there are five different heavy chains (γ, α, μ, δ, and ϵ) that determine the five immunoglobulin classes (IgG, IgA, IgM, IgD, and IgE). The basic properties of the immunoglobulins are shown in Table 9.1. In addition, there are four subclasses of IgG (IgG1, IgG2, IgG3, IgG4) and two subclasses of IgA (IgA1, IgA2). There are two light chain types (κ and λ). IgA and IgM both occur as polymers of the basic unit facilitated by the addition of an additional peptide synthesized by the B cell, the J chain. In plasma, IgM occurs as a pentamer. IgA can occur as a dimer and this is the predominant form in secretions. A secretory piece is a glycoprotein synthesized by mucosal epithelial cells and integrated into the secreted IgA molecules to facilitate secretion, but it also makes the IgA more resistant to protein degradation within the mucosal environment.

Both the heavy and light chains are composed of repeating structural domains. The class (or subclass) of the heavy chains or type of light chains is determined by the amino acid sequences in areas of the molecule called the constant domains, of which there are three or four depending upon the class. These constant domains confer non-antigen-binding function to the immunoglobulin molecules. The light chains have a single constant domain. Both heavy chains and light chains have a variable domain within which there is considerable amino acid variability. The heavy and light chains are arranged so that the variable domains are adjacent, forming a groove in which antigen binding occurs. Each antigen binding site will recognize a specific sequence or pattern of determinants,

called the epitope, on the antigen. Most antibodies will show high-affinity binding for one or only a few epitopes, although some low-affinity cross-reactivity with unrelated epitopes may be found. Many thousands of antigens are encountered during a lifetime and each antigen is estimated to result in the production of over 1000 different antibodies. A segmental organization of the genes for the immunoglobulin chains enables enormous variability in the immunoglobulin antigen binding site to be generated.

Production of immunoglobulins

The structure of the immunoglobulin genes and their rearrangement during B-cell development is described in detail in Chapter 3. In humans, the gene for the production of the immunoglobulin heavy chain is located in chromosome 14 and the genes for the κ and λ light chains are located on chromosomes 2 and 22, respectively. Diversity of the variable region is generated by the large number of possible combinations between the V, D, and J, or V and J regions of the genes and by somatic mutation generated during the proliferation of B cells during immune responses. There are two copies of each chromosome, so each cell, theoretically, has two chances for each gene to be successfully rearranged. The immunoglobulin heavy-chain gene(s) is rearranged first followed by the κ gene rearrangement. In about 40% of cells, the κ rearrangements are abortive and the cell then proceeds to the λ gene rearrangement. A small excess of free light chains (polyclonal) is constantly being produced; this is an entirely normal part of the B-cell function. The immunoglobulin molecule is then assembled and expressed on the surface of B cells. The cell is now committed to a light-chain type and unique variable region specificity (also called the idiotype). The organization of the heavy-chain gene enables the variable region to be spliced on to a different heavy chain by the process of class switching. This occurs after interaction with antigen, when cells that show appropriate recognition of the antigen are driven to proliferate. Some cells will mature

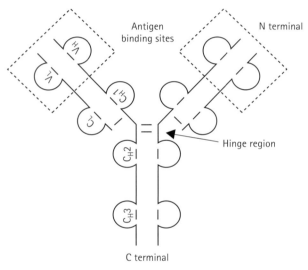

Figure 9.1 *Sketch of the basic monomeric immunoglobulin unit consisting of two identical heavy chains and two identical light chains arranged in a Y-shape. V_H, heavy-chain variable region; C_H, heavy-chain constant region (C_H1, C_H2, $C_H3 \pm C_H4$); V_L, light-chain variable region; C_L, light-chain constant region; ——, disulfide bonds (variable number in hinge region).*

Table 9.1 *The basic properties of the five classes of immunoglobulin*

	Molecular mass (kDa)	Half-life (days)	Usual molecular form	Subclasses	Approximate normal adult serum concentration (g/L)
IgG	150	23	Monomer	4	6.0–16.0
IgA	160 (monomer) 385 (secretory)	6	Monomer (circulating) Dimer (secretory)	2	0.8–4.0
IgM	950	5	Pentamer	–	0.5–2.0
IgD	180	3	Monomer	–	0.03–0.06
IgE	190	2.5	Monomer	–	<0.003

into memory cells, while others into end-differentiated plasma cells, and these are typically non-proliferative, have little membrane-bound immunoglobulin but produce large amounts of secreted immunoglobulin.

Under normal circumstances, there is enormous microheterogeneity amongst the immunoglobulin molecules. This results in 'polyclonal' immunoglobulins representing all classes, light-chain types, and a large number of different idiotypes produced by a large number of different B-cell clones. Monoclonal antibodies that consist of a single heavy-chain class, light-chain type, and idiotype result from the proliferation of a single clone of B cells. However, monoclonal B cells, especially those that have undergone malignant transformation, do not necessarily produce intact immunoglobulin. In approximately 20% of myeloma cases, they produce only monoclonal free light chains (Bence Jones protein). Almost all variations on the normal immunoglobulin molecules are possible; monoclonal monomeric (7S) instead of the normal pentameric IgM may be secreted, monoclonal fragments, e.g. free heavy chains (rarely seen in myeloma) and half molecules or truncated molecules can be seen. It is also possible to see combinations of immunoglobulin fragments and intact monoclonal immunoglobulin, with Bence Jones protein often detected in IgG, IgA, and IgD myeloma and in μ chain disease.

Any monoclonal protein or fragment will appear as a homogeneous compact band in electrophoretic separations and is termed a paraprotein. The term 'paraprotein' was first introduced in 1940 by Apitz to describe the proteins in blood, urine or tissues produced by myeloma cells and is synonymous with the terms 'monoclonal component' and 'M-protein'. Intact monoclonal immunoglobulin is most often found in the serum, although these proteins can 'leak' into the urine where there is renal damage. Low-molecular-weight fragments and Bence Jones protein pass readily through the glomerulus and into the urine. Clearly, these proteins must first pass through the blood compartment, where they may be found at low concentrations with normal renal function and at higher concentrations when their renal clearance is impaired.

INVESTIGATIONS OF MONOCLONAL COMPONENTS IN SERUM AND/OR URINE

The detection, typing, and quantification of monoclonal components in serum and urine are essential laboratory investigations in the diagnosis and monitoring of both malignant and non-malignant monoclonal B-cell expansions.[1] A serum paraprotein and/or urine Bence Jones protein is a highly sensitive tumor marker for certain B-cell malignancies, particularly myeloma (>95%) and Waldenström's macroglobulinemia (100%). A monoclonal component can also be found in other B-cell malignancies and in non-malignant diseases (see Table 9.2). It is important to note that the detection of a monoclonal protein does not necessarily indicate that the patient has myeloma or even a malignant transformation of B cells, nor does the absence of a paraprotein completely exclude the presence of myeloma or B cell malignancy. Fig. 9.2

Table 9.2 *Disorders associated with monoclonal immunoglobulin production*

- Malignant disorders
  - Multiple myeloma
  - Solitary plasmacytoma
  - Waldenström's macroglobulinemia
  - Non-Hodgkin's lymphoma
  - Chronic lymphocytic leukemia
- Clonal B-cell proliferation (not necessarily malignant)
  - Monoclonal gammopathy of unknown significance (MGUS)
  - AL amyloidosis[a]
  - Cryoglobulinemia/immune complex disease
  - Primary cold agglutinin disease
  - Peripheral neuropathy (generally a variant of MGUS)[a]
  - Dermatological disorders
    Lichen myxedematosus
    Pyoderma gangrenosum
- Transient
  - Post-infection
  - During regeneration after stem-cell transplantation

[a] Amyloidosis and neurological symptoms may also occur as complications in malignant disorders.

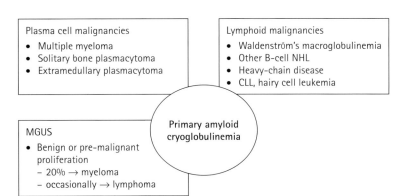

Plasma cell malignancies
- Multiple myeloma
- Solitary bone plasmacytoma
- Extramedullary plasmacytoma

Lymphoid malignancies
- Waldenström's macroglobulinemia
- Other B-cell NHL
- Heavy-chain disease
- CLL, hairy cell leukemia

MGUS
- Benign or pre-malignant proliferation
  - 20% → myeloma
  - occasionally → lymphoma

Primary amyloid cryoglobulinemia

Figure 9.2 *The disorders associated with paraproteins showing the overlap of AL amyloidosis and cryoglobulinemia with these diseases. CLL, chronic lymphocytic leukemia; NHL, non-Hodgkin's lymphoma.*

shows the major disorders associated with paraproteins, and indications for the investigation for the presence of a monoclonal immunoglobulin are shown in Table 9.3.

Samples and sample preparation

The types of samples appropriate for use in the various investigations discussed in this chapter are shown in Appendix B; however, if local laboratory protocols are available, they should be used.

SERUM

Serum samples are preferred for protein electrophoresis because the fibrinogen band in plasma can be mistaken for, or can mask, a paraprotein. Blood should be collected into tubes without anticoagulant and preferably without any additives (clot activator or gel separator). Serum should be allowed to clot, then centrifuged and separated and can be stored, in the short term, at 4 °C. If the samples are not contaminated with bacteria, then immunoglobulins, most monoclonal proteins, and most serum proteins are stable at 4 °C for at least 1 month. The exceptions to this are IgD monoclonal proteins and free heavy chains, which are both very susceptible to post-synthetic proteolytic degradation, and it is recommended that they should be analyzed as soon as possible after collection.

Table 9.3 *Indications for the investigation of serum and urine for a monoclonal immunoglobulin*

- Clinical symptoms
  - Backache
  - Lassitude
  - Recurrent infection
- Clinical syndromes
  - Renal failure
  - Nephrotic syndrome
  - Peripheral neuropathy
  - Hyperviscosity
  - Carpal tunnel syndrome
  - Malabsorption
- Radiological findings
  - Osteolytic lesions
  - Pathological fractures
- Hematological findings
  - Normochromic, normocytic anemia
  - Raised erythrocyte sedimentation rate
- Biochemical findings
  - Raised serum total protein
  - Raised serum globulin (total protein minus albumin)
  - Proteinuria
  - Abnormal renal function tests
  - Hypercalcemia
  - Subnormal immunoglobulin concentrations

The addition of sodium azide to a concentration of 1 mg/mL has been suggested as an antibacterial measure, but this practice is losing popularity owing to the safety issues of using sodium azide and also because azide can interfere with a number of immunoassays.[2] For longer-term storage, −40 °C to −70 °C is recommended. Storage at −20 °C should be discouraged because it is not the optimal temperature for protein stability. Repeated freezing and thawing of samples should always be avoided.

URINE

An early morning urine sample (usually the most concentrated of the day) should be used for the detection of Bence Jones protein in the urine. When Bence Jones protein excretion is to be used for monitoring disease, a timed collection is necessary. Unfortunately, 24-hour urine collections are notoriously inaccurate, so other approaches include the use of random urine samples with analytes corrected relative to albumin or creatinine concentration, or a timed 4- or 6-hour collection. The urine matrix renders proteins less stable than in serum and many of the problems associated with the interpretation of urine electrophoresis pattern are related to degradation on storage; urine should, therefore, be examined as soon as possible after collection. Near-patient testing for protein with, e.g. 'Dipstix' and 'Albustix,' will only detect urine albumin and cannot detect Bence Jones protein.

Protein electrophoresis

Protein electrophoresis is the only reliable method for the detection of paraproteins in serum or urine. Other methods have been proposed, such as the quantification of total (free and bound) κ and λ light chain concentrations or of free κ and λ light chains (see later), but no method has yet approached protein electrophoresis in terms of analytical specificity and sensitivity for the detection of monoclonal components. Once the abnormal band has been detected by electrophoresis, its concentrations can be determined by scanning densitometry. Immunofixation should be used to confirm clonality by typing of heavy and light chains. Immunofixation is also recommended for the sensitive detection of paraproteins where there is a strong suspicion but routine electrophoresis is negative.

Protein electrophoresis is most often done using agarose gel as a support medium, and both manual and automated systems are available. Increasingly automated capillary zone electrophoresis (CZE) systems are being introduced but, to date, the available dedicated laboratory systems have only been suitable for serum separations and have been unsuccessful in their adaptation to urine electrophoresis. Companies that make reliable electrophoresis systems are shown in Appendix C.

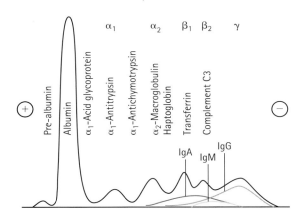

Figure 9.3 *The characteristic electrophoretic mobility of the major serum proteins at pH 8.6.*

SERUM ELECTROPHORESIS

Serum separated by electrophoresis at pH 8.6, both agarose and CZE systems, generates five major zones. Figure 9.3 shows the typical mobility of the major serum proteins. Ideally, agarose separations should be long enough (3–4 cm) to allow good separation of zones and show a good spread of the β–γ zone, which is achieved by properties of the agarose gel and buffer system that produce high endosmotic flow. The majority of serum paraproteins will be found in the β and γ zone, although paraproteins can be found anywhere on the electrophoretic separation between the α-1 zone and the post-γ region. Monoclonal heavy chains may show as diffuse zones running very anodally in the α2–β region of the electrophoretic separation. Representative examples of serum protein electrophoretic patterns are shown in Fig. 9.4.

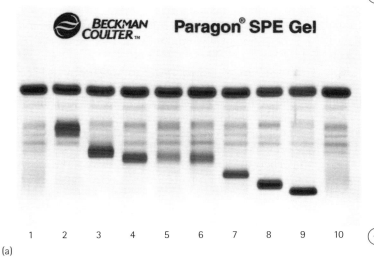

(a)

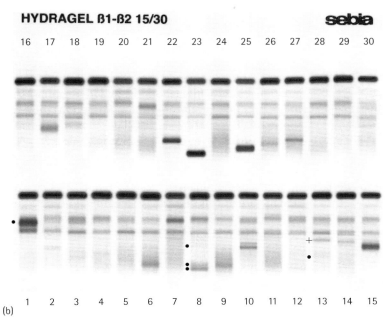

(b)

Figure 9.4 *Representative examples of serum protein electrophoretic patterns using two different gel electrophoresis systems. (a) Normal serum pattern in tracks 1 and 10. Samples in tracks 2–9 all show abnormal bands ranging from α_2 mobility to slow-γ mobility. Some of the samples are showing an additional lipoprotein band between the α_2 and β_1 zones (easily seen in track 10). Many of the samples are slightly aged and have lost the β_2 zone owing to degradation of the C3 complement component. (b) Normal serum pattern in track 28. Many of the samples show clear paraprotein bands, examples of less obvious paraproteins are seen in tracks 1, 8, and 13 and marked with •. Track 1 shows the same sample as track 2 in Fig. 9.4a. There is an IgA κ paraprotein band running in the α_2 region. Track 8 shows three small paraprotein bands (an IgG κ, an IgG λ, and an IgM κ) – an example of an oligoclonal response. Track 13 shows a diffuse 'zone' in the gamma – this is an IgD λ paraprotein band with a typically diffuse appearance. The sharp band in the β_2 region (+) is retained λ Bence Jones protein.*

Table 9.4 *Serum proteins that may be mistaken for monoclonal proteins*

- Fibrinogen in plasma or inadequately clotted samples results in an additional band in the fast γ region.
- Hemolysis during collection or processing of blood will result in a haptoglobin–hemoglobin complex that results in splitting of the normally homogeneous α_2 zone. Free hemoglobin runs in the β-region of the electrophoretic separation.
- Allotypic variants, e.g. α_1-antitrypsin, may result in two bands in a normally homogeneous region.
- Acute-phase protein increases, e.g. C-reactive protein, may result in additional bands being present.
- Lipoproteins may give distinct bands in the β region in agarose systems.

Paraproteins may be missed if they are present at low serum concentration ($<5.0\,g/L$), where the mobility coincides with other bands, such as β globulins, or where there is no suppression of normal background immunoglobulin concentrations. Problems occur most often with low-concentration IgM or IgA paraproteins. Whenever there is a raised concentration of IgA or IgM, with no clear increased staining in the β–γ region that would indicate a polyclonal increase, immunofixation should be done. IgD paraproteins and free heavy chains are susceptible to post-synthetic degradation, which results in diffuse paraprotein bands on electrophoresis, and these may be missed if present at low concentrations. Precipitation of paraproteins on cooling of blood samples (monoclonal cryoglobulins) and subsequent removal with the cell pellet can also result in failure to detect a significant paraprotein. Conversely, there are a number of proteins that can be mistaken for monoclonal protein in electrophoresis separations, which are summarized in Table 9.4.

URINE ELECTROPHORESIS

Urine should be checked in every patient in whom B-cell malignancy is being considered, including patients where no serum monoclonal component is detected. In patients where Bence Jones protein (BJP) has been detected in the urine, its concentration should be monitored. There is a small number of patients where BJP is not detected at presentation but does appear later ('Bence Jones escape') in the disease course; therefore, it is important to check urine regularly for BJP.

The presence of BJP provides a high index of suspicion for malignancy, although it does occur in apparently benign conditions. Even low concentrations ($10\,mg/L$) may be significant, so that high sensitivity electrophoresis of urine is essential. Sensitive stains for use with agarose gels are now available making the analysis of unconcentrated urine possible. Alternatively, the urine can

be concentrated at least 100-fold using concentration systems, where the water, ions, and low-molecular-weight peptides are separated from the higher-molecular-weight constituents by centrifugation across a semipermeable membrane. The molecular exclusion of these membranes should be between $11.5\,kDa$ and $13.0\,kDa$. There are comparable systems that do not require centrifugation where the water and low-molecular-weight molecules are pulled across the semipermeable membrane by osmosis. The companies making urine concentrators are shown in Appendix C. The urine concentrate can then be analyzed alongside serum in the agarose systems. A trace of albumin should be visible in every urine sample; failure to detect any albumin on the electrophoretic separation necessitates further concentration and reanalysis. Where a BJP is present in significant concentrations ($>100\,mg/L$) with no accompanying glomerular or tubular proteinuria, identification is straightforward. However, the renal damage associated with Bence Jones proteinuria frequently results in complex, non-standard patterns requiring immunofixation to resolve the possible presence of BJP.[3] Representative examples of urine protein electrophoretic patterns are shown in Fig. 9.5. A low concentration of BJP may also accompany significant glomerular proteinuria in patients with light-chain renal amyloidosis. Any urine with a marked glomerular proteinuria should be investigated by immunofixation even in the absence of a band suggestive of BJP.

There are a number of proteins that can be mistaken for monoclonal protein in urine electrophoresis separations, particularly where there is an element of tubular proteinuria; these are summarized in Table 9.5.

Typing of monoclonal immunoglobulin in serum and urine

Once a paraprotein band has been detected, it is important for the heavy- and light-chain components to be identified by immunofixation. This confirms monoclonality and the paraprotein type may give the clinician additional information about the underlying tumor and prognosis. Other indications for immunofixation are shown in Table 9.6. The distribution of heavy chain classes in B-cell dyscrasias is shown in Table 9.7.[4–7] The light-chain distribution of the common paraproteins is similar to that of the normal polyclonal immunoglobulin with a predominance of κ to λ (about 2:1). IgD paraproteins are usually of λ light chain type, although κ may be found and the few reported IgE paraproteins have all been of κ light chain type.

The electrophoretic pattern may change during the course of a patient's disease or treatment, e.g. some patients may start producing BJP during the course of the disease. Complete disappearance of a paraprotein is rare with standard-dose chemotherapy but is occurring

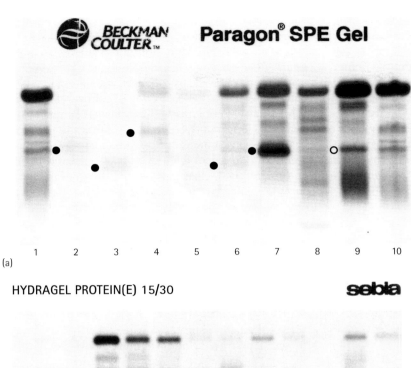

BECKMAN COULTER™   Paragon® SPE Gel

1 2 3 4 5 6 7 8 9 10
(a)

HYDRAGEL PROTEIN(E) 15/30   **sebia**

1 2 3 4 5 6 7 8 9 10 11 12 13
(b)

Figure 9.5 *Representative samples of urine protein electrophoretic patterns using two different gel electrophoresis systems. Samples in tracks 1 and 10 in (a) are normal serum. All other samples are urines that have been concentrated at least 100×. The majority of tracks show one or more protein bands in addition to albumin. Samples should be reconcentrated and rerun if no protein staining is seen, as in (b) 1–3. Clearly visible bands subsequently shown by immunofixation to represent Bence Jones protein (BJP) are indicated by closed circles. These bands vary in amount and mobility in the different samples. In all cases it is necessary to confirm that the bands represent BJP by performing immunofixation (IF). IF should also be performed in cases of strong clinical suspicion even if no clear band is visible on routine electrophoresis; for example urines (a) 5, (b) 7 and (b) 10 were all shown to contain BJP by IF. The pattern in track (a) 8 results from a tubular proteinuria and that in tracks (a) 9 and (b) 4 from a glomerular proteinuria. Bands of restricted mobility in the beta1globulin position in the latter samples, indicated by open circles, are due to transferrin. Note that BJP may also run in the beta1globulin position, as in samples (a) 2, (a) 7 and (b) 5.*

Table 9.5 *Urine proteins that may be mistaken for monoclonal proteins*

- α- and β-microglobulins
  - β_2-microglobulin, when present in high concentrations will give a very prominent band
- Lysozyme (migrating in the slow γ region)
- Degraded fragments of glomerular origin
- Seminal fluid proteins (very rare)

increasingly with treatment regimens using high-dose chemotherapy and bone marrow transplantation. Immunofixation is recommended for distinguishing between good partial remission and complete remission post hematopoietic stem cell transplantation for myeloma when no monoclonal component is seen on the electrophoretic separation. Immunofixation has also been shown to have comparable sensitivity to the detection of monoclonal immunoglobulin gene rearrangements.[8] An oligoclonal banding pattern is sometimes seen in patients after stem cell transplantation (see Fig. 9.8b, p. 135) and it is important to distinguish this from the original paraproteinemia.[9–12]

AGAROSE GEL IMMUNOFIXATION

Immunofixation has been the method of choice for the sensitive detection and typing of paraproteins in serum and urine for many years.[13] It is quick, flexible, and simple to interpret. Immunoelectrophoresis should not be used; abnormalities readily detected by immunofixation are missed by immunoelectrophoresis. Immunoisoelectric focusing, although reported to be more sensitive than immunofixation for the detection of paraproteins, has not gained general acceptance in diagnostic laboratories.[14]

Briefly, samples are separated by electrophoresis in a number of tracks of an agarose gel. Antiserum against each protein to be tested is layered on to the relevant protein separation and the gel incubated. (Companies producing reliable antisera are shown in Appendix C.) Insoluble immune complexes are formed, which precipitate, i.e. become 'fixed' into the matrix of the gel. The gels are then washed to remove any unreacted antibody and all the soluble protein in the sample that is not part of the immune complex, leaving the precipitated immune complex to be visualized by protein staining. This technique enhances the sensitivity of gel electrophoresis by both removing background staining and selectively increasing the amount of protein (by adding antibodies) in the band of interest. Representative examples of serum and urine immunofixation patterns are shown in Figs 9.6 and 9.7, and serial samples from one patient are shown in Fig. 9.8 (p. 135).

Table 9.6 *Major indications for immunofixation of serum or urine*

- To confirm clonality of a band detected by electrophoresis: Routinely test for the α, γ, or μ heavy chains, and the κ and λ light chains. Test for the δ and ε heavy chains where a serum shows monoclonal light chains without a corresponding α, γ, or μ heavy chain.
- To exclude low-concentration monoclonal components even where no band is apparent on electrophoresis but with clinical indications, e.g. AL amyloid.
- To exclude the presence of monoclonal IgA or IgM, if the sample is showing raised concentrations without obvious β–γ fusion, indicating a polyclonal increase.
- To positively identify other proteins that may be mistaken for monoclonal immunoglobulins, e.g. fibrinogen, C-reactive protein, β_2-microglobulin, and complement components, to exclude paraproteinaemia.
- Confirmation of complete remission following therapy when no monoclonal component is seen on the electrophoretic separation.

Serum immunofixation

Some large aggregated IgM paraproteins may precipitate on to the gel before immunofixation, fail to be removed during the washing stage, and thus give a reaction in all antiserum lanes. The true identity of the immunoglobulin can usually be revealed by mild sulfhydryl reduction (brief details of the method are shown in Appendix D) prior to electrophoresis and immunofixation. Free heavy chains usually show as diffuse zones that react only with antiserum to one of the heavy chains but not with antiserum to light chains. However, the conformational arrangement of some IgA or IgD paraproteins results in the 'hiding' of the reactive epitopes of the light chains and the failure of the light chain to react with the corresponding antiserum, and this can be misinterpreted as the presence of free heavy chain. It is advisable to check any suspected lone heavy chain found on immunofixation by immunoselection or by molecular weight analysis. We have also found the liquid-phase assays (immunonephelometry) for total κ and total λ light chains are able to detect the light chains even if they are folded into the quaternary structure of the immunoglobulin molecule.

Urine immunofixation and Bence Jones protein

The antisera most often used for immunofixation react with both free and bound immunoglobulin heavy or light chains. The presence of free light chains is assumed if no heavy chain reaction is present. Antisera to free κ and λ light chains are also available, and their popularity varies across the world. In some countries it is mandatory to use antiserum to free light chain to confirm the presence of BJP. However, in our experience, the quality of antiserum to total (free and bound) light chains is considerably better and using these with careful interpretation

Table 9.7 *Distribution of paraprotein types seen in various B-cell dyscrasias*

Monoclonal type	All paraproteins (%)	Myeloma (%)	Waldenström's macroglobulinemia (%)	Other B-cell diseases (NHL/CLL) (%)	MGUS (%)
G	53.2	53[a]	–	40	60
A	21.9	22[b]	–	10	35
M	11.4	0.5	100[c]	50	5
D	1.3	1.5[d,e]	–	–	–
E	<0.001[f,g]	0.1	–	–	–
BJP	11.6	21	–	–	(+)
Non-secretory	–	1	–	–	–
Biclonal[h]	1.5	Unknown	–	–	–

[a] 60% also show BJP.
[b] 80% also show BJP.
[c] 24% also show BJP.
[d] 90% also show BJP.
[e] Usually λ light chain.
[f] Dfficult to quantify but considerably less than 1/1000 paraproteinemias.
[g] Usually κ light chain.
[h] Does not include intact immunoglobulin with BJP or multiple bands of the same paraprotein type.
BJP, Bence Jones protein; CLL, chronic lymphocytic leukemia; MGUS, monoclonal gammopathy of undetermined significance; NHL, non-Hodgkin's lymphoma.

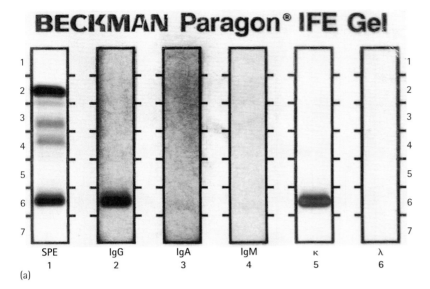

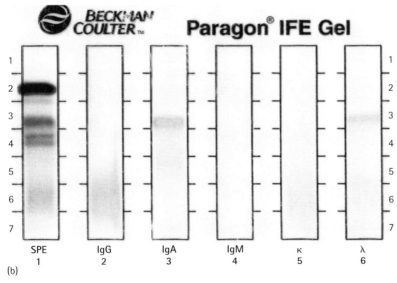

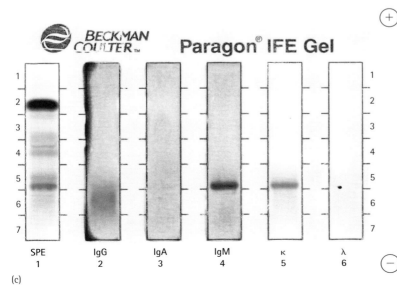

Figure 9.6 *Representative examples of serum immunofixation patterns. The tracks labelled SPE are the stained serum pattern, the remaining tracks are the immunofixation reactions. (a) A monoclonal IgG κ; (b) a monoclonal IgA λ running in the α_2 region; (c) a monoclonal IgM κ; (d) an IgD λ (very diffuse band) with a band of retained λ Bence Jones protein.*

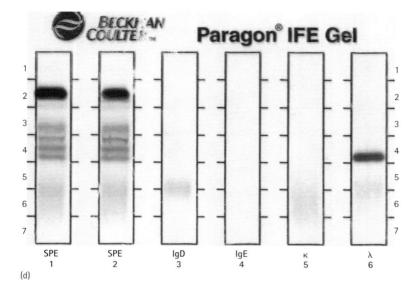

SPE 1   SPE 2   IgD 3   IgE 4   κ 5   λ 6

(d)

Figure 9.6 *(continued)*

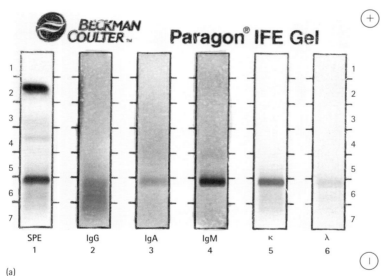

SPE 1   IgG 2   IgA 3   IgM 4   κ 5   λ 6

(a)

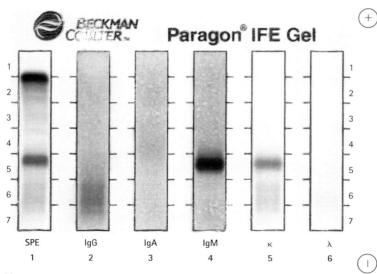

SPE 1   IgG 2   IgA 3   IgM 4   κ 5   λ 6

(b)

Figure 9.7 *An example of an immunofixation of a sample containing a large IgM κ paraprotein without and with treatment with dithiothreitol. The tracks labeled SPE are the stained serum pattern, the remaining tracks are the immunofixation reactions. (a) Clear reactions in the IgA, IgM, kappa, and lambda tracks are shown. This reaction across multiple tracks can be seen with high molecular immunoglobulin aggregates (immune complexes) and with large monoclonal proteins (especially IgMs). There is also polyclonal IgG with some IgG 'zoning.' (b) Immunofixation of the same sample but after treatment with dithiothreitol. The reactions in the IgA and λ tracks have disappeared, the polyclonal IgG with 'zoning' remains, and the paraprotein is clearly shown to be an IgM κ.*

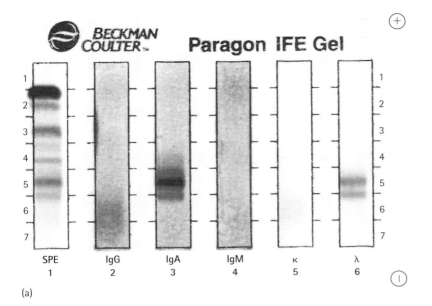

(a)

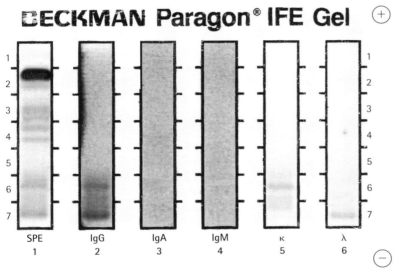

(b)

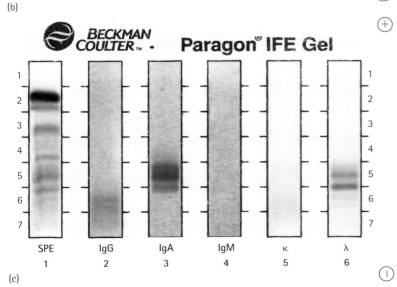

(c)

Figure 9.8 *Immunofixation of three samples from one patient during their treatment for myeloma. (a) This was taken at diagnosis and shows two IgA λ paraproteins (concentrations 20 g/L and 6 g/L). This immunofixation highlights the fact that this technique is not quantitative, with marked differences seen between the IgA and the λ staining for the same band (most noticeable in the most anodal band). (b) This was taken post-stem cell transplantation (25 months after diagnosis). The IgA λ paraprotein has disappeared, indicating complete remission, but there is an oligoclonal pattern with two IgG κ paraproteins and one IgG λ paraprotein. (c) This was taken 48 months after diagnosis. The oligoclonal pattern has disappeared and the original IgA λ paraproteins are clearly visible.*

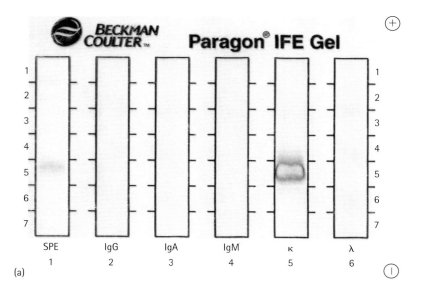

(a)

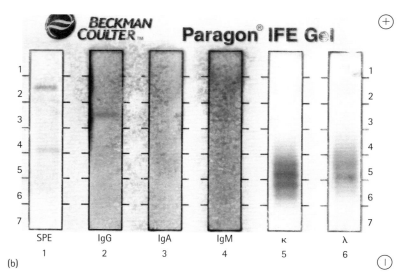

(b)

Figure 9.9 *Representative examples of urine immunofixation patterns. (a) A urine with κ Bence Jones protein (BJP). High concentrations of the BJP result in small soluble complexes that are washed out of the gel (prozone effect). Lower concentration of the BJP at the edges of the band results in large insoluble complexes that precipitate and therefore can be stained. (b) A pattern of light-chain banding seen in a tubular proteinuria. Multiple bands are seen in both κ and λ – but more often, the κ banding is the most prominent. The band seen in the IgG track without any corresponding light chain represents a fragment of catabolized IgG.*

of the immunofixation is a more reliable method for typing monoclonal components. On rare occasions, use of free light chain sera may be helpful, in particular where two monoclonal components are running very close together on the immunofixation and deciding whether the bands are intact immunoglobulin or free light chains is difficult. Immunofixation is not a quantitative method, with antiserum often showing greater binding to free light chains than to bound light chains. This can give the incorrect impression of disproportionately large amounts of BJP in comparison to the intact immunoglobulin.

A major problem with urine immunofixation is the distinction between monoclonal light chains and light-chain fragments generated from normal immunoglobulin catabolism, which result in a 'ladder-like' pattern, particularly in the immunofixation reaction with antiserum to κ light chains.[15,16] This 'κ banding' pattern is most often seen in

elderly patients with inflammatory conditions. Examples of BJP and κ banding are shown in Fig. 9.9.

Occasionally 'clonal' γ heavy chains are seen in urine and sometimes when an intact IgG monoclonal component is present in the serum. These proteins are typically seen in the α-2 region of the urine electrophoretic separation and are usually due to post-synthetic degradation of the monoclonal IgG often by bacterial contamination. In γ heavy-chain disease, the abnormal protein is always present in the serum and shows β–γ electrophoretic mobility.[17]

IMMUNOSUBTRACTION

The technique of immunofixation is not applicable in the automated CZE system. Immunosubtraction is a novel approach to paraprotein typing that was developed for CZE systems. Samples are incubated in wells, each well containing a different antiserum (to the α, γ, and μ heavy chains, and the κ and λ light chains) that has been coated on to sepharose beads. The antigen–antibody complexes form on the coated beads and these sediment in the well leaving a supernatant that should not contain the antigen corresponding to the antibody on the bead. The disappearance of a whole peak, part of a zone, or a change in shape of a zone may indicate the presence of a monoclonal protein. Figure 9.10 shows an example of immunosubtraction. Immunosubtraction works very well for the typing of large paraproteins superimposed on a γ zone of reduced intensity. In our experience, it is less satisfactory for typing small paraproteins, particularly with γ zones of normal intensity and for distinguishing polyclonal increases of the γ where one of the light-chain types predominates. To date, immunosubtraction reagents

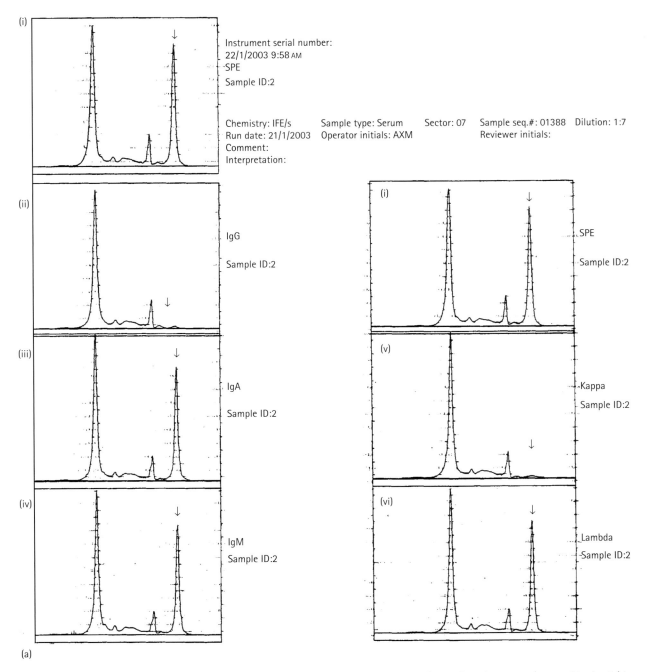

Figure 9.10 *Examples of immunosubtraction. (a) The paraprotein shown in the serum electrophoretic pattern (arrowed in chart i) is clearly removed by reaction with IgG antiserum (chart ii) and κ light-chain antiserum (chart v). (b) Similarly, a small diffuse paraprotein is shown to be an IgG κ (charts i, ii, and v).*

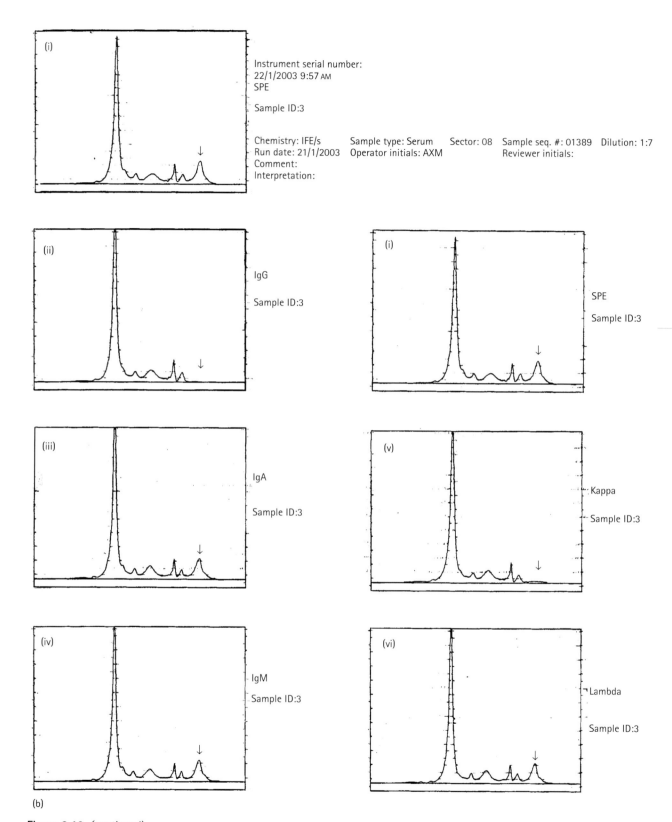

(i)

Instrument serial number:
22/1/2003 9:57 AM
SPE

Sample ID:3

Chemistry: IFE/s   Sample type: Serum   Sector: 08   Sample seq. #: 01389   Dilution: 1:7
Run date: 21/1/2003   Operator initials: AXM   Reviewer initials:
Comment:
Interpretation:

(ii)

IgG

Sample ID:3

(i)

SPE

Sample ID:3

(iii)

IgA

Sample ID:3

(v)

Kappa

Sample ID:3

(iv)

IgM

Sample ID:3

(vi)

Lambda

Sample ID:3

(b)

Figure 9.10 *(continued)*

are not available for typing IgD or IgE paraproteins, or other non-immunoglobulin proteins.

IMMUNOSELECTION

Immunoselection is a method that can be used to confirm the presence of free heavy (or free light) chains.[18] The technique is an adaptation of an electroimmunodiffusion method. The gels are not commercially available and the purpose-made gels are not readily adapted for use in modern dedicated electrophoresis sytems. There are probably only a handful of laboratories across the world that have the experience to make immunoselection plates and those same few laboratories will have stored positive controls for validation of the assays.

MOLECULAR WEIGHTS

The determination of molecular weights is most commonly done using gel filtration methods or sodium-dodecyl sulfate (SDS) polyacrylamide gel electrophoresis methods. Analytical ultracentrifuges are available but are they are limited to only a few major research laboratories. Checking molecular weights is mainly used for the detection or confirmation of the presence of heavy chains; however, it may also be used if considering high-molecular-weight aggregates, e.g. related to hyperviscosity syndromes. The high molecular weights result from aggregation, which occurs mainly with IgM and IgG paraproteins or from polymerization, which is more common with IgA and occasionally BJPs. Polymerization of BJP (most often into a tetramer) may result in molecules with molecular weighs of above 80 kDa, which, with normal renal function, result in the complete retention of the BJP in the serum.

MEASUREMENT OF κ:λ RATIOS FOR DETECTION AND TYPING OF MONOCLONAL IMMUNOGLOBULINS

The predominance of one light chain resulting from the presence of a monoclonal protein can cause the *ratio* of κ:λ light chains to fall outside the normal reference limits. Measurement of total (free and bound) κ and λ concentrations together with the total IgG, IgA, and IgM concentrations has been suggested as a method for both detecting and typing monoclonal components.[19,20] An abnormal κ:λ ratio suggests the presence of a monoclonal and whichever immunoglobulin has the concentration furthest above its reference range is inferred to be the heavy chain. However, our experience and that of others is that this approach is unable to detect reliably low concentrations (below 5 g/L) of monoclonal components, biclonal components, and polyclonal increases when one light chain predominates.[21] Measurement of the ratio of free κ and λ light chains has also been suggested as an automated 'screening' test for the presence of a monoclonal component in serum or urine. Neither total nor free κ:λ ratio methods have adequate specificity or sensitivity for monoclonal proteins to warrant them replacing good-quality serum and urine electrophoresis for the routine detection of monoclonal proteins.

IMMUNOGLOBULIN SUBCLASS TYPING

The subclass of IgG or IgA monoclonal proteins can be determined by techniques such as Ouchterlony (double immunodiffusion) or immunofixation using antibodies specific for each subclass.[22] Paraproteins of the IgA2 subclass are extremely rare. The subclass distribution of monoclonal IgG proteins is comparable to that of normal polyclonal IgG.[23] Overall, there seems to be little merit in subclass typing monoclonal proteins.

QUANTIFICATION OF MONOCLONAL COMPONENTS

The concentration of a monoclonal component is unable to predict tumor mass. Two patients presenting with similar paraprotein concentrations may have very different tumor burdens and the paraprotein concentration between patients at presentation can be highly variable. Table 9.8[4] shows the average paraprotein concentration at presentation with respect to the paraprotein type. The paraprotein concentration, within a patient, does reflect tumor mass and is, therefore, an essential component in the initial investigation and the assessment of the response to treatment of patients with B-cell malignancies.

SERUM

Immunochemical quantification of paraprotein bands is unreliable,[24] with impossibly high concentrations, spuriously low concentrations, and highly variable concentrations being reported. The only reliable method is to measure the percentage of the monoclonal protein (by scanning densitometry or from CZE readout) with respect to the total electrophoretic separation or to the globulin fraction. Representative examples of the densitometric scan of stained serum and urine protein electrophoretic

Table 9.8 *Average paraprotein concentration, by type, at presentation with myeloma*

Paraprotein type	Concentration (g/L)
IgG	43
IgA	28
IgD	14
IgM	19
IgE	30
Bence Jones only	5.4 g/24 hours (urine)

separations are shown in Fig. 9.11. In stained electrophoretic separations there is a differential dye binding between albumin and globulin; the most precise estimation of paraprotein is thus derived from the percentage of relative dye binding of the paraprotein band compared with the total globulin fraction rather than the total protein. This problem does not occur in the CZE measuring system because there is no staining step. At the 'exit' end of the capillaries, there is a ultraviolet detector system that continuously and directly reads the amount of protein passing before it. This method of protein detection also overcomes the second problem associated with dye binding, that of a non-linear relationship between dye binding and protein concentration at high paraprotein concentrations. Serum total protein is most often measured by Biuret-based methods.

It is useful to remember that the sum of the paraprotein and albumin plus an additional 10–15 g/L (to account for the other serum proteins) should be approximately equal to the measured serum total protein.

It is possible to reliably quantify a serum paraprotein down to a concentration of 1 g/L provided there is suppression of the background immunoglobulins. Monoclonal proteins with electrophoretic mobility in the β region can be difficult to quantify. However, the concentration of the β-proteins remains relatively stable; therefore, the paraprotein band, including the β-proteins, should be quantified and any major alterations in that concentration are likely to be due to changes in the concentration of the monoclonal component. While it is possible to 'delimit' a monoclonal peak, densitometric quantification should be reported, and once the concentration has fallen so that the peak cannot be clearly seen, immunochemical quantification of the relevant isotype can be used. The frequency of monitoring the concentration of the monoclonal components will depend upon the patient's clinical condition and treatment regimens (see Chapter 13).

With good laboratory practice, it is possible to measure the paraprotein concentration with coefficients of variation of below 5%. However, it is difficult to achieve this level of precision at low paraprotein concentrations, where the paraprotein is diffuse, or where it is superimposed on a γ region of normal or increased intensity; the significance of changes in concentration will depend on factors such as these. As a general rule, an increase or decrease of over 10% should be considered outside normal laboratory variability, although this does depend upon the baseline values. Changes, particularly increases, above this should be interpreted with respect to the clinical assessment. If there is inconsistency between increasing paraprotein concentration and clinical picture, a continuing upward trend on subsequent measurement after 1 month will increase suspicion of progressive disease. Cumulative reporting of paraprotein studies is invaluable in monitoring patients with myeloma and other paraproteinemias, and this is discussed further in Chapter 13.

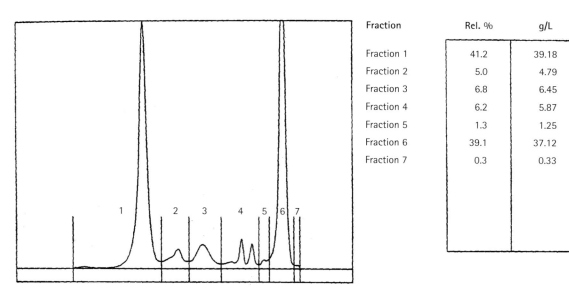

Fraction	Rel. %	g/L
Fraction 1	41.2	39.18
Fraction 2	5.0	4.79
Fraction 3	6.8	6.45
Fraction 4	6.2	5.87
Fraction 5	1.3	1.25
Fraction 6	39.1	37.12
Fraction 7	0.3	0.33

Figure 9.11 *An example of an electrophoretogram of a serum containing a monoclonal protein from the capillary zone electrophoresis system. A similar pattern should be generated by densitometric scanning of the stained serum electrophoretic separations. The various zones of the separation are usually delimited automatically based upon pre-determined positions or 'peak-to-trough' thresholds. This separation shows a large monoclonal component in fraction 6 with marked immune suppression and is, therefore, easily identified. Smaller monoclonals superimposed upon normal or polyclonally raised γ regions may need manual editing to delimit accurately and, therefore, quantify the monoclonal component.*

URINE

Unlike the volume of the vascular compartment, urine volume can be very variable and is influenced by factors such as fluid intake, renal function, state of hydration, and time of day. Quantification of BJP should start with the densitometric scan of the stained electrophoretic separation done in much the same way as serum paraprotein concentration. The band can be expressed as a percentage of the total protein but this can give misleading information, especially if the general background proteinuria is increased, making the percentage of BJP relatively lower. This percentage BJP can be used with the urine albumin or creatinine concentration to give grams of BJP per gram of albumin or per millimole of creatinine. It can also be used with the total protein concentration to generate a concentration in grams per liter and this result can be used with the 24-hour urine volume to generate a 24-hour excretion. There are both practical and analytical issues with no one method being ideal for all situations. Most importantly, a consistent approach should be taken to make it possible to compare results during the course of the disease. The International Federation of Clinical Chemists (IFCC) has published some guidelines for the investigation of urine for BJP.[25] Whichever approach is taken, the quantification of BJP is recommended as a criterion for response, progression, or relapse of multiple myeloma and in particular of Bence Jones-only myeloma.[8]

MEASUREMENT OF SERUM FREE LIGHT–CHAIN CONCENTRATIONS

The term 'free light chains' encompasses the slight excess of polyclonal free light chains produced during normal B-cell turnover, the larger excess of polyclonal free light chains produced during B-cell activation, and monoclonal free light chains associated with B-cell malignancies. The only way to distinguish monoclonal reliably from polyclonal free light chains is by electrophoresis and immunofixation.

Recently, antiserum recognizing free light chains only, suitable for automated methods on dedicated nephelometric or turbidimetric protein analyzers, has been produced.[26] It has been suggested that assays using this antiserum are useful in identifying and monitoring patients with Bence Jones and non-secretory myeloma.[27] Reference intervals for free κ and λ light chains have been established.[28] Free light-chain assays may be useful in detecting and monitoring low concentrations of free light chains seen in non-secretory myeloma and in AL amyloid.[29] It is also possible that the finding of very low concentrations of free light chains could be used to exclude Bence Jones proteinuria. It is essential that reliable antigen excess testing is part of the analytical process to avoid the risk of a very high concentration being incorrectly reported as low. However, there are limitations in using assays for free light chains: there is no national or international reference preparation for free light chains, the antiserum cannot directly determine clonality, biclonal gammopathies can give a κ:λ ratio within the reference range, and polyclonal free light chains may mask alterations in monoclonal free light chains. Considering these limitations, we would not recommend the introduction of these assays into routine laboratories. Additionally, they have neither the specificity nor the sensitivity to replace high-quality electrophoresis and immunofixation for detection and typing of monoclonal components.

Cerebrospinal fluid investigations

Occasionally, cerebrospinal fluid (CSF) will be analyzed in the investigation of cerebral involvement in B-cell malignancy. Immunofixation of CSF, treated similarly to urine, is usually successful. It is possible to quantify immunoglobulin concentrations in CSF by sensitive immunonephelometric or turbidimetric assays. Under normal circumstances, the CSF IgG is generated from the serum so, if a serum contains an IgG monoclonal component, it is likely that it will also appear in the CSF. The ratio of immunoglobulin to albumin within the CSF compared with that of a matched serum can indicate intrathecal synthesis of the monoclonal protein. The pattern seen on isoelectric focusing is characteristic with a series of harmonic bands that should be identical to the serum pattern and clearly distinguishable from an oligoclonal pattern. IgG oligoclonal banding detected only in the CSF by isoelectric focusing indicates intrathecal synthesis and is used in the investigation of diseases such as multiple sclerosis.

INVESTIGATIONS RELATED TO THE MONOCLONAL COMPONENT

Quantification of background immunoglobulins

Secondary immunodeficiencies are particularly associated with lymphoid malignancies. Immunosuppression in association with a paraprotein is strongly suggestive of a B-cell malignancy and the finding of low non-monoclonal-component immunoglobulin concentrations has a positive predictive value of 0.97 for malignancy.[30] The severity of the secondary immune suppression is related to the risk of infective complications and there have been attempts to reduce the risk of recurrent infections with intravenous immunoglobulin replacement.[31]

Serum immunoglobulin concentrations are most commonly measured by either immunonephelometry or immunoturbidimetry. These techniques are rapid (particularly if kinetic) and precise, typically running with coefficients of variation of below 5%. All methods use antiserum to polyclonal immunglobulins and are optimized to measure concentrations within a defined limit around the normal reference range. Samples with very high concentrations and those that do not obey the programmed reaction kinetics can give wildly aberrant values. It is, therefore, a fundamental requirement that the methods used for quantification of immunoglobulin have a reliable antigen excess check. The international reference preparation CRM470 has reduced interlaboratory variation considerably. The analytical systems used for the measurement of serum immunoglobulin should be able reliably to detect concentrations of 0.1 g/L of IgA and IgM and 1 g/L of IgG. National quality assurance schemes exist to assess interlaboratory performances. In general, performance is good, confirming the robustness of these assays. Immunonephelometry and immunoturbidimetry are unsuitable methods for quantification of monoclonal proteins (see section on quantification of monoclonal components, p. 139). Companies that manufacture dedicated analyzers for the measurement of serum protein concentrations are shown in Appendix C.

QUANTIFICATION OF IgG SUBCLASSES

Quantification can be done by immunonephelometry and immunoturbidimetry, but these techniques suffer from the same problems as total immunoglobulin measurements. In a study of IgG monoclonal proteins, the concentration of residual non-paraprotein IgG was significantly decreased but only a small proportion of patients showed all three non-paraprotein IgG subclasses below the reference range, suggesting some selectivity of immunosuppression. Patients with IgG2 monoclonal proteins were more likely to have depressed residual IgG than patients with IgG3, IgG1, or IgG4 monoclonal IgG proteins. Residual IgG1 was disproportionately reduced followed by residual IgG2, IgG3, and IgG4.[32] Overall, there seems to be little merit in measuring IgG subclass concentrations in patients with monoclonal proteins.

FUNCTIONAL ANTIBODIES

As part of the assessment of immune status, it is possible to quantify antibodies (especially IgG antibodies) to a variety of infectious agents, including tetanus, *Pneumococcus*, and *Haemophilus influenzae* type B. Vaccination against *Streptococcus pneumoniae* is recommended for immunocompromised individuals, although myeloma patients make only poor responses to vaccination.[33]

Prognostic factors

β₂-MICROGLOBULIN

β₂-Microglobulin (β2M) is a low-molecular-weight (11.8 kDa) protein found on the surface of most nucleated cells. It forms the invariant chain of the HLA class I molecules and is released into the serum from cell turnover. In conditions where there is increased cell turnover, e.g. malignancy (particularly lymphoid), acquired immune deficiency syndromes, and inflammatory conditions, serum β2M concentrations increase. β2M is cleared by glomerular filtration followed by proximal tubular reabsorption and catabolism. Serum concentrations, therefore, reflect both cell turnover and renal function, and serum β2M is an important prognostic indicator in myeloma (see Chapter 12).[34] Interferon-α, used in maintenance therapy of myeloma, can induce marked increase in serum β2M concentrations and this should be taken into consideration when using β2M for the assessment of tumor response during interferon-α therapy.[35] Rapid immunoassays (turbidimetry, nephelometry, microparticle-enhanced enzyme immunoassays, and latex-enhanced turbidimetry and nephelometry) are mainly used. The interlaboratory variation in β2M is considerable, in part due to a lack of any international reference preparation. β2M is unstable in urine and should not be measured.

C-REACTIVE PROTEIN

C-reactive protein (CRP) is an acute-phase reactant that is produced by the liver under the control of inflammatory cytokines, such as interleukin-6 (IL-6), IL-1, and tumor necrosis factor α. The assays for CRP are robust (immunonephelometric or immunoturbidimetric) and there is a reliable international reference preparation (CRM470) to which most assays are calibrated. CRP concentrations have been reported to correlate with disease activity in myeloma and, when combined with β2M concentrations, are highly informative with respect to prognosis.[36] CRP concentrations will also increase in infection, and this is useful for detecting and monitoring infection in patients.[37]

LACTATE DEHYDROGENASE

Measurement of lactate dehydrogenase (LDH) activity has also been proposed as a prognostic factor in myeloma with raised concentrations associated with worst prognosis.[38] Raised LDH activities also result from treatment with granulocyte or granulocyte–macrophage colony-stimulating factors.[39] LDH activity can be measured on many standard biochemistry analysers.

EFFECTS OF MONOCLONAL COMPONENTS

Symptoms and syndromes associated with monoclonal gammopathy may be attributed either to effects of the underlying B-cell tumor or to properties of the paraprotein itself. A number of biochemical investigations are concerned with defining the physicochemical properties of certain paraproteins to explain unusual direct effects.

Viscosity

Hyperviscosity syndrome is relatively common in myeloma. It is related not only to the serum paraprotein concentration but also to the molecular characteristics of that protein, and to the packed red blood cell volume, aggregation of protein molecules, the presence of disease involving the small blood vessels, hematocrit level, cardiac output, and other factors related to the patients clinical condition. Hyperviscosity is commonly associated with IgM paraproteins (approximately 10%) but can occur with IgA or IgG (usually IgG3) paraproteins[40] at high concentrations or when they form high-molecular-weight aggregates. Paraprotein concentrations above 30 g/L are most often associated with hyperviscosity and small increments above this concentration result in rapid escalation of the viscosity owing to the steep curvilinear relationship of concentration to viscosity. The measurement of pre- and post-plasmapheresis viscosity is especially useful for assessing effectiveness and predicting the need for additional plasmapheresis treatment.

The absolute unit of plasma viscosity is milliPascal seconds (mPa.s). An average plasma viscosity is 1.24 mPa.s at 37 °C (serum viscosity is lower), although laboratories should establish their own reference intervals. Water can be used as a low standard (viscosity 0.692 mPa.s at 37 °C) and freshly prepared 28% w/v sucrose solution (viscosity 1.972 mPa.s at 37 °C) as a high standard. Viscosity measurement can also be expressed relative to water; such a ratio has the advantage of being temperature independent. A typical reference range for normal serum relative to water is 1.6–2.0. There is no particular viscosity above which symptoms occur, although they are often seen with values above 4.0 and more often with values above 6.0.

The whole blood, serum, or plasma viscosities can be measured by a variety of techniques. The simplest and maybe the most common is the capillary tube apparatus and the 'falling ball' apparatus; both are relatively crude but will indicate gross abnormalities in viscosity. There may be limitations of temperature control. These systems can be run in water baths or incubators, and this is recommended when measuring the viscosity of samples containing cryoproteins. More sophisticated is the rotational-type viscometer where a solid spindle is rotated at various speeds in a matched cylinder that contains the sample. The equipment is very expensive, and the matched pairs of spindle and cylinder usually have to be custom-made in a size small enough to be appropriate for human blood samples. These systems do have advantages: they are usually temperature-controlled and more accurately reflect the sample behavior at various shear rates. Plasma

and serum are normally Newtonian fluids so that their viscosity values do not vary with the rate of shear. An exception is the non-Newtonian behavior of certain paraproteins and cryoglobulins that form shear-dependent reversible aggregates. Rotational viscometers are recommended for viscosity measurements where a monoclonal component is present.[41]

Cryoproteins

Cryoglobulins are immunoglobulins that can aggregate on cooling of the serum and usually redissolve on warming to 37 °C. Careful sample collection is vital. Serum and plasma should be collected, transported, and separated at 37 °C. Failure to do this may result in significant cryoproteins being lost with the cell pellet. Details of the collection protocol are shown in Appendix E. A sample containing a monoclonal cryoprotein is shown in Fig. 9.12.

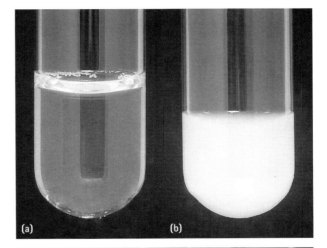

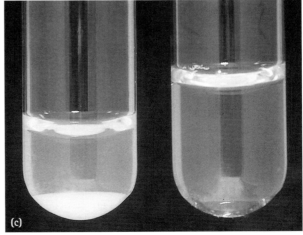

Figure 9.12 *An example of cryoprecipitation. The sample containing an IgM κ paraprotein was incubated at 37 °C where the sample remains a clear liquid (a) and at 4 °C where a cryoprecipitate has formed (b). The cryoprecipitate can be separated for further investigation by centrifugation at 4 °C (c).*

A cryoprotein will show particular thermal profile characteristics that influence the clinical significance. Monoclonal proteins that precipitate at temperatures close to 4 °C may not cause any significant symptoms, while those that precipitate close to 37 °C will cause the most significant symptoms, irrespective of relative concentrations. The thermal profile of a cryoprotein may be useful when the symptoms associated with a cryoprotein seem more severe than the concentration would suggest (brief method details are shown in Appendix E).

CLASSIFICATION OF CRYOPROTEINS

Type I cryoglobulins

Type I cryoglobulins are monoclonal immunoglobulins and account for approximately 25% of all cases. They occur predominantly with IgM paraproteins (6% of all macroglobulinemias and are especially associated with lymphoma). Cryoprecipitation may also be seen with IgG monoclonals (particularly of the IgG3 subclass) but only occasionally with IgA monoclonals. There have also been reports of cryoprecipitable BJP but these are exceptionally rare.[4] The monoclonal component is often present at high concentrations (greater than 30 g/L), although significant cryoprecipitation may occur with concentrations as low as 5 g/L. Cryoprecipitation occurs most readily in the microvasculature of the periphery (fingers, toes, ear lobes, nose) simply because these areas get the coldest.

These monoclonal cryoproteins tend to precipitate rapidly and 24-hour incubation is usually adequate for their detection.

Type II cryoglobulins

Type II cryoglobulins contain a monoclonal component (usually IgM κ) that shows rheumatoid factor activity with polyclonal IgG. These are most often associated with viral hepatitis (hepatitis B and C), may occur with other infections, e.g. mycoplasma pneumonia, and also can be seen in autoimmune diseases and in lymphoproliferative diseases. They are usually present at concentrations of less than 5 g/L.

Type III cryoglobulins

Type III cryoglobulins contain polyclonal rheumatoid factor (IgM) and polyclonal IgG or IgA. These are seen most often in association with autoimmune rheumatic diseases and persistent infections and only occasionally with lymphoproliferative diseases.

Type II and type III cryoproteins are associated with high-molecular-weight immune aggregates and often need up to 72 hours at 4 °C for any precipitate to form. The symptoms seen with these cryoproteins are linked more to their ability to deposit in tissue as immune complexes than their tendency to precipitate in the cold. Type II and type III cryoproteins are both associated with

neuropathies, vasculitis, and nephropathies. Immune complex or cryoprotein deposition in tissue is likely to cause activation of the classical complement cascade. Low complement concentrations (particularly C4) are a good marker of active immune complex disease and measurement of these components is an important part of the investigation of possible cryoproteinemia.

In addition to cryoprecipitating immunoglobulins, fibrinogen may precipitate in the cold. Cryofibrinogen may occur in inflammatory, malignant, and thromboembolic diseases. It can be investigated in exactly the same way as cryoglobulins but on an EDTA or sodium citrate plasma sample.

Immune complexes

Immune complexes are high-molecular-weight aggregates of immunoglobulin with antigen (which may be immunoglobulin itself). Production of immune complexes is a normal part of the immune response; however, excessive generation or failure to clear the immune complexes can result in their deposition (e.g. in the kidneys or skin), complement activation, and ultimately tissue damage. Rheumatoid factor activity, and cryoprecipitation are properties of immune complexes and there are specific methods for their investigation. There are other methods for detecting circulating immune complexes (CIC). The most commonly used are based on the ability of CIC to bind C1q or to aggregate platelets. The major problem is that CIC vary considerably in aggregate size and different assays detect preferentially small or large complexes.[42] There is also poor correlation between detection of complexes by any method and clinical manifestations. In general, they are poorly characterized assays lacking any standardization.

Autoantibodies

Some monoclonal components display autoantibody activity and give rise to associated clinical disorders. These autoantibodies include cold agglutinins, rheumatoid factors, anticardiolipin, and antimyelin-associated glycoprotein antibodies. Antibody activity to other antigens has also been described, e.g. dextran,[43] streptolysin O,[44] nucleic acid,[45] actin,[46] and antibiotics.[47]

COLD AGGLUTININS

IgM antibodies that are directed against I or i antigenic determinants of red blood cells will agglutinate red cells at 4 °C but very poorly or not at all at 37 °C *in vitro*. The presence of these antibodies is usually associated with low-grade intravascular hemolysis but effective red cell removal by the reticuloendothelial system occurs owing to C3 fixation by the antigen–antibody complex on the cell surface. Small amounts of polyclonal cold agglutinins may occur in inflammatory conditions or following infection with *Mycoplasma pneumoniae*[48] or viruses.[49] In primary cold agglutinin disease the antibody is classically a monoclonal IgM κ. It is most often associated with non-malignant disease but may also occur in lymphoma patients.[5,49,50]

Samples for the investigation of cold agglutinins should be collected and separated as described for cryoglobulins. The red cells will be Coombs' test positive when cold agglutinins are present.

RHEUMATOID FACTOR

Rheumatoid factors are antibodies that have activity against the Fc portion of IgG molecules. They are most often of the IgM class, but can be IgG or IgA, and will form high-molecular-weight aggregates or immune complexes. Rheumatoid factor activity is seen in about 3% of all IgM paraproteins, and these may result in cryoprecipitation or the presence of circulating immune complexes. Monoclonal components that have rheumatoid factor activity can stick or smear around the application point in the gel-type protein electrophoresis systems; this can result in an immunofixation pattern showing a false-positive reaction with all antibody types. This problem can usually be solved by treating the serum for 20 minutes prior to electrophoresis with 1 mg/mL dithiothreitol (see Appendix D). This treatment serves to reduce disulfide bridges so that large aggregates or immune complexes are dissociated.

ANTIPHOSPHOLIPID AND ANTICARDIOLIPIN ANTIBODIES

Antibodies to phospholipid components of cell membranes (particularly of endothelium and platelets) are associated with recurrent arterial or venous thrombosis. These antibodies are usually polyclonal with specificities to antigens, such as cardiolipin, phosphatidyl serine, and β_2-glycoprotein-1.[51] There are reports of monoclonal proteins associated with other abnormalities of the coagulation system,[52,53] including activity against proteins of the coagulation system, most often factor VIII.[54,55]

ANTIBODIES TO MYELIN-ASSOCIATED GLYCOPROTEIN

Myelin-associated glycoprotein (MAG) is a minor glycoprotein component of the peripheral and central nervous systems. Anti-MAG antibodies associated with peripheral neuropathy are usually monoclonal IgM and, rarely, IgG or IgA monoclonal components.[56,57] There are no generally accepted or standardized techniques for detection or quantification of anti-MAG antibodies. They can be demonstrated by immunoblotting against crude myelin extracts and measured semiquantitatively by enzyme-linked immunosorbant assay (ELISA). Neither technique is ideal, and it is likely that using both will give the best combination of specificity and sensitivity.[58]

ANTIBODIES TO C1 ESTERASE INHIBITOR

The complement component C1 esterase inhibitor is a protease inhibitor that is active in the early part of the classical complement cascade and also has activity in the clotting cascade. Hereditary angioedema, resulting from an inherited deficiency of this protein or non-functional form of it, is well described, and readily diagnosed by measuring total serum concentrations of complement components C3, C4, and C1 esterase inhibitor. Normal C3 concentrations with low C4 and C1 esterase inhibitor characterize the disease. Additionally, there are acquired forms of C1 esterase inhibitor deficiency that are associated with monoclonal gammopathies. A reaction between the idiotype of the monoclonal immunoglobulin and anti-idiotypic antibodies can result in increased consumption of C1Q and of the C1 inhibitor producing similar symptoms to the hereditary disease.[59] In this form of the disease, decreased levels of C1-inhibitor function with variable decreases in C1-inhibitor concentration are seen. The C4 concentration will still be low owing to its uncontrolled consumption, but the total C1 esterase inhibitor may be normal but with reduced functional activity due a cleavage.[60] In this situation, measurement of functional C1 esterase inhibitor is essential. This can be done by commercially available immunoassay. There is no international standard or national validation scheme for this test.

OTHER INVESTIGATIONS

General clinical biochemistry profile

The 'general biochemistry' profile is an important component of both the initial assessment and the monitoring of patients with myeloma. The typical analyses included under this heading are the electrolytes sodium and potassium, urea, creatinine, calcium, phosphate, albumin, and bone and liver enzymes. For all these analytes there are recommended methods, international reference preparations and external validation schemes. It is important to remember that abnormalities may be related to the disease or disease process, and abnormal results may also occur due to interference in the assays by the monoclonal components.

ELECTROLYTES

Pseudohyponatremia, seen with very high concentrations of paraprotein, is the best described abnormality, and is due to a combination of increased viscosity and the 'occupation' of a set volume of plasma by large amounts of monoclonal protein. Together, these cause an incorrectly low volume of the plasma to be delivered to the measuring system and a falsely low concentration is measured. This phenomenon is most apparent with the sodium where values may well fall below the lower limit of the reference interval. It is also seen with potassium but generally will not cause values to fall outside the reference limits.

UREA, CREATININE, CREATININE CLEARANCE, AND ASSESSMENT OF RENAL FUNCTION

Renal impairment is a common feature of myeloma and accurate assessment of renal function is vital. Creatinine is an endogenous substance produced and released during muscle metabolism. The rate of production is fairly constant and it is removed from the body mainly by glomerular filtration. Serum creatinine concentrations are rather insensitive for detecting mild renal impairment needing a fall in the glomerular filtration rate of over 30% before the serum creatinine increases above the reference range. Recently, formulae for calculating creatinine clearances from the plasma creatinine concentration have been suggested. The Cockcroft and Gault formula, which uses plasma calcium concentration, patient age (in years), and patient weight in kilograms, is the best known.[61] Plasma urea concentrations are still widely used but have many disadvantages and, in general, are less reliable markers of renal function than plasma creatinine concentrations or creatinine clearance values.

CALCIUM AND PHOSPHATE

Hypercalcemia is a common and occasionally life-threatening occurrence in patients with myeloma, both at presentation and during the course of the disease. The regulation of serum calcium concentrations is complex and mainly involves the bones, gut, and kidney, and is controlled by parathyroid hormone and vitamin D. In myeloma, the typical bony lesions result from osteoclast activation without concomitant osteoblast activation. The osteoclast-activating factors include the cytokines IL-1, tumor necrosis factor α, IL-6, and RANK-ligand (Chapter 6). Renal impairment, a common complication of myeloma, is another significant cause of hypercalcemia. Ionized calcium is approximately 50% of the total plasma calcium and it is now possible to measure this physiologically important portion of the serum calcium by ion selective electrodes. Total plasma calcium (both the ionized fraction and the fraction bound to albumin) can be measured by colorimetric methods. This concentration may then be used, along with the serum albumin

concentration, to calculate the ionized calcium. This method is, at best, only an approximation and the inaccuracies can be compounded by the presence of monoclonal components, which can bind large amounts of calcium but will not be accounted for in the calculation.[62]

Serum phosphate concentration is usually measured at the same time as the calcium concentration. It is likely to be raised when there is renal impairment, although there are more useful markers of renal function. The presence of monoclonal proteins can influence serum phosphate measurement, making it falsely high.[63]

ALBUMIN

Serum albumin concentration is routinely measured as part of a liver or bone profile, and must be considered when interpreting serum calcium concentration. It does reflect nutritional status but the relatively long half-life (approximately 20 days) makes it slow to respond to changes in nutrition. In myeloma, a serum albumin concentration below 30 g/L is associated with poor survival (Chapter 12).

LIVER FUNCTION TESTS AND ALKALINE PHOSPHATASE

In 96% of patients with myeloma, the plasma alkaline phosphatase is within the normal range and this, in the presence of hypercalcemia, is a useful marker to distinguish it from bony metastases associated with other malignant diseases. Raised alkaline phosphatase concentrations do not exclude myeloma because they may be associated with other pathological processes, e.g. obstructive liver disease and other bone disease. It is also worth remembering that enzymes can polymerize with other plasma proteins, e.g. a monoclonal component. These macroenzymes have reduced renal clearance and can give a persistently raised concentration.[64] The concentration of bilirubin and the activity of the aminotransferases may also be measured as part of these profiles. Abnormalities can be seen when there is hepatic involvement in the disease process and with the use of hepatotoxic drugs.

URIC ACID

Patients with myeloma may have raised plasma uric acid concentrations owing to a combination of increased cell turnover related to the tumor, cell destruction associated with chemotherapy, dehydration, and renal impairment. Urate may deposit in the kidneys as calculi that may further contribute to the renal disease.[65] Uric acid concentrations can be measured alongside the other 'general clinical biochemistry' analyses.

Other assays

CYTOKINES

A complex network of cytokines plays a fundamental role in the growth and proliferation of malignant cells. Cytokines affect cells by interacting with specific receptors on the cell membrane, and this connection between cytokine and receptor starts a signal transduction process within the cell that ultimately influences its survival or proliferation. IL-6 acts through a gp130 signal transduction receptor that is shared by other cytokines, e.g. oncostatin, ciliary neurotropic factor, leukemia inhibitory factor, and IL-11. Serum cytokine concentrations are influenced by many factors. Cytokines are rapidly sequestered by high-affinity receptors on cell surfaces; these receptors are often upregulated in inflammation and malignancy. The serum contains soluble receptors that may also be upregulated and these will bind to cytokines released into the circulation. Cytokines are rapidly cleared by renal filtration and, finally, both the soluble receptors and the cytokine millieu can further modulate the action of an individual cytokine. All these limitations must be considered when planning to measure serum cytokine concentrations.

Serum samples, collected into endotoxin-free tubes (to prevent stimulation of cytokine production by monocytes *in vitro*), are preferred for cytokine measurements. If this is not possible, clotted samples that are separated within 1 hour of collection or samples collected in EDTA can be used.[66] Techniques available for detecting or measuring cytokines include immunoassays, enzyme-linked immune spot assays (ELISPOT), fluorescence-activated cell sorting (FACS), *in situ* hybridization, and reverse transcription polymerase chain reaction (RT-PCR). However, bioassay and immunoassay are most commonly used for measurement of cytokine concentrations in biological fluids. Bioassays are technically demanding and very labor-intensive, and are best left to those who have real expertise. Bioassays most accurately reflect biological activity. There are many commercially available immunoassays for the quantification of cytokines but, overall, there is enormous variation in the quality of the assays. The problems of cytokine measurement by immunoassay has been reviewed.[67] Standard reference preparations are available from national standardization organizations but there is astonishing variability between the commercial kits. Clearly establishing international reference preparations will be an important step towards reducing this variability and the World Health Organization is addressing this.[68]

The use of cytokine measurements in clinical practice remains controversial but, in general, it has not lived up to the high expectations of the 1980s and 1990s. In myeloma, biologically active IL-6 levels were shown to be a prognostic factor,[69] but the complexity of the analytical process limit its routine use. An alternative approach would be to measure the concentration of C-reactive protein (see section on C-reactive protein above), an acute-phase protein that is produced by hepatocytes on activation by cytokines, particularly IL-6.

MARKERS OF BONE METABOLISM

Bone lesions are an important cause of morbidity in myeloma. There have been a number of attempts to monitor the bone resorption and bone formation using biochemical markers of bone turnover. Pyridinoline and deoxypyridinoline are mature covalent cross-links of collagen that are excreted into the urine and can be measured by methods, such as high-performance liquid chromatography (HPLC) and ELISA. Results should be expressed as a ratio to the urine creatinine concentration to account for any variations in urine volume. The amino- or carboxy-terminal propeptides on type I collagen can also be measured as markers of osteoblast collagen formation. These can be measured in the serum by immunoassay. Osteocalcin and bone alkaline phosphatase are also markers of bone formation that can be measured by immunoassay. There are suggestions that these analytes could be used as markers of bone 'activity.'[70] They may be better indicators of bone disease than skeletal X-rays in myeloma patients[71] and have been used to 'titrate' the dose of bisphosphonate therapy; however, at present, there is no clear routine clinical application for any of these tests.

Immunoassays are available but calibration between the kit manufacturers is variable. The demand for these assays is very limited so only a few specialist laboratories offer the service.

OTHER MARKERS

There are many other biochemical markers that have been measured in patients with myeloma. Some of these are summarized in Table 9.9,[72–80] although as yet they do not have a defined role in the investigation or management of patients.

Monoclonal proteins as interfering substances

Raised total protein concentration due to either polyclonally raised immunoglobulins or the presence of paraproteins has the capacity to influence analytical techniques adversely. The plasma viscosity may be increased and this may lead to improper sampling. Paraproteins may precipitate when they come into contact with strong acids or alkalis. This seems to be more of a problem in continuous flow analyzers than in the

Table 9.9 *Putative markers and their suggested contribution to the management of myeloma*

Analyte	Suggested use	Reference
Cystatin C	Index of glomerular filtration rate in preference to serum creatinine	72, 73
Neopterin	To distinguish bacterial infection from viral infection and graft-versus-host disease in patients post-bone marrow transplant	74,75
Drugs	To achieve therapeutic dosage but limit adverse effects	Consult company producing the relevant drugs
Parathyroid hormone-related protein (PTH-rP)	Implicated as a major factor responsible for hypercalcemia of malignancy, although not usually in myeloma	76–79
Nutritional markers	To assess and monitor nutritional status	80

newer discrete analyzers. There are some interferences that are method specific; for example, paraproteins have been reported to interfere with the *o*-phthalaldehyde method for urea but not with the urease conductivity method.[81] Immunoglobulins, particularly those at high concentration, can bind to other analytes, e.g. IgG can complex with enzymes, such as creatine kinase, lactate dehydrogenase, and amylase, creating a complex with a longer circulating half-life than the native enzymes and a consequent increase in serum activity.[82] High concentrations of immunoglobulin – either monoclonal or polyclonal – can cause major interferences in autoantibody tests. The immunoglobulin, most often IgG, nonspecifically binds to the antigen on ELISA plates or in tissue sections, and this is detected by the antihuman IgG detection system. Considerable caution must be exercised in the interpretation of autoantibody results in the presence of monoclonal proteins.

scanning densitometry) with respect to the total electrophoretic separation or the globulin fraction.
- Important prognostic biochemical factors to investigate are β_2-microglobulin, C-reactive protein, and lactate dehydrogenase.
- Important biochemical investigations are concerned with the physicochemical properties of certain paraproteins, such as viscosity, cryoproteins, immune complexes, and autoantibodies.
- A general biochemical profile is an important component and should include, among other investigations, electrolytes, urea, creatinine, calcium, albumin, liver function tests, and uric acid.

KEY POINTS

- The detection, typing, and quantification of monoclonal components in serum and urine are essential biochemical investigations in the diagnosis and monitoring of myeloma.
- Protein electrophoresis is the only reliable method for the detection of paraprotein in serum or urine.
- Immunofixation should be used for confirmation of clonality, typing and detection of minimal residual disease, and complete remission post-treatment.
- The only reliable method to quantify the monoclonal paraprotein is to measure the percentage of the monoclonal protein (e.g. by

REFERENCES

● = Key primary paper
◆ = Major review article

●1. Riches PG, Hobbs JR. Laboratory investigation of paraproteinaemia. *J Clin Pathol* 1988; **41**:776–85.
2. Seth J, Sturgeon C, Ellis A. *Annual report of the UK NEQAS for peptide hormones.* Edinburgh: UK NEQAS for Peptide Hormones, 1995.
●3. Beetham R. Detection of Bence-Jones protein in practice. *Ann Clin Biochem* 2000; **37**:563–70.
●4. Hobbs JR. Immunoglobulins in clinical chemistry. *Adv Clin Chem* 1971; **14**:219–317.
5. Hobbs JR, Carter PM, Cook KB, Foster M, Oon CJ. IgM paraproteins. *J Clin Pathol* 1975; **28**(Suppl. 6):54–64.
6. Kohn J, Srivastave PC. Paraproteinaemia in blood donors and the aged: benign and malignant. *Protides Biol Fluids* 1973; **20**:257–61.

7. Gore ME, Riches PG, Kohn J. Identification of the paraproteins and clinical significance of more than one paraprotein in serum of 56 patients. *J Clin Pathol* 1979; 32:313–17.

●8. Blade J, Samson D, Reece D, Apperley J, Bjorkstrand B, Gahrton G, *et al*. Criteria for evaluating disease response and progression in patients with multiple myeloma treated by high-dose therapy and haematopoietic stem cell transplantation. *Br J Haematol* 1998; 102:1115–23.

9. Zent CS, Wislon CS, Tricot G, Jagannath S, Siegel D, Desikan KR, *et al*. Oligoclonal protein bands and Ig isotype switching in multiple myeloma treated with high-dose therapy and hematopoietic cell transplantation. *Blood* 1998; 91:3518–23.

10. Mitus AJ, Stein R, Rappeport JM, Antin JH, Weinstein HJ, Alper CA, *et al*. Monoclonal and oligoclonal gammopathy after bone marrow transplantation. *Blood* 1989; 74:2764–8.

11. Hovenga S, de Wolf JT, Guikema JE, Klip H, Smit JW, Sibinga CT, *et al*. Autologous stem cell transplantation in multiple myeloma after VAD and EDAP courses: a high incidence of oligoclonal serum Igs post transplantation. *Bone Marrow Transplant* 2000; 25:723–8.

12. Bouko Y, Goldschmidt H, Feremans W, Bourhis J-H, Szydlo R, Greinix H, *et al*. Oligoclonal reconstitution after high-dose therapy with PBPCT in myeloma patients: implications for assessment of remission status. *Bone Marrow Transplant* 2002; 29(Suppl. 2):S102.

●13. Ritchie RF, Smith R. Immunofixation III. Application to the study of monoclonal proteins. *Clin Chem* 1976; 22:1982–5.

14. Sinclair D, Kumararatne DS, Forrester JB, Lamont A, Stott DI. The application of isoelectric focusing to routine screening for paraproteinaemia. *J Immunol Meth* 1983; 64:147–56.

●15. Harrison HH. The 'ladder light chain' or 'pseudo-oligoclonal' pattern in urinary immunofixation electrophoresis (IFE) studies: a distinctive IFE pattern and an explanation hypothesis relating to free polyclonal light chains. *Clin Chem* 1991; 37:1559–64.

16. MacNamara EM, Aguzzi F, Petrini C, Higginson J, Gasparro C, Bergami MR, *et al*. Restricted electrophoretic heterogeneity of immunoglobulin light chains in urine: a cause for confusion with Bence Jones protein. *Clin Chem* 1991; 37:1570–4.

17. Charles EZ, Valdes AJ. Free fragments of gamma chain in the urine: a possible source of confusion with gamma heavy-chain disease. *Am J Clin Pathol* 1994; 101:462–4.

18. Gale DSJ, Versey JMB, Hobbs JR. Rocket immunoselection for detection of heavy-chain disease. *Clin Chem* 1974; 20:1292–4.

19. Fifield R, Keller I. An immunochemical evaluation (ICE) using heavy and light chain measurements for the identification and typing of monoclonal proteins. *Ann Clin Biochem* 1990; 27:327–34.

20. Whicher JT, Wallage M, Fifield R. Use of immunoglobulins heavy and light chain measurements compared with existing techniques as a means of typing monoclonal immunoglobulins. *Clin Chem* 1987; 33:1771–3.

21. Jones RG, Aguzzi F, Bienvenu J, Bianchi P, Gasparro C, Bergami MR, *et al*. Use of immunoglobulin heavy-chain and light-chain measurements in a multicenter trial to investigate monoclonal components: I. Detection. *Clin Chem*. 1991; 37:1917–21.

22. Riches PG, Walker SA, Plebani A, Porta G. The use of monoclonal subclass specific antibodies in the investigation of paraproteins in human serum. *Clin Chim Acta* 1985; 146:207–13.

23. Hamilton RG. Human IgG subclass measurements in the clinical laboratory. *Clin Chem* 1987; 33:1707–25.

●24. Riches PG, Sheldon J, Smith AM, Hobbs JR. Overestimation of monoclonal immunoglobulin by immunochemical methods. *Ann Clin Biochem*. 1991; 28:253–9.

25. Graziani M, Merlini G, Petrini C. Guidelines for the analysis of Bence Jones protein. *Clin Chem Lab Med* 2003; 41:338–46.

26. Bradwell AR, Carr-Smith HD, Mead GP, Tang LX, Showell PJ, Drayson MT, *et al*. Highly sensitive automated immunoassay for immunoglobulin free light chains in serum and urine. *Clin Chem* 2001; 47:673–80.

27. Drayson M, Tang LX, Drew R, Mead GP, Carr-Smith HD, Bradwell AR. Serum free light chain measurements for identifying and monitoring patients with non-secretory myeloma. *Blood* 2001; 97:2900–2.

28. Katzmann JA, Clark RJ, Abraham RS, Bryant S, Lymp JF, Bradwell AR, *et al*. Serum reference intervals and diagnostic ranges for free κ and free λ immunoglobulin light chains: relative sensitivity for detection of monoclonal light chains. *Clin Chem* 2002; 49:1437–44.

29. Bradwell AR, Tang LX, Drayson MT, Drew RL. Immunoassays for detection of free light chains in sera of patients with non-secretory myeloma. *Blood* 2000; 96: p271b:4906.

30. Whicher JT. Monoclonal proteins. In: Holborow EJ, Reeves WG (eds) *Immunology in medicine*, 2nd edn. London: Academic Press, 1983:531–57.

31. Chapel HM, Lee M, Hargreaves R, Pamphilon DH, Prentice AG. Randomised trial of intravenous immunoglobulin as prophylaxis against infection in plateau-phase multiple myeloma. The UK group for Immunoglobulin Replacement Therapy in Multiple Myeloma. *Lancet* 1994; 343:1059–63.

32. Papadea C, Reimer CB, Check IJ. IgG subclass distribution in patients with multiple myeloma or with monoclonal gammopathy of undetermined significance. *Ann Clin Lab Sci* 1989; 19:27–37.

33. Robertson JD, Nagesh K, Jowitt SN, Dougal M, Anderson H, Mutton K, *et al*. Immunogenicity of vaccination against influenza, *Streptococcus pneumoniae* and *Haemophilus influenzae* type B in patients with multiple myeloma. *Br J Cancer* 2000; 82:1261–5.

●34. Cuzick J, Cooper EH, MacLennan ICM. The prognostic value of serum β2 microglobulin compared with other presentation features in myelomatosis (a report to the Medical Research Council's Working Party on Leukaemia in Adults). *Br J Cancer* 1985; 52:1–6.

35. Tienhaara A, Remes K, Pelliniemi T. Alphainterferon raises serum β microglobulin in patients with multiple myeloma. *Br J Haematol* 1991; 77:335–8.

36. Bataille R, Boccadoro M, Klein B, Durie B, Pileri A. C-reactive protein and beta-2 microglobulin produces a simple and powerful staging system. *Blood* 1992; 80:733–7.

37. Walker SA, Rogers TR, Riches PG, White S, Hobbs JR. Value of serum C-reactive protein in the management of bone marrow transplant recipients. Part I: early transplant period. *J Clin Pathol* 1984; 37:1018–21.

38. Kyle RA. Prognostic factors in multiple myeloma. *Stem Cells* 1995; 13 (Suppl 2):56–63.

150 Biochemical and immunological investigations

39. Sarris AH, Majlis A, Dimopoulos MA, Younes A, Swann F, Rodriguez MA, et al. Rising serum lactate dehydrogenase often caused by granulocyte- or granulocyte-macrophage colony stimulating factor and not tumor progression in patients with lymphoma or myeloma. Leuk Lymphoma 1995; 17:473–7.

40. Capra JD, Kunkel HG. Aggregation of γG3 proteins:relevance of the hyperviscosity syndrome. J Clin Invest 1970; 49:610–21.

41. International Committee for Standardisation in Haematology (Expert Panel on Blood Rheology). Guidelines on selection of laboratory tests for monitoring the acute phase response. J Clin Pathol 1988; 41:1203–12.

42. WHO Scientific Group. The role of immune complexes in disease. Technical Report. Geneva: World Health Organization, 1977:606.

43. Shimm DS, Cohen HJ. Transient monoclonal immunoglobulin G with anti-dextran activity. Acta Haematol (Basel) 1978; 59:99–103.

44. Kalliomaki JL, Granfors K, Toivanen A. An immunoglobulin G myeloma with anti-streptolysin activity and a lifelong history of cutaneous Streptococcal infection. Clin Immunol Immunopathol 1978; 9:22–7.

45. Intrator L, Andre C, Chenal C, Sultan C. Monoclonalmacroglobulin with anti-nuclear activity. J Clin Pathol 1979; 32:450–4.

46. Dighiero G, Guilbert B, Fermand J-P, Limberi P, Danon F, Avrameas S. Human monoclonal immunoglobulins with antibody activity against cytoskeleton proteins, thyroglobulin, and native DNA: immunologic studies and clinical correlations. Blood 1983; 62:264–70.

47. Del Carpio J, Espinoza LR, Lauter S, Osterland CK. Transient monoclonal proteins in drug hypersensitivity reactions. Am J Med 1979; 66:1051–6.

48. Janney FA, Lee LT, Howe C. Cold hemagglutinin cross-reactivity with Mycoplasma pneumoniae. Infect Immunol 1978; 22:29–33.

49. Pruzanski W, Shumak K. Biologic activity of cold-reacting autoantibodies. Second of two parts. N Engl J Med 1977; 297:583–9.

50. Pruzanski W, Shumak KH. Biologic activity of cold reacting autoantibodies (first of two parts). N Engl J Med 1977; 297:538–42.

51. Milford Ward A, Wild GD, Riches PG, Sheldon J (eds) SAS Protein Reference Unit handbook of autoimmunity. Sheffield: PRU Publications, 2001.

52. Bellotti V, Gamba G, Merlini G, Montani N, Bucciarelli E, Stoppini M, et al. Study of three patients with monoclonal gammopathies and 'lupus-like' anticoagulants. Br J Haematol 1989; 73:221–7.

53. Gastineau DA, Kazmier FJ, Nichols WL, Bowie EJW. Lupus anticoagulant: an analysis of the clinical and laboratory features of 219 cases. Am J Haematol 1985; 19:265–75.

54. Bovill EG, Ershler WB, Golden EA, Tindle BH, Edson JR. A human myeloma-produced monoclonal protein directed against the active subpopulation of von Willebrand factor. Am J Clin Pathol 1986; 85:115–23.

55. Thiagarajan Pshapiro SS, De Marco L. Monoclonal immunoglobulin M coagulation inhibitor with phospholipid specificity. Mechanism of lupus anticoagulant. J Clin Invest 1980; 66:397–405.

56. Latov N, Hays AP, Sherman WH. Peripheral neuropathy and anti-MAG antibodies. Crit Rev Neurobiol 1988; 3:301–32.

57. Nobile-Orazio E, Manfredini E, Carpo M, Meucci N, Monaco S, Ferrari S, et al. Frequency and clinical correlates of antineural IgM antibodies in neuropathy associated with IgM monoclonal gammopathy. Ann Neurol 1994; 36:416–24.

58. Pestronk A, Li F, Bieser K, Choksi R, Whitton A, Kornberg AJ, et al. Anti-MAG antibodies: major effects of antigen purity and antibody cross-reactivity on ELISA results and clinical correlation. Neurology 1994; 44:1131–7.

59. Geha RS, Quinti I, Austen KF, Cicardi M, Sheffer A, Rosen FS. Acquired C1-inhibitor deficiency with antiidiotypic antibody to monoclonal immunoglobulins. N Engl J Med 1985; 312:534–40.

60. Alsenz J, Bork K, Loos M. Autoantibody-mediated acquired deficiency of C1-inhibitor. N Engl J Med 1987; 316:1360–6.

61. Cockcroft DW, Gault MH. Prediction of creatinine clearance from serum creatinine. Nephron 1976; 16:31–41.

62. Annesley TM, Burritt MF, Kyle RA. Artefactual hypercalcemia in multiple myeloma. Mayo Clin Proc 1982; 57:572–5.

63. Oren S, Feldman A, Turkot S, Lugassy G. Hyperphosphatemia in multiple myeloma. Ann Haematol 1984; 69:41–3.

64. Owen MC, Pike LS, George PM, Barclay ML, Florkowski CM. Macro-alkaline phosphatase due to IgG k complex: demonstration with polyethylene glycol precipitation and immunofixation. Ann Clin Biochem 2002; 39:523–5.

65. Halabe A, Sperling O. Uric acid nephrolithiasis. Miner Electrolyte Metab 1994; 20:424–31.

66. Riches P, Gooding R, Millar BC, Rowbottom AW. Influence of collection and separation of blood samples on plasma IL1, IL6 and TNF concentrations. J Immunol Meth 1992; 153:125–33.

67. Banks RE. Measurement of cytokines in clinical samples using immunoassays: problems and pitfalls. Crit Rev Clin Lab Sci 2000; 37:131–82.

68. Wadhwa M, Thorpe R. Standardisation and calibration of cytokine immunoassays: meeting report and recommendations. Cytokine 1997; 9:791–3.

69. Bataille R, Jourdan M, Zhang XG, Klein B. Serum levels of interleukin-6 a potent myeloma cell growth factor as a reflection of disease activity in plasma cell dyscrasias. J Clin Invest 1989; 84:2008–11.

70. Clark R, Flory A, Ion E, Woodcock B, Durham B, Fraser W. Biochemical markers of bone turnover following high-dose chemotherapy and autografting in multiple myeloma. Blood 2000; 96:2697–701.

71. Carlson K, Larsson A, Simonsson B, Turesson I, Westin J, Ljunghall S. Evaluation of bone disease in multiple myeloma: a comparison between the resorption markers urinary deoxypyridinoline/creatinine (DPD) and serum ICTP, and an evaluation of the DPT/osteocalcin and ICTP/octeocalcin ratios. Eur J Haematol 1999; 62:300–6.

72. Newman DJ, Cystatin C A personal view. Ann Clin Biochem 2002; 39:89–104.

73. Norlund L, Fex G, Lanke J, Von Schenck H, Nilsson JE, Leksell H, et al. Reference intervals for the glomerular filtration rate and cell proliferation markers: Cystatin C and serum beta2 microglobulin.cystatin C ratio. Scand J Clin Lab Invest 1997; 57:463–70.

74. Hausen A, Fuchs D, Grunewald K, Huber H, Konig K, Wachter H. Urinary neopterine in the assessment of lymphoid and myeloid neoplasia, and neopterine levels in haemolytic anaemia and benign monoclonal gammopathy. Clin Biochem 1982; 15:34–7.

75. Sheldon J, Riches PG, Soni N, Jurges E, Gore M, Dadian G, *et al.* Plasma neopterin as an adjunct to C-reactive protein in the assessment of infection. *Clin Chem* 1991; **37**:2038–42.

76. Suva LJ, Winslow GA, Wettenhall RE, Hammonds RG, Moseley JM, Diefenbach-Jagger H, *et al.* A parathyroid hormone-related protein implicated in malignant hypercalcemia: cloning and expression. *Science* 1987; **237**:893–6.

77. Suzuki A, Takahashi T, Okuno Y, Tsuyuoka R, Sasaki Y, Fukumoto M, *et al.* Production of parathyroid hormone-related protein by cultured human myeloma cells. *Am J Hematol* 1994; **45**:88–90.

78. Zeimer H, Firkin F, Grill V, Slavin J, Zhou H, Martin TJ. Assessment of cellular expression of parathyroid hormone-related protein mRNA and protein in multiple myeloma. *J Pathol* 2000; **192**:336–41.

79. Otsuki T, Yamada O, Kurebayashi J, Sakaguchi H, Yata K, Uno M, *et al.* Expression and in vitro modification of parathyroid hormone-related protein (PTHrP) and PTH/PTHrP-receptor in human myeloma cells. *Leuk Lymphoma* 2001; **41**:397–409.

80. Haider M, Saider SQ. Assessment of protein-calorie malnutrition. A review. *Clin Chem* 1984; **30**:1286–99.

81. Pierce GF, Garrett NC, Koenig J, Lichti DA, Chan K-M. Interference by monoclonal proteins in the o-phthalaldehyde method for blood urea nitrogen. *Clin Chim Acta* 1986; **154**:233–6.

82. Pudek MR, Nanji AA. Antibody interference with biochemical tests and its clinical significance. *Clin Biochem* 1983; **16**:275–80.

APPENDIX A

National quality assurance schemes

Many countries have national quality assurance schemes. Laboratories should participate in these schemes to ensure comparability of results with other laboratories and general good laboratory performance.

In the UK, the United National External Quality Assessment Schemes runs the following schemes that may be relevant:

- specific proteins (includes quantification of immunoglobulins in serum);
- general clinical chemistry (includes electrolytes, urea, creatinine, calcium, liver, and bone enzymes).

Wolfson EQA Laboratory
PO Box 3909
Birmingham
B15 2UE
Tel: + 44 121 414 7300
Fax: + 44 121 414 1179
Email: queries@ukneqas.org.uk

- monoclonal proteins (includes detection and quantification of monoclonal components in serum and urine);
- C-reactive protein;
- β_2-microglobulin.

UKNEQAS
PO Box 894
Sheffield S5 7TY
Tel: + 44 121 414 7300
Fax: + 44 121 414 1179
Email: office@ukneqas.org.uk

In the USA, the College of American Pathologists runs the validation schemes:

- electrophoresis (serum total protein, albumin, monoclonal identification and quantification, and immunoglobulin quantification);
- diagnostic immunology (includes immunoglobulins, complement C3 and C4, and C-reactive protein);
- tumor markers (includes β_2-microglobulin);
- general clinical chemistry.

College of American Pathologists
325 Waukegan Road
Northfield
Illinois 60093-2750
Tel: 800 323 4040
Website: www.cap.org

APPENDIX B

Samples

Suggested samples to be used in the investigation of myeloma.

Investigation	Suggested sample
Immunoglobulins, protein electrophoresis, and typing of monoclonal protein in blood	Serum preferred (blood taken into tubes without additive)
Urine electrophoresis and Bence Jones protein (BJP) detection	Early-morning urine, random urine, 24-hour, or timed urine collection
β_2-microglobulin	Serum
IgG subclasses	Serum
Functional antibodies	Serum
Immunoglobulin glycosylation	Serum
Viscosity	Plasma – blood taken into EDTA or lithium heparin
Cryoproteins	Clotted blood and EDTA plasma collected at 37 °C (syringes, needles, and tubes warmed to 37 °C and blood centrifuged at 37 °C)
Immune complexes	Serum
Autoantibodies	Serum
Electrolytes	Serum or lithium heparin
Calcium	Serum or lithium heparin
Albumin	Serum or lithium heparin
Liver function tests and alkaline phosphatase	Serum or lithium heparin
Uric acid	Serum or lithium heparin
C-reactive protein	Serum or lithium heparin
Cytokines	Blood collected into endotoxin-free tubes or serum or EDTA separated immediately after collection
Cystatin C	Serum
Lactate dehydrogenase	Serum
Neopterin	Serum or lithium heparin
Serum amyloid A	Serum or lithium heparin
Drugs	Usually serum but suggest consult laboratory
Nutritional markers	Serum or lithium heparin
Markers of bone metabolism	Serum or urine depending marker – suggest consult laboratory

APPENDIX C

Equipment and reagents

This includes a list of companies that produce equipment of reagents that in our experience or to our knowledge perform satisfactorily. Inclusion in this list is not an endorsement of any of the products. Other products may be available but are not listed here because we have no specific knowledge or experience of them.

Electrophoresis systems (includes equipment, reagents, antiserum, etc.)

Beckman Coulter
Sebia
Helena

Additional antiserum

Dako (high-titer and reliable antisera for detection of IgD, IgE, κ, and λ light chains)

Urine concentration systems

Sartorius Collodion bags
Intersep concentrators
Amicon concentrators

Dedicated protein analyzers

Dade Behring
Beckman Coulter
Roche, Boehringer Mannheim

Miscellaneous

Chemicals, stains, etc. can be bought from BDH or Sigma

APPENDIX D

Mild sulfhydryl reduction of 'sticky' IgM paraproteins

1   Dilute the serum sample as recommended in your standard electrophoresis procedure.
2   Add dithiothreitol (Cleland's reagent) to a concentration of 1 mg/mL of the diluted sample.
3   Incubate at room temperature for 10 minutes.
4   Run the electrophoresis or immunofixation, according to your normal protocol.

APPENDIX E

Investigation of cryoproteins

COLLECTION OF SPECIMENS FOR CRYOPROTEINS

Blood must be collected into tubes that have been warmed to 37 °C and transported to the patient in a warm vacuum flask. Increasingly, vacuum-type tubes are being used but, if a syringe-based system is being used, then these must also be warmed to 37 °C and transported in the vacuum flask to the patient. Serum (tube with no anticoagulant and no additives) and plasma samples (EDTA or sodium citrate) should be collected so both cryoglobulins and cryofibrinogen may be detected. For laboratories doing a significant number of cryoinvestigations, we suggest that a thermos flask, blood collection tubes, and syringes, if necessary, are kept ready to use in a 37 °C incubator. Once the samples have been taken, they should be returned to the warm vacuum flask and transported back to the laboratory. The serum should be allowed to clot at 37 °C for approximately 1 hour, and then both serum and plasma centrifuged at 37 °C, preferably in a temperature-controlled centrifuge. Laboratories without these facilities can still do cryoprotein investigations using a temperature-maintained water bath, thermos flasks, and warmed centrifuge buckets. The serum and plasma should each be separated into two aliquots, one of each to be incubated at 37 °C and the other aliquots incubated at 4 °C.

DETECTION OF CRYOPROTEINS

1   Cryoproteins can precipitate (or dissolve) very quickly, so you must try to maintain the samples at their appropriate temperatures throughout any procedures. For automated procedures, we usually allocate the sample to a position early on the run and load it at the last possible moment. In manual techniques, once the samples have been diluted, the cryoprotein is less likely to precipitate. However, it is important to be vigilant, and changes in the appearance of the samples between the start and end of the assay should be noted.
2   The serum sample that has been kept at 37 °C should be analyzed after 24 hours' incubation for total protein, IgG, IgA, IgM, C3, C4, CRP, and rheumatoid factor.
3   Serum protein electrophoresis should be done on all four samples (serum at 37 °C and at 4 °C, and the plasma samples at 37 °C and at 4 °C) after 24 hours incubation. At this stage, inspect all four samples. Look for cloudiness, visible precipitates, or any difference in appearance between the samples at 37 °C and those at 4 °C.

4 If no precipitation was noted at 24 hours, re-examine after 72 hours' total incubation time.

5 If there is any doubt:
(a)   centrifuge of the samples at 4 °C in a temperature-controlled centrifuge at 4 °C – this may make any precipitate more readily visible;
(b)   try to 'redissolve' the precipitate by warming the tube to 37 °C.

6 If you decide that a cryoprotein is present, it is important that it should be identified.

IDENTIFICATION OF CRYOPROTEINS

These instructions apply to serum and/or plasma.

1 Cool the centrifuge to 4 °C.
2 Cool approximately 20 mL of 0.9% sodium chloride (normal saline) to 4 °C.
3 Centrifuge the sample at 4 °C for 15 minutes at approx. 2000*g*.
4 Carefully remove the supernatant into a labeled tube, measure and record its volume – this is the *supernatant 4 °C* and will be used in step 7.
5 Add 1 mL of the cold saline to the precipitate. Mix it thoroughly (preferably on a vortex mixer), then centrifuge at 4 °C for 15 minutes at approx. 2000*g*.
6 Give the cryoprecipitate two more washes (remove the supernatant – and discard – and resuspend the precipitate in cold saline, mix and centrifuge). At the end of the final centrifugation, resuspend the precipitate in 1 mL of 0.9% sodium chloride (normal saline) that is at room temperature. Mix this thoroughly and put the 'washed' cryoprecipitate at 37 °C to redissolve.
7 Run electrophoresis on the sample at 37 °C, the supernatant at 4 °C and the redissolved cryoprecipitate at 37 °C.

8 If there is a visible band in the redissolved cryoprecipitate, this can be identified by immunofixation (including fibrinogen, if you have investigated a plasma sample).

Establishing the thermal profile of a cryoprotein

This can be an important element in the investigation of a cryoprotein. The sample should be put into a water bath or incubator warmed to 37 °C and the temperature gradually reduced (approx. 5 °C at a time). The sample must be allowed to equilibrate at each temperature, and the operator has to agitate the sample to ascertain whether it is getting more viscous and look very carefully for signs of cloudiness. When the general temperature of the precipitation has been reached, the temperature can be adjusted in smaller steps around this point.

Estimation of the amount of cryoprotein

The cryoprotein can be estimated proportionately by the 'cryocrit' method. Take two small centrifuge tubes (approx. 1 cm diameter that will hold approx. 2–5 mL of sample). Put the sample in one of the tubes and label it appropriately. Place an equal volume of water into the second tube and calibrate this roughly into 10% intervals (using a ruler and marker pen). Both tubes are then centrifuged at 4 °C for 30 minutes and the approximate proportion of cryoprotein is estimated by comparison with the calibrated balance tube.

10

The role of imaging in multiple myeloma

BRIAN G.M. DURIE

INTRODUCTION

Bone destruction is the most important clinical feature of multiple myeloma.[1] As discussed in Chapter 6, myeloma can induce localized bone destruction in the form of lytic bone lesions and/or diffuse loss of bone integrity in the form of osteoporosis. Both these types of bone lesions can weaken bone, resulting in bone fractures or collapse of bones, such as vertebrae.

The primary goal of imaging techniques is the early detection of myeloma-associated bone destruction as a basis for treatment and subsequent monitoring. Secondary goals of imaging include discrimination between active or symptomatic myeloma with bone destruction and other disease states, such as monoclonal gammopathy of undetermined significance (MGUS). Imaging can also contribute to the assessment of prognosis and to determining

the need for treatment in early stage myeloma (see Chapters 12 and 13).

A summary of the uses of imaging is shown in Table 10.1, and the imaging technologies currently available are shown in Table 10.2. In this chapter, the role of each of these technologies in achieving the primary and secondary imaging goals will be summarized and discussed.

STANDARD RADIOLOGY

In 1903, Weber first noted that myeloma lytic lesions are evident on radiographs.[2] Over the years since then, X-rays have been used to identify myeloma-related bone disease. Despite 100 years of experience, there are still drawbacks in the use of standard radiology, in terms of both sensitivity and specificity (see Table 10.3). Some areas are not well visualized, e.g. the ribs, sternum and scapulae, and the pedicles of the vertebrae. Other imaging techniques may, therefore, be required for adequate

Table 10.1 *The role of imaging in multiple myeloma and related disorders*

- Diagnosis and differential diagnosis
  - MM vs. MGUS
  - SPB vs. early MM
- Indentification of high-risk myeloma lesions
  - Fractures/impending fractures
  - Spinal cord/nerve compression
- Evaluation of extent of disease
  - Staging and assessment of prognosis
  - As a baseline against which to assess subsequent changes
- Assessment of need for treatment in asymptomatic myeloma

MGUS, monoclonal gammopathy of undetermined significance; MM, multiple myeloma; SPB, solitary plasmacytoma of bone.

Table 10.2 *Currently available imaging techniques*

- Standard radiology (X-ray)
- Computed axial tomography (CT scanning)
- Magnetic resonance imaging (MRI)
- Nuclear imaging techniques including:
  - standard bone scintigraphy (bone scan)
  - MIBI scanning
  - FDG/PET scanning
- Bone densitometry measurement

FDG/PET, fluorodeoxyglucose positron emission tomography; MIBI, (technetium) 2-methoxy-isobutyl-isonitrile.

assessment of such areas. Standard radiology is not well equipped for the detection of early lytic bone disease, as at least 30% of bone mineral content must be lost before this is detectable on X-ray. Again, newer computer imaging techniques can be used to help with this type of assessment. Similarly, standard radiology may fail to detect diffuse osteopenia, which is the only impact upon the skeleton in 20% of myeloma patients. It cannot discriminate between osteopenia due to myeloma and that due to other causes, such as steroid-induced or post-menopausal osteopenia, and it is not able to detect resolution of disease, as healing is extremely rare (see later). Nevertheless, standard radiology remains the mainstay of imaging technique for diagnosis and management in most cases. Recommendations for the use of standard radiology are summarized in Table 10.4.

Diagnosis

Myeloma bone lesions are typically osteolytic and occur predominantly in the axial skeleton, i.e. skull, spine, rib cage, and pelvis, plus the proximal areas of the arms and legs (see Fig. 10.1 and Plate 4). A 'full skeletal survey' is the standard requisition to assess for the presence or absence of lytic disease. It is important to include all the sites of active marrow in the adult, comprising the cervical, thoracic and lumbar spine, skull, chest, pelvis, humeri, and femora.[3] A careful protocol is required. For example, the lateral skull X-ray must always compare the same side of the skull. Multiple views are required to assess the inner table of the bone cortex adequately where early lesions occur. The early crescent-shaped erosions can be easily missed. Approximately 50% of the cortex needs to be

Table 10.3 *Limitations in the use of standard radiology (see text for further discussion)*

- Some areas are not well-visualized
- Not sensitive for the detection of early lytic bone disease or diffuse osteopenia
- Cannot discriminate between osteopenia due to myeloma and that due to other causes
- Not able to detect resolution of disease

Table 10.4 *Use of standard radiography in myeloma*

- *Baseline evaluation* of patients with monoclonal protein in the serum and/or urine. *Full skeletal survey should include*: skull, spine (lateral and AP views of cervical, thoracic and lumbar spine), chest, shoulders and humeri, pelvis, hips, and femora.
- *In symptomatic patients,* additional imaging may be required for biopsy, radiotherapy, surgery, and/or other therapeutic interventions.
- *If standard radiology* is negative for lytic disease and/or osteopenia, additional imaging can be considered, especially in symptomatic patients.

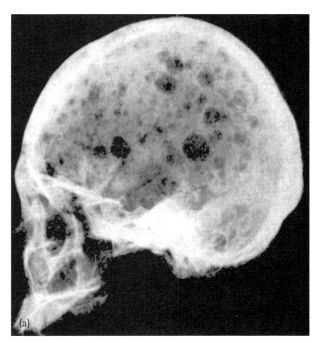
(a)

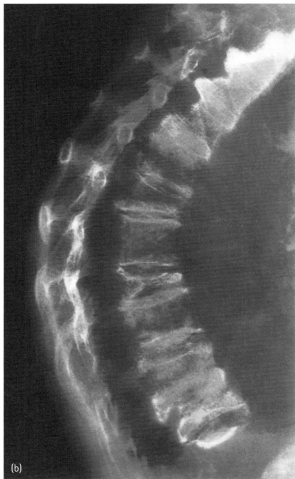
(b)

Figure 10.1 *Standard X-rays of (a) skull, showing lytic lesions, and (b) spine, showing osteoporosis and vertebral collapse.*

eroded to have good visualization. For optimal visualization of the vertebral bodies and the pedicles, both lateral and anteroposterior (AP) views of the spine are advised.

The presence of lytic lesions is a major criterion for diagnosis. However, the limitations of standard radiology in diagnosis include limited sensitivity (failure to detect early disease, whether lytic or osteopenic), lack of specificity (steroid-induced or sex hormone deficiency osteopenia versus myeloma), and poor visualization of occult sites.

X-rays are still the first step: the 'gold standard.' If lytic lesions are detected, then the full skeletal survey is sufficient. In the absence of lytic disease, further imaging may be advisable. If there is diffuse osteopenia in the absence of lytic disease, magnetic resonance imaging (MRI; see later) is recommended to determine whether the osteopenia is due to bone marrow disease. For example, MRI of the spine can help clarify whether osteopenia with collapse of a vertebra is myeloma-related or due to post-menopausal osteopenia. In patients with either normal X-rays or abnormalities that are not definitively myeloma related, MRI of the spine (with and without gadolinium) is recommended to assess the predilection for bone damage and to complete the staging assessment. Areas of bone pain negative on X-ray can be evaluated by MRI and/or computed tomography. This is particularly critical for back pain, which can be an indication of spinal cord compression. Since plasma cell disease can be partially or completely extramedullary, MRI and/or nuclear imaging can prove essential to fully diagnose medically urgent disease.

Differential diagnosis

The demonstration of lytic bone disease on X-ray clearly assists in differentiating myeloma from MGUS and solitary plasmacytoma. Newer imaging techniques are also helpful in this regard, as discussed below, and can also more definitely allow diagnosis of MGUS[4] (with no bone disease) and/or solitary plasmacytomata with no additional lesions in bone or in extramedullary sites (see Chapter 27). Standard X-rays can, however, be sufficient to reveal bony sclerosis associated with POEMS syndrome (polyneuropathy, organomegaly, endocrinopathy, monoclonal gammopathy, and skin changes).[5,6]

Determination of the extent of bone disease

There are several reasons for exactly characterizing myeloma bone disease as summarized in Table 10.1. Confirming the diagnosis and identifying impending fractures are obvious advantages. Even if myeloma bone disease is demonstrated on X-ray of a symptomatic area, a full skeletal survey should still be performed to detect areas that may be at risk of fracture and, therefore, require intervention. Carefully documenting the extent of

myeloma bone disease at the start of treatment is also a critically important baseline for future monitoring. The use of MRI, where available, in addition to standard X-rays may be helpful. Reserving MRI or other imaging 'until later' may seem cost-effective but can frequently detract from future decision-making, because it is not clear whether a new lesion on MRI is truly new.

The extent of lytic bone disease on standard radiology is a key criterion in the Durie–Salmon staging system (see Chapter 12). However, the use of standard radiology alone for staging purposes has always been difficult. Firstly, it is observer-dependent. Secondly, it is technology-dependent with a risk of understaging. In addition, reproducibility between radiology departments is remarkably difficult to achieve. Conversely, one is unlikely to miss clinically important disease in the absence of pain.[1] Plus the situations in which there is true confusion and misclassification of stage based upon X-rays alone are rather few.[7] When traditional staging is combined with use of other prognostic factors, such as serum β_2-microglobulin, serum albumin, age, performance status, and bone marrow cytogenetics, prognostic classification becomes rather precise.

Follow-up and monitoring

It is very rare for lytic bone lesions to recalcify:[8] even in patients in complete remission after high-dose therapy bone healing is only observed in 29%.[9] Radiological assessment does not, therefore, form part of the standard criteria for assessing response to treatment in myeloma.[10] On the other hand, radiological evidence of new bone lesions or definite increase in size of existing lesion(s) is sufficient to define progressive disease.[10]

COMPUTED TOMOGRAPHY

Computed tomography (CT) is very helpful[11–13] for the visualization of soft tissue involvement and for more detailed evaluation of bones in myeloma (see Fig. 10.2). It is generally cumbersome to image large segments of the body, but with newer rapid axial technologies, much more can be accomplished. For example, rapid CT of the chest is highly feasible and informative. The advantage of CT used in this fashion versus MRI is that one can assess the impact of bone marrow myeloma infiltration upon cortical bone that is precisely imaged by CT. Any soft tissue extension, if present, is also well visualized. However, the traditional use of CT is to image small areas of particular concern, such as the pedicle of a vertebra or an area of myeloma involvement close to a joint. CT is helpful as a basis for radiation therapy planning plus port assignment, as well as in preparation for surgical intervention to delineate the anatomic architecture as precisely as possible (see Fig. 10.3).

In comparison with standard X-ray, CT scanning rarely changes staging determinations. However, CT is particularly helpful in the documentation of the soft tissue extension of lytic lesions affecting the rib cage or pelvis. It is important also for CT-guided needle biopsy of lesions that are non-palpable and/or are in hard to reach locations. The use of CT is summarized in Table 10.5.

MAGNETIC RESONANCE IMAGING

Magnetic resonance imaging (MRI) has been widely available for the evaluation of myeloma for over 15 years (see Fig. 10.4).

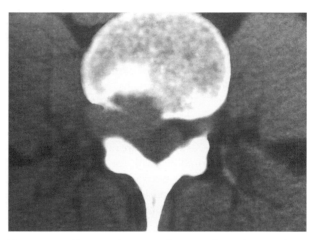

Figure 10.2 *Computed tomography scan of a lumbar vertebra illustrating a destructive lytic lesion posteriorly to the left compressing the nerve root. This lesion was not well visualized on standard radiographs.*

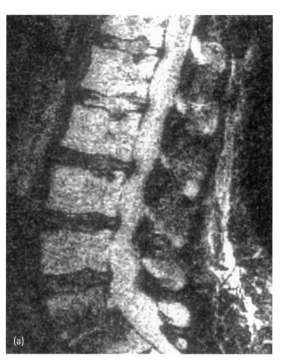

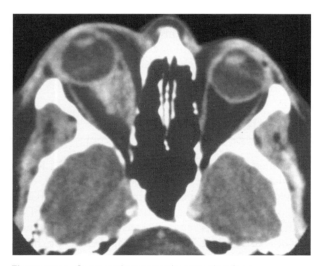

Figure 10.3 *Computed tomography scan showing a retro-orbital plasmacytoma behind the left orbit. This study served as the basis for a guided biopsy.*

Table 10.5 *Use of computed tomography (CT) scanning in myeloma*

- Detailed evaluation of areas of concern
- Radiotherapy planning
- CT-guided needle biopsy

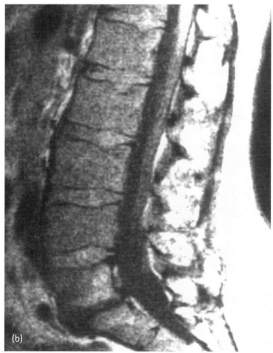

Figure 10.4 *(a) T1-weighted magnetic resonance (MR) image of the lumbar spine showing diffuse plus focal myeloma. The areas of disease are hypointense. (b) T2-weighted MR image.*

During this time, several specific advantages have emerged, as summarized in Table 10.6. First, the axial skeletal areas primarily affected by myeloma can be well imaged. If all the areas are to be imaged, then a special 'screening MRI' protocol must be used as a first step to avoid the enormous time and cost of full wide-field MRI imaging (see Fig. 10.5). Many myeloma specialists perform MRI of the entire spine or major parts of the spine as a baseline and/or to clarify the nature or extent of myeloma involvement, although the availability of MRI is variable in different parts of the world and cost implications currently limit its more widespread use.

Second, taking advantage of the various technical aspects of MRI can be most helpful in definitively identifying myeloma.[14–23] The MRI sequences that are most informative are shown in Table 10.7.

Third, the disease states in which MRI can be helpful have been evaluated. In patients with stage I myeloma and who are asymptomatic and have negative standard radiographs, MRI of the spine is useful.[24] Presence of an abnormal pattern occurs in 30–50% of such patients and indicates an increased likelihood of progression within the next 2 years. In contrast, patients with MGUS have negative MRI patterns.[25] In patients with known active stage II–III myeloma, serial monitoring can be useful to assess response to treatment. It is not clear whether different abnormal patterns, such as focal, diffuse, or mixed patterns of marrow involvement, confer a different prognosis either at baseline or over time.

Fourth, specific clinical scenarios have been identified in which MRI is uniquely important (see Table 10.8).

MRI is, therefore, frequently used for clinical decision-making rather than for formal staging and/or prognostic classification. As a clinical tool, MRI is enormously useful. The major disadvantages are the difficulties with wide-field screening and the non-discrimination between stable and active myeloma. The latter is an important clinical aspect. MGUS is negative by MRI. However, stage I and indolent or smoldering myeloma is frequently positive,

Table 10.6 *Specific advantages of magnetic resonance imaging*

- Excellent imaging of axial skeleton
- T1-weighted-, STIR, and gadolinium-enhanced sequences allow discrimination of myeloma from normal marrow, fat, and other pathologies
- Greater sensitivity compared with standard radiology
- Unique utility in clinical management (see Table 10.8)

STIR, sagittal T1-weighted inversion recovery.

Table 10.7 *Interpretation of magnetic resonance images*

Image	Interpretation
• T1-weighted	• Increased signal with fatty replacement • Focal myeloma lesions *hypo*intense
• T2-weighted with fat suppression • STIR	• Focal myeloma lesions *hyper*intense • Fatty replacement is *hypo*intense • Focal myeloma lesions *hyper*intense
• With gadolinium, T1-weighted with fat suppression	• Focal myeloma lesions enhance with gadolinium

STIR, sagittal T1-weighted inversion recovery.

Table 10.8 *Clinical scenarios identified in which magnetic resonance imaging (MRI) is uniquely important*

- Spinal cord and/or nerve root compression
- Soft tissue extension with organ/tissue injury
- Head and neck myeloma/plasmacytomata in both bone and soft tissue
- Evaluation of cardiac amyloidosis and/or soft tissue amyloid deposits[26]
- Hip MRI to identify avascular necrosis versus other pathologies
- Discrimination between hemangiomata and other pathologies
- Assessment of radiation effects on bone marrow

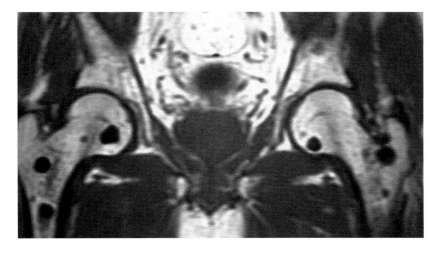

Figure 10.5 *Example of 'wide-field' magnetic resonance image showing multiple hypointense lesions in the femora and pelvis.*

but this positivity is *not* an indicator of need for immediate therapy. As noted above, such patients can remain stable for 2 years or longer. Likewise, for patients monitored during and after treatment who have residual disease, this residual 'MRI-positive myeloma' is not necessarily active disease that requires treatment. Distorted anatomy, including scar tissue or fibrosis, may also occur as part of what appears to be residual disease post-therapy.

NUCLEAR MEDICINE IMAGING

This has been used in an effort to improve the sensitivity of detection of myeloma bone disease as well as overcome some of the drawbacks with other technologies.

Although traditional technetium bone scintigraphy is highly sensitive for detection of solid tumor metastases to bone, that is not the case for myeloma or plasmacytomata. Conventional radiographs detect more lytic lesions (74–82%) versus bone scintigraphy (37–60%).[27,28] Bone scintigraphy is, therefore, not recommended. Nonetheless, it is worth noting that fractured rib lesions and very aggressive destructive lesions do image with bone scintigraphy, and such findings can be occasionally helpful and/or prognostically important.

Likewise, gallium-67 nuclear scans have been reported to be helpful to identify aggressive disease and/or extra-osseous involvement.[29] Sesta MIBI (technetium-2-methoxy-isobutyl-isonitrile; ^{99m}Tc-MIBI) scanning has also been used in the evaluation of myeloma.[30] The sensitivity of MIBI scanning is similar to standard radiology for the detection of lytic disease. Although MIBI uptake indicates presence of myeloma versus treated or healed lesions, as in the case of MRI, this does not necessarily indicate aggressive or active disease. MIBI scanning can be helpful to assess disease status post-therapy, especially in patients with non-secretory disease or unclear disease markers.

POSITRON EMISSION TOMOGRAPHY

Positron emission tomography (PET) scanning using ^{18}F glucose (FDG) is a new technology for evaluation of myeloma (see Fig. 10.6).[31–40] Since 1996, a large experience with whole-body FDG/PET has been accumulated at the Cedars Sinai Comprehensive Cancer Center.[31] Over 100 patients have been scanned with over 5 years of follow-up for the early patients. The initial experience has recently been published. Results are summarized in Table 10.9.

The particular advantages of whole body FDG/PET are several. It is more sensitive than standard radiology in that 25% of patients with positive scans have negative X-rays. However, unlike MRI, FDG/PET does not necessarily detect the early anatomic distortion in the bone marrow

found in patients with asymptomatic stage I disease with negative X-rays. Both MRI and FDG/PET are negative in MGUS, which is very helpful for confirmation of MGUS. MRI can detect early indolent marrow involvement. Whole-body FDG/PET detects early active myeloma, typically stage II or III with other evidence of disease progression. The poor-risk subgroup of patients with extramedullary disease is detected with whole body FDG/PET. Although MRI also reveals such disease, it is very cumbersome to perform wide-field MRI screening to encompass the potential areas of involvement.

The particular advantage of whole-body FDG/PET is the rapid screening of the entire skeletal areas at risk both at baseline and for serial monitoring. For early detection of residual or relapsing disease post-stem-cell transplantation and/or in patients with non-secretory or hyposecretory disease, this ability to monitor disease status objectively is most helpful. Areas of residual disease can be biopsied for special studies, such as genetic analysis. An unexpected adjunct to the use of FDG/PET is the detection of other malignancies with whole-body FDG/PET. Thus far, previously unknown renal, pancreatic, uterine, and prostate carcinoma have been diagnosed in patients with MGUS or early myeloma.

Additional studies are required to assess and confirm the overall clinical utility of whole-body FDG/PET.

DUAL–HEAD BONE DENSITOMETRY

Bone densitometry is useful to clarify the severity of diffuse osteopenia that is felt to be myeloma related.[41,42] Serial monitoring of patients receiving bisphosphonate therapy can be used to quantify improvement. With successful therapy, it is not unusual to document 5–10% improvement over a 6-month period. Since newer, more powerful bisphosonates are now available, failure to achieve benefit may trigger a switch to one of the newer agents.

SUMMARY

The various technologies discussed are complementary to each other in the evaluation of plasma cell disorders. The major advantages of each type are summarized in Table 10.10. Skeletal bone survey is mandatory for overall disease assessment. Clinically important disease is detected by X-ray. However, early focal and/or diffuse myeloma and soft tissue disease are often missed or not well delineated. CT scanning is ideal for detailed evaluation and treatment planning. MRI is excellent for wider-field assessment of the axial skeleton, when further information is required for clinical decision-making. Whole-body FDG/PET scanning is a new technology that should

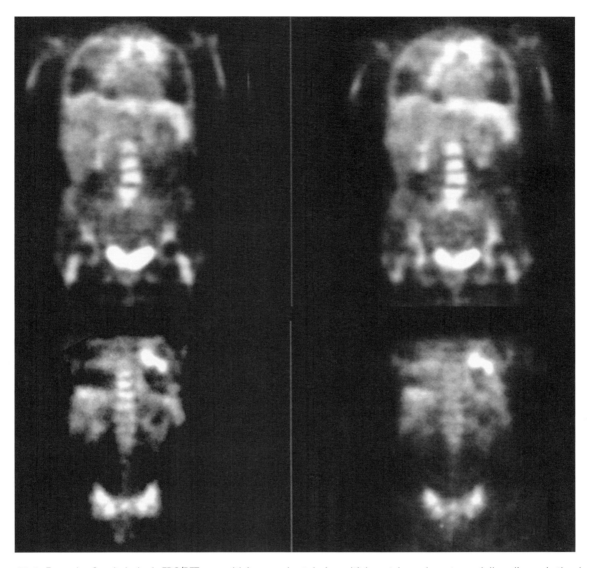

Figure 10.6 *Example of a whole-body FDG/PET scan with increased uptake in multiple vertebrae plus extramedullary disease in the chest.*

Table 10.9 *Whole-body FDG/PET scan results*

Disease state	Results
• MGUS	• Negative
• Myeloma	
At diagnosis	Usually positive
	• Usually multiple focal lesions evident
	• 25% have negative X-rays
	• 25% have extramedullary disease
Remission	Usually negative
	• Usually negative or with minimal uptake
	• Residual disease predicts early relapse
Relapse	Usually positive
	• Reliably detects relapse
	• Extra medullary disease is a poor prognostic sign

FDG/PET, fluorodeoxyglucose positron emission tomography; MGUS, monoclonal gammopathy of undetermined significance.

Table 10.10 *Summary of imaging technologies*

Technology	Clinical utility
• Standard radiology (skeletal survey)	• Still baseline gold standard for diagnosis and staging
• CT scanning	• Ideal for detailed evaluation of local areas of bone destruction with/without soft tissue extension
• MRI	• Excellent for evaluation of axial skeleton in presence of symptoms and/or if X-rays are negative
• Whole-body FDG/PET	• A new technology that can prove valuable for whole-body assessment of disease activity

CT, computed tomography; FDG/PET, fluorodeoxyglucose positron emission tomography; MRI, magnetic resonance imaging.

prove most helpful for identifying the presence and location of active myeloma incorporating deoxyglucose.

Since bone destruction is the cause of the most disabling problems, careful baseline and serial assessment of bone disease is essential to achieve the best quality of life for myeloma patients.

KEY POINTS

- Standard radiology remains the gold standard for imaging bone disease in myeloma but has limitations in terms of sensitivity and specificity.
- Computed tomography (CT) scanning is useful for imaging areas that are poorly visualized on X-ray, for demonstrating soft tissue disease, for CT-guided biopsy, and for planning radiotherapy.
- Magnetic resonance imaging (MRI) is the optimum technique for demonstrating the site of spinal cord or nerve root compression and is an essential investigation in the diagnosis of solitary plasmacytoma.
- Standard radionucleide bone scanning is relatively insensitive in myeloma but newer techniques, such as FDG/PET scanning, are helpful in visualizing occult sites of disease.

REFERENCES

● = Key primary paper
◆ = Major review article
* = Paper that represents the first formal publication of a management guideline

1. Durie BGM, Salmon SE. A clinical staging system for multiple myeloma. *Cancer* 1975; **36**:842–54.
2. Kyle RA. History of multiple myeloma. In: Wiernik PH, Canellos GP, Kyle RA, Schiffer CA (eds) *Neoplastic diseases of the blood*, 3rd edn. New York: Churchill Livingstone, 1996:325–32.
*3. UK Myeloma Forum. Diagnosis and management of multiple myeloma, *Br J Haematol* 2001; **115**:522–40.
4. Kyle RA, Therneau TM, Rajkumar SV, Offord JR, Larson DR, Plevak MF, *et al.* A long-term study of prognosis in monoclonal gammopathy of undetermined significance. *N Engl J Med* 2002; **346**:564–69.
5. Davies ML, Elson DL, Hertz D, McMillin JM. Syndrome of plasma cell dyscrasia, polyneuropathy, and diabetes mellitus. *West J Med* 1990; **152**:257–60.
6. Miralles GD, O'Fallon JR, Talley NJ. Plasma cell dyscrasia with polyneuropathy: the spectrum of POEMS syndrome. *N Engl J Med* 1992; **327**:1919–23.
7. Durie BGM, Bataille R. Therapeutic implications of myeloma staging. *Eur J Haematol.* 1989; **43**:111–16.

8. Cohen HJ, Siberman HR, Tornyos K, Bartolucci AA. Comparison of two long-term chemotherapy regimens, with or without agents to modify skeletal repair, in multiple myeloma. *Blood* 1984; **63**:639–48.
9. Cunningham D, Pas-Ares L, Gore ME, Malpas J, Hickish T, Nicolson M, *et al.* High-dose melphalan for multiple myeloma: long-term follow-up data. *J Clin Oncol* 1994; **12**:764–8.
10. Blade J, Samson D, Reece D, Apperley J, Bjorkstrand B, Gahrton G, *et al.* Criteria for evaluating disease response and progression in patients with multiple myeloma treated by high-dose therapy and haemopoietic stem cell transplantation. Myeloma Subcommittee of the EBMT. European Group for Blood and Marrow Transplant. *Br J Haematol* 1998; **102**:1115–23.
◆11. Kyle RA, Schreiman J, McLeod R. Computed tomography in diagnosis of multiple myeloma and its variants. *Arch Intern Med* 1985; **145**:1451–60.
◆12. Schreiman JS, McLeod RA, Kyle RA, Beabout JW. Multiple myeloma: evaluation by CT. *Radiology* 1985; **154**:483–6.
●13. Vogler JB, Murphy WA. Bone marrow imaging: state of the art. *Radiology* 1988; **168**:679–86.
14. Dimopoulos MA, Moulopoulos A, Smith T. Risk of disease progression in asymptomatic multiple myeloma. *Am J Med* 1993; **94**:57–61.
◆15. Moulopoulos LA, Dimopoulos MA, Alexanian R, Leeds NE, Libshitz HI. Multiple myeloma: MR patterns of response to treatment. M.D. Anderson Cancer Center, *Radiology* 1994; **193**:441–6.
16. Van de Berg BC, Lecouvet FE, Michaux L, Labaisse M, Malghem J, Jamart J, *et al.* Stage I multiple myeloma: value of MR imaging of the bone marrow in the determination of prognosis. St Luc University Hospital. *Radiology* 1996; **201**:243–6.
●17. Kusumoto S, Jinnai I, Itoh, K, Kawai N, Sakata T, Matsuda A, *et al.* Magnetic resonance imaging patterns in patients with multiple myeloma. *Br J Haematol* 1997; **99**:649–55.
●18. Mariette X, Zagdanski AM, Guermazi A, Bergot C, Arnould A, Frija J, *et al.* Prognostic value of vertebral sesions detected by magnetic resonance imaging in patients with stage I multiple myeloma. *Br J Haematol* 1999; **104**:723–9.
19. Moulopoulos LA, Varma DGK, Dimopoulous MA, Leeds NE, Kim EE, Johnston DA, *et al.* Multiple myeloma: spinal MR imaging in patients with untreated newly diagnosed disease. *Radiology* 1992; **185**:833–40.
20. Lecouvet FE, Vande Berg BC, Michaux L, Malghem J, Maldague BE, Jamart J, *et al.* Stage III multiple myeloma: clinical and prognostic value of spinal bone marrow MR imaging. *Radiology* 1998; **209**:653–60.
21. Angtuaco EJ, Avva R, Munshi CN, *et al.* MR skeletal survey of the axial skeleton: a predictor of patient survival in multiple myeloma? *Radiology* 1999; **213**(Suppl): 294 (Abstract 845).
22. Lecouvet FE, Vande Berg BC, Maldague BE, Michaux L, Laterre E, *et al.* Vertebral compression fractures in multiple myeloma. Part I. Distribution and appearance at MR imaging. *Radiology* 1997; **204**:195–9.
23. Lecouvet FE, Malghem J, Michaux L, Michaux JL, Lehmann F, Maldague BE, *et al.* Verterbal compression fractures in multiple myeloma. Part II. Assessment of fracture risk with MR imaging of the spinal bone marrow. *Radiology* 1997; **204**:201–5.

●24. Moulopoulos LA, Dimopoulos MA, Smith TL, Weber DM, Delasalle KB, Libshitz HI, *et al.* Prognostic significance of magnetic resonance imaging in patients with asymptomatic myeloma. *J Clin Oncol* 1995; **13**:251–6.

25. Bellaiche L, Laredo JD, Liote F, Koeger AC, Hamze B, Ziza JM, *et al.* Magnetic resonance appearance of monoclonal gammopathies of unknown significance and multiple myeloma. *Spine* 1997; **22**:2551–7.

26. Fattori R, Rocchi G, Celletti F, Bertaccini P, Rapezzi C, Gavelli G. Contribution of magnetic resonance imaging in the differential diagnosis of cardiac amyloidosis and symmetric hypertrophic cardiomyopathy. *Am Heart J* 1998; **136**:824–30.

27. Woolfenden JM, Pitto MJ, Durie BGM. Comparison of bone scintigraphy and radiography in multiple myeloma. *Radiology* 1980; **134**:726–31.

28. Wahner HW, Kyle RA, Beabout JW. Scintigraphic evaluation of the skeleton in multiple myeloma. *Mayo Clin Proc* 1980; **55**:739–46.

29. Waxman AD, Siemsen JK, Levine AM, Holdorf D, Suzuki R, Singer FR, *et al.* Radiographic and radionuclide imaging in multiple myeloma: the role of gallium scintigraphy: concise communication. *J Nucl Med* 1981; **22**:232–6.

30. Tirovola EB, Biassoni L, Britton KE, Kaleva N, Kouykin V, Malpas JS. The use of ^{99m}Tc-MIBI scanning in multiple myeloma. *Br J Cancer* 1996; **74**:1815–20.

31. Durie BGM, Waxman AD, D'Agnolo A, Williams CM. Whole-body FDG/PET scanning identifies high risk myeloma. *J Nucl Med* 2002; **43**:1457–63.

32. Strauss LG, Conti PS. The applications of PET in clinical oncology. *J Nucl Med.* 1991; **32**:623–48.

33. Conti PS, Lilien DL, Hawley K, Kippler J, Grafton ST, Bading JR. PET and [^{18}F]-FDG in oncology: a clinical update. *Nucl Med Biol* 1996; **23**:717–35.

34. Grossman SJ, Griffeth LK, Hanson PC. PET emerges as clinical oncologic tool. *Oncol Issues* 1999; **14**:16–19.

35. Tucker R, Coel M, Ko J, Morris P, Druger G, McGuigan P. Impact of fluorine-18 fluorodeoxyglucose positron emission tomography on patient management: first year's experience in a clinical center. *J Clin Oncol* 2001; **19**:2504–8.

36. Carrasquillo JA. Clinical indications for FDG positron emission tomography scanning – Part I. *Principles Pract Oncol* 2001; **15**:1–16.

37. Carrasquillo JA. Clinical indications for FDG positron emission tomography scanning – Part II. *Principles Pract Oncol* 2001; **15**:1–16.

38. Schirrmeister H, Buchmann I, Traeger H, Reske SN. Bone marrow imaging with F-18-Fluorodeoxyglucose-PET in patients with multiple myeloma [abstract]. *J Nucl Med* 1999; **40**:211.

39. El-Shirbiny AM, Yeung H, Imbriaco M, Michaeli J, Macapinlac H, *et al.* Technetium-99m-MIBI versus fluorine-18-FDG in diffuse multiple myeloma. *J Nucl Med* 1997; **38**:1208–10.

●40. Orchard K, Barrington S, Buscombe J, Hilson A, Prentice HG, Mehta A. Fluoro-deoxyglucose positron emission tomography imaging for the detection of occult disease in multiple myeloma. *Br J Haematol.* 2002; **117**:133–5.

41. Mariette X, Bergot C, Ravaud P, Roux C, Laval-Jeantet M, Brouet JC, *et al.* Evolution of bone densitometry in patients with myeloma treated with conventional or intensive therapy. *Cancer* 1995; **76**:1559–63.

42. Abildgaard N, Brixen K, Kristensen JE, Vejlgaard T, Charles P, Nielsen JL. Assessment of bone involvement in patients with multiple myeloma using bone densitometry. *Eur J Haematol* 1996; **57**:370–6.

11

Innovative approaches for diagnosis and monitoring

FAITH E. DAVIES AND GARETH J. MORGAN

INTRODUCTION

Recent years have seen major changes in the diagnostic use of genetics-based technologies. The current challenge is applying these technologies to improve treatment approaches in myeloma with the overall aim of individualizing myeloma therapy and improving patient survival. Although this is not feasible currently, within the next decade it is possible to see how strategies based on genetic technologies can be developed and applied in the clinical setting (see Table 11.1). Using these approaches, physicians will be able to not only predict outcome but also determine whether a patient will respond to a given treatment, an approach that is becoming more relevant with the introduction of effective new therapeutic agents.

NOVEL DIAGNOSTICS

Background

The application of novel diagnostic technology has to be within the framework of our current understanding of the pathogenesis of myeloma. The main phenotypic features of myeloma plasma cells include abnormal localization within the bone marrow with the replacement of normal bone elements and dysregulation of immunoglobulin secretion. In normal B-cell development, after encountering its cognate antigen, a virgin B cell migrates to a germinal center. It is thought that the initial event in the development of monoclonal gammopathy of undetermined significance (MGUS) is immortalization of

Table 11.1 *Innovative techniques used in diagnosis and monitoring*

Technique	Application
Molecular cytogenetics	Characterization of molecular events Prognosis Minimal residual disease detection
Gene profiling (tumor and host)	Understanding biology of tumor Prognosis
Expression microarrays	Diagnosis and classification Class prediction
Proteomics	Direct analysis of gene function

such a cell, which is then at an increased risk of developing chromosomal translocations into the immunoglobulin heavy-chain (IgH) switch region and which is genetically unstable. MGUS is a clonal pre-myelomatous condition in which there is a continual passage of clonally related cells through the germinal center, where they acquire mutations within their IgH regions. These cells subsequently migrate to the bone marrow and differentiate into plasma cells. The development of myeloma is associated with the independent growth of one such clone that proliferates within the bone marrow. During the early phases of the disease, the myeloma cells are predominately located in the bone marrow but are in equilibrium with a small population within the peripheral blood. In the later stages of the disease, changes in adhesion molecules may result in a more leukemic phase, which is associated with the acquisition of p53 and RAS mutations.

Despite the advances in our understanding of the pathogenesis of myeloma, most current prognostic and staging systems utilize relatively simple clinical data (see Chapter 12). However, a major criticism of these systems is that they rely on surrogate markers for predicting the behavior of the tumor. Thus, they are not capable of defining distinct biological groups and cannot, therefore, be used to define clinically meaningful subgroups or to predict response to specific treatments. Outlined below are a number of variables that may define important biological subgroups and consequently prove important clinically.

Molecular cytogenetics

Classical cytogenetics has taught us a great deal about the distinct subtypes of myeloma. The routine application of cytogenetics is hampered by the need to generate tumor-specific metaphases. Such approaches have been difficult in myeloma because of problems in reliably obtaining metaphases in an indolent tumor where only 1–2% of cells are in cycle. An abnormal karyotype is present in 30–50% of patients and numerous studies have demonstrated an increased incidence of cytogenetic abnormalities later in the disease process. These findings suggest that chromosomal abnormalities are fundamental in the disease pathogenesis and that they could be used prognostically (see Chapter 4 and Table 11.2).[1–5]

FLUORESCENT *IN SITU* HYBRIDIZATION (FISH)

In order to circumvent the need for metaphase analysis, fluorescent techniques applicable to interphase cells have been developed. Many of the results obtained with cytogenetics have now been confirmed using FISH.[6–8] In particular, chromosome 13q deletions are an important independent adverse prognostic factor with an incidence of approximately 50%.[9–11] However, no minimally deleted region in the 13q arm has been identified and consequently no tumor suppressor genes have yet been identified that are important in disease pathogenesis. Although cytogenetics and interphase and metaphase FISH have different

sensitivities for identifying abnormalities of this area (detection rates range from 15% to 50% depending on technique used), abnormalities of 13q have prognostic significance regardless of the technique used. FISH has also been used to determine the prognostic value of aneuploidy and showed that trisomies of chromosome 6, 9, and 17 are associated with a prolonged survival whereas monosomy 13 is associated with a poor overall survival.[12] With advances in the FISH technique, it appears that the incidence of chromosome 14 switch translocations has been grossly underestimated and that they actually occur in over 80% of cases. To date, 18 partner chromosomes have been identified, although in approximately 30–50% of cases the translocation partner remains unknown. The most frequently identified partners include t(11;14)(q13;q32) in 22–28%, t(4;14)(p16;q32) in 21%, t(8;14)(q24;q32) in 4–10%, t(7;14)(q32;q32) in 5%, t(6;14)(q25;q32) in 1%, and t(14;16)(q32;q23) in 1%.[13–19] These translocations result in a number of proto-oncogenes being juxtaposed to the IgH gene including *cyclin D1*, *fgfr3*, c-*myc*, *mum1/irf4*, and c-*maf*. Correlation of the translocations with prognosis and survival information from large trials suggests the translocations represent distinct disease entities.[20,21] It also appears that 14q32 and 13q chromosomal abnormalities are not randomly distributed, but correlate with presentation variables and prognostic factors (see Table 11.2).[22]

OTHER FISH–BASED APPROACHES

In order to improve the detection rate of chromosomal abnormalities, the basic FISH method has been adapted in a number of ways. Fiber FISH utilizes stretched DNA fibers to determine the position of chromosomal translocations. A mixture of labeled cosmids creates a 'bar code' for the region of interest, resulting in the breakage of the bar code when a breakpoint is present. A panel of myeloma cell lines has been examined using this technique and the results demonstrated that abnormalities

Table 11.2 *Molecular abnormalities detected by conventional cytogenetics and fluorescence* in situ *hybridization (FISH)*

	Detection method	Abnormality	Clinical effect
Numerical	Cytogenetics	Hyperdiploidy/pseudodiploidy/ hypodiploidy Commonly 3, 7, 9, 11, 13, and X	Hyperdiploidy associated with a survival advantage Monosomy 13, confers poor prognosis
	FISH	Trisomy 6, 9, 17 Monosomy 13	Survival advantage Controversial prognostic importance
Structural	Cytogenetics	Translocations and deletions of 1, 6, 16, 19 Del 13 and 11q	No effect Poor survival
	FISH	t(11;14) t(4;14) 14q and del 13	Better response to treatment and improved survival Poor outcome Correlates with clinical outcome

including the chromosome 14 region are very complex, with cryptic insertions of chromosome 14 material into other chromosomes, chromosome 14 deletions, and more than one chromosome 14 rearrangement simultaneously in one cell.[18] This is a difficult technique to perform, has important applications in the research setting, but is not routinely applicable to diagnostic samples.

Chromosomal paints are another useful way of identifying changes in both chromosome number and translocations, although the sensitivity of the technique is poor. Multicolor spectral karyotyping (SKY) is an adaptation of this technique and offers an exciting way to identify both translocation partners and aneuploidy. Using 24 fluorescently labeled 'chromosome paints,' simultaneous visualization of each of the chromosomes in a different color is accomplished. This technique is more sensitive than normal G-banding karyotyping; however, it does not overcome the problems of obtaining adequate metaphases from myeloma cases. As each chromosome is labeled in a unique color, it offers a way of directly visualizing translocation partners without designing specific probes to the regions. Two studies have been published using the SKY technique in myeloma.[23,24] Both studies demonstrated complex karyotypes and identified new translocations involving the immunoglobulin heavy-chain area. These translocations were t(12;14)(q24;q32), t(14;20)(q32;q11), and t(9;14) (p13;q32). The latter translocation is interesting, as it results in the deregulation of the *pax5* gene. This has not previously been identified in myeloma, although it has been described in Waldenström's macroglobulinemia. The other common translocations involving 14q32 were also identified, including t(14;16)(q32;q22), the *c-maf* translocation. This translocation was noted as being more frequent, occurring in six out of 50 cases, suggesting that the incidence of translocations may be dependent on the detection method used.

MATRIX COMPARATIVE GENOMIC HYBRIDIZATION

Hybridization of whole chromosome preparations, as performed by comparative genomic hybridization (CGH) has proved to be a useful tool for the detection of quantitative genomic alterations, i.e. gains and losses of chromosomal regions. Labeled tumor DNA and control DNA are hybridized in a competitive reaction to normal metaphases, and the resulting color ratios measured. The main advantage of this technique, especially in myeloma, is that abnormal tumor metaphases are not required, although samples with a high tumor content are needed (e.g. more than 30% plasma cells). The technique is relatively insensitive as only regions with loss or gain of greater than 10 Mb are detectable. A number of 'hot spots' have been identified, including chromosomal gains in 1q, 8q, and 11q, and losses in 13q, 6q, and 16q.[25,26] The use of CHIP-based solid-phase approaches to detect

chromosomal losses or gains has recently been developed, with the aim of improving resolution of traditional CGH and simplifying the analysis procedure.[27] This is achieved by substituting the target chromosomes with nucleic acid preparations consisting of defined sequences, such as sequence pools representative of whole chromosomes or chromosome arms down to the relevant fragment cloned in a YAC, BAC, PAC, cosmid, or other vectors. The resulting platform consists of a glass slide with immobilized target DNA arrayed in small spots. Using this method, both low and high copy number gains and losses are readily identified with the minimal size of deletions detectable being approximately 100 kb. The introduction of methods like these provides the basics for the development of automated diagnostic procedures with biochips with the ultimate aim of developing a chip-based technique to detect all of the genetic changes associated with myeloma.

POLYMERASE CHAIN REACTION (PCR)-BASED APPROACHES FOR CHARACTERIZING CHROMOSOMAL TRANSLOCATIONS

While the majority of the work characterizing switch translocations involving chromosome 14 has used Southern blotting, given the large amount of DNA required for this test, it is not readily applicable to patient material.[13–17] A vectorette PCR method has been developed to identify novel translocation partners in patient material.[28] The switch regions are several kilobases in length, located upstream (5′) to each of the constant heavy-chain (C_H) genes and consist of tandemly repeated G/C sequences within which the breakpoints for the switch rearrangements are found. The legitimate recombination between an upstream switch region (generally $S\mu$) and a downstream switch region results in the deletion of the intervening DNA, normally in the form of a circle, and the repositioning of an unchanged VDJ region in front of a new constant region. Point mutations, insertions, and deletions occur during this process near the site of recombination and indicate that an error-prone DNA synthesis mechanism is part of the process. The addition of the vectorette system to the PCR allows DNA fragments to be amplified when the sequence of only one end is known, for example 3′ primers recognizing the switch region sequences may be used. The method, therefore, offers advantages over the Southern blot, as it is more simple and rapid to perform and allows the simultaneous detection and isolation of the recombinant breakpoint regions.

PCR can also be used to look for specific known translocations, which occur relatively frequently in multiple myeloma (MM). The t(4;14) translocation is found in approximately 10% of myeloma patients and results in the deregulation of at least two genes, *mmset* and *fgfr3*, with the formation of a fusion product between *mmset* and IgH and overexpression of *fgfr3* expression.[16] Given the potential prognostic importance of this translocation, a PCR-based approach to detect the presence of the translocation in patient material has been developed. Using a reverse transcripton (RT)-PCR method, the presence of the IgH MMSET fusion product can also be identified and importantly correlated with an overexpression of FGFR3 expression as measured by RT-PCR.[29] This technique is highly sensitive and also offers an alternative method for minimal residual disease detection.

Genetic profiling

OF THE TUMOR

Characterization of mutations and, more recently, gene expression differences based on epigenetic silencing of defined genes offers an exciting way of looking at prognosis by characterization of the tumor cell. Many studies have been carried out over the years looking at the genetic changes acquired within the malignant plasma cell. These have been discussed in other chapters; however, these studies would suggest that mutations within oncogenes and tumor suppressor genes as well as tumor suppressor gene loss, as distinct from mutation, are rare events at presentation in multiple myeloma limiting their use as prognostic variables. They are, however, frequently detected in patients with endstage disease, which suggests they may play a part in disease progression rather then being key events in the initial pathogenesis.

In addition to gene deletion and mutation as a mechanism for tumor suppressor gene inactivation, methylation is also a relevant clinical mechanism. Approximately 40% of myeloma patients show methylation of p16 at diagnosis, whereas methylation of p15 is less frequent.[30,31] The presence of p16 hypermethylation correlates with other known poor prognostic factors and with a short progression-free and overall survival.[32] The use of methylation-sensitive PCR and chip-based strategies for the detection of gene inactivation may be a relevant technology.

OF THE PATIENT

The characterization of inherited genetic variation, and its effect on tumor response and the side effects of chemotherapy, have become more relevant since the completion of the human genome project. Single nucleotide polymorphisms (SNPs) within important genes can alter the function of the gene, particularly if they occur within promotor or functional coding regions. Until recently, the detection and characterization of SNPs was laborious, usually involving restriction fragment length polymorphism (RFLP) techniques. Real-time PCR has facilitated the rapid and accurate detection of SNPs. Taqman and

minor groove binding (MGB) probes are the current optimum approach but other high-throughput platforms are being developed. These techniques include single nucleotide extension combined with mass spectrometry detection and chip-based approaches.

A number of studies have explored the use of these techniques to look at the etiology and outcome of myeloma. Genetic variants within tumor necrosis factor (TNF) can affect the pro-inflammatory response and it has been suggested that they may influence the risk of developing myeloma and the outcome after treatment. Thalidomide exerts some of its effects via modulation of TNF and, interestingly, it has been suggested that these genetic variants may also affect the likelihood of responding to thalidomide.[33] Despite these encouraging results investigating the effects of TNF variants,[34] variants at the interleukin-6 (IL-6) locus,[35] a gene of central importance in myeloma, have not been shown to be relevant clinically. Variants at the GSTP1 locus are, however, clinically relevant.[36] This is a xenobiotic metabolizer gene, which metabolizes environmentally encountered alkylating agents and many of the therapeutic agents used in myeloma. Underactive variants of this gene are associated with increased risks of developing secondary leukemia and can also affect the response to treatment. Although in its infancy, this area of pharmacogenetics is likely to be an area of intense activity in the next years. Progress in this area will depend upon the availability of large banks of DNA from patients on known treatment regimes.

EXPRESSION MICROARRAYS

Perhaps the most important new approach for the subclassification of myeloma currently under development is the CHIP-based approach. Expression microarrays produce high-density ordered arrangements of immobilized nucleic acid spots on a solid substrate. These immobile probes are then exposed to the cDNA target that is hybridized to the array, following its synthesis by reverse transcribing tumor mRNA. The miniaturization of cDNA chips requires high-resolution detection and, therefore, fluorescence is the system of choice, the level of gene expression being equivalent to the level of fluorescence. The data are analyzed using sophisticated statistical packages algorithms that are able to handle the complex data generated (see Fig. 11.1).[37–39]

Although there are several different methods for producing DNA microarrays, most researchers use one of two platforms, cDNA or oligonucleotide microarrays. With cDNA arrays, PCR products of cDNA libraries representing genes of interest are robotically spotted on to nitrocellulose filters or glass. Fluorescence analysis of the arrays utilizes a hybridization approach analogous to CGH, where two samples, each fluorescently labeled, are hybridized to the chip. The samples used are a control reference RNA

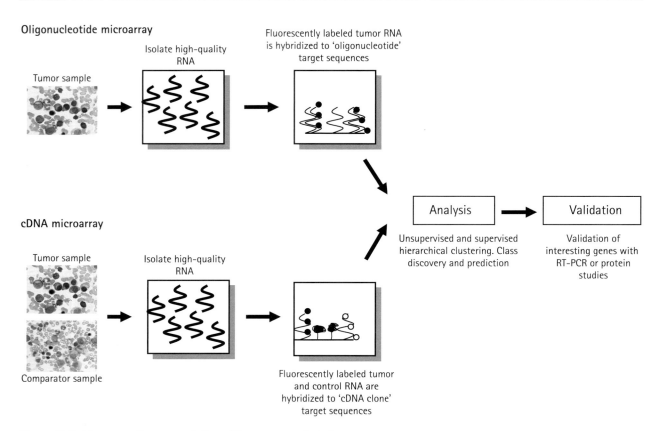

Figure 11.1 *Diagrammatic representation of the gene array technique.*

sample, usually the normal tissue counterpart, and target RNA from the tumor. Expression values are reported as ratios between two fluorescent values. This allows a comparative analysis of individual gene expression between the two samples, thus identifying upregulation or downregulation of genes in the tumor sample.

Oligonucleotide microarrays differ, as, although the oligonucleotide probes can be spotted on to the chip, they can also be synthesized directly on the surface of the chip using photolithographic chemistry. Fluorescence analysis of oligonucleotide microarrays uses only one target sample the tumor cDNA as each chip contains housekeeping genes, allowing comparison following normalization. The most commonly used system (Affymetrix) uses a single-color fluorescent label, where experimental mRNA is enzymatically amplified, biotin-labeled for detection, hybridized to the wafer, and detected through the binding of a fluorescent compound (streptavidin–phycoerythrin).

In both cDNA and oligonucleotide approaches, a digital image of the chip is obtained using a scanning laser microscope. The image is then processed by various densitometric analysis algorithms to produce a table of measurements for each element on the array. The major benefit of cDNA arrays is that they can be made by individual researchers in their laboratories, are easily customizable, are cheaper than oligonucleotide microarrays, and do not

require a prior knowledge of cDNA sequence. Although oligonucleotide chips are more expensive, they have greater specificity as oligonucleotides can be tailored to minimize chances of cross-hybridization. Despite the advantages and disadvantages of both techniques, the data generated by the two methods are relatively concordant.

Microarray experiments require between 10 and 40 g of high-quality RNA. Hence, obtaining sufficient RNA for gene array analysis from myeloma samples can be challenging. This has led to the development of methods for amplification of starting RNA. The amplification method needs to be linear and representative, which can be a problem, as some methods tend to overexpress the smaller segments. Newer methods, including the switch mechanism at the 5'-end of RNA transcripts (SMART) technique and Eisens *in-vitro* transcription (IVT) method, overcome some of these concerns and are now widely used.[40,41] Tumor cell heterogeneity can also complicate the interpretation of array data, and in myeloma, where plasma cells may only constitute 10% of the total nucleated cells, tumor cell selection is required. This can be done in two ways: the first utilizes flow sorting and the second magnetic microbeads. The most commonly used antibody used in both these approaches is anti-CD138. A theoretical limitation of focusing only on malignant tumor components relates to the growing appreciation that interactions between myeloma cells and marrow stromal cells, endothelial cells, and cells of the immune system play critical roles in tumor biology.

The analysis of gene expression data is complicated owing to the large number of data points generated from a single experiment. One of the important initial aspects of the analysis is the normalization of the data within the experiment and across experiments, thus allowing for hybridization artifacts on individual chips and variations in IVT and hybridization between different chips. It is important to consider what change in RNA expression level should be considered significant. To date, the majority of studies have reported the change in expression as 'fold change,' considering a gene with either a twofold increase or decrease as significant. As with all data sets, there is a background variability between different chip experiments and a statistical approach to define significant changes is important. This type of analysis is built into programs, such as dCHIP, which applies algorithms to the analysis of the data distribution.[39] However, there needs to be a degree of care taken with this approach, as a small change in mRNA expression may lead to a small but biologically significant change in protein expression. Alternatively, large changes in mRNA expression may not translate to biologically significant changes in protein expression.

The computational analysis of gene expression data has centered on two approaches: supervised and unsupervised learning. Unsupervised learning approaches include hierarchical clustering, where samples are split into subgroups based purely on the similarity and differences between their gene expression patterns. These are usually represented in a pictorial fashion called a 'hierarchical clustering map.' Samples are initially clustered on the horizontal axis with the samples being most similar next to each other. In a similar fashion, genes are clustered on the vertical axis. A dendrogram is generated and drawn on each axis, and represents the similarities and differences between samples/genes and splits the samples into different subgroups. Traditionally, red squares represent an upregulated gene and blue squares represent a downregulated gene (Fig. 11.2, Plate 5). In contrast, supervised learning approaches such as 'self-organizing maps' and 'supervised machine learning' incorporate the knowledge of sample biology or clinical features to find genes of interest linked to a particular disease entity, phenotype, or experimental treatment. In order to validate the list of genes more thoroughly, a 'training data' set is initially used to select genes that make the best distinction between subgroups. These features are then applied to an independent test data set to validate the ability of selected features to make that distinction.

This technology can be applied to both class discovery and class prediction. Class discovery is the identification of previously unrecognized subtypes of the disease based on gene expression, whereas class prediction is the use of

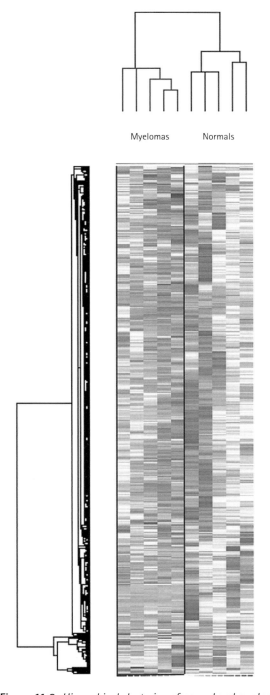

Figure 11.2 *Hierarchical clustering of normal and myeloma samples. Samples are initially clustered on the horizontal axis with the samples being most similar next to each other. In a similar fashion, genes are clustered on the vertical axis. A dendrogram is generated and drawn on each axis, and represents the similarities and differences between samples/genes and splits the samples into different subgroups. Traditionally, red squares represent an upregulated gene and blue squares represent a downregulated gene (see Plate 5). In this example, normal and myeloma samples clearly have a different gene expression pattern.*

technology to assign a particular patient to an already defined class. These approaches are well illustrated in the published studies of diffuse large B-cell lymphoma (DLBCL). Gene expression patterns can split DLBCL into a number of subgroups, representing different stages of B-cell differentiation, each with prognostic significance over and above traditional prognostic stratification using the international prognostic index (IPI).[42,43] Interpreting the patterns seen often requires additional experimental evidence. For large-cell lymphomas, comparisons have been made with B cells at different stages of development in relationship to the germinal center. Additional information can also be provided by artificially expressing a known gene and looking at the change in gene expression that occurs. This has recently been done using the B-cell transcription factor BLIMP1.

Similar studies in MM are also under way, although a little further behind because of technical difficulties in obtaining adequate RNA from bone marrow plasma cells. To date, a number of groups have identified genes that can accurately discriminate normal and malignant plasma cells.[44,45] These include genes involved in adhesion, apoptosis, cell cycle, drug resistance, growth arrest, oncogenesis, signaling, and transcription. The most striking feature is that the majority of genes are downregulated, suggesting that negative transcriptional regulators may be important. The number of genes distinguishing normal plasma cells from MGUS plasma cells is quite high compared with the small number of genes distinguishing MGUS plasma cells from MM plasma cells. Using oligonucleotide microarrays, one group has reported the identification of four distinct subgroups of myeloma patients each. The expression pattern of MM1 patients was similar to normal plasma cells and MGUS, whereas MM4 patients were similar to MM cell lines. Clinical parameters linked to poor prognosis, such as abnormal karyotype and high serum β-microglobulin levels, were most prevalent in MM4 group. Genes involved in DNA metabolism and cell-cycle control were also overexpressed in MM4 in comparison to MM1. These initial studies demonstrate that this approach offers the potential of developing an accurate staging and prognostic system based on gene expression.

Prediction of response to therapeutic agents is a potentially important use of this technology, and RNA expression analysis may be used to further delineate pathways involved in drug-induced apoptosis and resistance. A lot has been learnt about dexamethasone-induced apoptosis and resistance, using a dexamethasone-sensitive and resistant cell line model. Gene expression analysis using this model has further defined a number of genes involved in cell defence and repair that are induced transiently and early following exposure to dexamethasone.[46] Other genes induced later, both known and novel, mediate cell death, and repress growth and survival-related genes.

This kind of study dissecting drug pathways will allow for the improved use of drugs based on targeting genes that regulate MM cell growth and survival. If the drug-resistant phenotype can be determined, future studies will allow for the accurate prediction of whether patients will respond to treatment, depending on the gene expression pattern.

One further important potential use of this technology is in increasing the understanding of basic myeloma cell biology. Gene expression analysis has highlighted a number of important genes controlling the differentiation of normal B cells to normal plasma cells.[47] An increase in Blimp-1 expression, following relief from *bcl-6* repression in germinal center B cells, leads to direct repression of several essential B-cell transcription factors, including c-*myc*, CIITA, Id3 *pax5*, and Spi-B, and subsequent repression of several mature B-cell functions as well as proliferation. In this way, Blimp-1, along with the transcription factor XBP-1, drives B cells to become terminally differentiated plasma cells. Studies are under way examining the role of some of these genes in the differentiation of malignant plasma cells.

A number of groups have used myeloma cell lines models to address specific questions regarding control of cell growth, drug-induced apoptosis, and resistance. In one study, a myeloma-specific microarray was created with 4300 sequenced cDNAs spotted on glass slides and used to analyze cell lines.[48] A defined subset of 34 upregulated and 18 downregulated genes were able to differentiate myeloma from non-myeloma cell lines. These genes included those involved in B-cell biology, such as *syndecan 1*, *bcma*, *pim2*, *mum1/irf4*, and *xbp1*, and novel uncharacterized genes matching sequences in public databases. A further study has taken a similar approach and identified genes that are overexpressed in myeloma cells compared with autologous B-lymphoblastoid cell lines.[49] The genes included those that code for the oncogenic tyrosine kinase receptor Tyro3, the heparin-binding epidermal-like growth factor (HB-EGF; an epithelial autocrine tumor growth factor), the thrombin receptor (linked to HB-EGF and syndecan-1 processing, and to cell invasion), chemokine receptors (CCR1 and CCR2), the Wnt pathway actor frizzled related protein (FRZB), and the notch receptor ligand, jagged 2. Although these studies are in their infancy, they do provide a platform for identifying genes that are important in myeloma biology. Further studies will be required to characterize the role of each gene and to confirm that these genes are also significant in primary patients' material.

PROTEOMIC APPROACHES

Proteomics, the investigation of the expressed protein complement of a cell, is expanding rapidly into many aspects of post-genomic biology and medicine. The global qualitative and quantitative analysis of the pattern of proteins expressed at any particular time in any system provides important information about the effects of environmental factors on a genome. Proteins displaying changes in expression levels can be implicated in and linked to changes in cellular state, including alterations in signal transduction pathways, metabolic changes, effects of disease, or drug intervention.

Proteomics effectively combines the well-established procedures of high-resolution protein separation by two-dimensional polyacrylamide gel electrophoresis (2D-PAGE) with high-throughput protein identification involving mass spectrometry (MS) (see Fig. 11.3).[50]

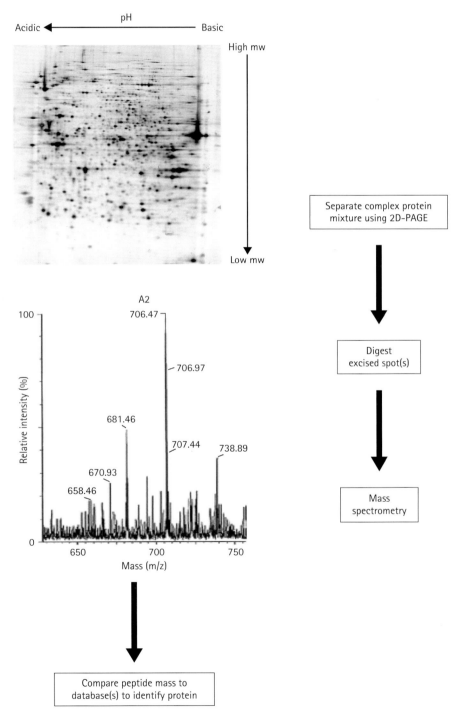

Figure 11.3 *Diagrammatic representation of the proteomic technique.*

Typically, complex protein mixtures can be resolved by 2D-PAGE to give patterns of up to 1000–2000 protein spots. By utilizing various physical or chemical methods to subfractionate the source material and a variety of conditions for 2D-PAGE, a much greater total number of proteins can be resolved over a number of gels. For example, the tissue may be fractionated by ultracentrifugation into subcellular compartments (cytosol, nuclei, mitochondria, plasma membrane, and intracellular membranes) or proteins may be subdivided into water-soluble, peripheral membrane proteins and integral membrane proteins. The conditions used for 2D-PAGE separation can then be varied by using wide or narrow pH gradient strips for the isoelectric focusing step (3–10, 3–6, 5–8, 6–11) or varying the porosity of the sodium dodecyl sulfate (SDS)-PAGE stage to enhance the numbers of protein spots displayed.

Following visualization of gel spots, by staining with silver or Sypro RUBY, the gel is scanned (using a laser densitometer or fluorimager), and a digital image is created and archived. Sophisticated image analysis software can then be used to analyze and compare multiple images to establish a 'basic' protein expression profile and identify changes that occur in different situations. Protein spots identified as being of interest owing to a change in expression level are then excised from the 2D gels and subjected to proteolysis using trypsin and the peptide digests are analyzed by MS. Usually this involves a first-pass screen using matrix-assisted laser desorption ionization/time of flight (MALDI/TOF)-MS, which measures the mass of each peptide in the mixture and generates a 'mass map' unique to the parent protein. This mass map is used to search protein sequence databases, in which each sequence has been digested *in silico* to produce theoretical mass maps. Comparison of observed and theoretical mass maps produces a hit list of potential matches for the parent protein. Relating probability scores to the biology then enables confident assignment of protein identity. This approach works very well for organisms that have been subjected to genome sequencing projects, which have led to the deposition of complete sequence information in public domain databases. In other cases, or where the mass maps produced are inadequate (e.g. few peptides, heavy post-translational modification), further MS is required. The second stage, which typically involves quadrupole time of flight (QTof)-MS/MS, aims to generate partial sequences for each of the peptides in the mixture. These 'sequence tags' provide additional information to enhance database searches and enable protein identification or, where still unsuccessful, provide *de novo* sequence information for future use in homology searches and cloning.

Currently, this technology is time-consuming, cumbersome, and extremely expensive. New high-throughput technology is becoming available with robotics facilities for sample manipulation. In conjunction with this, bioinformatic techniques are also improving, including sophisticated image analysis software, allowing for quicker interrogation of the peptide databases. Another approach in its infancy is protein chips. Proteins can be arrayed either on flat solid phases or in capillary systems, and binding can be covalent (via chemical linkers) or non-covalent (via hydrophobic, ionic, or other interactions). As with traditional proteomic techniques, charge, viscosity, membrane pore size, pH, and binding capacity play an essential role. Detection is similar to cDNA array methods using fluorescent intensity. Although in its infancy, these methods build on the DNA microarray technology and represent the next level of diagnostic tools, allowing direct analysis of gene function.

MOLECULAR MONITORING AND RESIDUAL DISEASE DETECTION

Background

Many patients who receive high-dose therapy (HDT) for myeloma achieve a complete remission by conventional criteria; however, with current therapy, all patients eventually relapse, as a consequence of residual disease. In order to develop effective maintenance strategies, aimed at prolonging the residual disease states, it is important to be able to monitor this stage of disease closely. Current approaches to measurement of residual disease levels are based on morphological assessment of bone marrow biopsies and use a number of electrophoretic approaches to detect changes in the serum and urine paraprotein levels. These, together with a number of clinical criteria, can be used to define response; these have been formalized in the criteria of the European Bone Marrow Transplant/International Bone Marrow Transplant Registry (EBMT/IBMTR) and have been discussed elsewhere.[51] Complete remission (CR) is currently defined as the absence of the original monoclonal paraprotein in serum and urine by immunofixation as well as <5% plasma cells in the bone marrow. Using these criteria, a number of studies have shown that patients who achieve a CR have an improved progression-free and possibly also overall survival compared with partial or non-responders.[10,52] Monitoring is always a function of the sensitivity and practicality of the test being used, and will, of course, change with time owing to developments in technology. Developments in this area and, in particular, how they affect monitoring in the minimal residual disease setting are discussed below (see Table 11.3).

PCR analysis

Numerous PCR strategies have been applied for residual disease monitoring in myeloma, with some showing an improved outcome for those achieving a minimal residual disease (MRD)-negative status, and some showing no difference. In myeloma there are a number of potential targets for the detection of clonality by PCR, including IgH rearrangements, light-chain rearrangements, κ deleting element rearrangements, partial rearrangements, and chromosome 14 translocations. Using these approaches, it is possible to obtain a marker of clonality in the majority of cases. Using consensus primers for IgH rearrangement, only 60–70% of patients have a detectable rearrangement as there is a high degree of somatic hypermutation in the neoplastic cells. A recent European Union Sponsored Biomedical project has facilitated the development of a set of oligonucleotide primers able to identify clonal rearrangements in a much higher percentage of patients with myeloma. These primers utilize sequence motifs within the IgH κ, λ, and κ deleting elements.[53]

The principle of consensus PCR-based approaches relies upon amplification of the rearranged V region using a consensus JH region primer and one of a number of potential V region primers. In the presence of a polyclonal population, either a smear or a fingerprint is seen after electrophoresis. In the presence of a clonal population, a single band of a specific size is seen that is unique to the clone (see Fig. 11.4). The ability to demonstrate clonal IgH rearrangements depends on the PCR strategy used, as a number of different primers spanning the IgH locus can be used with different pick-up rates.[54–57] These either are based on consensus sequences between the differing V family members or rely upon family-specific primers based on the framework 1 leader sequences (see Table 11.4). There are a number of methods used for detection of the clonal rearrangement; fluorescent PCR analysis has emerged as the system of choice and can be used to monitor residual disease with a consistent sensitivity of 1 in 10^4. Fluorescent dyes specifically label standards and PCR products, allowing for accurate sizing of the products to within a single base, which greatly facilies the identification of clonal rearrangements when they are present within a polyclonal background. A polyclonal B-cell pattern produces a fingerprint electrophoretogram, i.e. peaks in a normal distribution separated by three base pairs, whereas clonal rearrangements appear as distinct peaks (see Fig. 11.4).

Table 11.3 *Techniques and their application in minimal residual disease monitoring*

Technique	Sensitivity	Comments
Consensus PCR	10^{-4}	Technically difficult and time consuming
Clonospecific PCR	10^{-6}	Only applicable in 60%
Flow cytometry	10^{-4}	Simple, applicable to >90%
Serum free light chain assay	Not established	May be useful in non-secretory disease; limited data available

PCR, polymerase chain reaction.

Table 11.4 *Percentage pick-up rate of clonal IgH rearrangement with differing primer combinations*

V region primers	JHcon (%)
Fr3	59
Fr1f	59
Fr3 + Fr1f	77
Fr1 con	48
Fr2	48
Fr1con + Fr2	63
Total	**80**

Fr, framework; f, family; con, consensus.

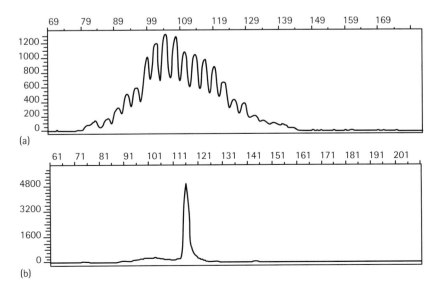
(a)

(b)

Figure 11.4 *Fluorescent polymerase chain reaction using consensus primers for the framework 3 region of the IgH locus. A polyclonal B-cell pattern produces a fingerprint electrophoretogram, i.e. peaks in a normal distribution separated by three base pairs (a), whereas clonal rearrangements appear as distinct peaks (b).*

Allele-specific oligonucleotide (ASO) PCR is undoubtedly the most sensitive approach for the detection of residual disease with the majority of studies reporting sensitivities of one tumor cell in 10^{5-6} normal cells. PCR products are generated as outlined above and, following sequence analysis, clonospecific primers or probes are designed for use in hybridization experiments. The increased sensitivity is the consequence of the detection of only tumor-specific immunoglobulin sequences and the lack of contaminating signal from the polyclonal background of normal B-cells. However, designing optimum oligonucleotides for this purpose can be difficult and normal B-cell sequences are often detected, leading to quite wide variations in the sensitivity of this approach. Consequently, for each probe/primer synthesized, it is important to validate its sensitivity.

One of the major requirements for a test aimed at detecting residual disease is an ability to quantify the level of disease. Clonospecific PCR can be modified to be semiquantive and this has been improved by the application of limiting dilutional approaches.[58] In this technique, multiple dilutions in normal DNA are made and the level of disease is calculated by a determination of the number of positive results in the dilutions. This approach is, however, complicated in myeloma because of the lack of 100% tumor DNA at presentation, and the development of real-time PCR technology has superseded this approach.[59,60] Detection of target DNA is based on the cleavage of fluorescently labeled probes by the 5′ to 3′ exonuclease activity of Taq DNA polymerase. The advantage of this approach is that quantitative data are obtained by using the number of cycles at which fluorescence crosses the baseline, the C_T value; however, clonospecific oligonucleotides are still required, which are time-consuming and expensive.

An important question that needs to be fully addressed is whether the application of PCR-based technology can provide additional useful information compared with simple monitoring of serum or urinary paraprotein levels.[52,61] A recent report has demonstrated that cases that were immunofixation negative were also IgH PCR negative, using a fluorescent consensus PCR with a sensitivity of 1 in 10^4, suggesting that this technique offers little advantage to conventional disease assessment methods.[52] A more sensitive ASO-PCR able to detect one tumor cell in 10^6 has been used to detect residual disease in a number of other studies.[62–64] These studies demonstrate that about 50% of patients in an immunofixation-negative CR have detectable disease with clonospecific PCR. Of note, the percentage of patients achieving a molecular CR is higher in patients receiving an allograft compared with those receiving an autograft.[64] Although the number of cases in these studies are small, there is a suggestion that PCR-positive patients have a shorter progression-free survival compared with those patients who become PCR negative. The data regarding the ability of sequential monitoring to predict relapse are few, presumably owing to a reluctance to perform frequent bone marrow aspirates; however, if this approach were to be successful, monitoring would probably have to be done at 3-monthly intervals.[54,59–61]

FLOW CYTOMETRY

A flow cytometry method has recently been described that is able to identify plasma cells with a sensitivity of 0.01% and is applicable to over 98% of patients.[65,66] The assay can distinguish neoplastic plasma cells from their normal counterparts based on their CD19 and CD56 expression, even if both cell types are present within the same sample (see Fig. 11.5). The method is more sensitive than immunofixation, and even in immunofixation-negative cases two groups of patients can be identified. Patients with normal sustainable plasma cell levels tend to recover normal immunoglobulin levels and have a prolonged progression-free survival. In contrast, patients with neoplastic cells 3–6 months after high-dose therapy have a much poorer progression-free and overall survival, and should, therefore, be considered for further treatment, such as further HDT, low-intensity conditioning allogeneic transplantation, or experimental strategies.

SERUM FREE LIGHT CHAIN ASSAYS

A new technique for measuring serum free light chains has recently been described, which uses a latex-enhanced immunoassay with antibodies specific for κ and λ light chains in free form, not bound to the heavy chain. The technique can detect 1.0 mg/L κ or λ paraprotein compared with 150–500 mg/L of paraprotein by immunofixation and 500–2000 mg/L by serum protein electrophoresis.[67] A recent report highlights the potential use of this technique in non-secretory myeloma.[68] Currently, the only way to assess response to treatment and the maintenance of MRD states in this form of myeloma is by frequent bone marrow aspirates. Serum free light chain levels can show altered κ:λ ratios in 67% of non-secretory patients and levels change with disease activity. Another study reports the use of serum free light chains in patients with urinary Bence Jones protein.[69] Traditionally, 24-hour urine collection has been used to measure response in this group of patients. These collections are cumbersome and prone to inaccuracies because of incomplete collection, and measurement of urinary light chain by electrophoresis is difficult. Although serum free light chain does not quantitatively match urinary M protein, changes in the serum free light-chain ratios over a period of time correlate with changes in the amounts of urinary paraprotein. These preliminary data would, therefore, suggest that this technique could be a sensitive and more convenient method of assessing response in myeloma

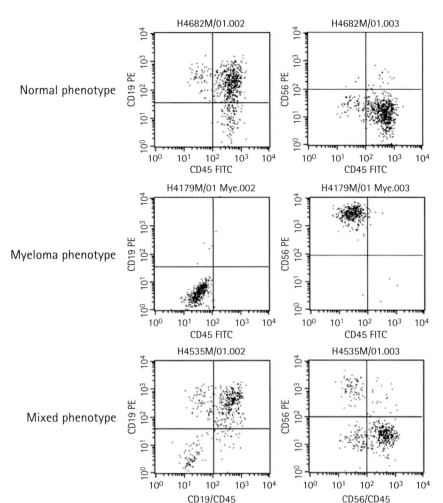

Figure 11.5 *Minimal residual disease flow cytometry. Neoplastic plasma cells can be distinguished from their normal counterparts based on their CD19 and CD56 expression, even if both cell types are present within the same sample. This method is more sensitive than immunofixation and may be used prognostically following autologous transplantation.*

patients. Further studies are currently under way comparing this technique with other sensitive methods for MRD detection in myeloma patients post-autologous transplantation.

ACKNOWLEDGMENTS

FED is supported by the Department of Health, UK, and GJM is supported by the Leukaemia Research Fund, UK. We would like to thank Dr A.C. Rawstron, Dr K. Rees, A.M. Dring, and A. Levine for help with the illustrations.

KEY POINTS

- A number of new technologies have been developed to improve the characterization of cytogenetic events in myeloma, including fiber fluorescence *in situ* hybridization, spectral karyotyping, matrix comparative genomic hybridization, and polymerase chain reaction for translocations.
- Inherited genetic variations in key cytokine and drug metabolizer genes may affect the predisposition to myeloma as well as response to treatment and side effects of chemotherapy.
- Genetic microarrays offer the opportunity to examine the expression of 10 000 genes in one experiment. Gene expression profiles may be helpful in identifying key genes involved in the pathogenesis of myeloma and drug resistance and in identifying subgroups of myeloma with different clinical outcomes.
- Although proteomic techniques are currently time-consuming and cumbersome, new high-throughput approaches represent the next level of diagnostic tools, allowing direct analysis of gene function.
- The current challenge is to apply these technologies in order to individualize patient therapy and improve outcome, i.e. personalized medicine.

REFERENCES

● = Key primary paper

◆ = Major review article

* = Paper that represents the first formal publication of a management guideline

1. Lai JL, Zandecki M, Mary JY, Bernardi F, Izydorczyk V, Flactif M, et al. Improved cytogenetics in multiple myeloma: a study of 151 patients including 117 patients at diagnosis. *Blood* 1995; **85**:2490–7.

2. Philip P, Drivsholm A, Hansen NE, Jenson MK, Kilman SA. Chromosomes and survival in multiple myeloma: a banding study of 25 cases. *Cancer Genet Cytogenet* 1980; **2**:243–57.

3. Sawyer JR, Waldron JA, Jaganath S, Barlogie B. Cytogenetics findings in 200 patients with multiple myeloma. *Cancer Genet Cytogenet* 1995; **82**:41–9.

4. Weh HJ, Gutensohn K, Selbaach J, Kruse R, Wacker-Baackhaus G, Seeger D, et al. Karyotype in multiple myeloma and plasma cell leukaemia. *Eur J Cancer* 1993; **29A**:1269–73.

5. Smadja NV, Louvert C, Isnard F, Dutel JL, Grange MJ, Varette C, et al. Cytogenetic study in multiple myeloma at diagnosis: comparison of two techniques. *Br J Haematol* 1995; **90**:619–24.

6. Flactif M, Zandecki M, Lai JL, Bernardi F, Obein V, Bauters F, et al. Interphase fluorescent in-situ hybridisation (FISH) as a powerful tool in the detection of aneuploidy in multiple myeloma. *Leukaemia* 1995; **9**:2109–14.

7. Tabernero D, San Miguel JF, Garcia-Sanz R, Najera L, Garcia-Isidoro M, Perez-Simon JA, et al. Incidence of chromosome numerical changes in multiple myeloma. *Am J Pathol* 1996; **149**:153–61.

8. Garcia-Sanz R, Orfao A, Gonzaalez M, Moro M, Hernaadez JM, Ortega F, et al. Prognostic implications of DNA aneuploidy in 156 untreated multiple myeloma patients. *Br J Haematol* 1995; **90**:106–12.

9. Tricot G, Barlogie B, Jaganath S, Bracy D, Mattox S, Vesole D, et al. Poor prognosis in multiple myeloma is associated only with partial or complete deletions of chromosome 13 or abnormalities involving 11q and not with other karyotype abnormalities. *Blood* 1995; **86**:4250–6.

10. Barlogie B, Jagannath S, Desikan KR, Mattox S, Vesole DH, Siegel G, et al. Total therapy with tandem transplants for newly diagnosed multiple myeloma. *Blood* 1999; **93**:55–65.

● 11. Fonseca R, Harrington D, Oken MM, Dewald GW, Bailey RJ, Van Wier SA, et al. Biological and prognostic significance of interphase fluorescence in situ hybridisation detection of chromosome 13 abnormalities (delta13) in multiple myeloma: an eastern cooperative oncology group study. *Cancer Res* 2002; **62**:715–20.

● 12. Perez-Simon JA, Garcia-Sanz R, Tabernero MD, Almeida J, Gonzalez M, Fernandez-Calvo J, et al. Prognostic value of numerical chromosome aberrations in multiple myeloma: a FISH analysis of 15 different chromosomes. *Blood* 1998; **91**:3366–71.

◆ 13. Bergsagel PL, Chesi M, Nardini E, Brents LA, Kirby SI, Kuehl WM. Promiscuous translocations into immunoglobulin

heavy chain switch regions in multiple myeloma. *Proc Natl Acad Sci USA* 1996; **93**:13931–6.

14. Bergsagel PL, Nardini E, Brents L, Chesi M, Kuehl WM. IgH translocations in multiple myeloma; a nearly universal event that rarely involves c-myc. *Curr Top Microbiol Immunol* 1997; **224**:283–7.

15. Chesi M, Bergsagel PL, Shonukan OO, Martelli MI, Brents LA, Chen T, et al. Frequent dysregulation of the c-maf proto-oncogene at 16q23 by translocation to an Ig locus in multiple myeloma. *Blood* 1998; **91**:4457–63.

16. Chesi M, Nardini E, Lim RSC, Smith KD, Kuehl WM, Bergsagel PL. The t(4;14) translocation in myeloma dysregulates both FGFR3 and a novel gene, MMSET, resulting in IgH/MMSET hybrid transcripts. *Blood* 1997; **92**:3025–34.

17. Iida S, Rao PH, Butler M, Corradini P, Boccadoro M, Klein B, et al. Deregulation of MUM1/IRF4 by chromosomal translocation in multiple myeloma. *Nat Genet* 1997; **17**:226–30.

18. Kuipers J, Vaandrager JW, Weghuis DO, Pearson PL, Scheres J, Lokhorst HM, et al. Fluorescence in situ hybridisation analysis shows the frequent occurrence of 14q32.3 rearrangements with involvement of immunoglobulin switch regions in myeloma cell lines. *Cancer Genet Cytogenet* 1999; **109**:99–107.

19. Nishida K, Tamura A, Nakazawa N, Ueda Y, Abe T, Matsuda F, et al. The Ig heavy chain gene is frequently involved in chromosomal translocations in multiple myeloma and plasma cell leukaemia as detected by in situ hybridisation. *Blood* 1997; **90**:526–34.

● 20. Fonseca R, Blood EA, Oken MM, Kyle RA, Dewald GW, Bailey RJ, et al. Myeloma and the t(11;14)(q13;q32); evidence for a biologically defined unique subset of patients. *Blood* 2002; **99**:3735–41.

21. Moreau P, Facon T, Leleu X, Morineau N, Huyghe P, Harousseau JL, et al. Recurrent 14q32 translocations determine the prognosis of multiple myeloma, especially in patients receiving intensive chemotherapy. *Blood* 2002; **100**:1579–83.

● 22. Avet-Loiseau H, Facon T, Grosbois B, Magrangeas F, Rapp MJ, Harousseau JL, et al. Oncogenesis of multiple myeloma: 14q32 and 13q chromosomal abnormalities are not randomly distributed, but correlate with natural history, immunological features, and clinical presentation. *Blood* 2002; **99**:2185–91.

● 23. Rao PH, Cigudosa JC, Ning Y, Calasanz MJ, Iida S, Tagawa S, et al. Multispectral karyotyping identifies new recurring breakpoints and translocations in multiple myeloma. *Blood* 1998; **92**:1743–8.

24. Sawyer JR, Lukacs JL, Munshi N, Desikan KR, Singhal S, Mehta J, et al. Identification of new nonrandom translocations in multiple myeloma with multicolor spectral karyotyping. *Blood* 1998; **92**:4269–78.

25. Avet-Loiseau H, Andree-Ashley LE, Moore D, Mellerin MP, Feusner J, Bataille R, et al. Molecular cytogenetic abnormalities in multiple myeloma and plasma cell leukaemia measured by comparative genomic hybridisation. *Genes Chromosomes Cancer* 1997; **19**:124–33.

● 26. Cigudosa JC, Rao PH, Calasanz J, Odero D, Michaeli J, Jhanwar SC, et al. Characterisation of nonrandom chromosomal gains and losses in multiple myeloma by comparative genomic hybridisation. *Blood* 1998; **91**:3007-10.

●27. Solinas-Toldo S, Lampel S, Stilgenbauer S, Nickolenko J, Benner A, Dohner H, *et al.* Matrix-based comparative genomic hybridisation: biochips to screen for genomic imbalances. *Genes Chromosomes Cancer* 1997; **20**:399-407.

28. Proffitt J, Fenton J, Pratt G, Yates Z, Morgan GJ. Isolation and characterisation of recombination events involving immunoglobulin heavy chain switch regions in multiple myeloma using long distance vectorette PCR. *Leukaemia* 1999; **13**:1100-7.

29. Sibley K, Fenton JA, Dring AM, Ashcroft AJ, Rawstron AC, Morgan GJ. A molecular study of the t(4;14) in multiple myeloma. *Br J Haematol* 2002; **118**:514-20.

30. Uchida T, Kinoshita T, Ohno T, Ohashi H, Nagai H, Saito H. Hypermethylation of p16INK4A gene promoter during the progression of plasma cell dyscrasia. *Leukemia* 2001; **15**:157-65.

31. Gonzalea M, Mateos MV, Garcia-Sanz R, Balanzategui A, Lopez-Perez R, Chillon MC, *et al.* De novo methylation of tumor suppressor gene p16INK4A gene is a frequent finding in multiple myeloma patients at diagnosis. *Leukemia* 2000; **14**:183-7.

32. Mateos MV, Garcia-Sanz R, Lopez-Perez R, Balanzategui A, Gonzalez MI, Fernandez-Calvo J, *et al.* p16INK4A gene inactivation by hypermethylation is associated with aggressive variants of monoclonal gammopathies. *Hematol J* 2001; **2**:146-9.

33. Neben K, Mytilineos J, Moehler TM, Preiss A, Kraemer A, Ho AD, *et al.* Polymorphisms of the tumor necrosis factor alpha gene promoter predict for outcome after thalidomide therapy in relapsed and refractory multiple myeloma. *Blood* 2002; **100**:2263-5.

34. Davies FE, Rollinson SJ, Rawstron AC, Roman E, Richards S, Drayson M, *et al.* High producer haplotypes of TNFα and LTα are associated with an increased risk of myeloma and have an improved progression free survival after treatment. *J Clin Oncol* 2000; **18**:2843-51.

35. Dring AM, Davies FE, Rollinson SJ, Roddam PL, Rawstron AC, Child JA, *et al.* Interleukin 6 polymorphisms in monoclonal gammopathy of uncertain significance and multiple myeloma. *Br J Haematol* 2001; **112**:249-50.

36. Dasgupta RK, Davies FE, Rollinson S, Rawstron A, Fenton JAL, Child JA, *et al.* Underactive genetic variants of glutathione s-transferase P1 (GSTP1). Modulate survival in multiple myeloma. *Blood* 1998; **92**(Suppl 1):abstract 680.

◆37. Lockhart DJ, Winzeler EA. Genomics, gene expression and DNA arrays. *Nature* 2000; **405**:827-36.

38. Golub TR, Slonim DK, Tamayo P, *et al.* Molecular classification of cancer: class discovery and class prediction by gene expression monitoring. *Science* 1999; **286**:531-7.

39. Li C, Wong WH. Model-based analysis of oligonucleotide arrays: expression index computation and outlier detection. *Proc Natl Acad Sci USA* 2001; **98**:31-6.

40. Zhumabayeva B, Diatchenko L, Chenchik A, Siebert PD. Use of SMART-generated cDNA for gene expression studies in multiple human tumors. *Biotechniques* 2001; **30**:158-63.

41. Phillips J, Eberwine JH. Antisense RNA Amplification: a linear amplification method for analyzing the mrna population from single living cells. *Methods* 1996; **10**:283-8.

●42. Alizadeh AA, Eisen MB, Davis RE, Ma C, Lossos IS, Rosenwald A, *et al.* Distinct types of diffuse large B-cell lymphoma identified by gene expression profiling. *Nature* 2000; **403**:503-11.

43. Shipp MA, Ross KN, Tamayo P, Weng AP, Kutok JL, Aguiar RC, *et al.* Diffuse large B-cell lymphoma outcome prediction by gene-expression profiling and supervised machine learning. *Nat Med* 2002; **8**:68-74.

●44. Zhan F, Hardin J, Kordsmeier B, Bumm K, Zheng M, Tian E, *et al.* Global gene expression profiling of multiple myeloma, monoclonal gammopathy of undetermined significance, and normal bone marrow plasma cells. *Blood* 2002; **99**:1745-57.

45. Davies FE, Dring AM, Li C, Rawstron AC, Shammas MA, O'Connor SM, Fenton JA, *et al.* Insights into the multistep transformation of MGUS to myeloma using microarray expression analysis. *Blood* 2003; **102**:4504-11.

46. Chauhan D, Auclair D, Robinson EK, Hideshima T, Li G, Podar K, *et al.* Identification of genes regulated by dexamethasone in multiple myeloma cells using oligonucleotide arrays. *Oncogene* 2002; **21**:1346-58.

47. Shaffer AL, Lin KI, Kuo TC, Yu X, Hurt EM, Rosenwald A, *et al.* Blimp-1 orchestrates plasma cell differentiation by extinguishing the mature B cell gene expression program. *Immunity* 2002; **17**:51-62.

48. Claudio JO, Masih-Khan E, Tang H, Goncalves J, Voralia M, Li ZH, *et al.* A molecular compendium of genes expressed in multiple myeloma. *Blood* 2002; **100**:2175-86.

49. De Vos J, Couderc G, Tarte K, Jourdan M, Requirand G, Delteil MC, *et al.* Identifying intr acellular signalling genes expressed in malignant plasma cells by using complementary DNA arrays. *Blood* 2001; **98**:771-80.

◆50. Banks RE, Dunn MJ, Hochstrasser DF, Sanchez JC, Blackstock W, Pappin DJ, *et al.* Proteomics: new perspectives, new biomedical opportunities. *Lancet* 2000; **18**:1749-56.

*51. Blade J, Samson D, Reece D, Apperley J, Bjorkstrand B, Gahrton G, *et al.* Criteria for evaluating disease response and progression in patients with multiple myeloma treated by high dose therapy and haemopoietic stem cell transplantation. Myeloma Subcommittee of the EBMT. *Br J Haematol* 1998; **102**:1115-23.

52. Davies FE, Forsyth PD, Rawstron AC, Owen RG, Pratt G, Evans PAS, *et al.* The impact of response following high dose melphalan and autologous transplantation for multiple myeloma. *Br J Haematol* 2001; **112**:814-20.

●53. Gonzalez D, Balanzategui A, Garcia-Sanz R, Gutierrez N, Seabra C, van Dongen JJ, *et al.* Incomplete DJH rearrangements of the IgH gene are frequent in multiple myeloma patients: immunobiological characteristics and clinical implications. *Leukemia* 2003; **7**:1398-403.

54. Owen RG, Johnson RJ, Rawstron AC, *et al.* Assessment of IgH PCR strategies in multiple myeloma. *J Clin Pathol* 1996; **49**:672-5.

55. Aubin J, Davi F, Nguyen-Salomon F, Leboeuf D, Debert C, Taher M, *et al.* Description of a novel FR1 IgH PCR strategy and its comparison with three other strategies for the detection of clonality in B cell malignancies. *Leukemia* 1995; **9**:471-9.

56. Welterlin V, Debecker A, Tschieb D, Zanetti C, Lange W, Henon PR, *et al.* Improvement of clonality detection rate in multiple myeloma using fluorescent IgH PCR with different sets of primers. *J Hemather Stem Cell Res* 2000; **9**:983-91.

57. Gleissner B, Maurer J, Thiel E. Detection of immunoglobulin heavy chain genes rearrangements in B-cell leukemias, lymphomas, multiple myelomas, monoclonal and polyclonal gammopathies. *Leuk Lymphoma* 2000; **39**:151–5.

58. Vescio RA, Han EJ, Schiller GJ, Lee JC, Wu CH, Cao J, *et al.* Quantitative comparison of multiple myeloma tumor contamination in bone marrow harvest and leukapheresis autografts. *Bone Marrow Transplant* 1996; **18**:103–10.

59. Rasmussen T, Poulsen TS, Honore L, Johnsen HE. Quantitation of minimal residual disease in multiple myeloma using an allele-specific real-time PCR assay. *Exp Hematol* 2000; **28**:1039–45.

●60. Ladetto M, Donovan JW, Harig S, Trojan A, Poor C, Schlossnan R, *et al.* Real-time polymerase chain reaction of immunoglobulin rearrangements for quantitative evaluation of minimal residual disease in multiple myeloma. *Biol Blood Marrow Transplant* 2000; **6**:241–53.

61. Gupta D, Bybee A, Cooke F, Giles C, Davis JG, McDonald C, *et al.* CD34+ selected peripheral blood progenitor cell transplantation in patients with multiple myeloma: tumour cell contamination and outcome. *Br J Haematol* 1999; **104**:166–77.

62. Corradini P, Voena C, Tarella C, Astolfi M, Ladetto M, Palumbo A, *et al.* Molecular and clinical remissions in multiple myeloma: role of autologous and allogeneic transplantation of hematopoeitic cells. *J Clin Oncol* 1999; **17**:208–15.

63. Martinelli G, Terragna C, Zamagni E, Ronconi S, Tosi P, Lemoli RM *et al.* Molecular remission after allogeneic or autologous transplantation of hematopoietic stem cells for multiple myeloma. *J Clin Oncol* 2000; **18**:2273–81.

●64. Corradini P, Cavo M, Lokhorst H, Martinelli G, Terragna C, Majolino I, *et al.* Molecular remission after myeloablative allogeneic stem cell transplantation predicts a better relapse-free survival in multiple myeloma. *Blood* 2003; **102**:1927–9.

◆65. Rawstron AC, Davies FE, Dasgupta R, Ashcroft AJ, Patmore R, Drayson MT, *et al.* Flow cytometric disease monitoring in multiple myeloma: the relationship between normal and neoplastic plasma cells predicts outcome post-transplantation. *Blood* 2002; **100**:3095–100.

66. Davies FE, Rawstron AC, Owen RG, Morgan GJ. Minimal disease monitoring in multiple myeloma. *Best Pract Res Clin Haematol* 2002; **15**:197–222.

●67. Bradwell AR, Carr-Smith HD, Mead GP, Tang LX, Showell PJ, Drayson MT, *et al.* Highly sensitive, automated immunoassay for immunoglobulin free light chains in serum and urine. *Clin Chem* 2001; **47**:673–80.

68. Drayson M, Tang LX, Drew R, Mead GP, Carr-Smith H, Bradwell AR. Serum free light-chain measurements for identifying and monitoring patients with nonsecretory multiple myeloma. *Blood* 2001; **97**:2900–2.

69. Abraham RS, Clark RJ, Bryant SC, Lymp JF, Larson T, Kyle RA, *et al.* Correlation of serum immunoglobulin free light chain quantification with urinary Bence Jones protein in light chain myeloma. *Clin Chem* 2002; **48**:655–7.

12

Multiple myeloma: differential diagnosis and prognosis

JESÚS F. SAN MIGUEL AND RAMÓN GARCÍA-SANZ

INTRODUCTION

The diagnosis of multiple myeloma (MM) is based on the presence of bone marrow (BM) infiltration by plasma cells, together with a serum and/or urine monoclonal component and lytic bone lesions. Although the presence of clinical symptoms, such as bone pain, anemia, and renal insufficiency, may herald the diagnosis of MM, there are many cases in which the initial finding is limited to the presence of a high erythrocyte sedimentation rate or an M-component detected in an otherwise asymptomatic patient. The main challenge at diagnosis is to distinguish active MM, which requires treatment, from monoclonal gammopathies of undetermined significance (MGUS) and indolent myeloma, which do not. In addition, there are some forms of plasma cell dyscrasias (PCD) that may require specific diagnosis and treatment. In the following pages, we will first review the diagnostic criteria of MM and related disorders, with particular emphasis on those in which differential diagnosis is problematic.

DIAGNOSTIC CRITERIA OF MULTIPLE MYELOMA

Conventional morphological assessment of the proportion of plasma cells (PCs) in the BM is one of the major criteria for the diagnosis of MM, especially in differentiating it from MGUS and solitary plasmacytoma.[1-3] Thus, in MM there are usually more than 10% PCs, although, owing to the heterogeneous distribution of PCs in BM, this figure may vary depending on the site of sample aspiration. The use of BM biopsies would probably be a more accurate method for evaluation of PC infiltration, but it would require substantial standardization. As far as the M-component is concerned, a serum concentration greater than 20 g/L is suggestive of a plasma cell tumor, while it is rare to see benign monoclonal gammopathy with a serum monoclonal component higher than 30 g/L. In borderline cases, a sequential study will help to clarify the situation, since a rising M-component strongly favors the diagnosis of a malignant disease, while the observation of a stable serum level suggests a benign condition. Moreover, the excretion of more than 1 g/24 hour urine light chains is generally associated with a neoplastic condition, although, in this case, patients with benign idiopathic Bence Jones proteinuria must be differentiated.[4] The presence of lytic bone lesions is the third major criteria for diagnosis of MM, but it is very important to exclude other possible causes of bone disease, such as metastatic carcinoma, which can be also associated with an unrelated M-component.

In patients with unequivocal MM, the three criteria mentioned above (BM plasmacytosis, serum and/or urinary M-component, and lytic bone lesions) do not always coexist, and several diagnostic systems have been proposed for the diagnosis and classification of MM. The most extensively used systems in the past corresponded to the Chronic Leukemia-Myeloma Task Force[1] or Kyle and Greipp,[3,5] the Southwest Oncology Group (SWOG)[2] or Durie and Salmon, and the British Columbia Cancer Agency (BCCA)[6] systems (Table 12.1). The criteria used were very similar, with only slight differences in parameter combinations or in the thresholds used. Nevertheless, these slight differences may lead to the diagnosis of a patient as MM instead of MGUS or vice versa depending on which system is used. In a study carried out by the working party of the Comprehensive Cancer Center West held in Leiden, the Netherlands,[7] three classification systems – SWOG,[2] Kyle and Greipp,[3,5] and the BCCA[7] – were evaluated in a group of 157 patients with monoclonal PCD. A diagnosis could be made in only 80% of patients, and it was not always the same. Thus, the three systems concurred completely in only 64% of all patients, and in up to 7% of cases the diagnosis between all three systems was different. Most discrepancies involved the discrimination between stage I MM, indolent MM, and

smoldering multiple myeloma (SMM). This is why some institutions have decided to limit their guidelines for differential diagnosis of MM to recommendations on diagnostic criteria for MM. For example, the *Working Group of the UK Myeloma Forum* has recently (2001) drawn up guidelines on behalf of the *British Committee for Standards in Haematology* (BCSH)[8] in which the criteria favoring diagnosis of MM include >10% PC in BM and presence of bone lytic lesions, which are always absent in MGUS. As far as the concentration of M-component is concerned, its variability in MM means that no specific diagnostic levels are proposed, although it is common that for MGUS the IgG paraprotein is <20 g/L and the IgA <10 g/L.

Fortunately, this situation has changed with the publication of consensus criteria for the classification of MM and other gammopathies, which were agreed by an International Myeloma Working Group.[9] These criteria distinguish between MGUS, asymptomatic (smoldering) myeloma, and symptomatic myeloma (Tables 12.1 and 12.2). No specific level of M-component is required for the diagnosis of MM, but for the diagnosis of MGUS it must be <30 g/l, and BMPC must be <10%. The concept of

Table 12.1 *Diagnostic criteria of multiple myeloma according to different groups*

Chronic Leukemia–Myeloma Task Force[1,5]	Durie (SWOG)[2]	International Myeloma Working Group[9]
Paraprotein present in serum and/or urine together with one of the following: A. Bone marrow plasmacytosis >10%, without any condition associated with reactive plasmacytosis B. Presence of plasma cells in tissue biopsy C. Peripheral blood plasmacytosis >0.5 ×10⁹/L D. Lytic lesions without any other explanation	**Major criteria:** I. Plasmacytoma on tissue biopsy II. Bone marrow plasmacytosis with >30% plasma cells III. Monoclonal globulin spike on serum electrophoresis: >35 g/L (IgG), 20 g/L (IgA), or light-chain excretion on urine electrophoresis ≥1 g/24 hours in the absence of amyloidosis	1. **Presence of M-component** 2. **Bone marrow plasmacytosis >10%** 3. **Presence of myeloma–related organ tissue impairment (ROTI) or end–organ damage related to plasma cell proliferative process. One of the following:** • Anemia with hemoglobin 2 g/dL below the normal level or <10 g/dL • Serum calcium level >10 mg/dL (0.25 mmol/L) above normal or >110 mg/dL (2.75 mmol/L) • Lytic bone lesions or osteoporosis with compressive fractures • Renal insufficiency (creatinine >2 mg/dL or 173 μmol/L) • Symptomatic hyperviscosity • Amyloidosis • Recurrent bacterial infections (>2 episodes in 12 months).
If no monoclonal component can be demonstrated on serum or urine electrophoresis, diagnosis requires the presence of bone lytic lesions or tumors with one of the following: A. Bone marrow plasmacytosis >20% without any conditions known to be associated with reactive plasmacytosis (chronic infections, neoplastic disorders, collagenosis, agranulocytosis, chronic hepatic disorders, HIV infection, leishmaniasis) B. Plasma cell infiltration on tissue biopsy	**Minor criteria:** a. Bone marrow plasmacytosis with 10–30% plasma cells b. Monoclonal globulin spike present, but less than levels defined above c. Lytic bone lesions d. Decrease of normal immunoglobulins: IgG < 6 g/L, IgA < 1 g/L, and IgM < 500 mg/L The diagnosis of myeloma generally requires a minimum one of the following criteria: 1. I + b, I + c, I + d (I + a is not enough) 2. II + b, II + c, II + d 3. III + a, III + c, III + d 4. a + b + c, a + b + d	CRAB: calcium increase, renal impairment, anemia, and bone lesion For symptomatic multiple myeloma, a minimum level of M-component or bone marrow plasma cell infiltration (although usually it is >10%) is not required, provided that these two features co-exist with the presence of end-organ damage

HIV, human immunodeficiency virus; SWOG, Southwest Oncology Group.

Table 12.2 *Diagnostic criteria of smoldering multiple myeloma, indolent multiple myeloma, and monoclonal gammopathy of undetermined significance*

Kyle and Greipp[1,5]	Durie (SWOG)[2]	International Myeloma Working Group
Smoldering multiple myeloma A. Serum paraprotein (usually >30 g/L) and ≥10% bone marrow plasmacytosis B. No anemia, renal failure, or hypercalcemia attributable to myeloma C. No organ impairment, including: • Bone lesions absent on radiographic bone survey • Absence of plasmablasts • Normal β_2-microglobulin in the absence of renal insufficiency • Absence of isotype-specific plasma cells • Peripheral blood B-cell labeling index <0.5% • Absence of light-chain isotype suppression • Urinary light chain <0.5 g/24 hours • Stable paraprotein in serum or urine during follow-up **Monoclonal gammopathy of undetermined significance** A. Serum paraprotein (usually less than 30 g/L) B. No anemia, renal failure, or hypercalcemia C. <10% plasma cells in bone marrow without aggregates on biopsy D. No organ damage, including: • Bone lesions absent on radiographic bone survey • Absence of plasmablasts • Normal β_2-microglobulin in the absence of renal insufficiency • Absence of isotype-specific plasma cells • Peripheral blood B-cell labeling index <0.5% • Absence of light chain isotype suppression • Urinary light chain <0.5 g/24 hours • Stable paraprotein in serum or urine during follow-up	**Indolent multiple myeloma** Criteria of multiple myeloma as described above, with the following restrictions: • No bony lesions, or limited (≤3 osteolytic lesions), without compressive fractures • Monoclonal component not higher than IgA 50 g/L, IgG 70 g/L • Normal serum calcium • No infections • No symptoms, or if present, with the following restrictions – Karnofsky performance >70%, hemoglobin >10 g/dL, serum creatinine <3 mg/dL **Smoldering multiple myeloma** Criteria of indolent multiple myeloma as described above, with additional restrictions: • No demonstrable bone lesions • Bone marrow plasma cells 10–30% **Monoclonal gammopathy of undetermined significance** • Monoclonal component in serum IgA <20 g/L, serum IgG <35 g/L, and urine light-chain excretion <1 g/24 hours • Bone marrow plasma cells <10% plasma cells • No bone lytic lesions • No symptoms	**Asymptomatic myeloma (smoldering multiple myeloma; SMM)** A. ≥30 g/L in serum and/or present in urine or >10% plasma cells at bone marrow B. Absence of end-organ damage: • Anemia with hemoglobin 2 g/dL below the normal level or <10 g/dL • Serum calcium level >10 mg/dL (0.25 mmol/L) above normal or >110 mg/dL (2.75 mmol/L) • Lytic bone lesions or osteoporosis with compressive fractures • Renal insufficiency (creatinine >2 mg/dL or 173 μmol/L) • Symptomatic hyperviscosity • Amyloidosis • Recurrent bacterial infections (>2 episodes in 12 months) **Monoclonal gammopathy of undetermined significance** A. <30 g/L in serum and/or present in urine B. <10% plasma cells in bone marrow C. Absence of end-organ damage: • Anemia with hemoglobin 2 g/dL below the normal level or <10 g/dL • Serum calcium level >10 mg/dL (0.25 mmol/L) above normal or >110 mg/dL (2.75 mmol/L) • Lytic bone lesions or osteoporosis with compressive fractures • Renal insufficiency (creatinine >2 mg/dL or 173 μmol/L) • Symptomatic hyperviscosity • Amyloidosis • Recurrent bacterial infections (>2 episodes in 12 months)

end-organ damage is important in the distinction between MGUS, and asymptomatic MM and symptomatic MM. Myeloma-related organ or tissue impairment (ROTI) is defined as one or more of the following (CRAB):

• serum calcium level >10 mg/L (0.25 mmol/L) above normal or >110 mg/dL (2.75 mmol/L);
• renal impairment (creatinine >2mg/dL, 173 μmol/L);
• anemia with 2 g/dL below the normal level or <10 g/dL;

• lytic bone lesions or osteoporosis with compressive fractures;

as well as symptomatic hyperviscosity, amyloidosis, or recurrent bacterial infections (more than two episodes in 12 months). Accordingly, symptomatic MM would be considered in patients with a serum and/or urine M-component (no level specified), BM plasmacytosis (>10%), or plasmacytoma and end-organ damage.

DIAGNOSTIC CRITERIA OF INDOLENT MYELOMA AND SMOLDERING MYELOMA

The majority of patients with myeloma require active treatment because of symptomatic disease at presentation. By contrast, asymptomatic patients should not receive cytostatic therapy, which is why it is important to identify this group of patients. Smoldering multiple myeloma was characterized by Kyle and Greipp in 1980 as a myeloma with a high serum M-protein ($>30\,g/L$) and a high bone marrow plasmacytosis ($>10\%$), but without bone pain or lytic lesions, anemia, hypercalcemia, renal insufficiency, or recurrent bacterial infections (Table 12.2).[10] These criteria were later refined by the same authors, with the addition of the plasma cell labeling index, defined to be less than 1% in these myelomas (Table 12.2).[3,5] In the criteria proposed by the International Myeloma Working Group, asymptomatic (smoldering) MM is recognized by the presence of $>30\,g/L$ serum M-protein and/or $>10\%$ bone marrow plasmacytosis in the absence of end-organ damage.[9]

The SWOG criteria defined SMM in a similar way, but they also identified another subgroup of MM, named *indolent myelomas*.[2] The diagnostic criteria for the latter subgroup were similar to those of SMM, but a small degree of organ impairment was allowed, such as moderate anemia (hemoglobin $> 10\,g/dL$) or renal insufficiency (creatinine $\leq 3\,mg/dL$), or the presence of limited bone lesions (three or fewer lesions). In contrast, a high monoclonal peak (IgG $> 70\,g/dL$, IgA $> 50\,g/dL$) was considered to be a criterion for exclusion. In addition, the plasma cell labeling index should be low ($<0.5\%$). Indolent myeloma has been accepted less widely as an entity in its own right, but it probably corresponds to clinical conditions that have previously being defined using other names, such as *asymptomatic MM*,[11] or *non-responding, non-progressive MM*.[12–14] The International Myeloma Working Group criteria does not separate indolent MM from asymptomatic (smoldering MM).[9]

DIAGNOSTIC CRITERIA OF MONOCLONAL GAMMOPATHY OF UNDETERMINED SIGNIFICANCE

This condition, whose main characteristic is the presence of a monoclonal protein in serum and or urine without other evidence of a plasma cell malignancy, cannot actually be considered as a malignant disorder in itself. It was initially named as benign or essential monoclonal gammopathy,[15] but now it is preferable to avoid the former name, since it is not always associated with a good (benign) prognosis.[16,17] Criteria used to define MGUS are shown in Table 12.2. The criteria of the International

Myeloma Working Group are an M-component $<30\,g/L$ and BMPCs $<10\%$ with no end-organ damage.

The incidence increases with age (1.5% in subjects older than 50 years, 3% in those over 70 years, and 10% in those over 80).[18,19] It can be associated with various other diseases, sometimes as a transitory abnormality, but it can also be seen without any underlying disease.[20] In this case, it is very important to distinguish it from MM, especially early-stage MM, since the therapeutic approach will be totally different.

However, some MGUS patients can progress to a malignant disease in a relatively short period of time. Up to 1.2% of cases of MGUS progress to overt MM every year.[21] This evolution has been reported to be associated with a number of prognostic factors, including high levels of monoclonal component, low numbers of residual normal plasma cells, or low levels of polyclonal immunoglobulins (see later).

OTHER SPECIAL FORMS OF PLASMA CELL DYSCRASIAS

In addition to the previously defined forms, there are some special forms of PCD that can require a different therapeutic approach and that can cause diagnostic problems. The diagnostic criteria for these disorders agreed by the International Myeloma Working Group are shown in Table 12.3.

Plasma cell leukemia

Plasma cell leukemia was initially described by Kyle in 1974 as a plasma cell disorder characterized by a relative peripheral blood plasmacytosis of more than 20% of total nucleated cells or an absolute number higher than 2×10^9 plasma cells per liter.[22] However, some authors have considered these criteria as arbitrary,[23] and the terminology is still under debate, since the French-American-British (FAB) group[24] suggested that the term 'plasma cell leukemia' should be restricted to a *de novo* presentation in leukemic phase, while others have also used it to describe patients whose MM evolves into a leukemic phase.[22,25]

It is important to recognize plasma cell leukemia, since its clinical course is usually very aggressive, and resistant to melphalan and prednisone.[26,27] The availability of new diagnostic tools, such as flow cytometry and cytogenetics (see later), may contribute to a refinement in the diagnosis, prognostic evaluation, and management of plasma cell leukemia.[26,27]

Solitary plasmacytoma of bone

The existence of a solitary plasmacytoma has been recognized in up to 3% of patients with PCD, usually in the

Table 12.3 *International Working Group diagnostic criteria for the monoclonal gammopathies*[9]

	Monoclonal gammopathy of undetermined significance	Asymptomatic myeloma (smoldering myeloma)	Symptomatic multiple myeloma
M-component	>30 g/L in serum **and**	≥30 g/L in serum[b] **and/or**	Present in serum and /or urine **and/or**
Percentage of bone marrow plasma cells	<10%	<10%	>10%[c]
	and	**and**	**and**
End-organ damage[a]	Absent	Absent	Present

[a] Myeloma-related organ or tissue impairment (end-organ damage) related to plasma cell proliferative process: anemia with hemoglobin 2 g/dL below the normal level or >10 g/dL, or serum calcium level >10 mg/L (0.25 mmol/L) above normal or >110 mg/dL (2.75 mmol/L), or lytic bone lesions or osteoporosis with compressive fractures, or renal insufficiency (creatinine >2 mg/dL or 173 mmol/L), (CRAB: calcium increase, renal impairment, anemia, and bone lesion) or symptomatic hyperviscosity, amyloidosis, or recurrent bacterial infections (>2 episodes in 12 months).
[b] Small amounts of M-protein may be present in the urine.
[c] For symptomatic multiple myeloma, a minimum level of M-component or bone marrow plasma cell infiltration (although usually it is >10%) is not required, provided the plasma cells are shown to be clonal and that these two features co-exist with the presence of end-organ damage.

	Non–secretory myeloma	Solitary plasmacytoma of bone	Extramedullary plasmacytoma
M-component	Absent (negative immunofixation) **and**	Absent or small **and**	Absent or small **and**
Percentage of plasma cells in bone marrow	≥10% or plasmacytoma	Normal	Normal
	and	**and**	**and**
End-organ damage	Present	Absent	Absent
Other		**and** Single area of bone destruction due to plasma cells Normal skeletal survey Normal magnetic resonance imaging, if done	**and** Extramedullary tumor of (clonal) plasma cells Normal skeletal survey Normal magnetic resonance imaging, if done

vertebral column. The diagnostic criteria require the existence of a solitary plasma cell tumor in which the biopsy confirms plasma cell histology, no additional lesions on skeletal survey, absence of plasma cell infiltration in a random bone marrow sample (<10% plasma cells), and no evidence of anemia, hypercalcemia, or renal impairment.[9,27–30] It is also recommended that an magnetic resonance image of the spine be obtained (Chapter 25).

Some groups suggest that patients in whom a paraprotein persists after the eradication of a plasmacytoma with local treatment should undergo a review of the diagnosis.[3,31] Despite the use of effective local radiotherapy, about two-thirds of patients with solitary bone plasmacytoma develop multiple myeloma at 10 years of follow-up, with a median time to progression of 2 years.[32]

Extramedullary plasmacytoma

In this situation, a plasma cell tumor arises outside the bone marrow most frequently in the upper respiratory tract (nose, paranasal sinuses, nasopharynx, and tonsils).[31–34] Other sites include the parathyroid gland, orbit,

lung, spleen, gastrointestinal tract, testes, and skin. In most cases the lesion is unique, although the presence of more lesions (multiple plasmacytomas) has also been reported. The diagnosis is based on the detection of the plasma cell tumor in an extramedullary site, in the absence of bone marrow plasma cell infiltration, bone lytic lesions, and other signs of MM (end-organ damage).

Non–secretory multiple myeloma

This specific type of MM requires particular attention, since it is very difficult to diagnose. The only way to make a definitive diagnosis is to demonstrate the presence of tissue infiltration (usually bone marrow) by cells with plasma cell morphology. However, plasma cell infiltration must be >10% and clonality must be assessed by immunophenotyping (demonstration of the presence of cytoplasmic immunoglobulins with restricted light chain: positive production without excretion). However, exceptional cases exist in which no monoclonal protein can be observed within the plasma cells.[35] In these cases, demonstration of the clonality through the study of the rearrangement status of the immunoglobulin genes is mandatory. Additional detection of aneuploid DNA content by flow cytometry or an abnormal clone by cytogenetics may be helpful. Recent evidence suggests that the serum free light-chain assay is able to detect raised levels of one or other light chain type in the majority of cases of non-secretory MM.[36]

IgM multiple myeloma

This exceptional form of myeloma has been reported very rarely[37] and must be distinguished from Waldenström's macroglobulinemia. The morphology and immunophenotype of the infiltrating cells will give the definitive diagnosis, as well as the existence of osteolytic lesions, which are very rare or absent in Waldenström's macroglobulinemia.[38]

NEW CRITERIA FOR DIFFERENTIAL DIAGNOSIS

Despite all previously mentioned diagnostic criteria, it is not rare to find cases in which differential diagnosis is problematic. The most frequent problem is to find a case with criteria for a certain diagnosis upon using one classification system but different criteria using another system. Another problem presents itself in patients in whom some variables could be attributed to associated problems (e.g. MGUS associated with renal insufficiency – including anemia). In the following sections we will review several new markers that may contribute in the differential diagnosis of PCD and that will probably be included in future diagnostic evaluation.

Morphological and cytochemical characteristics of plasma cells

The morphological characteristics of plasma cells do not contribute significantly to the differential diagnosis, although the observation of cytological pleomorphism and the presence of plasmablasts would be indicative of malignant forms of disease.[39,40] The cytochemical characteristics of PCs have not been closely reviewed in MM for diagnostic purposes, although some reports have suggested that acid phosphatase (AP) score can be of value in the diagnosis of PC disorders. However, neither AP nor α-naphthyl acetate esterase can comprehensively differentiate between MM and MGUS (stage I MM in particular displays low values similar to those found in MGUS).[41] The contribution of marrow morphology to diagnosis is reviewed in detail in Chapter 8.

Electrophoretic findings

As mentioned above, the quantity of the M-component is frequently used for differential diagnosis of MM and MGUS, since the latter condition usually shows a level of <30 g/L. In addition, those MGUS with a relatively high amount of M-component are more likely to progress to symptomatic forms of the disease. Thus, the risk of progression to MM or a related cancer 10 years after the diagnosis of MGUS is 6% for an initial monoclonal protein value of 5 g/L or less, 7% for a value of 10 g/L, 11% for 15 g/L, 20% for 20 g/L, 24% for 25 g/L, and 34% for 30 g/L. This relationship is also maintained at 20 years, or even increased.[21] It was for this reason that the International Myeloma Working Group agreed that a level of >30 g/L should be considered as asymptomatic MM rather than MGUS. In contrast, it should be noted that many MM patients have a monoclonal component of <30 g/L and there are MM cases with a very high monoclonal component that display an indolent course. The additional information provided by the analysis of other proteins besides the M-component can be of help, since low levels of polyclonal immunoglobulins or albumin favor the diagnosis of MM. Thus, in most MM patients the levels of normal or uninvolved Igs are reduced. However, in approximately 30% of patients with MGUS, there is also a decrease in uninvolved Igs,[42,43] which hampers the use of this parameter as a tool for differential diagnosis. Regarding the value of this criteria as a predictor for the risk of transformation from MGUS to MM, Baldini et al.[43] have reported that the risk is higher in MGUS patients with reduced serum polyclonal Igs, while Kyle et al.[42] have shown that a quarter of their MGUS patients had a decrease in normal Igs at diagnosis but remained stable during a median follow-up of 22 years.

Hematological parameters

Moderate normochromic normocytic anemia (hemoglobin below normal but >9 g/dL) is present in around half of MM patients, and it can be severe (Hb < 8 g/dL) in 20%. Anemia should not be present in MGUS and, if it is observed, therefore, the existence of an underlying disease should be confirmed; the diagnosis of MGUS must be questioned. By contrast, in the most aggressive forms of PCD (e.g. plasma cell leukemia), the presence of anemia is more frequent, and usually with low hemoglobin levels (<8 g/dL).

Peripheral blood (PB) examination may occasionally show circulating PC, but the incidence of these cases is low and usually associated with advanced disease. In MM, excluding PCL, only 2% of cases have >5% of circulating PC.[44] Nevertheless, if more sensitive techniques, such as immunophenotyping or PCR, are used, the incidence of MM cases with circulating PC rises to 80%.[45,46] The presence of these cells has also been reported in MGUS and SMM, but at much lower levels than in MM (0.02% in MGUS and SMM vs. 0.24% in MM, $P < 0.05$).[47] Interestingly, in SMM, the presence of circulating PC is associated with high risk of disease progression; thus, Witzig et al.[48] have shown that 66% of patients with circulating PC progress within 12 months, while only 8% of patients remaining stable had PC in PB.

Biochemical markers and cytokines

β_2-microglobulin (β2M) has demonstrated great value as a prognostic factor in MM (see later), but an elevated value cannot be considered specific for the diagnosis of MM. Nevertheless, β2M serum levels higher than 3 mg/L in a patient with a monoclonal component and no renal insufficiency strongly suggests the presence of MM.[49]

About one-quarter of all MM patients display high serum thymidine kinase (TK) levels.[50] However, determination of serum TK is not helpful to distinguish MGUS from MM, since usually only stage III MM cases show significantly increased values as compared with MGUS.[51]

Serum C-reactive protein (CRP), an acute-phase reactant protein induced by interleukin-6 (IL-6), is elevated in 40% of MM cases (>6 mg/L) but in only 8% of MGUS patients.[52] Moreover, MM patients who remain in remission display significantly lower CRP values than those cases that relapse, suggesting that this marker may be of help for disease monitoring. However, CRP is not a specific marker of disease activity in MM and it may increase due to many factors. IL-6 also influences the hepatic synthesis of other acute reactant phase proteins, such as α_1-antitrypsin and orosomucoid, which are increased in 40% and 20% of MM patients, respectively. However, the use of these proteins in differential diagnosis of monoclonal gammopathies is not well established.[53–55]

Serum IL-6 levels are increased in 30–50% of MM patients.[52,56–58] Although IL-6 levels in MM are higher than in patients with MGUS, the serum IL-6 level does not have a significant predictive value for discrimination between MM and MGUS, since the levels in early-stage MM and MGUS overlap.[52,56] Moreover, a small fraction of MGUS patients may display increased IL-6 values. Along the same lines, serum levels of IL-6 receptor (s-IL-6R) are also elevated in 25–50% of MM patients,[40,57,58] but, once again, it is not a reliable marker for differential diagnosis with MGUS.[57]

Several other cytokines, such as IL-2, IL-4, and IL-10, have also been analyzed in MM. However, they have not shown a clear value either in the differential diagnosis with MGUS or for the prognostic evaluation in MM patients. Nevertheless, Blade et al.[59] suggested that tumor

necrosis factor-α (TNFα) could help to predict the risk of transformation of MGUS into overt MM.

Bone disease

As previously mentioned, bone disease is one of the main criteria for diagnosis of MM. Up to now, it has been evaluated using plain skeletal radiographs in which the presence of lytic bone lesions is almost exclusive of MM. Magnetic resonance imaging (MRI) is being increasingly used for assessment of bone disease in patients at early stages of the disease without evident lytic lesions. Some reports have shown that in asymptomatic and early-stage MM, the presence of an abnormal vertebral pattern is associated with early progression.[60–63] Thus, up to 40% of stage I MM patients have specific lesions by MRI, which are not present in MGUS.[62]

Several biochemical markers have also become available for the specific evaluation of bone metabolism.[64–66] The pyridinium cross-links – pyridinoline (PYD/Pyr) and deoxypyridinoline (DPD/DPyr) – of collagen have been established as specific urinary markers of bone resorption. Patients with advanced MM show significantly higher levels of urinary excretion of PYD and DPD than healthy individuals and patients with MGUS.[64] However, these parameters are not helpful for discriminating MGUS from early-stage MM (I, II). Serum bone sialoprotein provides similar results, since it is significantly increased in stage III MM, but it does not discriminate between MGUS and stage I MM.

Serum osteocalcin and bone alkaline phosphatase have been used for a long time as markers of bone formation but, since the alteration of bone formation is a late phenomenon in MM,[60] they are not very useful in the distinction between MM and MGUS. Thus, although these markers are decreased in cases in advanced clinical stage, especially if there is extensive bone disease,[66–68] the levels are similar between normal individuals, MGUS, and stage I MM.[60]

Immunophenotypic studies

Several groups have identified differences in the phenotypic characteristics of myelomatous PC and normal PC. These differences are mainly based on a different pattern of CD19 and CD56 expression.[69–71] Accordingly, malignant PC display a strong reactivity for CD56, usually associated with the lack of positivity for CD19 (CD19$^-$/CD56^{++}). This phenotype is never present in BM PC from healthy individuals. In addition, myelomatous PC usually express slightly lower levels of CD38, as well as higher flow cytometry light scatter values, than normal PC.[72] The α-chain of the IL-6 receptor (CD126) is another marker that is expressed by neoplastic but not normal plasma cells, so it can be used to distinguish them.[73] This differentiation is very important because it can be useful for differential diagnosis. We have found that the presence of residual polyclonal (normal) PC is a constant finding in MGUS patients, while it is a rare event in MM (22% of cases). In addition, if normal PCs are present in MM, their frequency is significantly lower (<3% of total PCs) than that observed in MGUS.[71,72] On multivariate analysis, we found that the ratio of normal/neoplastic PCs was the main independent variable for differential diagnosis between MGUS and MM. Accordingly, quantification of normal and myelomatous PCs is a new important criterion for differential diagnosis of MM versus MGUS.

MM patients have reduced numbers of CD4$^+$ cells with significantly decreased CD4$^+$/CD8$^+$ ratios.[74–76] Moreover, a correlation has been reported between the number of peripheral blood CD4$^+$ T cells and different stages of MM, since the number descends as the stage increases.[77,78] The reduced levels of the CD4$^+$/CD8$^+$ ratio are seen only in patients with MM, not in MGUS patients, and, therefore, could represent a useful parameter for differential diagnosis between the two entities.[78]

Cytogenetic and FISH investigations

Cytogenetics is not useful for the differentiation of MM and MGUS, since similar chromosome abnormalities have been found in both disorders.[79–85] Thus, not only numerical gains of some chromosomes such as chromosomes 3, 6, 7, 9, and 11, but also monosomy 13/13q− have been observed in MGUS as well as in MM patients.[79,86,87] Nevertheless, our group has recently observed that some FISH patterns may help to discriminate these two disorders (co-existence of monosomy 13 together with gains of chromosome 6 and/or chromosome 9 was exclusively found in MM patients). Moreover, we have found that in a high proportion of MGUS patients (67%), two or more cytogenetically different PC clones co-existed, while this occurred in only 19% of MM patients (Rasillo et al., unpublished data). Avet-Loiseau et al.[87] have suggested that specific patterns of genetic abnormalities could favor development of MGUS into MM. Accordingly, they reported a higher incidence of monosomy 13, but not a different incidence of 14q32 rearrangements, among MM cases who had a prior history of MGUS; a more detailed analysis of both abnormalities showed that the combination of t(4;14) – but not t(11;14) – and monosomy 13/13q was shared by a significant proportion of MGUS and MM patients.

DNA ploidy studies

Flow cytometric assessment of cell DNA content provides rapid and objective information about global DNA abnormalities per cell. Using a highly sensitive method with simultaneous staining for PC and DNA, we have observed that, in 62% of MM cases, all PCs display an aneuploid DNA content.[72,88,89] By contrast, in MGUS patients, two clearly different PC subsets can be discriminated in 73% of the cases: one of them shows a DNA index of 1.00 (polyclonal PC), while the second one displays a DNA index >1.00 (clonal PC).[72,90] The presence of these two PC populations with different DNA content could be useful in differentiating between MM and MGUS, since in MM there is only one PC population – either aneuploid or diploid. These results are consistent with the immunophenotypic data described above.

Molecular genetic techniques

MONOCLONAL IMMUNOGLOBULIN GENE REARRANGEMENTS

At present, polymerase chain reaction (PCR)-based techniques can identify tumor-related DNA sequences based on the unique N region generated during V(D)J assembly. In addition, in MM, somatic mutations add more specificity to the V(D)J region, especially because no intraclonal variations have been described.[91,92] This aspect may be relevant because, although somatic mutations have also been reported in MGUS, intraclonal variations have been recognized[93,94] so could represent a difference between MM and MGUS. Accordingly, the target cell in MGUS would be a follicular-center-derived cell that has not switched off the mutational machinery, while the target cell in MM would be a post-follicular cell in which this machinery is already switched off.

Investigation of the CDR3 sequence has also been used to demonstrate the clonal involvement of circulating B cells in myeloma. Accordingly, it has been reported that a small subset of BM and peripheral blood B lymphocytes displayed the same rearrangement pattern as myelomatous PC in 50% and 25% of MM cases, respectively.[95] Moreover, the number of PB clonotypic B cells could help to discriminate a group of MGUS with a higher risk of malignant transformation, since the risk of transformation to MM in MGUS patients with an excess of PB clonal B lymphocytes was found to be greater than in cases without such an excess (53% vs. 17%).[96]

ONCOGENES AND TUMOR SUPPRESSOR GENES

Disregulation of oncogenes and tumor suppressor genes plays an important role in the pathogenesis of MM. Some of these genetic abnormalities could have prognostic value but are of relatively little help in distinguishing between MM and MGUS, since many of the genetic abnormalities are present in both entities.

The t(8;14) has been described in less than 5% of MM, but DNA rearrangements involving the c-myc gene (8q24) or the 20 kb downstream MLVI-4 locus may be present in up to 10–20% of all MM patients.[97,98] Moreover, expression of c-*myc* mRNA and c-myc protein is commonly increased in MM cells and MM derived cell lines.[99–101] No data concerning its role in MGUS are available.

The t(11;14) has been identified in 25–40% of MM patients, with a different breakpoint from that observed in mantle cell lymphoma,[102,103] although it also promotes enhanced expression of cyclin D1. This translocation seems to be associated with lymphoplasmacytic cell morphology,[104–106] and to date it has not been observed in MGUS. The fibroblast growth factor receptor 3 gene (*fgfr3*) is deregulated by the t(4;14)(p16;q32) in ~25% of newly diagnosed MM and myeloma cells, and in a similar number of patients.[107–110] No particular clinical forms have been described for patients with this abnormality and, although the translocation has not been described in MGUS, this could be due to the lack of studies as yet carried out.

Mutations of N- and K-*ras* are not present in MGUS, but they have been found in 9–30% of MM.[111] The incidence increases (up to 70%) in progressive terminal MM and plasma cell leukemia patients.[112] p53 mutations occur only in ~5% of early-stage MM, but its incidence increases with disease progression and reaches up to 40% in plasma cell leukemia.[113] Again, the presence of this alteration favors the diagnosis of MM versus MGUS, but its lack of specificity impairs its use as a definitive diagnostic tool.

The retinoblastoma (Rb) tumor suppressor gene is located in chromosome 13, which is deleted or partially deleted in approximately 30% of abnormal MM karyotypes.[114–117] By Southern blot or interphase FISH analysis, monoallelic detection of Rb gene has been reported in about 30–60% of MM patients and cell lines,[113,118,119] although without changes in pRb expression.[119] It was initially thought that this alteration could be useful for differential diagnosis, since it is present in virtually all plasma cell leukemia cases.[27] However, several studies have already observed the presence of 13 deletions in MGUS.[83,84]

Altered inhibitors of cyclin-dependent kinases p16, p15, p21WAFI, and MDM2 have also been described in monoclonal gammopathies.[120–124] However, few data are available concerning its usefulness in the differential diagnosis between MM and MGUS. The only available data refer to p16 gene. In our experience, this is frequently hypermethylated in MM but not in MGUS,[125] but these data have not been confirmed by others.[124]

Plasma cell labeling index

Apart form its indubitable prognostic value, the plasma cell labeling index (PCLI) may be of help in differentiating among patients with MM, MGUS, and, especially, smoldering myeloma.[126] Accordingly, it has been shown that in patients with M-component, an elevated PCLI (assessed by the incorporation of bromodeoxyuridine) constitutes a good indication that either MM is already present or symptomatic myeloma will soon develop. However, more than one-third of patients with symptomatic MM have a normal PCLI,[127] and we have observed that some MGUS patients can have a high S-phase value.[72] Obviously, this hampers the specificity of the PCLI for differential diagnosis between MGUS and MM.

PROGNOSTIC FACTORS: CONTRIBUTION TO CLINICAL MANAGEMENT

The survival duration of patients with MM ranges from a few months to more than 10 years. This heterogeneity relates mainly to specific characteristics of the tumor itself and of the host. The identification of those characteristics associated with either a good or poor prognosis are most important not only for doctors but also for patients, in order to obtain more individualized information about disease outcome, instead of simply offering a general median survival rate. For the past 30 years many groups have reported on their investigations into the clinical and biological disease characteristics influencing survival. In fact, there is a disassociation between the large body of information generated in this field and its translation into clinical practice. The main reason for studying prognostic factors should be the identification of risk groups in order to adapt patient treatment according to the expected outcome. This would be particularly important for the evaluation of new therapeutic strategies.

In the first part of this review, we will be discussing the most relevant prognostic factors reported in the literature, which have usually been identified upon analyzing symptomatic MM patients treated with conventional chemotherapy.[126–129] Then we will briefly review two other situations for which evaluation of prognostic factors is required: in asymptomatic MM and in patients undergoing high-dose therapy.

Prognostic factors can be classified into three major categories: (1) host factors; (2) factors that reflect the specific characteristics of the malignant clone; and (3) a series of factors resulting from the interaction between the tumor clone and the host, which mainly reflect the tumor, burden, and disease complications (Fig. 12.1).

Host factors

Among host factors, the favorable influence of a good performance status (ECOG ≥2) and of young age are well established. Thus, an age lower than 60 or 70 years is associated with prolonged survival. Moreover, it has been

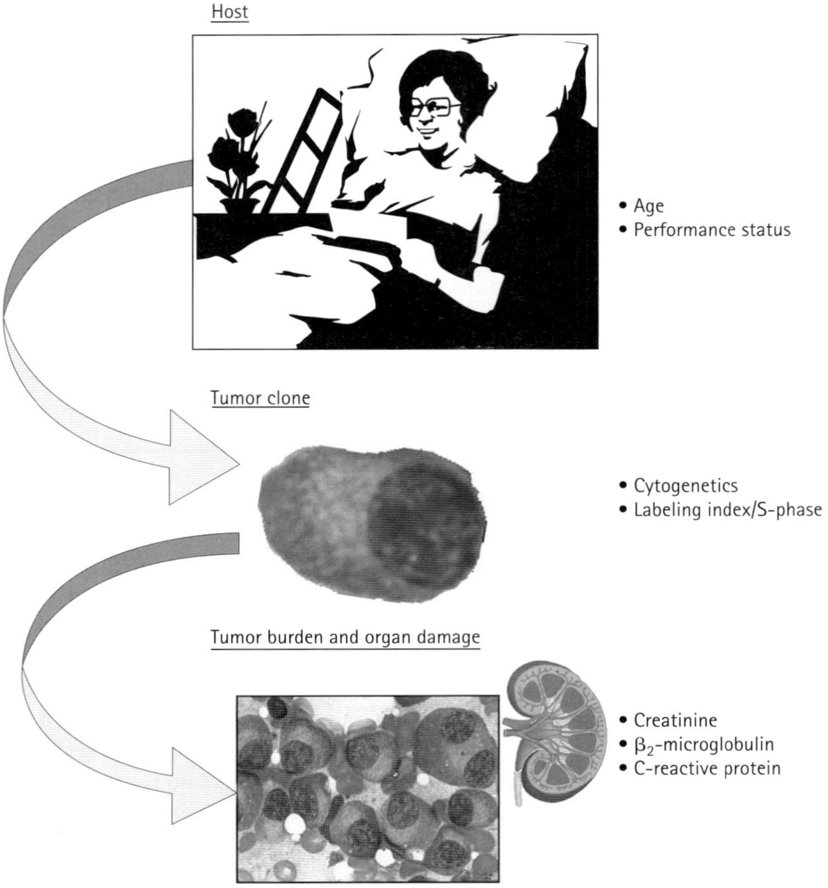

Host

- Age
- Performance status

Tumor clone

- Cytogenetics
- Labeling index/S-phase

Tumor burden and organ damage

- Creatinine
- β_2-microglobulin
- C-reactive protein

Figure 12.1 *Prognostic factors in myeloma.*

reported that patients under 40 years of age and with normal renal function and low β2M have a median survival of over 8 years.[130] As far as race is concerned, the Southwest Oncology Group has published a study showing that survival is similar in black and white patients.[131] We are not aware of any similar studies comparing other ethnic groups.

The immune status of the patient may play an important role in tumor growth control. The role in immune surveillance of T and NK cells is well established. We have observed that the number of CD4 cells is significantly reduced in MM patients, particularly in those in advanced clinical stages, and that the reduction is due mainly to memory and not to naive CD4 cells. Moreover, patients with low CD4 levels ($<700 \times 10^6$ cells/L) display a significantly shorter survival, although this is not an independent prognostic factor.[75] Similar results on the impact of CD4 cells have been reproduced by the Eastern Cooperative Oncology Group (ECOG).[132] In addition, this group has shown that high levels of peripheral blood (PB) CD19$^+$ cells are positively associated with prolonged survival.[76] Within the NK cells lineage, several antigenic and functionally different NK cell subpopulations coexist, and this could help to explain the discrepant results

reported in the literature.[133,134] In our experience, the overall number of NK cells is significantly increased in patients with MM, but their distribution according to clinical stages differs depending on the type of NK subpopulation. Thus, the number of mature NK cells increases in the early stages of the disease – probably in an attempt to control the tumor growth – while in advanced stages, the number of PB mature NK cells decreases and the relative number of immature NK cells increases.[134]

To complete the picture concerning the prognostic influence of immune surveillance, it should be pointed out that myeloma patients may develop T-cell clones, which can recognize autologous idiotypic Ig structures as tumor-specific antigens. The occurrence of expanded T-cell clones, defined by the presence of rearrangements in the T-cell receptor (TCR) β-chain detected by Southern blot, is associated with an improved prognosis.[135] These clonal cytotoxic T cells reside in the CD8$^+$ CD57$^+$ CD28$^-$ compartment.[136]

Malignant clone factors

The second cohort of prognostic factors is those that reflect specific characteristics of myelomatous PC and includes morphology, immunocytochemistry, immunophenotyping, cytogenetics, oncogenes, multidrug resistance, and the proliferative activity of PC. Several groups, but particularly the German[137] and Mayo Clinic Groups,[40,138] have shown that immature/plasmablastic morphology is associated with a poor outcome and has independent prognostic significance. In spite of these data, little attention is as yet paid to the morphological characteristics of PC. This attitude is completely different from that observed in other hematological malignancies, such as acute leukemias and lymphomas, where the morphological features of the malignant cells are quite significant for classification and prognosis. Regarding immunocytochemistry, a study by the SWOG showed that low PC acid phosphatase levels are associated with poor survival (1.7 years for patients with low scores vs. 2.8 years for those with high scores).[139]

The prognostic influence of immunophenotyping has been extensively investigated.[140–144] Based on our experience and that of other groups, it can be concluded that the expression of CD20 and sIg, which identify immature PC, tend to be associated with poor prognosis.[140,141] Downregulation of CD56 and CD11a – adhesion molecules that favor the BM homing of PC – and higher expression of CD44 have been associated with extramedullary spreading of malignant PC.[142,143] The expression of CD28 has been related to disease activity, probably confined to highly proliferative accelerated phases of the disease.[142,145] The adverse prognostic influence initially attributed to myelomonocytic antigens expressed by PC was not later reproduced.[140] In any case, it is most probable that none of these antigens constitutes an independent prognostic factor and routine immunophenotyping should not be performed for prognostic evaluation purposes. In contrast, immunophenotypic studies can be of value for differential diagnosis between MGUS and MM,[69,72] as well as for investigation of changes in the PC compartment (tumor burden) induced by treatment.[71] The CD138 antigen (syndecan-1) is shed from the surface of PC and can be measured in serum. The Nordic Myeloma Study Group has reported that patients with high serum syndecan-1 ($\geq$1170 units/mL) display a short survival (20 months vs. 44 months).[146]

As occurs with acute leukemia, cytogenetics is emerging as one of the most important prognostic tools for MM. Therefore, investigation of cytogenetic changes should be mandatory in all patients with newly diagnosed MM. The Arkansas Group[114,147] has shown that, in patients with MM treated with intensive chemotherapy, either partial or complete deletions of chromosome 13 are associated with short survival. Several other groups, including our own,[117,148–150] have reported the same experience, but now in patients treated with conventional chemotherapy, in which monosomy 13 was analyzed by FISH. The Arkansas Group postulated that the prognostic influence of monosomy 13 detected by conventional cytogenetics is superior to that detected by FISH, since in the former, PC should display not only the cytogenetic abnormality but also a proliferative capacity high enough to yield good-quality mitosis. Nevertheless, several papers indicate that the detection of monosomy 13 by FISH has prognostic relevance not only for patients treated with standard chemotherapy[117] but also probably in those receiving high-dose therapy.[151] Other chromosomal changes associated with poor survival are t(4;14)(p16;q32), t(14;16)(q32;q23), and 17p13 deletion (p53), while t(11;14)(q13;q32) appears to have a favorable prognosis.[150] Moreover, the presence of complex as well as hypodiploid karyotypes is also associated with treatment failure. Other potential adverse cytogenetic features are abnormalities of chromosome 1p/1q and deletion of chromosome 22.[151,152] By contrast, trisomies of chromosomes 9, 11, and 17 tend to have a favorable prognostic influence.[117] In line with this latter observation, our results on DNA content analyzed by flow cytometry, also show that cases with hyperdiploid DNA cell content have a significantly better prognosis than diploid myelomas, although the prognostic value of this parameter is lost in multivariate analysis.[88]

Regarding oncogenes and tumor suppressor genes, it has become increasingly evident that their disregulation contributes to the pathogenesis of MM. The development and progression of the tumor clone implies a multistep process that requires the accumulation of sequential changes. In addition, it has been shown that some of these genetic abnormalities could have an impact on the prognosis of the disease. Thus, some oncogenic events, such as p53 mutations[113] or c-myc overexpression,[153] are associated with progressive disease and relapse and, therefore, could reflect disease aggressiveness and treatment refractoriness. The retinoblastoma gene is located on chromosome 13 and, accordingly, the adverse prognostic impact of Rb deletions parallels that of monosomy 13.[117,149,154] Patients who display K-ras mutations have significantly shorter survival as compared with those who do not (2 vs. 3.7 years).[111] In addition, we have observed that methylation of p16 is associated with high proliferative activity of PC and poor prognosis, but it is not an independent prognostic factor, owing to its relationship with the number of PC cells in S-phase.[125]

Multidrug resistance should in theory be a relevant prognostic factor in MM. However, it has not yet been included in a large-scale multivariate analysis. Resistance due to p-glycoprotein (MDR-1) is usually observed in patients who have been exposed to anthracyclines and vinca alkaloids.[155,156] Nevertheless, conflicting results have been reported regarding the independent prognostic value of MRD-1 expression.[157,158] These discrepancies may be related, at least in part, to technical pitfalls, since residual normal cells also display MRD activity and, therefore, appropriate internal controls are mandatory. Recent data suggest that lung-resistant protein (LRP) may afford more important information. It is expressed in 50% of patients and identifies a subgroup with low probability of response to conventional doses of melphalan, but this adverse influence disappears in patients treated with high-dose chemotherapy.[158]

Finally, the proliferative activity of the malignant PC, as assessed either by the labeling index (LI) with bromodeoxyuridine[159] or by flow cytometry with propidium iodide,[160] is one of the most important prognostic markers for MM. In our experience, the number of PC in S-phase together with cytogenetics, β2M, PS, and age, represents the best combination of disease characteristics for survival prediction.[117,144] Joshua et al.[161] have shown that the proliferative activity is almost entirely attributable to an increase in the LI of the primitive PC.

It is also worth mentioning that response to front-line therapy is an important prognostic factor, but we should also be aware that patients with rapid response may have a short duration of response and survival. This was suggested by Hansen et al.[162] 25 years ago and confirmed by Boccadoro and Pileri[163] through kinetic studies.

Prognostic factors associated with tumor burden and disease complications

Within this third group of prognostic factors, for which information is more abundant, are:

1 factors derived from the expansion of the malignant clone – tumor burden;
2 factors related to disease complications – anemia, renal insufficiency, skeletal lesions, etc.;
3 a wide array of biochemical markers, including some cytokines that reflect disease activity.

The tumor burden can be assessed by means of the Durie and Salmon classification (Table 12.4),[164] which was specifically obtained from mathematical models for the evaluation of tumor mass. Other prognostic factors that reflect the tumor burden are the proportion of PC in BM, the histopathological pattern of infiltration, and the presence of circulating PC. A high number of PC in BM as well as a diffuse pattern of infiltration are generally associated with a poor prognosis. However, these are not consistent prognostic factors, probably owing to the heterogeneous distribution of PC in BM (the areas with bone tenderness or lytic lesions are usually more heavily infiltrated). The detection of circulating PC, identified either by morphology or immunophenotyping, is associated with advanced disease, and it has been reported that the presence of high levels of circulating PC (>4% PC) is an independent adverse prognostic factor.[45]

For many years, it has been well established that some disease complications, such as anemia, thrombocytopenia, and particularly renal insufficiency, assessed either by urea or creatinine, have a relevant influence on disease outcome.[165] Skeletal lesions, which also have adverse impact on survival, have usually been evaluated by X-ray and, more recently, using markers of bone resorption such as pyridinoline (PYD) and deoxypyridinoline (DPD). Although the urinary levels of PYD and DPD are increased in patients with advanced clinical stages and progressive disease, and also correlate with CRP, creatinine, and albumin levels, the relationship with survival is apparently only marginal.[64] Serum bone sialoprotein is another biochemical marker of bone turnover and affords similar results to DPD.

Several biochemical markers, including some cytokines, that reflect disease activity may offer relevant prognostic information. The most important of these is the uncorrected β2M levels, which increase as a result of both tumor burden growth and renal function deterioration (it is actually a very sensitive indicator of glomerular filtration). Several threshold values (from 3 to

Table 12.4 *The Durie and Salmon staging system for myeloma*

Stage	Criteria	Tumor load (cells $\times 10^{12}/m^2$)
I	All of the following: 1. Hemoglobin > 10 g/dL 2. Serum calcium < 12 mg/dL 3. X-ray: no bone destruction (scale 0) or solitary plasmacytoma 4. Low paraprotein production: (a) serum IgG < 5 g/dL (b) serum IgA < 3 g/dL (c) urine light chain < 4 g/24 hours	Low (<0.6)
II	Laboratory and radiological parameters intermediate between stages I and II	Medium (0.6–1.2)
III	At least one of the following criteria: 1. Hemoglobin < 8.5 g/dL 2. Serum calcium > 12 mg/dL 3. X-ray: advanced lytic bone lesions (scale 3) 4. High paraprotein production: (a) serum IgG > 7 g/dL (b) serum IgA > 5 g/dL (c) urine light chain > 12 g/24 hours	High (>1.2)

Subclassification:
A Serum creatinine < 2 mg/dL
B Serum creatinine ⩾ 2 mg/dL

6 mg/dL) have been used to discriminate prognostic sub-groups,[144,166–169] but β2M level can also be used as a continuous variable since the higher the β2M value, the shorter the survival. Owing to its strong influence on disease outcome, the measurement of serum β2M levels at diagnosis is mandatory. In contrast, β2M is not helpful for monitoring the course of the disease, since there are patients who relapse without a previous increase in β2M levels, while others display levels in the upper normal limit without any evidence of disease progression.[169] Other markers of disease activity, such as thymidine kinase,[50] neopterin, and lactate dehydrogenase, do not usually remain independent prognostic factors in multivariate analysis.[169] IL-6 is the major PC growth factor and elevated serum levels are associated with short survival.[170,171] Similarly, high levels of its soluble receptor (s-IL-6R) correlate with poor prognosis.[129,172] Nevertheless, conflicting results have also been reported,[57] and neither of these two markers is generally used in clinical practice for prognostic evaluation of patients with MM. IL-6 also influences the hepatic synthesis of acute phase reactant proteins such as CRP, α_1-antitrypsin (α_1AT), and orosomucoid. In fact, serum CRP levels reflect IL-6 activity,[173] and they represent a surrogate marker for IL-6 concentration, and the same applies for α_1AT.[54] Moreover, since the measurement of these proteins is simpler and cheaper than that of IL-6, either α_1AT or particularly CRP can replace IL-6 as prognostic factors,[129] and together with BM constitute a very useful combination to predict survival in MM patients.[173] It should be noted that although CRP levels may be influenced by many factors different from myeloma activity, the presence at diagnosis of serum CRP values >6 mg/L constitutes an independent prognostic factor. This feature allowed Bataille et al.[173] to stratify MM patients into three groups according to CRP and β2M serum levels: (1) low-risk group CRP and β2M <6 mg/L (50% of patients); (2) intermediate-risk group CRP or β2M ≥ to 6 mg/L (35% of patients); (3) high-risk group CRP and β2M ≥ 6 mg/L (15% of patients). The median survival was 54, 27, and 6 months, respectively ($P < 0.0001$).

The SWOG has proposed a staging scheme based on β2M and albumin levels. Stage I, II, and III patients all have albumin >3 g/dL and they differentiate in the level of β2M (<2.5 mg/L, 2.5–5.5 mg/L, and >5.5 mg/L, respectively), while stage IV corresponds to cases with albumin <3 g/dL and β2M >5.5 mg/L.

Prognostic factors in asymptomatic myelomas

There has been an increase in the number of patients now being diagnosed as asymptomatic MM and, among these, a relatively high proportion have a young age at presentation.

Within asymptomatic MM patients, the identification of those cases at high risk of progression could help to select candidates for early treatment. The study conducted by Facon et al.[174] included 91 stage I asymptomatic MM patients, of whom 41 experienced disease progression at a median of 48 months. In multivariate analysis, the only significant factors influencing progression were Hb <12 g/dL, BM plasmacytosis >25%, and MC >30 g/L. Patients with two or three risk factors progressed within 6 months, while those without risk factors remained free of progression for >50 months. A second study, conducted at the MD Anderson,[175] included 101 asymptomatic patients without lytic lesions. In this series, the presence of two out of the following three factors identified a subgroup of patients at high risk of early progression: M-component >30 g/L, Bence Jones protein >50 mg/24 h, and IgA isotype. In addition, in patients with only one adverse factor, MRI proved to be a useful tool for the identification of cases at risk of progression. These data illustrate how these types of studies may help physicians in making clinical decisions for a difficult subset of MM patients in which treatment is controversial.

Prognostic factors in stem cell transplants

Another new situation in which an evaluation of prognostic factors is important is the availability of stem-cell transplantation as a therapeutic option for a large number of MM patients. This procedure appears to produce prolongations in both survival and quality of life. However, owing to its high cost, it is important to have models to predict which patients will benefit from transplants, thereby avoiding the financial and emotional burden imposed on those unlikely to respond. In this area, it would also be desirable to have predictive models to individualize the choice between allogeneic and autologous transplants in young patients.

An obvious question upon using high-dose chemotherapy is whether the influence of prognostic factors change from that observed under conventional chemotherapy. Preliminary data suggest that they are similar. The Arkansas Group[114,176] initially identified low β2M levels, less prior therapy, and Ig isotype different from IgA as independent favorable variables for overall survival (OS) and disease-free survival (DFS). In addition, age <50 years, ECOG <2, and stages I/II were also positive factors, but only in university analysis. The same group has shown that abnormalities in chromosome 11q and 13 were associated with poor outcome in patients receiving tandem autologous transplants: event-free survival (EFS) (21 months vs. 50 months, $P = 0.0001$) and OS (34 months vs. 62 months, $P = 0.001$).[147] Moreover, the presence of any type of translocation (unfavorable-complex karyotype) is a dominant adverse prognostic variable.[147] At the European

Bone Marrow Transplantaion (EBMT) group,[177] it was found that stage I, being in complete remission (CR) before transplant, one line of therapy, age <45 years, and low β2M levels were all favorable factors. Controversial results exist concerning the influence of LI, since the Arkansas group[178] has suggested that its adverse effect disappears under their total therapy program, while Gertz *et al.*[179] have shown that a high LI as well as the presence of circulating monoclonal PC in the blood stem cell harvest were all associated with shortened survival after transplantation. Interestingly, in both studies, β2M retained its adverse prognostic influence.

The Mayo Clinic Group[180] has postulated that the outcome of autologous stem-cell transplant is more dependent on biological variables, such as PCLI, than on response to transplant (complete vs. partial response). Nevertheless, several other studies have shown that achievement of CR is the most important prognostic factor.[181-183] One interesting additional issue is to examine variables associated with long-term (≥5 years) EFS after transplant. The Arkansas Group[184] has reported that the most favorable features are pre-transplant CRP < 4 mg/L, β2M < 2.5 mg/dL, prior therapy ≤12 months, and absence of adverse cytogenetic abnormalities. Regarding response to transplant, although attaining a CR was a favorable variable in univariate analysis, it was not an independent feature in multivariate analysis. This is consistent with the possibility of re-establishing a prolonged MGUS phase in some transplanted MM patients.

In the allogeneic BMT setting, the experience of Seattle[185] and of the EBMT[186] shows that β2M is again the most important prognostic factor, together with clinical stage, age, and lines of treatment before transplantation. It should be noted that neither the influence of the LI nor the cytogenetics was evaluated in any of these studies.

Prognostic factors: summary

In the previous pages we have discussed a large number of prognostic factors, but perhaps only a few of them have real independent value. A summary of the most important would include: (1) two host factors that reflect the ability of the patient to tolerate chemotherapy (*age and performance status*); and (2) two intrinsic characteristics of the malignant clone (*cytogenetics and proliferative activity LI*) together with two biochemical markers that reflect tumor burden/disease complications (*β2M and CRP*) (Fig. 12.1).

Currently, clinicians have a wide array of therapeutic options for MM patients and, as in other disorders, such as acute lymphoblastic leukemia and non-Hodgkin's lymphoma, an international classification for MM patients based on risk group categories has been defined

according to simple, objective, and independent prognostic factors. This International Staging System (ISS) is derived from a total of 11 171 patients compiled from American, Asian, and European cooperative groups and large individual institutions.[187] The ISS is based on the levels of β2M and albumin (Table 12.5), and it allows the discrimination of three risk groups regardless of age, geographic region, or standard or transplant therapy. This system would assist clinical decision-making and allow the individualization of treatment according to patients' characteristics. In addition, prognostic factors could represent a valuable tool for the evaluation of results of new treatment strategies. In this context, experimental therapies should be assayed on homogeneous cohorts of patients identified according to prognostic factors. Moreover, upon evaluating randomized trials, for the balance of the two arms it would be important to take into account not only the individual prognostic factors but also the possible additive effect of two or three prognostic factors within a particular therapeutic arm. This system will be a very useful tool for the future, although further efforts will have to be carried out in order to improve it with the inclusion of other parameters, such as cytogenetics and molecular markers.

Table 12.5 *International staging system for multiple myeloma*

Stage	Parameters	Median survival (months)
1	β2M < 3.5 mg/L and albumin > 3.5 g/dL	62
2	β2M < 3.5 mg/L and albumin < 3.5 g/dL, or β2M 3.5–5.5	44
3	β2M > 5.5 mg/L	29

β2M, β2-microgobulin.

KEY POINTS

- New criteria for the differential diagnosis of monoclonal gammopathy of undetermined significance (MGUS), asymptomatic myeloma, and symptomatic myeloma have been published by an International Myeloma Working Group.
- These place emphasis on the presence or absence of myeloma-related end-organ damage (ROTI) (see Table 12.3).
- Criteria for MGUS are M-protein in serum <30 g/L *and* <10% plasma cells in the marrow *and* no ROTI.

- Criteria for asymptomatic myeloma are M-component in serum >30 g/L *and/or* >10% plasma cells in the marrow *and* no ROTI.
- Criteria for symptomatic myeloma are M-component in serum or urine (any level) *and/or* clonal plasma cells in the marrow (no specific value required if ROTI present) *and* ROTI.
- Additional parameters that can aid in differential diagnosis include plasma cell labeling index, β_2-microglobulin level, plasma cell immunophenotype, presence of circulating plasma cells, levels of uninvolved immunoglobulins, and biochemical markers of bone disease.
- Prognosis in myeloma varies widely according to a number of prognostic factors, the most important of which are serum β_2-microglobulin level, serum albumin, and various cytogenetic abnormalities.

ACKNOWLEDGMENTS

This work has been partially supported by grants from 'Red Española de Mieloma' (G03/136) and F15.55 PI 02/0905.

REFERENCES

• = Key primary paper
◆ = Major review article
* = Paper that represents the first formal publication of a management guideline

1. Committee of the Chronic Leukemia-Myeloma Task Force, National Cancer Institute. Proposed Guidelines for protocol studies. II. Plasma cell myeloma. *Cancer Chemother Rep* 1973; **4**:145–58.
2. Durie BGM. Staging and kinetics of multiple myeloma. In: Wiernik PH, Canellos GP, Kyle RA, Schiffer CA (eds) *Neoplastic diseases of the blood*, 2nd edn. New York: Churchill Livingstone, 1991:439–51.
3. Greipp PR, Kyle RA. Clinical, morphological and cell kinetic differences among multiple myeloma, monoclonal gammopathy of unknown undetermined significance and smoldering myeloma. *Blood* 1983; **62**:166–71.
4. Kyle RA. Idiopathic Bence Jones proteinuria: a distinct entity? *Am J Med* 1973; **65**:222.
5. Greipp PR. Advances in diagnosis and management of myeloma. *Semin Hematol* 1992; **29**(Suppl 2):24–45.
6. Lymphoma Tumor Group. Plasma cell disorders. In: British Columbia Cancer Agency (ed.) *Cancer Treatment Policies*. Vancouver: British Columbia Cancer Agency, 1994:4–6.
7. Ong F, Hermans J, Noordijk EM, Kluin-Nelemans JC. Is the Durie and Salmaon diagnostic classification system for plasma cell discrasias still the best choice? *Ann Hematol* 1995; **70**:19–24.
*8. UK Myeloma Forum. Guideline: diagnosis and managements of multiple myeloma. *Br J Haematol* 2001; **115**:522–40.
9. International Myeloma Working Group. Criteria for the classification of monoclonal gammopathies, multiple myeloma and related disorders: a report of the International Myeloma Working Group. *Br J Haematol* 2003; **121**:749–57.
*10. Kyle RA, Greipp PR. Smoldering multiple myeloma. *N Engl J Med* 1980; **302**:1347–9.
11. Dimopoulos MA, Moulopoulos A, Delasalle K, Alexanian R. Solitary plasmacytoma and asymptomatic multiple myeloma. *Hematol Oncol Clin North Am* 1992; **6**:359–69.
12. Paccagnella A, Cartei G, Fosser V, *et al.* Treatment of multiple myeloma with M-2 protocol and without maintenance therapy. *Eur J Cancer Clin Oncol* 1983; **19**:1345–51.
13. Bladé J, Rozman C, Montserrat E, Cervantes F, Feliu E, Granena A, *et al.* Treatment of alkylating resistant multiple myeloma with vincristine, BCNU, doxorubicin and prednisone (VBAP). *Eur J Cancer Clin Oncol* 1986; **22**:1193–7.
◆14. San Miguel JF, Bladé J, García-Sanz R. Treatment of multiple myeloma. *Haematologica* 1999; **84**:36–58.
15. Waldenström J. Studies on conditions associated with disturbed gamma globulin formation (gammopathies). *Harvey Lect* 1961; **56**:211–21.
16. Kyle RA. Monoclonal gammopathies of undetermined significance. *Semin Hematol* 1989; **26**:176–200.
17. Kyle RA. Benign monoclonal gammopathies – after 20 to 35 years of follow-up. *Mayo Clin Proc* 1993; **68**:26–36.
18. Haller J. Frequency of abnormal serum immunoglobulins in the aged. *Acta Med Scand* 1963; **173**:737–45.
19. Saleun JP, Vicariot M, Deroff P, Morin JF. Monoclonal gammopathies in the adult population of Finistere, France. *J Clin Pathol* 1982; **35**:63–8.
20. Foerster J. Plasma cell disorders: General considerations. In: Lee GR, Foerster J, Lukens J, Paraskevas F, Greer JP, Rodgers GM (eds) *Wintrobe's clinical hematology*, 10th edn. Baltimore, MD: Williams and Wilkins, 1999:2613–30.
•21. Kyle RA, Therneau TM, Rajkumar SV, Offord JR, Larson DR, Plevak MF, *et al.* A long-term study of prognosis in monoclonal gammopathy of undetermined significance. *N Engl J Med* 2002; **346**:564–9.
22. Kyle RA, Maldonado JE, Bayrd ED. Plasma cell leukemia. Report on 17 cases. *Arch Intern Med* 1974; **133**:813–18.
23. Baim BJ: *Blood cells: a practical guide*. Oxford: Blackwell Science, 1995.
24. Bennet JM, Catowsky D, Daniel M-T, Flandrin G, Galton DAG, Gralnick H, *et al.* Proposals for the classification of chronic (mature) B and T lymphoid leukemias. *J Clin Pathol* 1989; **42**:567–84.
25. Noel P, Kyle RA. Plasma cell leukemia: an evaluation of response to therapy. *Am J Med* 1987; **83**:1062–8.
•26. García-Sanz R, Orfão A, González M, Tabernero MD, Bladé J, Ma J. *et al.* Primary plasma cell leukemia: clinical, immunophenotypical, DNA ploidy and cytogenetic characteristics. *Blood* 1999; **93**:1032–7.
27. Dimopoulos MA, Palumbo A, Delasalle KB, Alexanian R. Primary plasma cell leukaemia. *Br J Haematol* 1994; **88**:754–9.

28. Chack L, Cox RS, Bostwick DG, *et al.* Solitary plasmacytoma of bone. Treatment, progression and survival. *J Clin Oncol* 1987; **5**:1811–15.

29. Frassica DAM, Frassica FJ, Schray MF, Sim FH, Kyle RA. Solitary plasmacytoma of bone. *Int J Radiat Oncol Biol Phys* 1989; **16**:43–8.

30. Knowling MA, Harwood AR, Bergsagel DF. Comparison of extramedullary plasmacytomas with solitary and multiple plasma cells tumors of bone. *J Clin Oncol* 1983; **1**:255–62.

●31. Bataille R, Sany J. Solitary myeloma: Clinical and prognostic features of a review of 114 cases. *Cancer* 1981; **48**:845–51.

◆32. Dimopoulos MA, Kiamouris C, Moulopoulos A. Solitary plasmacytoma of bone and extramedullary plasmacytoma. *Hematol Oncol Clin North Am* 1999; **13**:1249–57.

33. Witshaw E. The natural history of extramedullary plasmacytoma and its relation to solitary myeloma of bone and myelomatosis. *Medicine (Baltimore)* 1976; **55**:217–38.

34. Corwin J, Lindberg RD. Solitary plasmacytoma of bones versus extramedullary plasmacytoma and their relationship to multiple myeloma. *Cancer* 1979; **43**:1007–13.

35. Franchi F, Seminara P, Teodori L, Adone G, Bianco P. The non-producer multiple myeloma. report of a case and review of the literature. *Blut* 1986; **52**:281–7.

36. Drayson M, Tang LX, Drew R, Mead GP, Carr-Smith H, Bradwell AR. Serum free light chain measurements for identifying and monitoring patients with nonsecretory multiple myeloma. *Blood* 2001; **7**:2900–2.

37. Sahota SS, Garand R, Mahroof R, Smith A, Juge-Morineau N, Stevenson FK, Bataille R. V(H) gene analysis of IgM-secreting myeloma indicates an origin from a memory cell undergoing isotype switch events. *Blood* 1999; **94**:1070–6.

38. García-Sanz R, Montoto S, Torrequebrada A, García de Coca A, Petit J, Sureda A, *et al.* Waldenström macroglobulinaemia: presenting features and outcome in a series with 217 cases. *Br J Haematol* 2001; **115**:1–9.

39. Schambeck CM, Bartl R, Hochtlen-Vollmar W, *et al.* Characterization of myeloma cells by means of labeling index, bone marrow histology and serum B$_2$-microglobulin. *Am J Clin Pathol* 1996; **106**:64–8.

●40. Greipp PR, Leong T, Bennett JM, Gaillard JP, Klein B, Stewart JA, *et al.* Plasmablastic morphology – an independent prognostic factor with clinical and laboratory correlates: Eastern Cooperative Oncology Group (ECOG) myeloma trial E9486 report by the ECOG Myeloma Laboratory Group. *Blood* 1998; **91**:2501–7.

41. Portero JA, Martin S, González M, San Miguel JF. Cytochemistry in the differential diagnosis of monoclonal gammopathies. *Br J Haematol* 1985; **60**:768–9.

42. Kyle RA. Monoclonal gammopathy of undetermined significance and solitary plasmacytoma: implications for progression to overt multiple myeloma. *Hematol Oncol Clin North Am* 1997; **11**:71–88.

43. Baldini L, Guffanti A, Cesana BM, Colombi M, Chiorboli O, Damilano I, *et al.* Role of different hematologic variables in defining the risk of malignant transformation in monoclonal gammopathy. *Blood* 1996; **87**:912–18.

44. Kyle RA, Bayrd ED. *The monoclonal gammopathies: multiple myeloma and related plasma-cell disorders.* Springfield, IL: Charles C. Thomas, 1976.

45. Witzig TE, Gertz M, Lust JA, Kyle RA, O'Fallon W, Greipp PR. Peripheral blood monoclonal plasma cells as a predictor of survival in patients with multiple myeloma. *Blood* 1996; **88**:1780–7.

46. Rawstron AC, Owen RG, Davies FE. Circulating plasma cells in multiple myeloma: characterization and correlation with disease stage. *Br J Haematol* 1997; **97**:46–55.

47. Billadeau D, Van Ness B, Kimlinger T, Kyle RA, Therneau TM, Greipp PR, Witzig TE. Clonal circulating cells are common in plasma cell proliferative disorders: a comparison of monoclonal gammopathy of undetermined significance, smoldering multiple myeloma and active myeloma. *Blood* 1996; **88**:289–96.

48. Witzig TE, Kyle RA, O'Fallon WM, Greipp PR. Detection of peripheral blood plasma cells as a predictor of disease course in patients with smoldering multiple myeloma. *Br J Haematol* 1994; **87**:266–72.

49. Kyle RA: Monoclonal gammopathy of undetermined significance and solitary plasmacytoma: Implications for progression to overt multiple myeloma. *Hematol Oncol Clin North Am* 1997; **11**:71–88.

50. Brown RD, Joshua DE, Nelson M, Gibson J, Dunn J, MacLennan CM. Serum thymidine kinase as a prognostic indicator for patient with multiple myeloma: results from the MRC (UK) V trial. *Br J Hematol* 1993; **84**:238–44.

51. Back H, Jagenburg R, Rodjer S, Westin J. Serum deoxythymidine kinase: no help in the diagnosis and prognosis of monoclonal gammopathy. *Br J Hematol* 1993; **84**:746–8.

52. Du Villard L, Guiguet M, Casanovas RO, *et al.* Diagnostic value of serum IL-6 level in monoclonal gammopathies. *Br J Haematol* 1995; **89**:243–9.

53. San Miguel J, Corrales A, Alberca I, Vicente V, Lopez Borrasca A. Acute phase reactant proteins in differential diagnosis of monoclonal gammopathy. *Neoplasma* 1983; **30**:57–62.

54. Pelliniemi TT, Irjala K, Mattila K, Pulkki K, Rajamaki A, Tienhaara A, *et al.* Immunoreactive interleukin-6 and acute phase proteins as prognostic factors in multiple myeloma. Finnish Leukemia Group. *Blood* 1995; **85**:765–71.

55. Merlini G, Perfetti V, Gobbi PG, Quaglini S, Franciotta DM, Marinone G, Ascari E. Acute phase proteins and prognosis in multiple myeloma. *Br J Haematol* 1993; **83**:595–601.

56. Schaar CG, Kaiser U, Snijder S, Ong F, Hermans J, Franck PF, *et al.* Serum interlukin-6 has no discriminatory role in paraproteinaemia nor a prognostic role in multiple myeloma. *Br J Haematol* 1999; **107**:132–8.

57. Ohtani K, Ninomiya H, Hasegawa Y, Kobayashi T, Kojima H, Nagasawa T, *et al.* Clinical significance of elevated soluble interleukin-6 receptor levels in the sera of patients with plasma cell dyscrasias. *Br J Haematol* 1995; **91**:116–20.

58. Pulkki K, Pelliniemi TT, Rajamaki A, Tienhaara A, Laakso M, Lahtinen R. Soluble interleukin-6 receptor as a prognostic factor in multiple myeloma. Finnish Leukaemia Group. *Br J Haematol* 1996; **92**:370–4.

59. Blade J, Filella X, Montoto S, *et al.* Clinical relevance of interleukin 6 (IL-6) and tumor necrosis factor alpha (TNF-α) serum levels in monoclonal gammopathy of undetermined significance (MGUS). *Br J Haematol* 1998; **102**:9–14.

60. Bataille R, Chappard D, Klein B. Mechanisms of bone lesions in multiple myeloma. *Hematol Oncol Clin North Am* 1992; **6**:285–95.

61. Moulopoulos LA, Dimopoulos MA, Smith TL. Weber DM, Delasalle KB, Libshitz HI, *et al.* Prognostic significance of magnetic resonance imaging in patients in asymptomatic MM. *J Clin Oncol* 1995; **131**:251–6.

62. Laroche M, Assoun J, Sixou L, Attal M. Comparison of MRI and computed tomography in the various stages of plasma cell disorders: correlations with biological and histological findings. Myelome-Midi-Pyrenees Group. *Clin Exp Rheumatol* 1996; **14**:171–6.

63. Mariette X, Zagdanski AM, Guermazi A, Bergot C, Arnould A, Frija J, *et al.* Prognostic value of vertebral lesions detected by magnetic resonance imaging in patients with stage I multiple myeloma. *Br J Haematol* 1999; **104**:723–9.

64. Pecherstorfer M, Seibel M.J, Woitge HW, Horn E, Schuster J, Neuda J, *et al.* Bone resorption in multiple myeloma and in monoclonal gammopathy of undetermined significance: quantification by urinary pyridinium cross-links of collagen. *Blood* 1997; **90**:3743–50.

65. Peest D, Deicher H, Feet W, Harms P, Braun HJ, Planker M, *et al.* Pyridinium cross-links in multiple myeloma: correlation with clinical parameters and use for monitoring of intravenous clodronate therapy – a pilot study of the German Myeloma treatment group (GMTG). *Eur J Cancer* 1996; **32**:2053–7.

66. Nawawi H, Samon D, Apperley J, Girgis S. Biochemical bone markers in patients with multiple myeloma. *Clin Chim Acta* 1996; **30**:61–77.

67. Bataille R, Delmas PD, Sany J. Serum bone gla-protein (osteocalcin) in multiple myeloma. *Cancer* 1987; **59**:329–34.

68. Bataille R, Delmas PD, Chappard D, Sany J. Abnormal serum gla-protein in multiple myeloma: crucial role of bone formation and prognostic implications. *Cancer* 1990; **66**:167–72.

69. Harada H, Kawano MM, Huang N, Harada Y, Iwato K, Tanabe O, *et al.* Phenotypic difference of normal plasma cells from mature myeloma cells. *Blood* 1993; **81**:2658–63.

70. Ocqueteau M, Orfao A, Garcia-Sanz R, Almeida J, Gonzalez M, San Miguel JF: Expression of the CD117 antigen (c-kit) on normal and myelomatous plasma cells. *Br J Haematol* 1996; **95**:489–93.

71. San Miguel JF, Almeida J, Mateo G, Blade J, López-Berges MC, Caballero MD, *et al.* Immunophenotypic evaluation of the plasma cell compartment in multiple myeloma: a tool for comparing the efficacy of different treatment strategies and predicting outcome. *Blood* 2002; **99**:1853–6.

●72. Ocqueteau M, Orfao A, Almeida J, Blade J, Gonzalez M, Garcia-Sanz R, *et al.* Immunophenotypic characterization of plasma cells from monoclonal gammopathy of undetermined significance patients. Implications for the differential diagnosis between MGUS and multiple myeloma. *Am J Pathol* 1998; **152**:1655–65.

73. Rawstron AC, Fenton JA, Ashcroft J, English A, Jones RA, Richards SJ, *et al.* The interleukin-6 receptor alpha-chain (CD126) is expressed by neoplastic but not notmal plasma cells. *Blood* 2000; **96**:3880–6.

74. Mills KH, Cawley JC. Abnormal monoclonal antibody-defined helper/suppressor T-cell subpopulations in multiple myeloma: relationship to treatment and clinical stage. *Br J Haematol* 1983; **53**:271–5.

75. San Miguel JF, Gonzalez M, Gascon A, Moro MJ, Hernandez JM, Ortega F, *et al.* Lymphoid subsets and prognostic factors in multiple myeloma. Cooperative Group for the Study of Monoclonal Gammopathies. *Br J Haematol* 1992; **80**:305–9.

76. Kay NE, Leong T, Kyle RA, Greipp P, Billadeau D, Van Ness B, Bone N, *et al.* Circulating blood B cells in multiple myeloma: analysis and relationship to circulating clonal cells and clinical parameters in a cohort of patients entered on the Eastern Cooperative Oncology Group Phase III E9486 Clinical Trial. *Blood* 1997; **90**:340–5.

77. Tienhaara A, Pelliniemi TT. Peripheral blood lymphocyte subsets in multiple myeloma and monoclonal gammopathy of undetermined significance. *Clin Lab Haematol* 1994; **16**:213–23.

78. San Miguel JF, Garcia-Sanz R, Gonzalez M, Orfao A. Immunophenotype and DNA cell content in multiple myeloma. *Baillieres Clin Haematol* 1995; **8**:735–59.

79. Drach J, Schuster J, Nowotny H, *et al.* Multiple myeloma: high incidence chromosomal aneuploidy as detected by interphase fluorescence in situ hybridization. *Cancer Res* 1995; **55**:3854–9.

80. Lee W, Han K, Drut RM, Harris CP, Meissner LF. Use of fluorescence in situ hybridizatiion for retrospective detection of anueploidy in multiple myeloma. *Genes Chromosomes Cancer* 1993; **7**:137–43.

81. Tabernero D, San Miguel JF, García-Sanz R, *et al.* Incidence of chromosome numerical changes in multiple myeloma. Fluorescence in situ hybridization analysis using 15 chromosome-specific probes. *Am J Pathol* 1996; **149**:153–61.

82. Drach J, Angerler J, Schuster J, Rothermundt C, Thalhammer R, Haas OA, *et al.* Interphase fluorescence in situ hybridization identifies chromosomal abnormalities in plasma cells from patients with monoclonal gammopathy of undetermined significance. *Blood* 1995; **86**:3915–21.

83. Ahmann GJ, Jalal SM, Juneau AL, Christensen ER, Hanson CA, Dewald GW, *et al.* A novel three-color, clone-specific fluorescence in situ hybridization procedure for monoclonal gammopathies. *Cancer Genet Cytogenet* 1998; **101**:7–11.

84. Konigsberg R, Ackermann J, Kaufmann H, Zojer N, Urbauer E, Kromer E, *et al.* Deletions of chromosome 13q in monoclonal gammopathy of undetermined significance. *Leukemia* 2000; **14**:1975–9.

85. Lloveras E, Sole F, Florensa L, Besses C, Espinet B, Gil M, *et al.* Contribution of cytogenetics and in situ hybridization to the study of monoclonal gammopathies of undetermined significance. *Cancer Genet Cytogenet* 2002; **132**:25–9.

86. Zandecki M, Lai JL, Genevieve F, Bernardi F, Volle-Remy H, Blanchet O, *et al.* Several cytogenetic subclones may be identified within plasma cells from patients with monoclonal gammopathy of undetermined significance, both at diagnosis and during the indolent course of this condition. *Blood* 1997; **90**:3682–90.

87. Avet-Loiseau H, Brigaudeau C, Morineau N, Talmant P, Lai JL, Daviet A, *et al.* High incidence of criptic translocations involving the immunoglobulin heavy chain gene in multiple myeloma as shown by fluorescence in situ hybridization. *Genes Chromosomes Cancer* 1999; **24**:9–15.

88. Garcia-Sanz R, Orfao A, Gonzalez M, Moro MJ, Hernandez JM, Ortega F, *et al.* Prognostic implications of DNA aneuploidy in 156 untreated multiple myeloma patients. *Br J Haematol* 1995; **90**:106–12.

89. San Miguel JF, Garcia-Sanz R, Gonzalez M, Orfao A. DNA cell content studies in multiple myeloma. *Leuk Lymphoma* 1996; **23**:33–41.

90. Almeida J, Orfao A, Ocqueteau M, Mateo G, Corral M, Caballero MD, et al. High-sensitive immunophenotyping and DNA ploidy studies for the investigation of minimal residual disease in multiple myeloma. *Br J Haematol* 1999; **107**:121–31.

●91. Bakkus MH, Heirman C, Van Riet I, Van Camp B, Thielemans K. Evidence that multiple myeloma Ig heavy chain VDJ genes contain somatic mutations but show no intraclonal variation. *Blood* 1992; **80**:2326–35.

92. Vescio RA, Cao J, Hong CH, Lee JC, Wu CH, Der Danielian M, et al. Myeloma Ig heavy chain V region sequences reveal prior antigenic selection and marked somatic mutation but not intraclonal diversity. *J Immunol* 1995; **155**:2487–93.

93. Zaccaria A, Tassinari A, Saglio G, Guerrasio A, Tura S. Immunoglobulin gene rearrangements in human multiple myeloma. *Br J Haematol* 1989; **73**:425–32.

94. Sahota SS, Leo R, Hamblin TJ, Stevenson FK. Ig VH gene mutational patterns indicate different tumor cell status in human myeloma and monoclonal gammopathy of undetermined significance. *Blood* 1996; **87**:746–55.

95. Van Riet Y, Heirman C, Lacor P, De Waele M, Thielemans K, Van Camp B. Detection of monoclonal B lymphocytes in bone marrow and peripheral blood of multiple myeloma patients by immunoglobulin gene rearrangement studies. *Br J Haematol* 1989; **73**:289–95.

96. Isaksson E, Björkholm M, Holm G, Johansson B, Nilsson B, Mellstedt H, et al. Blood clonal B-cell excess in patients with monoclonal gammopathy of undetermined significance (MGUS): association with malignant transformation. *Br J Haematol* 1996; **92**:71–6.

97. Palumbo AP, Boccadoro M, Battaglio S, Corradini P, Tsichlis PN, Huebner K, et al. Human homologue of Moloney leukemia virus integration-4 locus (MLVI-4), located 20 kilobases 3 of the myc gene, is rearranged in multiple myelomas. *Cancer Res* 1990; **50**:6478–85.

98. Muller JR, Janz S, Potter M. Differences between Burkitt's lymphomas and mouse plasmacytomas in the immunoglobulin heavy-chain c-myc recombinations that occur in their chromosomal translocations. *Cancer Res* 1995; **55**:5012–20.

99. Sumegi J, Hedberg T, Bjorkholm M, Godal T, et al. Amplification of the c-myc oncogene in human plasma-cell leukemia. *Int J Cancer* 1985; **36**:367–74.

100. Paulin FE, West MJ, Sullivan NF, Whitney RL, Lyne L, Willis AE, et al. Aberrant translational control of the c-myc gene in multiple myeloma. *Oncogene* 1996; **13**:505–13.

◆101. Hallek M, Bergsagel PL, Anderson KC. Multiple myeloma: increasing evidence for a multistep transformation process. *Blood* 1998; **91**:3–21.

102. Bergsagel PL, Chesi M, Nardini E, Brents LA, Kirby SL, Kuehl WM, et al. Promiscuous translocations into immunoglobulin heavy chain switch regions in multiple myeloma. *Proc Natl Acad Sci USA* 1996; **93**:1393–401.

103. Chesi M, Bergsagel PL, Brents LA, Smith CM, Gerhard DS, Kuehl WM, et al. Dysregulation of cyclin D1 by translocation into an IgH gamma switch region in two multiple myeloma cell lines. *Blood* 1996; **88**:674–80.

104. Athanasiou E, Kaloutsi V, Kotoula V, Hytiroglou P, Kostopoulos I, Zervas C, et al. Cyclin D1 overexpression in multiple myeloma. A morphologic, immunohistochemical, and in situ hybridization study of 71 paraffin-embedded bone marrow biopsy specimens. *Am J Clin Pathol* 2001; **116**:535–42.

105. Hoyer JD, Hanson CA, Fonseca R, Greipp PR, Dewald GW, Kurtin PJ. The (11;14)(q13;q32) translocation in multiple myeloma. A morphologic and immunohistochemical study. *Am J Clin Pathol* 2000; **113**:831–7.

106. Hoechtlen-Vollmar W, Menzel G, Bartl R, Lamerz R, Wick M, Seidel D. Amplification of cyclin D1 gene in multiple myeloma: clinical and prognostic relevance. *Br J Haematol* 2000; **109**:30–8.

107. Chesi M, Nardini E, Brents LA, Schrock E, Ried T, Kuehl WM, et al. Frequent translocation t(4;14)(p16.3;q32.3) in multiple myeloma is associated with increased expression and activating mutations of fibroblast growth factor receptor 3. *Nat Genet* 1997; **16**:260–4.

108. Richelda R, Ronchetti D, Baldini L, Cro L, Viggiano L, Marzella R, et al. A novel chromosomal translocation t(4; 14)(p16.3; q32) in multiple myeloma involves the fibroblast growth-factor receptor 3 gene. *Blood* 1997; **90**:4062–70.

109. Avet-Loiseau H, Li JY, Facon T, Brigaudeau C, Morineau N, Maloisel F, et al. High incidence of translocations t(11;14)(q13;q32) and t(4;14)(p16;q32) in patients with plasma cell malignancies. *Cancer Res* 1998; **58**:5640–5.

110. Chesi M, Nardini E, Lim RS, Smith KD, Kuehl WM, Bergsagel PL. The t(4;14) translocation in myeloma dysregulates both FGFR3 and a novel gene, MMSET, resulting in IgH/MMSET hybrid transcripts. *Blood* 1998; **92**:3025–34.

111. Liu P, Leong T, Quam L, Billadeau D, Kay NE, Greipp P, et al. Activating mutations of N- and K-ras in multiple myeloma show different clinical associations: analysis of the Eastern Cooperative Oncology Group Phase III Trial. *Blood* 1996; **88**:2699–706.

112. Corradini P, Ladetto M, Voena C, et al. Mutational activation of N- and K-ras oncogenes in plasma cell dyscrasias. *Blood* 1993; **81**:2708–15.

113. Corradini P, Inghirami G, Astolfi M, Ladetto M, Voena C, Ballerini P, et al. Inactivation of tumor suppressor genes, p53 and Rb1, in plasma cell dyscrasias. *Leukemia* 1994; **8**:758–67.

●114. Tricot G, Barlogie B, Jagannath S, Bracy D, Mattox S, Vesole DH, et al. Poor prognosis in multiple myeloma is associated only with partial or complete deletions of chromosome 13 or abnormalities involving 11q and not with other karyotype abnormalities. *Blood* 1995; **86**:4250–6.

115. Hernández JM, Gutiérrez NC, Almeida J, et al.: IL-4 improves the detection of cytogenetic abnormalities in multiple myeloma and increases the proportion of clonally abnormal metaphases. *Br J Haematol* 1998; **103**:163–7.

116. Cigudosa JC, Rao PM, Calasanz MJ, Odero MD. Characterization of non random chromosomal gains and losses in multiple myeloma by comparative genomic hybridization. *Blood* 1998; **91**:3007–14.

●117. Perez-Simon JA, Garcia-Sanz R, Tabernero MD, Almeida J, Gonzalez M, Fernandez-Calvo J, et al. Prognostic value of numerical chromosome aberrations in multiple myeloma: a FISH analysis of 15 different chromosomes. *Blood* 1998; **91**:3366–71.

118. Dao DD, Sawyer JR, Epstein J, Hoover RG, Barlogie B, Tricot G, et al. Deletion of the retinoblastoma gene in multiple myeloma. *Leukemia* 1994; **8**:1280–4.

119. Juge-Morineau N, Mellerin MP, Francois S, et al. High incidence of deletions but infrequent inactivation of the retinoblastoma gene in human myeloma cells. *Br J Haematol* 1995; **91**:664–70.

120. Teoh G, Urashima M, Ogata A, Chauhan D, DeCaprio JA, Treon SP, et al. MDM2 protein overexpression promotes proliferation and survival of multiple myeloma cells. *Blood* 1997; **90**:1982–92.

121. Urashima M, Teoh G, Ogata A, Chauhan D, Treon SP, Sugimoto Y, et al. Characterization of p16(INK4A) expression in multiple myeloma and plasma cell leukemia. *Clin Cancer Res* 1997; **3**:2173–9.

122. Gonzalez M, Mateos MV, Garcia-Sanz R, Balanzategui A, Lopez-Perez R, Chillon MC, et al. De novo methylation of tumor suppressor gene p16/INK4a is a frequent finding in multiple myeloma patients at diagnosis. *Leukemia* 2000; **14**:183–7.

123. Kim DK, Cho ES, Lee SJ, Um HD. Constitutive hyperexpression of p21(WAF1) in human U266 myeloma cells blocks the lethal signaling induced by oxidative stress but not by Fas. *Biochem Biophys Res Commun* 2001; **289**:34–8.

124. Guillerm G, Gyan E, Wolowiec D, Facon T, Avet-Loiseau H, Kuliczkowski K, et al. p16(INK4a) and p15(INK4b) gene methylations in plasma cells from monoclonal gammopathy of undetermined significance. *Blood* 2001; **98**:244–6.

125. Mateos MV, Garcia-Sanz R, López-Pérez R, Balanzategui A, González MI, Fernández-Calvo J, et al. p16/INK4a gene inactivation by hypermethylation is associated with aggressive variants of monoclonal gammopathies. *Hematol J* 2001; **2**:146–9.

126. Kyle RA. Why better prognostic factors for multiple myeloma are needed? *Blood* 1994; **83**:1713–16.

127. Kyle RA. Prognostic factors in multiple myeloma. *Stem Cells* 1995; **13**:56–63.

128. San Miguel JF. Overview of prognostic factors in multiple myeloma. *Cancer Res Ther Control* 1998; **6**:97–9.

129. Turesson I. Prognostic evaluation in multiple myeloma: an analysis of the impact of new prognostic factors. *Br J Haematol* 1999; **106**:1005–12.

130. Bladé J. Presenting features and prognosis in 72 patients with multiple myeloma who were younger than 40 years. *Br J Haematol* 1996; **93**:345–51.

131. Modiano MR, Villar-Werstler P, Crowley J, Salmon SE. Evaluation of race as a prognostic factor in multiple myeloma. An ancillary of Southwest Oncology Group Study 8229. *J Clin Oncol* 1996; **14**:974–7.

132. Kay NE, Leong TL, Bone N, Vesole DH, Greipp PR, Van Ness B, et al. Blood levels of immune cells predict survival in myeloma patients: results of an Eastern Cooperative Oncology Group phase 3 trial for newly diagnosed multiple myeloma patients. *Blood* 2001; **98**:23–8.

133. Österborg A, Nilsson B, Björkholm M. Natural killer cell activity in monoclonal gammopathies: relation to disease activity. *Eur J Immunol* 1990; **45**:153–7.

134. García-Sanz R, González M, Orfao A, Moro MJ, Hernandez JM, Borrego D, et al. Analysis of natural killer-associated antigens in peripheral blood and bone marrow of multiple myeloma patients and prognostic implications. *Br J Haematol* 1996; **93**:81–8.

135. Brown RD, Yuen E, Nelson M, Gibson J, Joshua D. The prognostic significance of T cell receptor beta gene rearrangements and idiotype-reactive T cells in multiple myeloma. *Leukemia* 1997; **11**:1312–17.

136. Sze DM, Giesajtis G, Brown RD, Raitakari M, Gibson J, Ho J, et al. Clonal cytotoxic T cells are expanded in myeloma and reside in the CD8(+)CD57(+)CD28(−) compartment. *Blood* 2001; **98**:2817–27.

137. Bartl R, Frisch B, Burkhardt R, Fateh-Moghadam A, Mahl G, Gierster P, et al. Bone marrow histology in myeloma: its importance in diagnosis, prognosis, classification and staging. *Br J Haematol* 1982; **51**:361–75.

138. Greipp PR. Advances in the diagnosis and management of myeloma. *Semin Hematol* 1992; **92** (Suppl 2):24–45.

139. Saeed SM, Stock-Novack D, Pohlod R, Crowley J, Salmon SE. Prognostic correlation of plasma cell acid phosphatase and beta-glucuronidase in multiple myeloma: a Southwest Oncology Group study. *Blood* 1991; **78**:3281–7.

140. San Miguel JF, González M, Gascón A, et al. Immunophenotype heterogeneity of multiple myeloma: influence on the biology and clinical course of the disease. *Br J Haematol* 1991; **77**:185–90.

141. Omede P, Boccadoro M, Fusaro A, Gallone G, Pileri A. Multiple myeloma: 'early' plasma cell phenotype identifies patients with aggressive biological and clinical characteristics. *Br J Haematol* 1993; **85**:504–13.

142. Pellat-Deceunynck C, Bataille R, Robillard N, Harousseau JL, Rapp MJ, Juge-Morineau N, et al. Expression of CD28 and CD40 in human myeloma cells: a comparative study with normal plasma cells. *Blood* 1994; **84**:2597–603.

143. Pellat-Deceunynck C, Barille S, Puthier D, Rapp MJ, Harousseau JL, Bataille R, et al. Adhesion molecules on human myeloma cells: significant changes in expression related to malignancy, tumour spreading and immortalization. *Cancer Res* 1995; **55**:3647–53.

●144. San Miguel JF, Garcia-Sanz R, Gonzalez M, Moro MJ, Hernandez JM, Ortega F, et al. A new staging system for multiple myeloma based on the number of S-phase plasma cells. *Blood* 1995; **85**:448–55.

145. Robillard N, Jego G, Pellat-Deceunynck C, Pineau D, Puthier D, Mellerin MP, et al. CD28, a marker associated with tumoral expansion in multiple myeloma. *Clin Cancer Res* 1998; **4**:1521–6.

146. Seidel C, Sundan A, Hjorth M, Turesson I, Dahl IM, Abildgaard N, et al. Serum syndecan-1: a new independent prognostic marker in multiple myeloma. *Blood* 2000; **95**:388–92.

147. Tricot G, Sawyer JR, Jagannath S, Desikan KR, Siegel D, Naucke S, et al. Unique role of cytogenetics in the prognosis of patients with myeloma receiving high-dose therapy and autotransplants. *J Clin Oncol* 1997; **15**:2659–66.

148. Zojer N, Konigsberg R, Ackermann J, Fritz E, Dallinger S, Kromer E, et al. Deletion of 13q14 remains an independent adverse prognostic variable in multiple myeloma despite its frequent detection by interphase fluorescence in situ hybridization. *Blood* 2000; **95**:1925–30.

149. Fonseca R, Oken MM, Harrington D, Bailey RJ, Van Wier SA, Henderson KJ, et al. Deletions of chromosome 13 in multiple myeloma identified by interphase FISH usually denote large deletions of the q arm or monosomy. Leukemia 2001; 15:981–6.

150. Fonseca R, Harrington D, Blood E, Rue M , Oken MM, Dewald GW, et al. A molecular clasiffication of multiple myeloma based on cytogenetic abnormalities detected by interphase FISH, is powerful in identifying discrete groups of patients with dissimilar prognosis. Blood 2001; 98:733a.

151. Worel N, Greinix H, Ackermann J, Kaufmann H, Urbauer E, Hocker P, et al. Deletion of chromosome 13q14 detected by fluorescence in situ hybridization has prognostic impact on survival after high-dose therapy in patients with multiple myeloma. Ann Hematol 2001; 80:345–8.

152. Segeren C, Beverloo B, Poddighe J, Slater R, van der Holt B, Steijaert M, et al. Abnormal chromosomes 1p/q and 13/13q are adverse prognostic factors for the outcome of upfront high-dose therapy in patients with multiple myeloma. Blood 2002; 98:159a.

153. Skopelitou A, Hadjiyannakis M, Tsenga A, Theocharis S, Alexopoulou V, Kittas C, et al. Expression of C-myc p62 oncoprotein in multiple myeloma: an immunohistochemical study of 180 cases. Anticancer Res 1993; 13:1091–5.

154. Drach J. Presence of a p53 gene deletion in patients with multiple myeloma predicts for short survival after conventional-dose chemotherapy. Blood 1998; 92: 802–9.

155. Grogan TM, Spier CM, Salmon SE, Matzner M, Rybski J, Weinstein RS, et al. P-glycoprotein expression in human plasma cell myeloma: correlation with prior chemotherapy. Blood 1993; 81:490–5.

156. Sonneveld P, Marie JP, Huisman C, Vekhoff A, Schoester M, Faussat AM, et al. Reversal of multidrug resistance by SDZ PSC 833, combined with VAD (vincristine, doxorubicin, dexamethasone) in refractory multiple myeloma. A phase I study. Leukemia 1996; 10:1741–50.

157. Gieseler F, Nussler V. Cellular resistance mechanisms with impact on the therapy of multiple myeloma. Leukemia 1997; 11(Suppl 5):S1–S4.

158. Raaijmakers HG, Izquierdo MA, Lokhorst HM, de Leeuw C, Belien JA, Bloem AC, et al. Lung-resistance-related protein expression is a negative predictive factor for response to conventional low but not to intensified dose alkylating chemotherapy in multiple myeloma. Blood 1998; 91:1029–36.

•159. Greipp PR, Lust JA, O'Fallon WM, Katzmann JA, Witzig TE, Kyle RA. Plasma cell labeling index and beta 2-microglobulin predict survival independent of thymidine kinase and C-reactive protein in multiple myeloma. Blood 1993; 81:3382–7.

160. Orfao A, Garcia-Sanz R, Lopez-Berges MC, Belen VM, Gonzalez M, Caballero MD, et al. A new method for the analysis of plasma cell DNA content in multiple myeloma samples using a CD38/propidium iodide double staining technique. Cytometry 1994; 17:332–9.

161. Joshua D, Petersen A, Brown R, Pope B, Snowdon L, Gibson J. The labelling index of primitive plasma cells determines the clinical behaviour of patients with myelomatosis. Br J Haematol 1996; 94:76–81.

162. Hansen OP, Jessen B, Videbaek A. Prognosis of myelomatosis on treatment with prednisone and cytostatics. Scand J Haematol 1974; 10:282–90.

163. Boccadoro M, Pileri A. Cell kinetics of multiple myeloma. Hematol Pathol 1987; 1:137–42.

164. Durie BGM, Salmon SE. A clinical staging system for multiple myeloma. Correlation of measured myeloma cell mass with presenting clinical features, response to treatment and survival. Cancer 1975; 36:842–54.

165. San Miguel JF, Sanchez I, Gonzalez M. Prognostic factors and classification in multiple myeloma. Br J Cancer 1989; 59:113–18.

166. Cuzick J, De Stavola BL, Cooper EH. Long-term prognostic value of serum B-2-microglobulin in myelomatosis. Br J Haematol 1990; 75:506–10.

167. Garewal H, Durie BGM, Kyle RA, Finley P, Bower B, Serokman R. Serum B2μmicroglobulin in the initial staging and subsequent monitoring of monoclonal plasma cell disorders. J Clin Oncol 1984; 2:51–7.

168. Bataille R, Greiner J, Sany J. Beta-2-microglobulin in myeloma: optimal use for staging, prognosis and treatment: a prospective study of 160 patients. Blood 1984; 63: 468–76.

169. Boccadoro M, Omede P, Frieri R. Multiple Myeloma: beta-2-microglobulin is not a useful follow-up parameter. Acta Haematol 1989; 82:122–5.

170. Bataille R, Jourdan M, Zhang XG, Klein B. Serum levels of interleukin 6, a potent myeloma cell growth factor, as a reflect of disease severity in plasma cell dyscrasias. J Clin Invest 1989; 84:2008–11.

171. Papadaki H, Kyriakou D, Foudoulakis A, Markidou F, Alexandrakis M, Eliopoulos GD. Serum levels of soluble IL-6 receptor in multiple myeloma as indicator of disease activity. Acta Haematol 1997; 97:191–5.

172. Pulkki K, Pelliniemi R.T, Rajamaki A, et al.: Soluble interleukin-6 receptor as a prognostic factor in multiple myeloma. Br J Haematol 1996; 92:370–4.

173. Bataille R, Boccadoro M, Klein B, Durie B, Pileri A. C-reactive protein and beta-2 microglobulin produce a simple and powerful myeloma staging system. Blood 1992; 80:733–7.

174. Facon T, Menard JF, Michaux JL, Euller-Ziegler L, Bernard JF, Grosbois B, et al. Prognostic factors in low tumour mass asymptomatic multiple myeloma: a report on 91 patients. The Groupe d'Etudes et de Recherche sur le Myelome (GERM). Am J Hematol 1995; 48:71–5.

175. Weber DM, Dimopoulos MA, Moulopoulos LA, Delasalle KB, Smith T, Alexanian R. Prognostic features of asymptomatic multiple myeloma. Br J Haematol 1997; 97:810–14.

176. Barlogie B, Jagannath S, Vesole D, Tricot G. Autologous and allogeneic transplants for multiple myeloma. Semin Hematol 1995; 32:31–44.

177. Bjorkstrand B, Ljungman P, Bird JM, Samson D, Brandt L, Alegre A, et al. Autologous stem cell transplantation in multiple myeloma: results of the European Group for Bone Marrow Transplantation. Stem Cells 1995; 13 (Suppl 2):140–6.

178. Shaughnessy J Jr, Barlogie B, McCoy JPJ, Sawyer J, Fassas A, Zangari M, et al. Early relapse after Total Therapy II for multiple myeloma is s gnificantly associated with

cytogenetic abnormalities of chromosome 13 (CA13) but not interphase FISH-del 13 or plasma cell labeling index (PCLI). *Blood* 2001; **98**:734a.

179. Gertz MA, Witzig TE, Pineda AA, Greipp PR, Kyle RA, Litzow MR. Monoclonal plasma cells in the blood stem cell harvest from patients with multiple myeloma are associated with shortened relapse-free survival after transplantation. *Bone Marrow Transplant* 1997; **19**:337–42.

180. Rajkumar SV, Fonseca R, Dispenzieri A, Lacy MQ, Witzig TE, Lust JA, *et al.* Effect of complete response on outcome following autologous stem cell transplantation for myeloma. *Bone Marrow Transplant* 2000; **26**:979–83.

181. Barlogie B, Jagannath S, Desikan KR, Mattox S, Vesole D, Siegel D, *et al.* Total therapy with tandem transplants for newly diagnosed multiple myeloma. *Blood* 1999; **93**:55–65.

182. Lahuerta JJ, de la Serna J, Blade J, Grande C, Alegre A, Vazquez L, *et al.* Remission status defined by immunofixation vs electrophoresis after autologous transplantation has a major impact on the outcome of multiple myeloma patients. *Br J Haematol* 2000; **109**:438–46.

183. Alexanian R, Weber D, Giralt S, Dimopoulos M, Delasalle K, Smith T, *et al.* Impact of complete remission with intensive

therapy in patients with responsive multiple myeloma. *Bone Marrow Transplant* 2001; **27**:1037–43.

184. Tricot G, Spencer A, Desikan KR, Badros A, Zangari M, Toor A, *et al.* Predicting long term (⩾5 YR) event-free survival (EFS) in multiple myeloma following tandem autotransplants (TT). *Blood* 2002; **98**:2787–93.

185. Bensinger WI, Buckner CD, Anasetti C, Clift R, Storb R, Barnett T, *et al.* Allogeneic marrow transplantation for multiple myeloma: an analysis of risk factors on outcome. *Blood* 1996; **88**:2787–93.

● 186. Gahrton G, Tura S, Ljungman P, Blade J, Brandt L, Cavo M, *et al.* Prognostic factors in allogeneic bone marrow transplantation for multiple myeloma. *J Clin Oncol* 1995; **13**:1312–22.

* 187. Greipp Ph, San Miguel JF, Fonsea R, Avet-Loiseau H, Jacobson JL, Rasmussen E, *et al.* On behalf of the International Myeloma Working Group plus Cancer Research and Biostatistics (CRAB). Development of an international prognostic index (IPI) for myeloma: report of the International Myeloma Working Group at the IXth International Workshop on Multiple Myeloma, Salamanca, Spain. May 23–27, 2003. *Hematol J* 2003; **4**(Suppl 1):S42.

PART 4

Treatment of myeloma

13

Principles of management

DIANA M. SAMSON

INTRODUCTION: THE AIMS OF TREATMENT

Multiple myeloma (MM) continues to present a therapeutic challenge. In spite of new approaches to treatment, MM at present remains incurable, with a median survival of between 3 and 4 years. Treatment produces a response in approximately two-thirds of patients, with a fall in paraprotein and improvement or resolution of clinical symptoms. However, complete remission (CR) is very rare, except after high-dose therapy, and in most patients the paraprotein falls but reaches a plateau after a few months of treatment. At this stage, the patient is said to be in 'plateau phase'. Sooner or later the paraprotein starts to rise again, indicating relapse, or there may be a recurrence of symptoms. Further treatment at this stage, perhaps with a different drug or drug combination, may again produce a response, but the duration of response is usually shorter than that of the initial remission. Eventually, the disease becomes refractory to treatment and the patient succumbs to infection, renal failure, or other disease complication.

High-dose therapy with autologous stem cell support prolongs remission and survival, but it is not curative and, at present, the only potentially curative treatment approach is allogeneic transplantation, which is an option for only a minority of patients. The most important aims of treatment are, therefore, to relieve symptoms and to prolong life without the treatment causing unacceptable side effects. The treatment-related side effects and risks that are considered acceptable will vary in different patient groups. In a young patient, the risk of allogeneic bone marrow transplantation (BMT) may be justified by the chance of long-term relapse-free survival, while in an elderly patient, the possible survival benefit of combination chemotherapy as compared with simple oral treatment may be outweighed by the increased toxicity.

WHEN TO START TREATMENT

Because myeloma is not curable with current therapy, treatment is not necessarily indicated immediately after diagnosis. Increasing numbers of patients are being found by chance investigations to have multiple myeloma, without any relevant symptoms and with no evidence of organ impairment. It is important to be sure that a patient does have multiple myeloma rather than monoclonal gammopathy of undetermined significance (MGUS) or solitary myeloma (see Chapter 12). Even where the diagnostic criteria for multiple myeloma are fulfilled, in some asymptomatic patients the disease will remain nonprogressive over a period of time, sometimes many years, without treatment.[1,2] The terms 'equivocal myeloma,' 'smoldering myeloma' and 'indolent myeloma' have variously been used to describe these patients, most of whom would be classified as stage IA on the Durie–Salmon staging system (see Chapter 12).

An observational study looked at the factors affecting the risk of disease progression in 95 patients with asymptomatic multiple myeloma seen at the MD Anderson Hospital over many years, who were initially untreated.[3] This study showed that patients who are asymptomatic but who have radiological evidence of bone disease (at least one lytic lesion) are at high risk of progression. At the

Table 13.1 *Risk of progression in asymptomatic multiple myeloma*

Study	Number of patients	Criteria	Significant adverse prognostic factors	Median time to progression
Dimopoulos *et al.* (1993)[3]	95	DS stage not stated; 17 had one or more lytic lesions	Lytic bone lesion Paraprotein level > 30 g/L BJP > 50 mg/24 hours	No factors: >61 months No lytic lesion and 1 other factor: 25 months Lytic lesion and/or both other factors: 10 months
Facon *et al.* (1995)[4]	91	DS stage I	Hb < 12 BM plasmacytosis > 25% Paraprotein level: (IgG > 30 g/L or IgA > 25 g/L)	No factors: >50 months 2/3 factors: 6 months
Weber *et al.* (1997)[5*]	101	DS stage not stated; patients with any lytic lesions excluded MRI performed in 43 patients	IgA isotype Paraprotein level > 30 g/L BJP > 50 mg/24 hours	0 factors: 95 months 1 factor: 39 months 2/3 factors: 6 months 1 factor and normal MRI: 57 months 1 factor and abnormal MRI: 21 months
Mariette *et al.* (1999)[6]	55	Asymptomatic DS stage I and negative skeletal survey MRI performed in all	BM plasmacytosis > 20% Abnormal MRI (β_2-microglobulin only significant on univariate analysis)	At 25 months median follow-up: Normal MRI: 2/38 progressed Abnormal MRI: 10/17 progressed

* 69 patients also in series of Dimopoulos *et al.* (1993).
BJP, Bence Jones protein; BM, bone marrow; DS, Durie–Salmon; Hb, hemoglobin; IgA, immunoglobulin A; IgG, immunoglobulin G; MRI, magnetic resonance imaging.

time of reporting, progression had occurred in 74 patients, after a median of 26 months, while 19 patients were still progression-free at a median follow-up time of 23 months. Factors that significantly predicted for earlier progression were the presence of a lytic bone lesion at presentation ($P < 0.01$; all patients progressed with a median of 8 months), serum paraprotein >30 g/L ($P < 0.01$), and light chain excretion >50 mg/24 hours ($P = 0.02$). These characteristics were used to define three risk groups: low risk – no risk factors; intermediate risk – no lytic lesion but one other factor; and high risk – lytic lesion and/or both other factors (Table 13.1). The presence and extent of abnormality revealed by magnetic resonance imaging (MRI) of the spine was also found to correlate with earlier progression.

There are a number of other studies looking at the time to progression of asymptomatic patients but these excluded patients with any evidence of bone disease (Table 13.1).[4–6] In general, these studies indicate that higher tumor burden is associated with shorter time to progression, with higher paraprotein levels and bone marrow (BM) plasmacytosis being associated with earlier progression, although β_2-microglobulin was only evaluable in one series. Two of these studies found that patients with no evidence of bone disease on standard X-rays but with abnormal bone marrow appearances on MRI examination of the spine are at higher risk of disease progression.[5,6] However, the prognostic effect of an abnormal MRI is

much less marked than that of lytic bone disease. In the study reported by Mariette *et al.*,[6] median time to progression had not been reached by 25 months even in patients with an abnormal MRI, while in the later MD Anderson study,[5] MRI was only discriminatory in patients with other adverse features – high levels of paraprotein or Bence Jones protein (BJP) excretion or IgA isotype. Taking these studies together, the following patients are at high risk of progression:

- patients with any evidence of bone disease on standard X-rays;
- patients with two of the following:
  - serum paraprotein > 25–30 g/L
  - BJP > 50 mg/24 hours or IgA isotype
  - BM plasmacytosis > 20–25%;
- patients with one of the above and abnormal marrow appearance on MRI.

In two of these studies,[3,4] it was observed that despite differences in time to progression, response rate and survival after starting chemotherapy were similar for all groups of patients. This suggests that early intervention might not be beneficial, except perhaps in those with adverse prognostic factors.

There have been two randomized studies comparing initial versus deferred treatment in asymptomatic stage I patients (Table 13.2). In a study from Scandinavia,[7] 50

Table 13.2 *Randomized trials of initial vs. deferred treatment in asymptomatic multiple myeloma*

Study	Number of patients	Criteria	Treatment	Median survival
Hjorth *et al.* (1993)[7]	50	Asymptomatic stage I with no bone lesions	Randomized to MP at diagnosis or progression	Initial treatment: 52 months Deferred treatment: 52 months
Riccardi *et al.* (2000)[8]	145	Asymptomatic stage I; 35 had a single lytic lesionand received local radiotherapy	Randomized to MP at diagnosis or progression	Initial treatment: 64 months Deferred treatment: 71 months (ns)

MP, melphalan–prednisone.

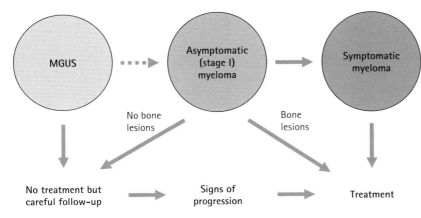

Figure 13.1 *Indications for starting treatment. MGUS, monoclonal gammopathy of undetermined significance.*

patients were randomized to receive MP either at diagnosis or at the time of disease progression. This study excluded stage I patients with a lytic lesion, as such patients were all treated at diagnosis. The median time from diagnosis to the start of treatment in the deferred treatment group was 12 months (range 2 months to 3 years), with one patient still untreated at over 6 years. It is of note that skeletal X-rays were not performed as part of routine follow-up, but only if there were relevant symptoms or other signs of progression, and nine patients progressed with symptomatic bone disease. Median survival was 52 months in both treatment groups. A subsequent study by an Italian Co-operative Group[8] also compared initial versus deferred treatment with MP in stage I patients, but included patients with a single lytic lesion and treated this with local radiotherapy. They too found no significant survival benefit for initial as compared with deferred treatment. (64 vs. 71 months; odds ratio 1.17 for death with deferred treatment).

The consensus view is, therefore, that asymptomatic patients with no evidence of bone disease should not be offered immediate chemotherapy, since treatment is not required to alleviate symptoms and has significant short-term and long-term side effects, including the development of secondary leukemia.[9] If in doubt as to whether treatment is indicated, it is better to wait 2–3 months and reassess rather than embark on possibly unnecessary chemotherapy without a clear indication. Indications to commence treatment would include development of

progressive disease (see later) or evidence of organ impairment attributable to MM.

However, where treatment is deferred, regular follow-up and monitoring of disease parameters is essential. While monitoring the level of serum paraprotein and/or urinary light chain excretion is essential, as well as regular checks of the blood count and routine biochemistry, it is also important to examine the patient at regular intervals and to advise them about reporting any new symptoms. It may also be appropriate to consider repeating the bone marrow and skeletal X-rays.

The following recommendations for the management of asymptomatic patients with MM were included in the UK Myeloma Forum Guidelines on Diagnosis and Management of Myeloma (see also Fig. 13.1).[10]

- Treatment should be delayed until there are signs of progression in patients with equivocal/indolent/ smoldering myeloma and no bone lesions. Such patients must, however, be carefully monitored by 3-monthly physical examination, and measurement of both serum and urinary paraprotein.
- Repeat bone marrow examinations and skeletal X-rays will be required less often or when new symptoms or signs develop.
- Patients with radiological evidence of bone disease should commence treatment immediately.
- MRI examination may be helpful in selected patients.

New approaches in asymptomatic patients

The consensus view that treatment should be deferred in asymptomatic patients is based on the benefits and risks of standard-dose chemotherapy. With the advent of new treatment approaches, the situation may change. Thus, it might be appropriate to consider a potentially curative option that had an acceptable risk, or a treatment that might defer progression and had few side effects. In younger patients with stage I myeloma, consideration should be given to storing stem cells at diagnosis and using granulocyte colony-stimulating factor (G-CSF) for mobilization, and, if there are features suggesting that the patient will soon progress, it may be appropriate to consider early treatment with a view to high-dose therapy. Based on favorable results obtained in patients with relapsed disease, clinical trials on the use of thalidomide in newly diagnosed patients have been commenced in both Europe and the USA. Some of these trials have included asymptomatic patients. Preliminary data on thalidomide alone in a small series of patients with smoldering MM treated at the Mayo Clinic showed a response rate that was comparable with that obtained in relapsed-refractory patients, whereas combined thalidomide–dexamethasone therapy for symptomatic MM produced responses in 65–70%.[11] A similar study from the MD Anderson Hospital yielded similar results.[12] However, there are, as yet, no data available to suggest whether progression was deferred by early treatment with thalidomide and no randomized studies have yet been published. Bisphosphonates are another class of drug that might have a role in early-stage MM.

APPROPRIATE SETTING FOR THE MANAGEMENT OF MYELOMA

Effective and high-quality care in myeloma requires a multispecialty and multidisciplinary team familiar with the range of clinical problems likely to be encountered. A hematologist or oncologist should lead the care of patients with multiple myeloma, and should be working within a setting that provides the core range of essential accessible expertise and services shown in Table 13.3. These may be available locally or in a neighboring hospital. There should be clear policies and protocols for access to these services.

AN INTEGRATED MANAGEMENT PLAN

The stages of treatment can be divided into induction, consolidation and/or maintenance and treatment at relapse (Table 13.4 and Fig. 13.2). Supportive care is an important part of treatment throughout the course of the disease. It is helpful to decide on an overall management

Table 13.3 *Range of services required for management of patients with multiple myeloma*

- Clinical pathology (diagnostic hematology, clinical biochemistry, immunology, histopathology)
- Diagnostic radiology and imaging
- Pharmacy facilities and expertise for dispensing cytotoxic drugs
- Renal services, including rapid access to hemodialysis
- Radiotherapy
- Neurosurgery
- Orthopedic surgery
- Physiotherapy/rehabilitation
- Specialist hematology/oncology nurses
- Access to accredited bone marrow/stem cell transplant center
- Primary care liaison
- Palliative care physicians/nurses
- Administrative support for case registration, audit, and clinical trials
- Social services and financial advice
- Written patient information
- Patient support group

strategy soon after diagnosis. In particular, the choice of initial chemotherapy will be influenced by whether the patient is a candidate for future high-dose therapy.

Choice of initial chemotherapy

The choice of initial therapy will be governed largely by the patient's age and general fitness, particularly the level of renal function. It is also essential to take into account at diagnosis the possibility of future autologous transplantation, so as to avoid the use of stem-cell-damaging drugs in patients where autografting is an option. Patients up to the age of at least 65 years should be considered as possible candidates for future autografting, and, in these patients, vincristine–Adriamycin–dexamethasone (VAD) or a VAD-type regimen should be used (see Chapter 14). Some patients over the age of 65 may also be suitable candidates for high-dose therapy (see Chapter 16). For most patients over 65 years, the choice currently lies between simple oral chemotherapy and standard combination regimens. Overall, there is little difference in long-term outcome between these options, and simple oral treatment, therefore, seems the most appropriate choice for older patients.[10]

For patients presenting with renal failure, VAD is the obvious choice and can be used in some older patients. Oral idarubicin and dexamethasone is an alternative, but, as yet, there are insufficient data on its use in patients to recommend its use without dosage modification in patients with renal failure. Melphalan and cyclophosphamide are both difficult to use in patients with renal impairment because myelosuppression is unpredictable even when the doses are reduced (see Chapter 22). Steroids

Table 13.4 *Treatment options in multiple myeloma*

Induction	Consolidation/maintenance	Refractory/relapsed disease
Simple alkylating agents: melphalan or cyclophosphamide ± prednisolone Combination chemotherapy: e.g. ABCM, VMCP/VBAP VAD-type regimens: VAD, VAMP, C-VAMP, Z-Dex Dexamethasone alone	High-dose therapy with stem cell support (autograft) Allogeneic BMT in selected patients Mini-allograft under trial Interferon maintenance Thalidomide maintenance under trial Vaccination strategies under trial	• Primarily refractory to alkylating agents: VAD or VAD-type regimen • Primarily refractory to VAD: intermediate or high-dose melphalan with stem cell support • Thalidomide ± dexamethasone Relapsed disease: • Any regimen used for induction • Thalidomide ± dexamethasone • Bortezomib • Steroids alone • DHBI New approaches under trial: • Thalidomide analogs • Other biological approaches • Monoclonal antibodies

ABCM, Adriamycin®, BCNU, cyclophosphamide, melphalan; BCNU, carmustine; BMT, bone marrow transplantation; C-VAMP, as VAMP with addition of weekly cyclophosphamide; DHBI, double hemi-body irradiation; VAD, infused vincristine and Adriamycin® with pulsed dexamethasone; VAMP, as VAD with methyl prednisolone in place of dexamethasone; VMCP/VBAP, vincristine, melphalan, cyclophosphamide, prednisolone/vincristine, BCNU, Adriamycin®, prednisolone; Z-Dex, oral idarubicin (Zavedos) with dexamethasone.

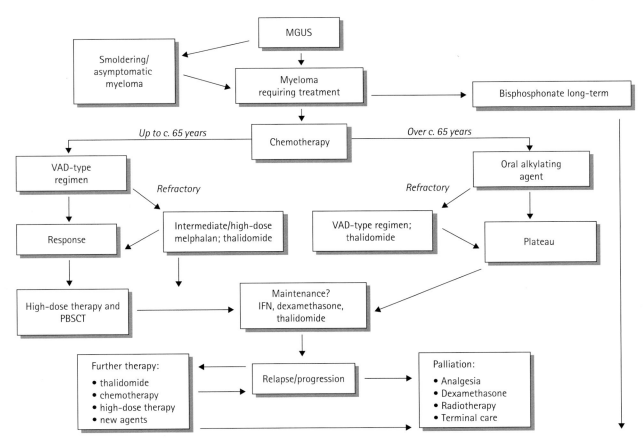

Figure 13.2 *Management pathways in multiple myeloma. IFN, interferon; MGUS, monoclonal gammopathy of undetermined significance; PBSCT, peripheral blood stem cell transplantation; VAD, vincristine–Adriamycin–dexamethasone.*

alone, e.g. pulsed high-dose dexamethasone, are very useful initial therapy in patients where there is an urgency to treat but in whom it is difficult to decide immediately on appropriate chemotherapy, e.g. those presenting with pancytopenia or patients with renal failure who may be unsuitable for intravenous therapy. Chemotherapy should be continued until the patient has reached plateau phase, i.e. observations have been stable for a period of 3 months, since there is no advantage to prolonging chemotherapy once plateau has been reached.[13] In patients who are proceeding to high-dose therapy and transplant as consolidation therapy, there is probably no advantage to continuing induction chemotherapy beyond the point of maximum response; this is usually no longer than 3–4 months when VAD-type regimens are used.

Planned high–dose therapy

Current evidence suggests that while high-dose therapy is not curative, it prolongs remission and survival as compared with conventional dose chemotherapy. High-dose therapy with autologous stem cell support is currently considered standard treatment in patients up to the age of about 65 years and may be suitable for some older patients (see Chapter 16). Selected patients may be offered allogeneic stem cell transplantation (see Chapter 17). The results of high-dose therapy are best when carried out in first remission, but it may also be worthwhile in patients with primary refractory or relapsed disease. The role of low-intensity allogeneic stem cell transplantation is currently being explored.

Maintenance

A number of studies indicate that there is no benefit from continuing chemotherapy once stable plateau phase is reached. However, maintenance therapy with α-interferon has a modest effect in prolonging response and survival (see Chapter 14). Studies looking at the role of thalidomide as maintenance therapy are in progress.

Options at relapse

There is currently no standard therapy for patients with relapsed disease. A wide variety of approaches are available. The disease may respond to the same chemotherapy as that used previously or to a different regimen or may prove refractory to treatment. For patients initially treated with oral chemotherapy, unless the relapse occurs soon after stopping treatment, it is worth trying the same regimen that induced the initial remission.[13,14] Over 50% of patients who responded initially to MP will respond again to MP at relapse.[13] Patients refractory to MP may still respond to cyclophosphamide. In younger patients, VAD is generally preferred at relapse, although the oral anthracycline-based regimens, Z-Dex (oral idarubicin and dexamethasone) and CIDEX (lomustine (CCNU), oral idarubicin, and dexamethasone) are suitable alternatives to VAD and other intravenous anthracycline-containing regimens.[15,16] For patients not responding to VAD, combinations of VAD with drug-resistance modifiers, such as cyclosporin or PSC833, have been used,[17,18] but with limited success. Patients relapsing after, or refractory to, more than one chemotherapy regimen may do well on steroids alone, and double hemi-body irradiation can also be useful in this situation (see Chapter 15). Thalidomide, with or without dexamethasone, is increasingly being used in the treatment of relapsed disease in patients of all ages[19] and there are also a number of other promising new biological approaches to therapy, including bortezomib and arsenic trioxide (see Chapter 19).

Primary refractory disease

At present, there is no standard approach to the management of patients with primary refractory disease. Younger patients failing to respond to VAD usually respond to intermediate or high-dose melphalan, while older patients failing to respond to oral alkylating agents may respond to an anthracycline-containing regimen (Fig. 13.2). Thalidomide is also effective in patients with primary refractory disease.

The role of supportive care

Optimal supportive care is fundamental and should be a key part of the overall care plan. Despite the importance of supportive care, there is little published research in this area. Table 13.5 summarizes the recommendations of the UK Myeloma Forum on supportive care in myeloma,[10] and this aspect of management is discussed in detail in Chapter 18. Patients should be informed appropriately about the condition, its potential complications, and the importance of supportive measures.

MONITORING DISEASE STATUS

Once the diagnosis has been established, regular monitoring is required to determine disease status and response to treatment. Changes in the level of serum paraprotein and/or urinary light-chain excretion form the basis of assessing response to therapy and monitoring the progress of the disease, but monitoring should involve regular measurement of paraprotein in serum and urine and checks of full blood count, renal function, and serum calcium. In non-secretory myeloma, serial bone marrow

Table 13.5 *General aspects of care in multiple myeloma*

Renal function	Maintain adequate hydration in all patients (fluid intake of at least 3 L/day). Avoid potentially nephrotoxic drugs
Hypercalcemia	Volume replacement with intravenous saline and an intravenous bisphosphonate (a loop diuretic is not of additional benefit unless there is volume overload)
Bone disease and pain management	*Analgesia*: a variety of analgesics may be used, including simple analgesics, opiates, and fentanyl patches. NSAIDs should be avoided in patients with renal impairment and used with caution in other patients *Chemotherapy and radiotherapy*: response to chemotherapy is a major factor in reducing progression of bone disease. Local radiotherapy may be of benefit in patients with localized severe pain *Orthopedic surgery*: fixation of long bones may be required to treat or prevent pathological fracture. Radiotherapy, if required, is better given post-operatively once healing has occurred rather than pre-operatively *Bisphosphonates*: all patients should receive a bisphosphonate long term *General measures*: it is important to maintain mobility, as immobility increases bone loss and the risk of infection as well as impairing quality of life. Physiotherapy and aids such as spinal supports may be useful
Hyperviscosity	Symptomatic patients should be treated urgently with plasma exchange; isovolemic venesection may be used if plasma exchange facilities are not immediately available. If transfusion is essential exchange transfusion should be performed. Chemotherapy should be instituted promptly
Spinal cord compression	Management requires emergency hospital admission and investigation with MRI scanning to define the site and extent of tumor. CT scanning may be used if MRI is unavailable or contraindicated. Dexamethasone should be commenced immediately. Local radiotherapy is the treatment of choice; there is no advantage in outcome for surgical treatment in the absence of spinal instability. Spinal surgery in myeloma patients may be difficult because of osteoporosis but may be indicated for spinal instability
Infection	Arrangements should be in place to ensure 24-hour access to specialist team advice. Admission for intravenous antibiotic therapy is usually needed for severe systemic infection. Influenza vaccination should be given to myeloma patients annually. Pneumococcal and *Haemophilus* vaccinations may be given, although there is no evidence of their efficacy in multiple myeloma patients
Anemia	Transfuse as appropriate or consider erythropoietin
Psychological problems	Depression and anxiety occur, and should be actively managed with referral where necessary to psychiatric/psychological services

CT, computed tomography; MRI, magnetic resonance imaging; NSAIDs, non-steroidal anti-inflammatory drugs.

aspirations are essential for the assessment of disease status, although the patchy nature of marrow involvement makes it difficult to interpret small changes in plasma cell numbers. Recent evidence suggests that serum free light chain assay is helpful in the diagnosis and monitoring of patients with non-secretory disease.[20] Radiological imaging (see Chapter 10) is important in the assessment of disease progression but is less helpful in assessing response because recalcification of lytic lesions, although occasionally documented,[21] is extremely unusual even with long-term remission. MRI scans may show improvement[22] but are difficult to assess without considerable experience.

Criteria for defining response

Response criteria were first developed by the Committee of the Chronic Leukaemia and Myeloma Task Force (CLMTF) of the US National Cancer Institute.[23] The main response parameter is a reduction in the paraprotein and/or urinary light chain excretion by at least 50% (Table 13.6). In 1972 the Southwest Oncology Group (SWOG)[24] defined 'objective response' as a reduction of at least 75% in the calculated serum paraprotein synthetic rate (rather than paraprotein concentration) and/or a decrease of at least 90% in urinary light-chain excretion, sustained for at least 2 months. The calculation of paraprotein synthetic rate depends on the serum level and fractional catabolic rate of the particular immunoglobulin isotype and subclass. The reason for this rather complicated analysis is that in some immunoglobulin (Ig) subclasses the fractional catabolic rate declines markedly once levels come down to below 30 g/L so that, below this level, changes in protein concentration alone will underestimate tumor reduction. However, the SWOG criteria have not been widely adopted by other groups, and most studies have used the Myeloma Task Force of the National Cancer Institute (MTF) criteria for objective response. In the Medical Research Council (MRC) myeloma trials, efficacy of treatment has been evaluated by the proportion of patients reaching a plateau.[25] Plateau phase consists of a period of stability after chemotherapy in which no further response occurs despite continuing treatment. The definition of

Table 13.6 *Criteria used to defined response in myeloma as defined by the Myeloma Task Force (MTF), the Southwest Oncology Group (SWOG), and the Medical Research Council (MRC)*

MTF	SWOG	MRC criteria for plateau
One or more of the following	All of the following criteria, sustained for at least 2 months	All of the following
Reduction of serum paraprotein level to 50% or less of pre-treatment value	Reduction of calculated synthetic rate of serum paraprotein to 25% or less of pre-treatment value	Stable or undetectable serum paraprotein for at least 3 months*
Reduction of light-chain excretion to 50% or less of pre-treatment value if originally <1.0 g/24 hours, or a fall to <1.0 g/24 hours if originally >1.0 g/24 hours	Reduction of light-chain excretion to less than 10% of pre-treatment value and to less than 0.2 g/24 hours	Stable or undetectable urinary light-chain excretion for at least 3 months*
Reduction of 50% in size of plasmacytomas	Improvement in bone pain and performance status	Few or no symptoms attributable to myeloma
Radiological evidence of skeletal healing	Correction of anemia and hypo-albuminemia, if attributed to multiple myeloma	No transfusion requirement

*6 months in Trials IV and V.

plateau does not require any specific degree of paraprotein reduction. The minimal period of stable observation required to define plateau was 6 months in the early MRC trials but in recent trials has been reduced to 3 months.

Complete remission

Complete response/complete remission rates – as assessed by routine electrophoresis – are seen in less than 10% of patients treated with conventional oral treatment, and neither the CLMTF nor the SWOG response criteria include a definition of CR. With the introduction of new regimens, such as VAD and high-dose melphalan, detectable paraprotein disappeared in a significant proportion of patients, and criteria for CR were first formulated.[26,27] As the use of high-dose therapy has increased, there has been a concomitant increase in the number of patients entering CR. Furthermore, the significance of CR after high-dose therapy appears different to that after conventional-dose therapy, in that it has been shown that achieving CR after high-dose therapy is correlated with improved remission duration and survival (see later). The accurate definition of CR is, therefore, crucial in patients treated with high-dose therapy. In initial reports a negative result on routine electrophoresis (EP) was accepted as sufficient to define CR, but there was then a gradual move towards a more stringent definition of CR requiring that paraprotein is also undetectable by immunofixation (IF). A group representing the European Group for Blood and Marrow Transplantation (EBMT), the International Bone

Marrow Transplant Registry (IBMTR), and the Autologous Blood and Marrow Transplant Registry (ABMTR) reviewed the existing response criteria and agreed new criteria for the definition for response and CR (Table 13.7).[28] These criteria were primarily intended for assessment of response in patients treated with high-dose therapy but are also applicable to other situations. Criteria for the definition of progression or relapse (from CR) were also agreed. It was decided that CR should be defined according to the most sensitive test in routine use, i.e. immunofixation. The definition of CR requires that the paraprotein is undetectable by immunofixation for a period of at least 6 weeks, and also that the definition of relapse from CR includes recurrence of detectable paraprotein on immunofixation. Regular immunofixation is, therefore, required to monitor patients in whom there is no paraprotein detectable on routine electrophoresis.

The presence of oligoclonal bands may complicate the assessment of remission status in patients following stem-cell transplant, particularly during the first year after transplantation. Transient paraproteins or oligoclonal bands on immunofixation of serum are frequently observed following stem-cell transplant in patients with a variety of diseases, not only myeloma.[29–31] These are attributed to asynchronous B-cell reconstitution. Where these bands include a protein of the same isotype as the original myeloma protein, it may be impossible to determine whether this represents the original clone. Careful follow-up can resolve the issue in some cases but, in one series, it was found that in about 10% of patients it remained impossible to be sure whether they were in complete remission.[32]

Table 13.7 *EBMT, IBMTR, and ABMTR criteria for response, relapse, and progression in patients with multiple myeloma treated with high-dose therapy and stem-cell transplantation*

Complete response (CR) requires all of the following:
1   Absence of the original monoclonal paraprotein in serum and urine by immunofixation, maintained for a minimum of 6 weeks. The presence of oligoclonal bands consistent with immune reconstitution does not exclude CR
2   <5% plasma cells in a bone marrow aspirate and also in trephine biopsy, if biopsy has been performed. If absence of monoclonal protein is sustained for at least 6 weeks, it is not necessary to repeat the bone marrow to confirm CR, except in patients with non-secretory myeloma, where the marrow examination must be repeated after an interval of at least 6 weeks to confirm CR
3   No increase in the size or number of lytic bone lesions on skeletal X-ray, if performed (it is not necessary to perform X-rays unless there is a clinical indication. Development of a compression fracture does not exclude PR)
4   Disappearance of soft-tissue plasmacytomas

Partial response (PR) requires all of the following:
1   ≥50% reduction in the serum monoclonal paraprotein maintained for a minimum of 6 weeks
2   Reduction in 24-hour urinary light-chain excretion either by ≥90% or to <200 mg, maintained for a minimum of 6 weeks
3   For patients with non-secretory myeloma only, ≥50% reduction in plasma cells in a bone marrow aspirate and also in trephine biopsy, if biopsy has been performed, maintained for a minimum of 6 weeks
4   ≥50% reduction in size of soft-tissue plasmacytomas
5   No increase in the size or number of lytic bone lesions on skeletal X-ray, if performed (it is not necessary to perform X-rays unless there is a clinical indication. Development of a compression fracture does not exclude CR)
Patients in whom some, but not all, of the criteria for PR are fulfilled and classified as minimal response (MR), providing the remaining criteria satisfy the requirements for MR

Minimal response (MR) requires all of the following:
1   25–49% reduction in the serum monoclonal paraprotein maintained for a minimum of 6 weeks
2   50–89% reduction in 24-hour urinary light-chain excretion, which still exceeds <200 mg/24 hours, maintained for a minimum of 6 weeks
3   For patients with non-secretory myeloma only, 25–49% reduction in plasma cells in a bone marrow aspirate and also in trephine biopsy, if biopsy has been performed, maintained for a minimum of 6 weeks
4   25–49% reduction in size of soft-tissue plasmacytomas
5   No increase in the size or number of lytic bone lesions on skeletal X-ray, if performed (it is not necessary to perform X-rays unless there is a clinical indication. Development of a compression fracture does not exclude MR)

No change (NC)
1   Not meeting the criteria of either minimal response or progressive disease

Relapse from CR requires at least one of the following:
1   Reappearance of serum or urinary paraprotein on immunofixation or on routine electrophoresis, confirmed by at least one further investigation and excluding oligoclonal reconstitution
2   >5% plasma cells in a bone marrow aspirate or on trephine biopsy
3   Development of new lytic bone lesions or soft-tissue plasmacytomas or definite increase in the size of residual bone lesions (development of a compression fracture does not exclude continued CR)
4   Development of hypercalcemia (corrected serum calcium >2.8 mmol/L) not attributable to any other cause

Progressive disease (for patients not in CR) requires at least one of the following:
1   >25% increase in the level of serum monoclonal paraprotein, which must also be an absolute increase of at least 5 g/L and confirmed by at least one repeat observation
2   >25% increase in 24-hour urinary light-chain excretion, which must also be an absolute increase of at least 200 mg/24 hours and confirmed by at least one repeat observation
3   >25% increase in plasma cells in a bone marrow aspirate or on trephine biopsy, which must also be an absolute increase of at least 10% of total nucleated cells.
4   Definite increase in size of existing bone lesions or soft-tissue plasmacytomas
5   Development of new lytic bone lesions or soft-tissue plasmacytomas of definite increase in the size of residual bone lesions (development of a compression fracture does not exclude continued response)
6   Development of hypercalcemia (corrected serum calcium >2.8 mmol/L) not attributable to any other cause

Response and survival

It might be expected that a greater degree of tumor response would lead to longer remission duration and improved survival, but the evidence for this is poor. In practice, patients who do not achieve conventional definition of response, but who do not progress, may have long survival,[33–36] and it does not appear that attaining any given degree of response is correlated with long-term outcome (with the exception of CR after high-dose therapy – see below). Although Alexanian et al.,[24] in one of the first studies of combination chemotherapy for myeloma, reported that the survival of patients treated with combination chemotherapy was directly correlated with the degree of reduction of M-protein synthesis, several subsequent studies reported a lack of correlation between the degree of response, whether defined by MTF or SWOG criteria, and subsequent survival.[33–36] Consistent with this is the observation that in trials comparing combination chemotherapy (CCT) with MP, response rates were higher with CCT but there was no survival advantage. A more recent study from the Finnish Leukaemia group[37] confirmed the lack of correlation between the level of response achieved and survival, and concluded that the primary goal of conventional chemotherapy should be stabilization of disease rather than the level of response.

This lack of correlation between degree of response and long-term outcome extends to patients achieving CR after conventional-dose therapy. Although approximately 20% of patients enter CR following treatment with VAD and related regimens,[26,27,38] this does not translate into improved remission duration. In a study of VAD as first-line therapy, remission duration was only 18 months, even in those patients entering CR.[26] Similar observations were made in relation to high-dose melphalan at a dose of 140 mg/m^2 without stem-cell support.[27]

In contrast, it appears that patients in CR after high-dose therapy and stem-cell transplant do have improved remission duration and survival as compared with those who enter or remain in partial remission (PR).[39–45] This cannot be entirely explained by the increasing use of more stringent criteria for CR in recent years, since, in some of these series, CR was based on negative routine electrophoresis without immunofixation.[39–41] It seems more likely that there is a difference in the quality of CR after conventional therapy and after high-dose therapy; in other words, the level of minimal residual disease is presumably lower in patients in CR post-transplant than in those who are in CR after conventional-dose therapy. Lahuerta et al.[44] observed that CR defined by a negative immunofixation result but not by negative routine electrophoresis conferred improved survival after autologous transplantation. Davies et al.[45] also observed a trend towards an improved progression-free survival (PFS) in patients who attained a CR with negative immunofixation after autologous transplantation compared with PR patients, a trend that was not seen when routine electrophoresis was used to define CR.

Minimal residual disease

It is evident that the majority of patients in CR have residual disease below the level of detection of immunofixation, as relapse eventually occurs in almost all cases. Residual tumor cells can be detected in over 50% of such patients using polymerase chain reaction (PCR) for the clone-specific IgH rearrangement, which affords a sensitivity of 10^{-4}–10^{-6} (0.001–0.00001%) depending on the technique used.[46–50] The technique can be adapted to provide quantitative results and there is some evidence that the level of minimal residual disease (MRD) in patients after high-dose therapy is predictive of outcome.[49] However, the technique is laborious and has a number of methodological problems.[50] In particular, the clone-specific rearrangement is unique to each patient, so that identification, sequencing, and design of specific primers are necessary for every patient. An alternative approach is the use of flow cytometry, based on expression of an abnormal immunophenotype.[50,51] This is applicable to all patients and can be performed rapidly. While the sensitivity is less than that of PCR-based methods (maximum sensitivity of 0.01%, if 200 000 events are acquired), it appears to provide results of prognostic significance.[50]

Problems in assessing response

NON–SECRETORY MYELOMA

In non-secretory myeloma, formal assessment of response is dependent on serial sampling of bone marrow. Because of the patchy nature of myeloma infiltration, accurate assessment of response is often difficult, and weight should also be given to improvement in symptoms and normalization of hematological and biochemical values. Recent data indicate that the levels of either κ or λ free light chain (FLC) in the serum are often raised in non-secretory disease even though there is no detectable paraprotein or urinary BJP, and that serum FLC assay may prove useful in monitoring these patients.[20]

SEVERE CHRONIC RENAL FAILURE

This is another situation where the assessment of response may be difficult. Most myeloma patients with chronic renal failure have Bence Jones-only myeloma and urinary light-chain excretion cannot be monitored in the presence of oliguria or anuria. Furthermore, changes in renal function can affect BJP excretion. Surprisingly, this problem has not been addressed in any of the published response criteria. In practice, such patients are generally monitored in the same way as those with non-secretory myeloma, by improvement in symptoms and normalization of hematological and biochemical values. FLC assay is likely to prove of particular help in monitoring these patients. Whereas BJP excretion will fluctuate with glomerular filtration rate and tubular reabsorption, serum FLC levels reflect the net effect of secretion from the neoplastic and non-neoplastic plasma cells and removal by glomerular filtration, and the serum $\kappa{:}\lambda$ ratio is not affected by changes in glomerular filtration rate (GFR).

Criteria for progression/relapse

Relapse is usually manifest by a rise in paraprotein, often in conjunction with a recurrence of symptoms. In a minority of patients, disease progression is manifested by increasing marrow or skeletal involvement, or development of other complications, without a rise in paraprotein or light-chain excretion. The EBMT/IBMTR/ABMTR response criteria also include definitions of relapse (from CR) and progression. Isolated extramedullary relapse is rare, but there are some data suggesting that it may be more common after high-dose therapy.[52,53] MRI or fluorodeoxyglucose positron emission tomography (FDG-PET) scanning is helpful in the diagnosis of these isolated relapses.[54]

QUALITY OF LIFE IN MYELOMA

Improving quality of life (QoL) is one of the most important aims of treatment in myeloma. Bone pain, fractures, and vertebral collapse are major problems for myeloma patients, as are anemia and fatigue. However, the efficacy of different approaches to treatment has traditionally been evaluated purely by tumor response, remission duration, and survival, and there was little evidence relating to the effect of therapy on QoL. More recently, there has been a general recognition of the need for evaluation of health-related QoL in cancer patients as an addition to the traditional endpoints. This has been highlighted by the need for better evaluation of therapeutic approaches that have frequent side effects (such as interferon) or are expensive (such as high-dose therapy). In addition, the development of drugs, such as the bisphosphonates and erythropoietin, which are primarily aimed at relieving symptoms rather than acting directly on the myeloma, places more emphasis on the assessment of QoL. Assessment of QoL contributes to pharmaco-economic evaluation of different treatments, so that outcomes can be expressed as cost per quality-adjusted life year gained.

Methods of assessing QoL

While it could be indirectly assumed that a treatment that reduces skeletal events or raises Hb level would also improve QoL, it is important to assess QoL formally. A number of assessment methods have been developed and validated, such as the QLQ-30 questionnaire developed by the European Organisation for Research and Treatment of Cancer (EORTC). The QLQ-30 is designed for all types of cancer. It contains a number of questions pertaining to physical, psychological, and social functioning, and some questions about specific symptoms. A number of disease-specific modules have also been developed to be used as supplements to QLQ-30, including a myeloma-specific module (QLQ-MY24), which is currently undergoing validation.[55] Another method of looking at QoL is Q-TWiST (quality-adjusted time without symptoms or toxicity) analysis.[56]

Studies assessing QoL

The Nordic Myeloma Study Group (NMSG) was the first to incorporate assessment of QoL into a clinical trial in myeloma patients and has since published a number of articles relating to QoL and pharmaco-economics in myeloma. Their initial study[57] evaluated the use of the EORTC QLQ-30 questionnaire in a series of 581 patients in a trial comparing MP with and without α-interferon (IFN) (NMSG 4/90), and confirmed that the questionnaire provided a valid and reliable method of assessing QoL. It was able to discriminate between patients with different clinical status and that changes in scores correlated with objective changes in disease. The group also observed that QoL assessed before and during chemotherapy was predictive of survival and, moreover, had a higher correlation with survival than did objective response rate.[58] At a 12-month landmark analysis, the relative risk of death for patients with physical functioning score 0–20 vs. 80–100 was 5.64, whereas the relative risk for patients without objective response to chemotherapy compared with those with at least a minor response was 2.32.

INTERFERON AND QoL

The results of the NMSG 4/90 trial showed that during the first 12 months on IFN, patients' QoL was decreased compared with those on placebo but that from 12 months onwards, there were no significant differences between the two groups.[59] However, taking into account the cost of IFN and the modest prolongation of survival when added to chemotherapy, it was concluded that IFN had an unfavorable cost–utility ratio, estimated at between $US50 000 and $US100 000 per quality-adjusted life-year gained.[60] A study from Canada[61] used Q-TWiST analysis in a study of IFN maintenance after MP and found that while patients on IFN gained an average of 5 months of survival, they suffered an average of 4.1 months of moderate or worse toxicity.

HIGH–DOSE THERAPY AND QoL

A cost–utility analysis comparing high-dose therapy with conventional chemotherapy in a non-randomized population-based study has been carried out by the Nordic Myeloma Study Group.[62] The intensive treatment yielded a significant increase in median survival time from 44 to 62 months, with a gain of 1.2 quality-adjusted life years (QALY). The cost per QALY gained was estimated at $27 000. The Nordic Group also looked at QoL in a trial of conventional vs. high-dose therapy in c. 350 patients.[63] They found that the high-dose therapy had lower QoL scores immediately after the transplant, but at 1 and 2 years there was no difference and by 3 years there was a trend towards improved QoL, as compared with patients in the conventional chemotherapy group. A co-operative French group[56] used Q-TWiST analysis to address the same issue in two trials of conventional vs. high-dose therapy. They found an average gain in TWiST of 5.5 months and 5.8 months in the high-dose group in the two studies as compared with the control group. Preliminary cost–utility analysis suggested a cost–utility ratio of $US30 000–40 000 per QALY gained. These results add weight to the argument for the adoption of high-dose therapy as the standard treatment for younger patients.

SUPPORTIVE CARE AND QoL

QoL assessment using patient questionnaires has also contributed towards the evidence in favor of erythropoietin (Epo) treatment of anemia in myeloma. QoL has been shown to correlate with anemia in cancer patients including those with myeloma,[64] and correction and randomized studies of Epo versus placebo have shown significant improvements in the hemoglobin (Hb) level, decreases in transfusion requirements, and improvements in patient-assessed QoL in myeloma patients receiving Epo.[65,66] To date there have been no trials using formal QoL assessments to evaluate bisphosphonate therapy, although reduction in pain scores and fracture rates can be taken as indirect measures of improvement in QoL.

CLINICAL TRIALS IN MYELOMA

The role of clinical trials

Since current treatment for myeloma remains unsatisfactory, it is clear that new treatment approaches must be developed. Well-designed clinical trials are essential to evaluating new approaches and comparing the results with existing treatments. Wherever possible, patients should be entered into clinical trials. This requires a significant time commitment on the part of the treating physician and the team, which should be recognized by the provision of support staff, in particular specialist nurses and assistance with data management.

Criteria for evaluation of treatment regimens

Criteria by which treatment regimens are usually evaluated include the proportion of patients achieving an objective response, i.e. a given degree of tumor reduction, the duration of the response, and survival, although QoL analysis is now assuming increasing importance. As discussed above, there is little correlation between response rate and long-term outcome. Response duration is the second measure of outcome that can be evaluated. It has most usually been used in evaluating maintenance therapy, e.g. with interferon. Response duration does not, however, necessarily correlate with survival, possibly because of variable response to treatment at relapse. Thus, interferon maintenance has a greater effect on prolonging remission duration than on survival. Survival is the ultimate measure of outcome but this also is not without problems of analysis. Firstly, in a disease affecting the elderly, a number of deaths will occur from unrelated causes and survival analyses do not always censor these deaths. Peest et al.[67] showed that median overall survival was 1 year shorter than median tumor-related survival in a series of 320 patients. Another problem in using survival as the endpoint to assess first-line therapy is the effectiveness of therapy given at relapse.

Interpreting trial results

The intrinsic variability of prognosis in myeloma is extremely important when attempting to compare the results of different treatment approaches. Results from non-randomized studies must be interpreted with caution. Even where randomized studies are concerned, randomization may not have been stratified for prognostic factors. The most important prognostic factors, serum β_2-microglobulin and deletion of chromosome 13, have only been available in more recent studies and the latter only in selected centres. Particularly in small studies, differences in outcome between different treatment arms may occur because of patient heterogeneity, and it is not surprising that many studies addressing the same question (e.g. whether interferon maintenance prolongs survival) have yielded different results. The problem of sample size can be overcome to a considerable extent by meta-analysis, as has been applied by the Myeloma Trialists' Collaborative Group.[68,69]

Another important consideration is that the results of trials may not be applicable to all patients. The survival in a trial population is influenced both by active and passive exclusions. Trials tend to exclude poor-risk patients and many trials exclude patients with significant renal impairment. A study from the NMSG[70] noted that during a 3-year period, only 180 of 314 newly diagnosed cases were entered into current clinical trials; some were notified but excluded, while others were not notified. Those patients not in the trial had a significantly shorter survival than that of the trial population.

Evidence–based guidelines

The process of development of evidence-based guidelines involves reviewing the published evidence, taking into account the above considerations and producing recommendations accordingly. The higher the level of evidence, the stronger is the relevant recommendation. In general, the results of a meta-analysis will carry more weight than those of a randomized study, which in turn are graded higher than those of a non-randomized study. The UK Myeloma Forum has written such evidence-based guidelines on the diagnosis and management of myeloma on behalf on the British Committee for Standards in Haematology.[10] A Canadian group has published guidelines on the role of high-dose therapy and stem-cell transplantation,[71] and the Cochrane collaboration and the American Society of Clinical Oncologists have both produced guidelines on the use of bisphosphonates in myeloma.[72,73] The UK Myeloma Forum has also recently published evidence-based guidelines on the

Table 13.8 *Sources of patient information and support*

Country	Organization	Website	Comment
USA/international	International Myeloma Foundation	www.myeloma.org	Information and support; helpline for USA and abroad
USA	Multiple Myeloma Research Foundation	www.multiplemyeloma.org	Information and list of local support groups
USA	Amyloidosis Support Network	www.amyloidosis.org	Information and support; telephone helpline
USA	National Cancer Institute	www.cancer.gov	Treatment and research information. Patient information booklet on multiple myeloma
USA	Leukemia and Lymphoma Society (USA)	www.leukaemia–lymphoma.org	Patient information booklet on myeloma
Canada	Canadian Cancer Society	www.cancer.ca	Information about myeloma on website
Australasia	Myeloma Australasia	www.myelomaaustralia.com	Links to support groups and information on treatment, care, and support
Denmark	Dansk myeloma forening	www.cancer.myelomatose.dk	Specifically for myeloma patients
Netherlands	Kontaktgroep Kahler patienten	www.kahler.nl	Specifically for myeloma patients
Norway	Den Norske Kreftforening	www.kreft.no/	For patients with hematological malignancies
Sweden	Swedish Cancer Foundation	www.cancerfonden.se	For all cancers
Switzerland	Myeloma Kontakt Gruppe Schweiz	www.multiples-myelom.ch	Information and support; telephone helpline
UK	International Myeloma Foundation – UK	www.myeloma.org.uk	Information and support; telephone helpline
UK	UK Myeloma Forum	www.ukmf.org.uk	Online information

diagnosis and management of solitary plasmacytoma and of AL amyloidosis.[74,75]

THE PATIENT'S PERSPECTIVE

Provision of information and support for patients and their carers is essential to assist patients in making informed choices on treatment options, as well as understanding the importance of compliance with treatment regimens, which, at times, can be very demanding. The diagnosis needs to be communicated honestly to the patient with the minimum of delay. Uncertainty about the condition is generally more distressing to a patient and his or her family. The information should be communicated in a quiet area with privacy, ideally in the company of a close relative and with the presence of a specialist nurse. Patients and their partners/carers should be given time to ask appropriate questions once they have been given the diagnosis; this may best be done after an interval of a few hours or days. It is important for patients and their families to understand that, although treatment is not curative, it will relieve symptoms and prolong survival and its quality; the positive aspects of treatment need to be stressed.

The management plan needs to be communicated simply to the patient and his/her carer and should be clearly written in the case record so that the information is readily accessible to other members of the multidisciplinary specialist team. Patients need to be informed of the names of the key members of the specialist team who are in charge of their care and given clear information on access to advice/support from the team.

The specialist team should be able to provide patients and their families with information on national and local support networks, whether these are specific to myeloma or in relation to cancer generally.

Information should also be available for the patient and family on availability of assistance with financial and social problems. Bone problems may result in long-term disability and preclude many patients returning to work. High-dose and conventional chemotherapy regimens also make employment impractical for periods of several months. Patients commonly need advice, therefore, on socioeconomic problems, which result from the condition and its treatment.

Useful information sources

There are a number of patient information and support organizations that produce excellent written information on myeloma and related disorders; some also provide support through telephone helplines and run seminars for patients (see Table 13.8).

KEY POINTS

- The aims of treatment in myeloma are to relieve symptoms, improve quality of life, and prolong survival.
- Quality care in myeloma requires an integrated multidisciplinary team, good supportive care, and provision of patient information and support.
- Patients with asymptomatic early-stage myeloma do not require immediate chemotherapy.
- With conventional dose therapy, the aim of treatment is to achieve stable plateau rather than any given degree of tumor response, whereas with high-dose therapy the aim is to achieve complete remission.
- Current criteria for the definition of complete remission and relapse require regular monitoring by immunofixation in appropriate patients.
- Wherever possible, patients should be entered into appropriate clinical trials.

REFERENCES

● = Key primary paper
◆ = Major review article
* = Paper that represents the first formal publication of a management guideline

1. Kyle RA, Greipp PR. Smoldering multiple myeloma. *N Engl J Med* 1980; **302**:1347–9.
2. Alexanian R. Localized and indolent myeloma. *Blood* 1980; **56**:521–5.
3. Dimopoulos MA, Moulopoulos A, Smith T, Delasalle KB, Alexanian R. Risk of disease progression in asymptomatic multiple myeloma. *Am J Med* 1993; **94**:57–61.
4. Facon T, Menard JF, Michaux JL, Euller-Ziegler L, Bernard JF, Grosbois B, *et al.* Prognostic factors in low tumour mass asymptomatic multiple myeloma: a report on 91 patients. The Groupe d'Etudes et de Recherche sur le Myelome (GERM). *Am J Hematol* 1995; **48**:71–5.
●5. Weber DM, Dimopoulos MA, Moulopoulos LA, Delasalle KB, Smith T, Alexanian R. Prognostic features of asymptomatic multiple myeloma. *Br J Haematol* 1997; **97**:810–14.
●6. Mariette X, Zagdanski AM, Guermazi A, Bergot C, Arnould A, Frija J, *et al.* Prognostic value of vertebral lesions detected by magnetic resonance imaging in patients with stage I multiple myeloma. *Br J Haematol* 1999; **104**:723–9.
●7. Hjorth M, Hallquist L, Holmberg E, Magnusson B, Rodjer S, Westin J. Initial versus deferred melphalan–prednisone therapy for asymptomatic multiple myeloma stage I: a randomised study of the Myeloma Group of Western Sweden. *Eur J Haematol* 1993; **50**:95–102.
8. Riccardi A, Mora O, Tinelli C, Valentini D, Brugnatelli S, Spanedda R, *et al.* Long-term survival of stage I multiple

myeloma given chemotherapy just after diagnosis or at progression of the disease: a multicentre randomised study. *Br J Cancer* 2000; **82**:1254–60.

9. Bergsagel DE, Bailey AJ, Langley GR, MacDonald RN, White DF, Miller AB, *et al.* The chemotherapy of plasma-cell myeloma and the incidence of acute leukaemia. *N Engl J Med* 1979; **301**:743–8.

*10. UK Myeloma Forum. Diagnosis and management of multiple myeloma. *Br J Haematol* 2001; **115**:522–40.

11. Rajkumar SV, Dispenzieri A, Fonseca R, Lacy MQ, Geyer S, Lust JA, *et al.* Thalidomide for previously untreated indolent or smoldering multiple myeloma. *Leukemia* 2001: **15**:1274–6.

12. Weber DM, Rankin K, Delasalle K, Gavino M, Alexanian R. Thalidomide alone and in combination for previously untreated myeloma. *Abstracts of the VIIIth International Myeloma Workshop*, Banff, Canada, 2001:109, abstract S66.

●13. Belch A, Shelley W, Bergsagel D, Wilson K, Klimo P, White D, *et al.* A randomised trial of maintenance versus no maintenance melphalan and prednisone in responding multiple myeloma patients. *Br J Cancer* 1988; **57**: 94–9.

14. Pacagnella A, Chiarion-Sileni V, Soesan M, Baggio G, Bolzonella D, de Besi P, *et al.* Second and third responses to the same induction regimen in relapsing patients with myeloma. *Cancer* 1991; **68**:975–80.

15. Cook G, Sharp RA, Tansey P, Franklin IM. A phase I/II trial of Z-Dex (oral idarubicin and dexamethasone), an oral equivalent of VAD, as initial therapy at diagnosis or progression in multiple myeloma. *Br J Haematol* 1996; **93**:931–4.

16. Parameswaran R, Giles C, Boots M, Littlewood TJ, Mills MJ, Kelsey SM, *et al.* CCNU (lomustine) idarubicin and dexamethasone (CIDEX): an effective oral regimen for the treatment of refractory or relapsed myeloma. *Br J Haematol* 2000; **109**:571–5.

17. Sonneveld P, Suciu S, Weijermans P, Beksac M, Neuwirtova R, Solbu G, *et al.* Cyclosporin A combined with vincristine, doxorubicin and dexamethasone (VAD) compared with VAD alone in patients with advanced refractory multiple myeloma: an EORTC-HOVON randomized phase III study (06914). *Br J Haematol* 2001; **115**:895–902.

18. Sonneveld P, Marie JP, Huisman C, Vekhoff A, Schoester M, Faussat AM, *et al.* Reversal of multidrug resistance by SDZ PSC 833, combined with VAD (vincristine, doxorubicin, dexamethasone) in refractory multiple myeloma. A phase I study. *Leukemia* 1996; **10**:1741–50.

19. Cavenagh J, Oakervee H. UK Myeloma Forum and the BCSH Haematology/Oncology Task Forces. Thalidomide in multiple myeloma: current status and future prospects. *Br J Haematol* 2003; **120**:18–26.

●20. Drayson M, Tang LX, Drew R, Mead GP, Carr-Smith H, Bradwell AR. Serum free light chain measurements for identifying and monitoring patients with nonsecretory multiple myeloma. *Blood* 2001; **7**:2900–2.

21. Rodriguez LH, Finkelstein JB, Shullenberger CC, Alexanian R. Bone healing in multiple myeloma with melphalan chemotherapy. *Ann Intern Med* 1972; **76**:551–6.

22. Moulopoulos MA, Dimopoulos MA, Alexanian R, Leeds HE, Libshitz HI. Multiple myeloma: MR patterns of response to treatment. *Radiology* 1994; **193**:441–6.

23. Chronic Leukaemia and Myeloma Task Force of the National Cancer Institute. Proposed guidelines for protocol studies. II Plasma cell myeloma. *Cancer Chemother Rep* 1973; **4**:145–58.

24. Alexanian R, Bonnet J, Gehan E, Haut A, Hewlett J, Lane M, *et al.* Combination chemotherapy for multiple myeloma. *Cancer* 1972; **30**:382–9.

25. MacLennan ICM, Chapman C, Dunn J, Kelly K. Combined chemotherapy with ABCM versus melphalan for treatment of myelomatosis. *Lancet* 1992; **339**:200–5.

26. Samson D, Gaminara E, Newland A, van de Pette J, Kearney J, McCarthy D, *et al.* Infusion of vincristine and doxorubicin with oral dexamethasone as first-line therapy for multiple myeloma. *Lancet* 1989; **2**:882–5.

27. Gore ME, Selby PJ, Viner C, Clark PI, Meldrum M, Millar B, *et al.* Intensive treatment of multiple myeloma and criteria for complete remission. *Lancet* 1989; **2**:879–82.

●28. Blade J, Samson D, Reece D, Apperley J, Bjorkstrand B, Gahrton G, *et al.* Criteria for evaluating disease response and progression in patients with multiple myeloma treated by high-dose therapy and haematopoietic stem cell transplantation. *Br J Haematol* 1998; **102**:1115–23.

29. Zent CS, Wislon CS, Tricot G, Jagannath S, Siegel D, Desikan KR, *et al.* Oligoclonal protein bands and Ig isotype switching in multiple myeloma treated with high-dose therapy and hematopoietic cell transplantation. *Blood* 1998; **91**:3518–23.

30. Mitus AJ, Stein R, Rappeport JM, Antin JH, Weinstein HJ, Alper CA, *et al.* Monoclonal and oligoclonal gammopathy after bone marrow transplantation. *Blood* 1989; **74**:2764–8.

31. Hovenga S, de Wolf JT, Guikema JE, Klip H, Smit JW, Sibinga CT, *et al.* Autologous stem cell transplantation in multiple myeloma after VAD and EDAP courses: a high incidence of oligoclonal serum Igs post transplantation. *Bone Marrow Transplant* 2000; **25**:723–8.

32. Bouko Y, Goldschmidt H, Feremans W, Bourhis J-H, Szydlo R, Greinix H, *et al.* Oligoclonal reconstitution after high-dose therapy with PBPCT in myeloma patients: implications for assessment of remission status. *Bone Marrow Transplant* 2002; **29**(Suppl 2): S102.

33. Palmer M, Belch A, Brox L, Pollock E, Koch M. Are the current criteria for response useful in the management of multiple myeloma? *J Clin Oncol* 1987; **5**:1373–7.

34. Baldini L, Radaelli F, Chiorboli O, Furnagalli S, Cro L, Segala M, *et al.* No correlation between response and survival in patients with multiple myeloma treated with vincristine, melphalan, cyclophosphamide and prednisone. *Cancer* 1991; **68**:62–7.

35. Marmont F, Levis A, Falda M, Resegotti L. Lack of correlation between objective response and death rate in multiple myeloma patients treated with oral melphalan and prednisone. *Ann Oncol* 1991; **2**:191–5.

36. Joshua DE, Penny R, Matthews JP, Laidlaw CR, Gibson J, Bradstock K, *et al.*, for the Australian Leukaemia Study Group. Australian Leukaemia Study Group Myeloma II: a randomised trial of intensive combination chemotherapy with or without interferon in patients with myeloma. *Br J Haematol* 1997; **97**:38–45.

37. Oivanen TM, Kellokumpu-Lehtinen P, Koivisto AM, Koivunen E, Palva I. Response level and survival after conventional chemotherapy for multiple myeloma: a

Finnish Leukaemia Group study. *Eur J Haematol* 1999; **62**:109–16.

38. Raje N, Powles R, Kulkarni S, Milan S, Middleton G, Singhal S, *et al.* A comparison of vincristine and doxorubicin infusional chemotherapy with methylprednisolone (VAMP) with the addition of weekly cyclophosphamide (C-VAMP) as induction treatment followed by autografting in previously untreated myeloma. *Br J Haematol* 1997; **97**:153–60.

39. Gahrton G, Tura S, Ljungman P, Belanger C, Brandt L, Cavo M, *et al.* Allogeneic bone marrow transplantation in multiple myeloma. European Group for Bone Marrow Transplantation. *N Engl J Med* 1991; **325**:1267–73.

40. Gahrton G, Tura S, Ljungman P, Blade J, Brandt L, Cavo M, *et al.* Prognostic factors in allogeneic bone marrow transplantation for multiple myeloma. *J Clin Oncol* 1995; **13**:1312–22.

41. Bjorkstrand B, Ljungman P, Bird JM, Samson D, Brandt L, Alegre A, *et al.* Autologous stem cell transplantation in multiple myeloma: results of the European Group for Bone Marrow Transplantation. *Stem Cells* 1995; **13**(Suppl. 2):140–6.

42. Attal M, Harousseau JL, Stoppa AM, Sotto JJ, Fuzibet JG, Rossi JF, *et al.* A prospective randomized trial of autologous transplantation and chemotherapy in multiple myeloma. *N Engl J Med* 1996; **335**: 91–7.

43. Barlogie B, Jagannath S, Vesole DH, Naucke S, Cheson B, Mattox S, *et al.* Superiority of tandem autologous transplantation over standard therapy for previously untreated multiple myeloma. *Blood* 1197; **89**:789–93.

●44. Lahuerta JJ, Martinez-Lopez J, Serna JD, Blade J, Grande C, Alegre A, *et al.* Remission status defined by immunofixation vs. electrophoresis after autologous transplantation has a major impact on the outcome of multiple myeloma patients. *Br J Haematol* 2000; **109**:438–43.

45. Davies FE, Forsyth PD, Rawstron AC, Owen RG, Pratt G, Evans PA, *et al.* The impact of attaining a minimal disease state after high-dose melphalan and autologous transplantation for multiple myeloma. *Br J Haematol* 2001; **112**:814–9.

46. Cavo M, Terragna C, Martinelli G, Ronconi S, Zamagni E, Tosi P, *et al.* Molecular monitoring of minimal residual disease in patients in long-term complete remission after allogeneic stem cell transplantation for multiple myeloma. *Blood* 2000; **96**:355–7.

47. Martinelli G, Terragna C, Zamagni E, Ronconi S, Tosi P, Lemoli RM, *et al.* Molecular remission after allogeneic or autologous transplantation of hematopoietic stem cells for multiple myeloma. *J Clin Oncol* 2000; **18**:2273–81.

48. Rasmussen T, Poulsen TS, Honore L, Johnsen HE. Quantitation of minimal residual disease in multiple myeloma using an allele-specific real-time PCR assay. *Exp Hematol* 2000; **28**:1039–45.

49. Lipinski E, Cremer FW, Ho AD, Goldschmidt H, Moos M. Molecular monitoring of the tumor load predicts progressive disease in patients with multiple myeloma after high-dose therapy with autologous peripheral blood stem cell transplantation. *Bone Marrow Transplant* 2001; **28**:957–62.

◆50. Davies FE, Rawstron AC, Owen RG, Morgan GJ. Minimal residual disease monitoring in multiple myeloma. *Best Pract Res Clin Haematol* 2002; **15**:197–222.

51. San Miguel JF, Almeida J, Mateo G, Blade J, Lopez-Berges C, Caballero D, *et al.* Immunophenotypic evaluation of the plasma cell compartment in multiple myeloma: a tool for comparing the efficacy of different treatment strategies and predicting outcome. *Blood* 2002; **99**:1853–6.

52. Alegre A, Granda A, Martinez-Chamorro C, Diaz-Mediavilla J, Martinez R, Garcia-Larana J, *et al.*; Spanish Registry of Transplants in Multiple Myelomas; Spanish Group of Hemopoietic Transplant (GETH); PETHEMA. Different patterns of relapse after autologous peripheral blood stem cell transplantation in multiple myeloma: clinical results of 280 cases from the Spanish Registry. *Haematologica* 2002; **87**:609–14.

53. Biagi JJ, Mileshkin L, Grigg AP, Westerman DW, Prince HM. Efficacy of thalidomide therapy for extramedullary relapse of myeloma following allogeneic transplantation. *Bone Marrow Transplant* 2001; **28**:1145–50.

●54. Orchard K, Barrington S, Buscombe J, Hilson A, Prentice HG, Mehta A. Fluoro-deoxyglucose positron emission tomography imaging for the detection of occult disease in multiple myeloma. *Br J Haematol* 2002; **117**:133–5.

55. Stead ML, Brown JM, Velikova G, Kaasa S, Wisloff F, Child JA, *et al.* Development of an EORTC questionnaire module to be used in health-related quality-of life assessment for patients with multiple myeloma. European Organisation for Research and Treatment of Cancer Study Group on Quality of Life. *Br J Haematol* 1999; **104**:605–11.

56. Porche R, Levy V, Fermand JP, Katsahian S, Chevret S, Ravaud P. Evaluating high-dose therapy in multiple myeloma: use of quality-adjusted survival analysis. *Qual Life Res* 2002; **11**:91–9.

●57. Wisloff F, Eika S, Hippe E, Hjorth M, Holmberg E, Kaasa S, *et al.* Measurement of health-related quality of life in multiple myeloma. Nordic Myeloma Study Group. *Br J Haematol* 1996; **92**:604–13.

58. Wisloff F, Hjorth M. Health-related quality of life assessed before and during chemotherapy predicts for survival in multiple myeloma. Nordic Myeloma Study Group. *J Clin Oncol* 1997; **97**:29–37.

59. Wisloff F, Gulbrandsen N. Health-related quality of life and patients' perceptions in interferon-treated multiple myeloma patients. Nordic Myeloma Study Group. *Acta Oncol* 2000; **39**:809–13.

60. Wisloff F, Hjorth M, Kaasa S, Westin J. Effect of interferon on the health-related quality of life of multiple myeloma patients: results of a Nordic randomized trial comparing melphalan-prednisolone with melphalan-prednisolone plus alpha-interferon. The Nordic Myeloma Study Group. *Br J Haematol* 1996; **94**:324–32.

61. Zee B, Cole B, Li T, Browman G, James K, Johnston D, *et al.* Quality-adjusted time without symptoms or toxicity analysis of interferon maintenance in multiple myeloma. *J Clin Oncol* 1998; **1**:2834–9.

62. Gulbrandsen N, Wisloff F, Nord E, Lenhoff S, Hjorth M, Westin J. Cost–utility analysis of high-dose melphalan with autologous blood stem cell support vs. melphalan plus prednisone in patients younger than 60 years with multiple myeloma. *Eur J Haematol* 2001; **66**:328–36.

63. Gulbrandsen N, Wisloff F, Brinch L, Carlson K, Dahl IM, Gimsing P, *et al.*; The Nordic Myeloma Study Group.

Health-related quality of life in multiple myeloma patients receiving high-dose chemotherapy with autologous blood stem-cell support. *Med Oncol* 2001; **18**:65–77.

64. Lind M, Vernon C, Cruickshank D, Wilkinson P, Littlewood T, Stuart N, *et al.* The level of haemoglobin in anaemic cancer patients correlates positively with quality of life. *Br J Cancer* 2002; **86**:1243–9.

65. Dammacco F, Castoldi G, Rodjer S. Efficacy of epoetin alfa in the treatment of anaemia of multiple myeloma. *Br J Haematol* 2001; **113**:172–9.

◆66. Littlewood TJ, Bajetta E, Nortier JW, Vercammen E, Rapoport B. Effects of epoetin alfa on hematologic parameters and quality of life in cancer patients receiving nonplatinum chemotherapy: results of a randomized, double-blind, placebo-controlled trial. *J Clin Oncol* 2001; **19**:2865–74.

67. Peest D, Coldewey R, Deicher H. Overall vs. tumour-related survival In multiple myeloma. *Eur J Cancer* 1991; **27**:672.

◆68. Myeloma Trialists' Collaborative Group. Combination chemotherapy versus melphalan plus prednisone as treatment for multiple myeloma: an overview of 6,633 patients from 27 randomized trials. *J Clin Oncol* 1998; **16**:3832–42.

◆69. Myeloma Trialists' Collaborative Group. Interferon as therapy for multiple myeloma: an individual patient data overview of 24 randomized trials and 4012 patients. *Br J Haematol* 2001; **113**:1020–34.

70. Hjorth M, Holmberg E, Rodjer S, Westin J. Impact of active and passive exclusions on the results of a clinical trial in multiple myeloma. The Myeloma Group of Western Sweden. *Br J Haematol* 1992; **80**:55–61.

71. Imrie K, Esmail R, Meyer M. The role of high-dose chemotherapy and stem cell transplantation in patients with multiple myeloma: a practice guideline of the Cancer Care Ontario Practice Guidelines Initiative. *Ann Intern Med* 2002; **136**:619–29.

*72. Djulbegovic B, Wheatley K, Ross J, Clark O, Bos G, Goldschmidt H, *et al.* Bisphosphonates in multiple myeloma. *Cochrane Database Syst Rev* 2001; (4):CD003188.

*73. Berenson JR, Hillner BE, Kyle RA, Anderson K, Lipton A, Yee GC, *et al.* American Society of Clinical Oncology Practice Guidelines: the role of bisphosphonates in multiple myeloma. *J Clin Oncol* 2002; **20**:3719–36.

*74. Soutar RL, Lucraft H, Jackson G, Reece A, Bird J, Low E, *et al.* Guidelines on the diagnosis and management of solitary plasmacytoma of bone (SBP) and solitary extramedullary plasmacytoma (SEP). www.ukmf.org.uk and *Br J Haematol* 2004 (in press).

*75. Bird J, Cavenagh J, Hawkins P, Lachmann H, Mehta A, Samson D, for the UK Myeloma Forum. Guidelines on the diagnosis and management of AL amyloidosis. www.ukmf.org.uk and *Br J Haematol* 2004 (in press).

14

Chemotherapy, steroids, and interferon

DIANA M. SAMSON

INTRODUCTION

Before the introduction of melphalan in 1958,[1] the average survival of myeloma patients was only a few months. Alexanian et al.[2] in 1969 first published the results of treatment with oral melphalan and prednisolone (MP), using different dosage regimens with or without prednisolone, and demonstrated prolongation of survival to between 17 and 24 months. Although there are now several promising new approaches to treatment, chemotherapy remains the mainstay of treatment in multiple myeloma (MM). Many patients will also require radiotherapy at some stage in their disease. This chapter will review the use of standard-dose chemotherapy, including the use of steroids and interferon, and will discuss options for management in different patient groups.

CHEMOTHERAPY

A summary of the most widely used chemotherapy regimes is given in Table 14.1, and the most important characteristics of frequently used cytotoxic agents[3,4] are shown in Table 14.2.

Melphalan ± prednisolone

Alkylating agents, such as melphalan, act principally by cross-linking of DNA strands, preventing replication of DNA and transcription of RNA, and are cell-cycle-non-specific. In the study of oral melphalon and prednisone

reported by Alexanian et al.[2] in 1969, different dosage regimens were compared with or without prednisone, producing median survival times of 17–24 months. Both continuous and intermittent melphalan were equally effective, but the intermittent schedule causes less myelosuppression and requires less dose modification and has become the accepted method of giving melphalan. Numerous other studies of oral melphalan or MP have confirmed a response rate in the order of 50%, with survival varying between 2 and 4 years.[5–8]

Melphalan is generally well tolerated and alopecia is rare. Mild degrees of nausea do occur. The major toxicity is myelosuppression, with platelets generally affected more severely than neutrophils. Melphalan should not generally be used in patients with platelets $<75 \times 10^9$/L or neutrophils $<1.0 \times 10^9$/L. There is a long-term risk of secondary acute myeloid leukemia (AML).[9,10]

Response to MP is typically gradual over a period of 3–6 months and it may take several months to reach maximal response. This may be a disadvantage for patients with aggressive disease. Complete remission, i.e. disappearance of the paraprotein with a normal number of plasma cells in the bone marrow, is exceptional. Most patients reach a stable plateau phase, defined as paraprotein level stable for at least 3 months and transfusion independent with minimal symptoms. Plateau phase usually lasts 18–24 months before relapse. Continuing chemotherapy after attainment of plateau phase does not prolong remission but many patients will respond again to MP at the time of first relapse.[11]

Recommendations on the use of oral melphalan are shown in Table 14.3. Since meta-analysis of published trials has shown no convincing survival benefit for

Table 14.1 *Chemotherapy regimens most frequently used in multiple myeloma (see text for references)*

Type of chemotherapy	Regimen	Drugs	Overall and complete response (CR) rates[a] (%)	Overall survival[a] (median)
Simple alkylating agents	MP C-weekly CWAP	Melphalan and prednis(ol)one Cyclophosphamide weekly (oral or IV) Cyclophosphamide weekly plus alternate-day prednis(ol)one	50–60% (5% CR)	2.5–3.5 years
Alkylator-based combination chemotherapy	VBMCP (M-2 protocol) VMCP/VBAP ABCM CIDEX	Vincristine, BCNU, melphalan, cyclophosphamide, prednis(ol)one Vincristine, melphalan, cyclophosphamide, and prednis(ol)one, alternating with vincristine, BCNU, Adriamycin, and prednis(ol)one Adriamycin and BCNU alternating with cyclophosphamide and melphalan CCNU, oral idarubicin, and dexamethasone	65–70% (10% CR) Not tested in newly diagnosed patients	2.5–3.5 years n/a
VAD-type regimens	VAD VAMP C-VAMP Z-Dex	Infused vincristine and Adriamycin with pulsed high-dose dexamethasone As VAD, with IV methyl prednisolone in place of dexamethasone As VAMP, with weekly IV cyclophosphamide Oral idarubicin and pulsed high-dose dexamethasone	70–75% (10–20% CR)	2.5–3.5 years when not followed by high-dose therapy
High-dose dexamethasone	HDDex	Pulsed dexamethasone as in VAD	65%	No data
Other combinations	EDAP DCEP CEVAD DT-PACE	Infused etoposide, cytosine arabinoside, and cisplatin with dexamethasone Cyclophosphamide, etoposide, and cisplatin with dexamethasone Cyclophosphamide, etoposide, vincristine, Adriamycin, and dexamethasone Thalidomide and dexamethasone with pulsed infusions of cisplatin, Adriamycin, cyclophosphamide, and etoposide	No published data on results of initial therapy in newly diagnosed patients	n/a

[a] In newly-diagnosed patients.
BCNU, 1,3-bis(2-chloroethyl)-1-nitrosourea [carmustine]; CCNU, 1-(2-chloroethyl)-3-cyclohexyl-1-nitrosourea [lomustine]; IV, intravenous; n/a, not applicable.

combination chemotherapy as compared with oral melphalan and prednisolone (see later), melphalan with or without prednisolone remains the treatment of choice for most patients in whom high-dose therapy is not planned, i.e. most elderly patients. Melphalan should be avoided in patients in whom it is planned to proceed to high-dose therapy (HDT), because toxicity to normal marrow stem cells may be cumulative and may compromise their subsequent harvest.[12–14]

MELPHALAN DOSAGE

Melphalan may be administered orally or intravenously. It is erratically absorbed (25–90%) from the gastrointestinal tract and the absorption is reduced by food so that it should be taken on an empty stomach. Typical doses of melphalan in different protocols have been 0.2–0.25 mg/kg per day or 7–9 mg/m^2 per day for 4 days every 4–6 weeks, with a range from 6 to 12 mg/m^2 per day.[15] There is some evidence to suggest that dose intensity of oral melphalan is correlated with outcome; Fernberg *et al.*[7] observed a correlation with cumulative melphalan dose and response. However, in a meta-analysis of trials comparing MP with combination chemotherapy, it was concluded that there was no evidence for a difference in outcome depending on melphalan dose intensity in patients receiving MP.[15]

Table 14.2 *Cytotoxic agents used in treating multiple myeloma[3,4]*

Drug	Route of administration	Metabolism	Main route of elimination	Predominant toxicities	Comments
Melphalan	Oral or IV	Spontaneous hydrolysis, conjugation to glutathione	Most non-renal; part renal	Myelosuppression	Absorption very variable. Toxicity increased in renal failure: reduce dose or avoid
Cyclophosphamide	Oral or IV	Metabolized by liver to active metabolites	Renal (parent drug and metabolites)	Myelosuppression; hemorrhagic cystitis	Maintain good hydration. Use MESNA with high doses. Reduce dose in severe renal failure
Carmustine (BCNU)[a]	IV	Metabolized by liver	Renal	Myelosuppression; pulmonary fibrosis	Myelosuppression can be long-lasting and cumulative
Lomustine (CCNU)[a]	Oral	Metabolized by liver	Renal	Myelosuppression; pulmonary fibrosis	Myelosuppression can be long-lasting and cumulative
Doxorubicin (Adriamycin)	IV	Metabolized by liver; doxorubicinol also active	Bile (doxo and doxol)	Myelosuppression; cardiomyopathy	No dose modification required in renal failure. Maximum recommended cumulative dose 450 mg/m^2
Idarubicin	Oral or IV	Metabolized by liver; idarubicinol also active	Bile; part renal (idarubicin and idarubicinol)	Myelosuppression; cardiomyopathy	Dose reduction of oral idarubicin may be advisable in renal failure. Maximum recommended cumulative dose not clearly established
Vincristine	IV	Metabolized by liver	Bile	Neuropathy	No dose modification required in renal failure
Etoposide	Oral or IV	Metabolized by liver	Renal; part in bile	Myelosuppression	Reduce dose in renal failure

[a] See footnote to Table 14.1.
IV, intravenous.

Table 14.3 *Recommendations on the use of oral melphalan (UK Myeloma Forum, 2001)[21]*

- Melphalan with or without prednisolone is the initial treatment of choice for most patients in whom high-dose therapy is not planned
- The neutrophil count should be $>1.0 \times 10^9$/L and the platelet count $>75 \times 10^9$/L before treatment. The dose should be modified if severe myelotoxicity occurs
- Treatment should be continued to plateau phase (paraprotein level stable for 3 months) and then stopped
- Melphalan should be used with caution in patients with renal impairment
- The evidence of benefit from steroids in standard doses is controversial. It is, therefore, reasonable not to include prednisolone, particularly in patients at risk of steroid-related side effects

Because absorption of oral melphalan is variable, it has been suggested that the dose be increased until there is evidence of myelosuppression.[8] However, there is no evidence that this produces benefit in practice, and in one trial hematological toxicity was similar in responders and non-responders.[7] (An equivalent dose given intravenously was not found to improve response rate or survival.[16])

MELPHALAN IN RENAL IMPAIRMENT

The majority of the drug is cleared by non-renal mechanisms but renal clearance is also important. In one study it was found that 21–34% of drug was excreted unchanged in the urine.[17] There is a negative correlation between the area under the curve of plasma melphalan concentration and renal function,[18] and myelosuppression is enhanced in patients with renal failure.[19] However, the extent of drug accumulation is variable in each individual and cannot be predicted from the degree of renal impairment.[20] It is, therefore, difficult to make accurate dose adjustments in patients with renal impairment. Initial doses should be reduced if the glomerular filtration rate (GFR) is below 40–50 mL/minute and titrated against bone marrow toxicity in subsequent courses. It is recommended that melphalan should not generally be used in patients where the GFR is below 30 mL/minute.[21]

THE ROLE OF PREDNISOLONE

In Alexanian's original study,[2] the best results were achieved with a combination of intermittent melphalan (0.25 mg/kg per day) together with prednisone (2 mg/kg per day) both for 4 days every 6 weeks. Objective response rate was 70% (Southwest Oncology Group (SWOG) criteria; see Chapter 13), as compared with 35% for intermittent melphalan alone and 19% for continuous daily melphalan. Median survival was 24 months in the prednisone group compared with 17–18 months with melphalan alone. Most subsequent studies using oral melphalan have also used predniso(lo)ne, although there are other randomized studies that do not support the conclusion that the addition of steroid to melphalan or combination chemotherapy improves long-term survival.[23–25] In two Medical Research Council (MRC) trials there was no benefit from the addition of standard doses of corticosteroids to oral melphalan or to the ABCM combination chemotherapy regimen.[26,27] Thus, it is reasonable to omit steroids if there are concerns about possible side-effects.[21]

INTERMEDIATE–DOSE INTRAVENOUS MELPHALAN

The first attempt to induce complete remission with HDT was with the use of high-dose melphalan, pioneered by McElwain and colleagues at the Royal Marsden Hospital. A single administration of melphalan at a dose of 140 mg/m^2 resulted in an encouraging 25% complete remission rate in previously untreated patients, but without stem cell or growth factor support there was significant treatment-related mortality.[28] For this reason, high-dose melphalan 140 mg/m^2 is usually only given with stem cell support, although the toxicity can be reduced significantly by the use of growth factors, provided there is adequate bone marrow reserve.[29]

In the past few years, several authors have investigated the use of intravenous melphalan at intermediate dosage (doses between 25 and 70 mg/m^2). Tsakanikas et al.[30] used a single dose of melphalan (50–70 mg/m^2) to treat 18 patients with advanced disease resistant to VAD. There was a 50% objective response rate with a median response duration of 6 months and median survival of 11.5

months. Three other groups have used serial courses of intravenous melphalan at a dose approximately equivalent to the dose that would be given orally in standard melphalan therapy. Petrucci et al.[31] treated 34 patients with relapsed or refractory myeloma using a dose of 20 mg/m^2 melphalan plus prednisolone every 4–6 weeks for 12 courses. Treatment was administered on an outpatient basis. A total of 35% of patients responded and the median duration of survival in these patients was not reached at 28 months of follow-up. The median duration of response was 16 months. A Swedish study[32] used a similar regime of 30 mg/m^2 every 4–6 weeks for up to 12 courses. Six of eight patients reached objective response after 1–5 courses. Schey et al.[33] reported an 82% response rate in newly diagnosed patients using melphalan 25 mg/m^2 with dexamethasone. There was moderate myelotoxicity in these studies, although there were no treatment-related deaths. While the response rate may be higher than with standard oral MP, this is not certain without a randomized study and it is not clear that long-term outcome is improved.

Cyclophosphamide ± steroids

In early placebo-controlled studies, oral cyclophosphamide given at a dose of 2–4 mg/kg per day continuously was found to prolong survival,[34,35] and cyclophosphamide was also found to be effective in melphalan-resistant patients.[36] Several randomized trials have shown that cyclophosphamide produces results similar to those of melphalan in terms of response rate and survival.[23,37,38] The third MRC myeloma trial showed no difference between MP and intravenous cyclophosphamide (600 mg/m^2 3-weekly).[26] The use of intravenous cyclophosphamide was further developed in the CWAP regimen – weekly intravenous cyclophosphamide (150–300 mg/m^2) with alternate-day prednisolone. This was found to be more effective than cyclophosphamide given every 4 weeks and produced responses in approximately 50% of patients with advanced disease, including patients who were resistant to melphalan and also some who had failed on oral cyclophosphamide therapy.[39,40] Weekly cyclophosphamide is considerably less myelotoxic than melphalan, and was used without prednisolone (C-weekly) in the MRC fifth myeloma trial for patients with cytopenia precluding combination therapy (ABCM) or oral melphalan.[25] There have been no randomized trials comparing C-weekly with MP, but cross-trial analysis of C-weekly with melphalan in the MRC Myeloma IV and V trials suggested similar efficacy. It is interesting that in the Myeloma V study, patients changing from ABCM to C-weekly because of myelosuppression actually survived at least as long if not longer than non-cytopenic patients continuing on ABCM. There is, however, no formal study of C-weekly as a first-line therapy. An oral equivalent of the IV C-weekly schedule is cyclophosphamide 600 mg/m^2 weekly. There are no data from randomized controlled trials on the effect of adding prednisolone to cyclophosphamide. However, since cyclophosphamide is used mainly in patients with cytopenia, there may be an advantage to the addition of steroids.

Recommendations on the use of cyclophosphamide are shown in Table 14.4. Cyclophosphamide is generally well tolerated, although it causes more alopecia than melphalan. The dose-limiting toxicity is myelosuppression, and neutrophils are generally more affected than platelets. However, it is less myelotoxic than melphalan and the C-weekly regimen was successfully used in the MRC Myeloma V trial in patients with cytopenia. There is a risk of hemorrhagic cystitis, although this is rare at conventional doses. It is generally recommended that cyclophosphamide be given in the morning so that the toxic metabolites do not remain in the bladder overnight. Patients should be encouraged to maintain a high fluid intake. When high doses are given, intravenous hydration and sodium 2-mercapto-ethane sulfonate (MESNA) are recommended.

CYCLOPHOSPHAMIDE IN RENAL FAILURE

Most of the parent compound is cleared by hepatic metabolism, but the kidney is the main route of excretion for the active metabolites of cyclophosphamide and there may be significant retention of these in patients with severe renal failure. However, dose adjustment does not appear to be necessary unless severe renal insufficiency is present.[41] The manufacturer's recommendations are that the dose should be reduced by 25% if the GFR is 10–50 mL/minute, and by 50% if the GFR is less than 10 mL/minute.

Alkylator–based combination chemotherapy regimens

Various combination regimens have been used in an attempt to improve the outcome obtained with simple alkylating agents. These regimens generally include cyclophosphamide and melphalan with two or more of the following drugs: vincristine (V), Adriamycin (A),

Table 14.4 *Recommendations on the use of cyclophosphamide (UK Myeloma Forum, 2001)*[21]

- Cyclophosphamide is suitable for patients who would otherwise be treated with melphalan or MP,[a] but in whom the neutrophil and/or platelet counts are below the required level
- Treatment should be continued to plateau phase (paraprotein level stable for 3 months) and then stopped
- Cyclophosphamide should be used with caution in patients with renal impairment

[a] See Table 14.1.

prednisolone (P), and BCNU (B). In an early SWOG study, patients receiving V had survival times longer than those in any previous SWOG study.[42] V alone given after initial chemotherapy produced a further reduction in tumor mass in some responding patients,[43] possibly because cells were recruited into the cell cycle when the tumor mass was reduced by prior chemotherapy. A Cancer and Leukaemia Group B (CALGB) study compared melphalan, BCNU, and CCNU as initial single-agent therapy and found the three drugs to be equally effective in terms of response rate, myelotoxicity, and survival.[44] Alberts et al.[45,46] reported the effectiveness of Adriamycin and combined Adriamycin/BCNU in relapsed patients resistant to melphalan. Several multidrug regimens have been developed incorporating some or all of these agents. The most widely used have been the VBMCP regimen (a minor modification of the M-2 protocol) used by the Eastern Cooperative Oncology Group (ECOG) and the VMCP/VBAP protocol developed by the SWOG. The relative contribution of the various components to overall efficacy remains unclear, particularly in the case of vincristine, since the IV MRC myeloma trial failed to show any advantage for bolus injections of vincristine in addition to MP.[47]

These combination regimens are more complicated to administer than single alkylating agents. They require intravenous delivery of some of the drugs and more frequent hospital attendance. They are also more toxic (e.g. more myelosuppression, vomiting, alopecia, cardiotoxicity, infection). Combinations that include melphalan or nitrosoureas may prejudice subsequent stem-cell harvesting.[12–14]

THE VBMCP (M–2) PROTOCOL

The use of the M-2 protocol in myeloma was first published by Case et al.,[48] who reported results in 73 patients. Over 80% of previously untreated and 13/26 previously treated patients obtained objective responses (50% tumor reduction). Projected median survival in the previously untreated patients was over 3 years, which compared favorably with historical controls treated with MP in whom median survival was 22 months. The ECOG subsequently carried out a large randomized study comparing VBMCP with MP.[49,50] This confirmed higher response rate and longer remission duration and, although there was no long-term survival benefit, the VBMCP regimen has continued to be the basis for ECOG studies and has also been used by other groups. MOCCA is a similar regimen, incorporating methyl prednisolone, vincristine (O), cyclophosphamide, CCNU, and melphalan (A: Alkeran).[51,52]

VMCP AND VMCP/VBAP

The VMCP/VBAP regimen, using the same drugs as VBMCP plus Adriamycin, was a development from early studies at the MD Anderson Hospital in which the following combinations were evaluated: VMCP, VCAP, VBAP,

CAP, and VCP.[42] Response rates (SWOG criteria) were 55–64% for all the four-drug combinations, but only 14% for VCP and 45% for CAP. Thus, inclusion of both V and A gave a higher response rate. The next step was to evaluate alternating combinations, including all the available drugs known to be active in myeloma – VMCP/VCAP and VMCP/VBAP. The response rates for both these alternating regimens were the same, and were not significantly different from those achieved in the earlier study using any of the three four-drug regimens.[53] However, the SWOG adopted the alternating combination including BCNU, i.e. VMCP/VBAP, for several subsequent studies and it has become one of the most widely used of the standard combination chemotherapy regimens.

ABCM

The ABCM regimen used by the MRC in the Myeloma V and VI studies is similar in many ways to VMCP/VBAP, since it includes four of the same drugs and alternates drug combinations at 3-weekly intervals (AB alternating with CM; see Table 14.1). It differs in that both V and P are omitted, since neither had been shown to improve survival in previous MRC studies.[23,47,54] Data from cross-trial analysis comparing results of the MRC trials using ABCM (V and VI) and SWOG studies suggest that ABCM and VMCP/VBAP are similarly effective.[55]

OTHER ALKYLATOR-BASED COMBINATIONS

There are a number of other similar standard-dose combination chemotherapy regimens, including VBAMDex and VBAD.[56,57]

Is alkylator-based combination chemotherapy more effective than a single alkylating agent with prednis(ol)one?

Over 20 randomized trials have been carried out comparing such regimens with melphalan or MP (see Myeloma Trialists' Collaborative Group[15] for references). While many of the studies found an increased response rate as compared with MP, and a complete remission (CR) rate up to 10%, only two studies observed a significant survival benefit. The first of these was an early SWOG study comparing VMCP/VBAP with MP,[58,59] a benefit not confirmed in later studies.[60,61] The other was the MRC Myeloma V trial, which compared ABCM and melphalan alone.[25] This is the largest randomized study reported and produced a highly significant benefit for survival in patients treated with ABCM; median survival of 32 vs. 24 months ($P < 0.0001$). Significant survival benefit was observed in all prognostic subgroups, stratified either by β_2-microglobulin level or by the Cuzick index.[62] The magnitude of the survival advantage was, however, relatively modest in clinical terms, with median survival

being prolonged by only a few months, and less than 25% of patients in the ABCM arm surviving at 5 years.

A meta-analysis of 6633 patients in 27 randomized trials comparing combination chemotherapy (CCT) with MP was undertaken by the Myeloma Trialists' Collaborative Group.[15] They found that taking the results of all the trials together, response rates were significantly higher than with MP (60% vs. 53.2%, $P < 0.00001$). However, there was no significant difference in mortality between CCT and MP (Fig. 14.1). These results confirmed the findings of an earlier meta-analysis of 18 trials.[63] This earlier study had suggested that CCT might be better than MP in patients with a poor prognosis, but the larger meta-analysis failed to find any group where there was a significant difference in outcome; in particular, there was no evidence that poor-risk patients benefited more from CCT. A small number of studies have subsequently been published confirming the lack of benefit of CCT.[64–66] It can be concluded that there is no significant survival benefit for combination chemotherapy either for patients overall or in any prognostic subgroup.

The position regarding ABCM is rather unusual. The results of the MRC Myeloma V study were not included in either of the two meta-analyses. The results were not

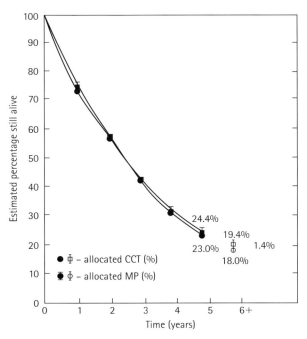

Figure 14.1 *Overall survival of patients in trials of combination chemotherapy (CCT) vs. melphalan and predniolone. From a meta-analysis of 4930 patients in 20 trials carried out by the Myeloma Trialists' Collaborative Group.[15] Reproduced from Myeloma Trialists' Collaborative Group, combination chemotherapy versus melphalan plus prednisone as treatment for multiple myeloma: an overview of 6633 patients from 27 randomized trials, J Clin Oncol 1998; 16:3822–42, with permission from Lippincott, Williams and Wilkins.*

Table 14.5 *Recommendations on the use of alkylator-based combination chemotherapy (UK Myeloma Forum, 2001)*[21]

- Combination chemotherapy regimens offer no clear advantage over single alkylating agents, but may be considered as an alternative to melphalan or MP[a] for patients in whom it is not planned to proceed to high-dose therapy
- The ABCM[a] regimen is recommended, if combination chemotherapy is to be used[b]
- Possible benefits should be balanced against the increased side effects, particularly in patients over the age of 65
- Treatment should be continued to plateau phase and then stopped
- These regimens should be used with caution in patients with renal impairment

[a] See Table 14.1.
[b] See text for discussion.

yet available at the time of the earlier analysis and it was not included in the Myeloma Trialists' Collaborative Group meta-analysis because the standard arm was melphalan alone rather than MP. Although a cross-trial comparison suggested the efficacy of ABCM regimen did not differ significantly from that of regimens such as VMCP/VBAP[55] as noted, this was one of the few trials to show a significant benefit for combination chemotherapy. For this reason, the UK Myeloma Forum guidelines recommend the use of the ABCM regimen in preference to other combination regimens (Table 14.5). Although some investigators feel that the benefit of ABCM in the Myeloma V study was due to a suboptimal standard arm, cross-trial analysis with previous MRC studies showed that results of M7 were similar to those of the M and P or MVP.

VAD and similar regimens

VAD

The first of these regimens to be introduced was the VAD regimen, developed by Barlogie *et al.*[67] It is a combination of vincristine (V), Adriamycin (A), and dexamethasone (D), but differs from conventional regimens in that the V and A are given not as bolus injections but by continuous infusion over 4 days. The rationale for the slow infusion was to expose the myeloma cells to the cytotoxic drugs over a longer period. Modifications of the regimen include VAMP, where methyl prednisolone replaces dexamethasone, and MOD, where mitoxantrone is substituted for Adriamycin. The VAD regimen was found to be more effective than any previously described regimen in relapsed patients with a response rate of approximately 40% and a survival of over 1 year in responding

patients.[67] These results were confirmed in other studies.[68–71]

In newly diagnosed patients, VAD is associated with a high response rate of 60–80% and an appreciable CR rate of between 10 and 25%.[72–74] Response is rapid, with 90% of maximum response reached after two courses of treatment.[72] Some patients respond more slowly, but if there is no evidence of response after two courses, the patient is unlikely to respond and treatment should be changed.

Unfortunately, the remissions achieved with VAD are not durable, lasting on average only 18 months, even in patients who achieve CR.[72] In an attempt to improve the duration of the remission, one group has given MP in between VAD cycles,[75] and others have used either concurrent or maintenance interferon.[74,76] Neither of these approaches appears to result in more durable responses. For many patients, therefore, VAD is not superior to other chemotherapy combinations and, in the only published study comparing VAD with other first-line therapy, there was no benefit of VAD over VBMCP in terms of response rate or survival.[77]

Nevertheless, the VAD regimen has advantages in certain situations. Since none of the drugs are renally excreted, it can be given without dosage modification in patients in severe renal failure, including those on dialysis.[72,78] It produces almost no myelosuppression, and so is particularly useful in patients presenting with neutropenia or thrombocytopenia. It is also an ideal initial cytoreductive therapy for patients in whom it is planned to proceed to stem cell harvest. The rate of response is dramatic, with most patients achieving 90% of their maximum response within 6 weeks, an advantage in patients who require rapid tumor reduction, e.g. those with rapidly progressive bone disease. The cardiotoxicity of Adriamycin is reduced by giving it as a continuous infusion.[79] The main disadvantages are the necessity for a central venous line for administration, and the high incidence of steroid-related side effects.

Recommendations for the use of VAD are shown in Table 14.6. When used as induction prior to high-dose therapy, there is probably no advantage to giving more than three to four courses, as most patients reach maximal cytoreduction by this stage.[72]

MODIFICATIONS OF VAD

It is not entirely clear whether the method of administration, i.e. by continuous slow infusion, is essential for the effectiveness of the VAD regimen. One non-randomized study where V and A were infused over 2 hours suggested that response rates were lower than expected with standard VAD.[80] However, another non-randomized study in 139 newly diagnosed patients, where VA was administered by rapid infusion, observed a response rate of 67%.[81] A recent study has used liposomal doxorubicin

Table 14.6 *Recommendations on the use of VAD-type regimens and high-dose dexamethasone (UK Myeloma Forum (2001)[21]*

- A VAD[a]-type regimen should be used as primary chemotherapy for patients in whom it is intended to offer high-dose therapy (updated recommendations in preparation indicate that HDDex[a] may be considered as an alternative)
- VAD is appropriate chemotherapy for patients presenting with renal failure and for patients in whom a rapid response is required
- HDDex alone is recommended for initial treatment in patients in whom cytotoxic chemotherapy is contraindicated, e.g. those with severe pancytopenia or those requiring extensive local radiotherapy
- HDDex is useful as initial therapy in patients presenting with renal failure
- No recommendation can be made on current evidence as to specific subsequent therapy after initial dexamethasone alone

[a] See Table 14.1.

in order to reduce the risk of cardiotoxicity in elderly patients.[82] The results were promising, with 11 of 12 patients responding, including three entering CR.

The original VAD regimen contained three 4-day pulses of dexamethasone in every cycle.[67] Subsequent studies have used various modifications of the steroid dose in an attempt to reduce steroid-related toxicity. For example, the Riverside Haematology Group study[72] used three pulses in alternate courses with only one pulse in the intervening courses. Some current trials are using three pulses of dexamethasone in the first course and only one pulse in subsequent courses. There are no randomized studies comparing these different dose schedules of dexamethasone.

VAMP AND C-VAMP

In these regimens, high-dose dexamethasone is replaced by intravenous methyl prednisolone with a view to reducing steroid-related toxicity. C-VAMP includes weekly intravenous cyclophosphamide between courses of VAMP. There have been no randomized trials comparing VAMP, C-VAMP, and VAD. Overall response and CR rates appear similar.[83,84] In a non-randomized study comparing VAMP and C-VAMP, C-VAMP was associated with a higher CR rate than VAMP (24% vs. 8%),[84] but it should be noted that the CR rate with VAD has varied from 7% to 28% in different non-randomized series.[72,74] There are no data indicating whether steroid-related toxicity is in fact lower with methyl prednisolone than with dexamethasone.

MOD, NOP, AND NOP–BOLUS

In these regimens, mitoxantrone is used instead of Adriamycin. Potential advantages include less cardiotoxicity

and less alopecia. MOD is a true variant of VAD in that both M (melphalan) and O (vincristine) are given by continuous infusion. A randomized study of MOD versus VAD in relapsed patients showed VAD and MOD to be equally effective.[85] MOD is, therefore, a useful regimen in patients who would be suitable for a VAD-type regimen but in whom there is reduced cardiac function or in whom the accepted total Adriamycin dosage has already been reached. NOP is a variant where the vincristine is given by infusion but the mitoxantrone (N) is given by bolus injection, and in NOP-bolus both drugs are given as a bolus. In non-randomized studies of NOP and NOP-bolus in relapsed patients, there was a 20–25% response rate, rather lower than with other studies using VAD.[86,87] A randomized study of NOP-bolus versus MP in newly diagnosed patients suggested that NOP was inferior as primary treatment, with no survival advantage and a number of toxic deaths.[88]

ORAL IDARUBICIN WITH DEXAMETHASONE

Initial studies of oral idarubicin showed activity in myeloma, either as a single agent or in combination with steroids.[89–91] Oral equivalents of the VAD regimen were subsequently developed. The Z-Dex regimen[92] comprises idarubicin (Zavedos[TM]) 10 mg/m^2 daily for 4 days together with pulsed high-dose dexamethasone. The VID regimen[93] contains idarubicin and dexamethasone at the same doses as in Z-Dex, but also includes IV vincristine, given as a bolus on day 1. In a phase I/II study, 80% of newly diagnosed patients responded with a CR rate of 7%. Responses appeared to be as rapid as those observed with VAD. Stem-cell harvesting was not affected by this regimen.[94] There are no data on long-term outcome. Note that in the original report, three pulses of dexamethasone were given with every cycle, but the authors have subsequently reduced the dexamethasone to three pulses in the first course and only one pulse in subsequent courses (personal communication).

On the basis of current evidence, it is not possible to make a firm recommendation for the use of Z-Dex; however, the regimen appears to offer a suitable alternative to VAD as initial therapy prior to stem-cell harvest and HDT. It avoids the need for a central line with associated risk of complications. It is also suitable for the treatment of relapsed disease. A similar regimen incorporating oral CCNU (CIDex) was studied in relapsed patients, and found to produce responses in 56% of patients with untested relapse and 31% of those with refractory relapse.[95]

Caution is recommended in the use of oral idarubicin in patients with severe renal impairment. Idarubicin and the active metabolite idarubicinol are mainly excreted by the biliary route, but some is cleared by the kidney. More idarubicinol is formed after oral than intravenous dosing and idarubicinol has a long half-life. Idarubicin toxicity is, therefore, potentially increased in patients with renal impairment receiving oral idarubicin. Most available data are on patients with creatinine levels below 200 μmol/L. A number of current trials allow inclusion of patients with higher levels of serum creatinine, and toxicity did not appear to be increased in patients with severe renal failure included in the CIDex study,[95] but there are presently insufficient data to recommend routine use of oral idarubicin or to guide dose modification in patients with creatinine levels above 200 μmol/L.

OTHER COMBINATION CHEMOTHERAPY REGIMENS

More recently, new combinations have been evaluated in relapsed patients, including drugs such as cytosine,[96,97] etoposide,[97–102] ifosfamide,[98] teniposide,[103] epirubicin,[104] and cisplatinum.[97,105] Etoposide, in particular, appears to be useful, since Barlogie et al.[97] showed that response to a combined infusional regimen of etoposide, dexamethasone, ara-C, and cisplatin (EDAP) was significantly more effective than DAP alone in relapsed patients. The combination of dexamethasone, cyclophosphamide, etoposide, and cisplatin (DCEP) and the CEVAD regimen (etoposide, vincristine, Adriamycin, and dexamethasone) has also produced responses in 30–50% of selected patients with relapsed and refractory disease.[101,105] However, these regimens are intensive and the responses frequently short-lived in the context of refractory relapsed disease.

Newer cytotoxic agents

It is disappointing in view of their activity in Waldenström's disease that the new purine analogues (fludarabine, 2-chlorodeoxyadenosine (2-CDA) and deoxycoformycin) have shown little evidence of activity in MM.[106–108] A number of other new cytotoxic agents have been tested and the only one that appears to have useful activity in myeloma is arsenic trioxide (ATO). In preliminary results of phase I/II trials of ATO in patients with relapsed or refractory disease, over 50% achieved minor responses or stabilization of disease.[109,110] Toxicities included leucopenia, abdominal pain, and diarrhea, fever, and fatigue. Paclitaxel and topotecan have been tested and found to have only limited activity.[111,112] All trans retinoic acid (ATRA) inhibits growth of some human MM cell lines but clinical trials have been disappointing.[113,114]

The role of steroids

Steroids are useful in myeloma because of their lack of myelotoxicity. The incidence of infection is, however, increased in patients receiving steroids and other steroid-related side effects are common.

CONVENTIONAL–DOSE STEROIDS

Steroids are active against myeloma cells while sparing normal bone marrow and hence form a useful part of the therapeutic repertoire. The addition of steroids in moderate doses to conventional chemotherapy regimens can increase the speed of response and reduce myelosuppression, although it is not clear whether there is a long-term survival benefit. In the first report of Alexanian et al.[2] in 1969 comparing intermittent oral melphalan, continuous oral melphalan, and intermittent melphalan with prednisone (1 mg/kg alternate days throughout, or 2 mg/kg/day for 4 days for 6 weeks), the inclusion of prednisone was found to increase response rate (61% vs. 17% for continuous melphalan and 32% for intermittent melphalan; SWOG criteria) and improve survival (median survival 24 months vs. 17–18 months for either melphalan schedule). The addition of prednisone or later prednisolone to conventional alkylating agent regimens has subsequently been almost universal.

However, the second MRC Myelomatosis trial,[23] comparing melphalan, melphalan/prednisolone, and cyclophosphamide, found that the addition of prednisolone did not improve survival; median survival was identical at 20 months for both melphalan and melphalan/prednisolone. The Finnish Leukaemia Group also failed to demonstrate a benefit of conventional-dose steroid (methyl prednisolone 0.8 mg/kg per day for days 1–7) added to a combination regimen comprising VCR, CCNU, C, and M (methyl prednisolone, vincristine, cyclophosphamide, lomustine, melphalan (MOCCA) vs. cyclophosphamide, vincristine, lomustine, melphalan (COLA[24])). The response rate was 72% with steroid and 62% without (ns), while survival was 56 months vs. 61 months (ns). In addition, there was an 8% early death rate in the steroid arm and 0% in the other arm. Preliminary results from the MRC Myeloma VI trial showed no survival benefit of adding pulsed prednisolone (60 mg/m² for 4 days) during initial therapy with ABCM.[27] In contrast, the results of a SWOG study[115] comparing VMCP/ VBAP with or without addition of prednisone showed a benefit of the additional steroid on both response rate and survival. Response rate was 49% with additional prednisone and 36% in the control arm, while median survival was 42 months compared with 23 months ($P = 0.04$).

Thus, the evidence is unclear as to whether there is any benefit of steroids in conventional doses, although there is no doubt that, in individual cases, the addition of conventional dose steroid can reduce myelosuppression, allowing chemotherapy to be more easily administered, and can also improve well-being. However, care must be taken about increased risk of infection.

HIGH–DOSE DEXAMETHASONE

More recently, following the success of the VAD regimen, there has been renewed interest in the role of steroids, and it has become clear that, when used at high dosage, steroids alone can produce rapid and extensive responses, both in untreated and relapsed patients. Alexanian et al.[116] had already demonstrated the effectiveness of pulsed prednisolone therapy in refractory patients. Historical comparison of the results in treating refractory patients with dexamethasone alone or with VAD suggested that dexamethasone alone is responsible for much of the efficacy of VAD. Alexanian et al.[117] treated 49 refractory patients (relapsed on treatment or primary refractory) with high-dose dexamethasone (HDDex) alone, giving three 4-day pulses of 40 mg/day every 36 days, and compared their results with a historical group of 39 refractory patients treated with the VAD regimen. In the patients who were refractory to initial treatment, there was little difference in response: 27% and 32% for HDDex and VAD, respectively (SWOG criteria). In relapsed patients, however, the response rate to HDDex was only 21% vs. 65% with VAD. Thus, responses were achieved with dexamethasone alone, but the additional vincristine and Adriamycin more than doubled the response in relapsed patients. However, the median survival was the same in patients treated with HDDex or with VAD – 12 months overall and 22 months in responders.

In a non-randomized trial using the same schedule of dexamethasone, HDDex alone was found to induce responses in 43% of newly diagnosed patients.[118] Responses were rapid and the incidence of serious side effects was only 4% compared with 27% in a historical control group of patients receiving VAD. Responding patients were then given interferon maintenance. Follow-up was not sufficient for accurate assessment of response duration or survival, although survival appeared similar to that achieved with VAD.

Friedenberg et al.[119] also used single-agent HDDex in relapsed/refractory patients, using a more intensive schedule of 40 mg daily for 4 days/week every week for 8 weeks. Those who responded were then maintained on the same dose at 2-weekly intervals. There were 40% objective responses, but 55% had moderate to severe side effects, including central nervous system effects, gastrointestinal bleeding, and infection, with one treatment-related death. Median survival was shorter than in Alexanian's study – 31 weeks in the responders. Norfolk and Child[120] reported the use of pulsed oral prednisolone 60 mg/m^2 for 5 days every 14 days in 17 patients with relapsed or refractory myeloma. There were ten responses and eight patients reached stable plateau. The median survival for all patients was 19–20 months.

High-dose steroids, particularly HDDex, therefore, are very effective at inducing rapid responses with a marked degree of cytoreduction. Approximately 40% of de novo patients and 20–25% of relapsed/refractory patients will achieve objective responses to single-agent dexamethasone. It has the major advantage of lack of myelosuppression and is not associated with secondary leukemia, but infection is a significant risk. However, the long-term remission duration is not likely to be better than that observed with VAD, i.e. about 18 months in previously untreated patients. Thus, it is an ideal agent to use alone or in combination to achieve rapid cytoreduction as an initial treatment, but it would probably need to be followed by some form of chemotherapy and/or interferon to act on residual myeloma cells. A schedule of dexamethasone 40 mg daily for 4 days every 2 weeks until response occurs, then reducing to 4-weekly, is widely used. Recommendations on the use of HDDex are shown in Table 14.6. More recently, data have been presented from the Mayo Clinic suggesting that dexamethasone alone is as effective an initial induction regimen as VAD for patients in whom subsequent high-dose therapy is planned.[121] A total of 63% of patients treated with HDDex alone entered PR after initial induction as compared with 73% of historical controls receiving VAD ($P = 0.25$), and there was no difference in the proportion of patients achieving objective response after the subsequent high-dose therapy (94% and 100%). Since HDDex alone is simpler to administer, and avoids the need for catheter placement and the risk of neutropenic infections and thrombotic events seen with cytotoxic therapy, there is a case for using HDDex alone as induction prior to high-dose therapy.

INTERFERON–α

The interferons are a family of compounds produced by leucocytes, fibroblasts, and T lymphocytes and that have antiproliferative activity against viruses and human tumor cells. The interferons also have immune-modulating effects. The therapeutic effects of interferon-α (IFN) have been assessed in myeloma patients at induction, at plateau phase, following high-dose therapy, and in patients with relapse/refractory disease, both as monotherapy and combined with chemotherapy. Most studies have been with recombinant IFN; the two main types (α2a and α2b) appear clinically indistinguishable. IFN is administered by subcutaneous injection.

Most patients experience some side effects, which are significant in up to one-third. Flu-like symptoms are

Table 14.7 *Randomized studies of maintenance therapy with interferon and/or steroids in newly diagnosed patients*

Study	Prior therapy	Randomization	Number of patients randomized	Remission duration (median)	Survival (median)
Italian (Mandelli et al.[128])	MP[a] or VMCP[a]	IFN vs. nil	101	26 vs. 14 months ($P < 0.0002$)	50 vs. 42 months (ns)
Nordic (Westin et al.[129])	MP	IFN vs. nil	125	15 vs. 6 months ($P < 0.0001$)	35 vs. 36 months (ns)
Canadian (Browman et al.[130])	MP	IFN vs. nil	176	18 vs. 13 months ($P < 0.003$)	44 vs. 33 months ($P = 0.05$)
Australian Leukaemia Study Group (Joshua et al.[131])	Alkylator-based combination therapy	IFN vs. nil (IFN also given with induction in IFN arm)	113	17 vs. 13 months ($P = 0.5$)	45 vs. 30 months ($P = 0.14$)
MRC (Drayson et al.[132])	Various, including MP, ABCM[a], VAD[a]	IFN vs. nil	284	16.9 vs. 12.7 months ($P = 0.2$)[b]	41.2 vs. 34.5 months ($P = 0.57$)[b]
SWOG (Salmon et al.[115])	Alkylator-based combination therapy	IFN vs. nil	193	12 vs. 11 (ns)	32 vs. 38 months (ns)
UCLA (Berenson et al.[142])	VAD with prednisone ± quinine	Prednisone 50 mg alternate days vs. 10 mg alternate days	125	14 vs. 5 months ($P = 0.003$)	Median 37 vs. 26 months ($P = 0.05$)
SWOG (Salmon et al.[133])	VAD	IFN plus prednisone vs. IFN alone	89	19 vs. 9 months ($P = 0.008$)	57 vs. 46 months ($P = 0.36$)
MD Anderson (Alexanian et al.[144])	Melphalan and dexamethasone	IFN vs. dexamethasone	84	10 months in both arms	Not reported; better response to re-induction in IFN group

[a] See Table 14.1.
[b] In the MRC trial, the median values were at the widest point of separation of the curves and, overall, the curves were not significantly different between the two arms.
IFN, interferon-α; MRC, Medical Research Council; ns, not significant; SWOG, Southwest Oncology Group; UCLA, University of California, Los Angeles.

common a few hours after each of the initial injections; this generally resolves after the first 2–3 weeks of therapy. The symptoms will respond to paracetamol, which should be taken at the time of each initial injection. Fatigue and depression are recognized side effects of longer-term interferon therapy. Other less common problems include hypothyroidism, peripheral neuropathy, ocular side effects, arrhythmias, diarrhea, abnormal liver function, and nephritis. Interferon may cause myelosuppression with reduction of neutrophil and platelet counts. Some 20–25% of patients may prove intolerant to interferon therapy. Most side effects will resolve on cessation of interferon.

IFN in induction

Interferon-α is active as a single agent in MM but response rates are lower than with standard chemotherapy.[122] IFN has been combined with standard induction chemotherapy in a number of studies. Higher response rates have

been observed with the addition of IFN but a survival benefit has been harder to demonstrate. Some studies have observed no survival benefit[123] and the data are conflicting.[124] The Myeloma Trialists' Group has published a meta-analysis of individual patient data from 4012 patients in 12 induction trials and 12 maintenance trials.[125] In the induction trials, complete (17% vs. 14%; $P = 0.08$) and complete plus partial (58% vs. 53%; $P = 0.01$) response rates were slightly better with IFN, and response duration in responders was significantly better with IFN (30% vs. 25% at 3 years, log-rank $P = 0.0005$). However, there was no statistically significant survival benefit for IFN in induction (odds reduction 8%). A meta-analysis using published data rather than individual patient data yielded similar results, with improvement in response rates with IFN and prolongation of median progression-free survival (PFS) by about 5 months, but an overall survival benefit of only 2–3 months.[126] In a large randomized study, the Nordic

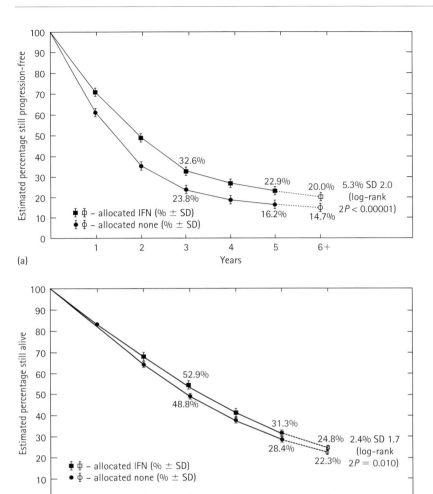

Figure 14.2 *Progression-free (a) and overall survival (b) of patients in trials of interferon vs. none. From a meta-analysis of 4012 patients in 24 trials carried out by the Myeloma Trialists' Collaborative Group.[125] This analysis includes trials where interferon-α was given in induction, as maintenance, or both. Reproduced from Myeloma Trialists' Collaborative Group, Interferon as therapy for multiple myeloma: an individual patient data overview of 24 randomized trials and 4012 patients, Br J Haematol 2001; 113:1020–34, with permission.*

myeloma group showed no gain in survival for patients receiving IFN in induction and maintenance;[127] this study also showed a significant reduction in quality of life during the first year of therapy for patients receiving IFN. In the absence of a survival benefit, the use of IFN in induction is not generally recommended.

IFN as maintenance therapy

A number of studies have examined the therapeutic role of IFN maintenance therapy following induction chemotherapy[115,128–132] and autologous transplantation (see Table 14.7).[133,134] The meta-analysis from the Myeloma Trialists' Group evaluated individual patient data on 1543 patients in 12 maintenance trials.[125] Progression-free survival was, again, significantly improved in IFN-treated patients ($P = 0.00001$), with a prolongation of about 6 months in median PFS ($P = 0.0001$), and there was also a significant prolongation of overall survival (OS) in the

maintenance studies; median OS was also prolonged by about 7 months (Fig. 14.2). Similar results were obtained in the meta-analysis of published data on IFN trials,[126] which found that median PFS was prolonged by 4 months and OS by 7 months. In this study, the additional costs of IFN maintenance per 1-year gain in survival were $18 968. Retrospective case-controlled data from the European Group for Blood and Marrow Transplantation (EBMT) registry have suggested significant gains in PFS and OS for interferon-treated patients; however, such data are non-randomized and subject to selection bias.[135]

Overall, the data do not show significantly better response or survival in any particular patient groups. Trials generally show a greater gain in PFS than in OS, suggesting that survival following relapse/progression is shorter among interferon-treated patients. Dosages of IFN-α have varied, but no benefit has been shown for doses greater than 3 MU/m² given 3 times/week. There are no data on duration of therapy. Recommendations on the use of interferon should also take into account the side effects.

Table 14.8 *Recommendations on the use of interferon (UK Myeloma Forum, 2001)*[21]

- Interferon therapy is not indicated during induction therapy
- Interferon therapy has activity as maintenance therapy during plateau phase following conventional chemotherapy or following high-dose therapy, but the balance between expected small survival benefit and side effects precludes generalized treatment recommendations
- Careful consideration should be given as to whether interferon should be continued in the face of side effects that impair quality of life

A study by Ludwig *et al.*[136] looking at the preferences of patients found that approximately 50% of patients would accept an unidentified treatment with the profile of IFN if an improvement in remission duration and/or survival of 6 months could be expected. Recommendations are shown in Table 14.8.

CHOICE OF INITIAL CHEMOTHERAPY

The choice of initial therapy will be governed largely by the patient's age and general fitness, particularly the level of renal function. It is also essential to take into account at diagnosis the possibility of future autologous transplantation, so as to avoid the use of stem-cell-damaging drugs in patients where autografting is an option.

Younger patients

Patients up to the age of at least 65 years, and some older patients, should be considered as possible candidates for future autografting, even if performance status is initially poor or if they present with acute renal failure. In these patients VAD or a VAD-type regimen should be used, or alternatively high-dose dexamethasone alone, which appears to be as effective as VAD in this setting.[121] The use of thalidomide and dexamethasone as initial treatment is currently under evaluation (see Chapter 19). In patients who are proceeding to high-dose therapy and transplant as consolidation therapy, there is probably no advantage to continuing induction chemotherapy beyond the point of maximum response; this is usually no longer than 3–4 months when VAD-type regimens are used.

Older patients

For most patients over 65–70 years, the choice lies between simple oral chemotherapy and standard combination regimens. As discussed, there is little difference in long-term outcome between these options and the MRC

Myeloma V trial in fact showed no benefit for ABCM in patients over 65 years. Simple oral treatment, therefore, seems the most appropriate choice for older patients. Chemotherapy should be continued until the patient has reached plateau phase, i.e. observations have been stable for a period of 3 months, since there is no advantage to prolonging therapy once plateau has been reached. Thalidomide and dexamethasone as initial treatment is also being evaluated in older patients.

Patients with renal failure

For patients presenting with renal failure, VAD is the obvious choice, and can be used in some older patients. Oral idarubicin and dexamethasone is an alternative but, as yet, there are insufficient data on its use in patients to recommend its use without dosage modification in patients with renal failure. Melphalan and cyclophosphamide are both difficult to use in patients with renal impairment, since myelosuppression is unpredictable even when the doses are reduced. Steroids alone, e.g. pulsed high-dose dexamethasone, are also useful for patients with renal failure, who may be unsuitable for intravenous therapy.

MAINTENANCE THERAPY

Maintenance chemotherapy

In the majority of responding patients, paraprotein level tends to reach a plateau and does not fall any further, even if treatment is continued. The question of whether continuing chemotherapy at this stage offers any advantage in terms of preventing relapse has been addressed in a number of studies. An early SWOG study[137] showed no benefit for maintenance with either MP or BCNU plus prednisolone given 6-weekly after an initial six cycles of MP-based induction therapy. Comparison with a control group given no maintenance showed no difference in response duration or survival between the three arms. The incidence of pneumonia and Herpes zoster was, however, increased in the maintenance groups. The third MRC myeloma trial[126] randomized patients in plateau after induction with either MP or cyclophosphamide to receive no further treatment or maintenance with intermittent induction courses alternating with azathioprine and vincristine. Survival was slightly better in the maintenance arm but the difference was not significant. In the MRC IV myeloma trial, patients reaching plateau after MP with or without vincristine were randomized to continue the same therapy for a further year or to stop treatment. In contrast to the previous study, at the time of reporting there was a small but not significant survival advantage for those receiving no maintenance. Long-term follow up of the IV trial[54] confirmed no significant difference in survival.

Belch et al.[11] randomized patients who had reached stable plateau (at least 4 months) with MP induction to continue MP to relapse or to stop treatment. Time to relapse was significantly shorter in the no maintenance group (median 23 vs. 31 months), but many of these patients responded to restarting MP and the time to final progression on MP was actually longer in the no-maintenance arm (39 vs. 31 months). Median survival was not significantly different. They concluded that maintenance offered no advantage to patients who had reached stable plateau phase. A small Norwegian study[138] also reported no differences in patients randomized to maintenance or no maintenance with continued induction therapy, which was either MP or VBMCP. None of these studies, therefore, indicates any benefit from continuing chemotherapy once stable plateau phase is reached.

Interferon maintenance

As discussed above, modest increases in PFS and OS of up to 6 months are identified in meta-analysis, most clearly observed for patients receiving maintenance therapy following chemotherapy or autologous transplant. However, published data suggest that only 5–10% of myeloma patients achieve a significant gain in survival from IFN,[139] and cost–utility analysis of IFN therapy suggests a cost of $50 000–100 000 per quality-adjusted life year gained.[140,141] Potential benefits must also be balanced against possible toxicity. There are, unfortunately, no clear data indicating which patients are most likely to benefit, nor on optimum dose or duration of therapy.

Steroids in maintenance

Berenson et al.[142] reported the results of a study of alternate day prednisone as maintenance therapy in patients who had responded to VAD (Table 14.7). They compared two doses, 10 mg and 50 mg, and found that the higher dose was associated with improved remission duration and survival. Perhaps surprisingly, they did not report any problems with osteoporosis in the group receiving the higher dose. Consistent with this observation, the SWOG found a significantly longer remission duration in patients receiving IFN plus prednisone 50 mg on alternate days than in those on IFN alone.[143] A direct comparison of IFN with steroid maintenance was reported from the MD Anderson hospital.[144] They compared IFN with intermittent high-dose dexamethasone (20 mg/m2 for 4 days every month) in patients who were initially treated with intermittent melphalan and pulsed dexamethasone (MD). They found no difference in remission duration,

which was 10 months in both arms, but observed that when relapsing patients were retreated with MD, patients who had received IFN maintenance were much more likely to respond. Both regimens were associated with a similar incidence of side effects. It is difficult to draw firm conclusions from these different studies, but there may be a rationale for combining IFN with steroids as maintenance therapy.

Thalidomide

The use of thalidomide in myeloma is discussed in Chapter 19. Its role in maintenance therapy is currently being evaluated.

REFRACTORY AND RELAPSED DISEASE

Primary refractory disease

There is a lack of evidence from randomized controlled trials on the optimum approach to treating primary refractory disease. Patients refractory to alkylating agents may respond well to VAD-type regimens.[67] As most patients initially treated with alkylating agents will be in the older age group, oral anthracycline-containing regimes, such as Z-Dex or CIDEX, may be more suitable. Oral idarubicin alone was found to be associated with a low proportion of response is advanced disease.[145] Patients with primary refractory disease may also respond well to thalidomide or thalidomide with dexamethasone.[146]

Younger patients treated with VAD as primary therapy, and who fail to respond prior to planned stem cell transplant (SCT) may still respond to intermediate or high-dose melphalan.[147,148] Stem cells should be harvested prior to high-dose melphalan. A single high-dose procedure can be performed. An alternative approach, which has been used at our institution, is to give an initial intermediate to high dose of melphalan (80–120 mg/m^2) to achieve remission, followed by a standard autograft. This depends on the ability to harvest sufficient stem cells to support two procedures, as it is usually difficult to harvest adequate peripheral blood stem cells (PBSCs) after high-dose melphalan. The advent of thalidomide provides an alternative approach, since many patients refractory to VAD will respond to thalidomide, and this has the advantage of not damaging normal stem cells, so that PBSCs can be harvested after the patients has responded rather than while still in a refractory state.[149]

Relapsed/progressive disease

Since almost all patients with myeloma will relapse, the overall management strategy should include plans to treat relapse. In most cases, the therapeutic objectives will still be to achieve disease control, ameliorate symptoms, improve quality of life, and prolong survival. Early relapse carries a poor prognosis and is likely to respond poorly to most chemotherapy. Patients who relapse or progress after a long stable plateau phase are likely to respond well to further treatment.

Possible treatment regimens for relapsed myeloma, therefore, include no further antineoplastic treatment, further chemotherapy with the same or an alternative regimen, or high-dose therapy. Thalidomide has already become an established and effective treatment for relapsed disease, and there are a number of other novel and experimental therapies available, which are discussed in Chapter 19.

Available evidence suggests that if the patient was initially treated with MP and achieved stable plateau, MP is appropriate treatment, as a further response can be achieved in 50% patients.[11] Patients who have been treated previously with alkylating agents may respond well to VAD or related regimens[67] or an idarubicin-based regimen.[92,95] High-dose therapy and stem cell transplantation may be considered in patients who have not had a prior stem cell transplant. A second HDT may also be appropriate in selected patients who relapse after an initial autograft (those with a low β_2-microglobulin, one prior transplant and late relapse).[150–152] Thalidomide alone or with dexamethasone has been shown to produce responses in 30% of relapsed/refractory patients, and higher response rates have been reported with the combination of thalidomide and dexamethasone.[143] Double hemi-body irradiation is useful in some late-stage patients with widespread bone pain who are refractory to chemotherapy and steroids.[153] Caution is required as it can cause significant myelosuppression.

Drug resistance in myeloma

Resistance to chemotherapy is a common problem in myeloma. In many cases, drug resistance is associated with expression of the mdr-1 phenotype. The product of the mdr-1 gene is a 170-kDa glycoprotein, P-glycoprotein (or PgP), which is overexpressed in the cell membrane and which functions as a drug efflux pump. It confers resistance to a number of different chemotherapeutic agents including Adriamycin, vincristine, and etoposide. The extent of over expression of PgP in myeloma is correlated with resistance to chemotherapy[154–156] and also with exposure to Adriamycin and/or vincristine.[156]

Several drugs can reverse PgP function *in vitro*, probably by competitive binding. These include verapamil and quinidine, cyclosporin A, and the cyclosporin analog PSC833. However, in general, the doses required for *in vitro* effect cannot be achieved *in vivo* without significant toxicity and clinical results have been disappointing.[157,158] A randomized study from the Hovon group comparing VAD plus cyclosporin A with VAD alone in 75 patients with refractory disease found no effect of cyclosporin A on the overall response rate, PFS, and overall survival with VAD, while preliminary data on the use of PSC833 in combination with VAD have not suggested marked improvement in response rate in refractory patients.

THE FUTURE

Over the past few years it has become apparent that conventional chemotherapy is unable to achieve long-term disease control in myeloma, despite the introduction of new chemotherapeutic agents and more complex regimens. Improvements in outcome in recent years are the result of other approaches, including high-dose therapy and biological response modifiers, as discussed in subsequent chapters. Thalidomide alone or in combination with dexamethasone has become an accepted alternative to standard-dose chemotherapy in relapsed disease and is being increasingly used in newly diagnosed patients. At the same time, high-dose dexamethasone alone is being increasingly used as an alternative to VAD for initial induction in patients going on to high-dose therapy. It is, therefore, likely that the standard chemotherapy regimens that have hitherto been the mainstay of treatment will be used less often in the future than in the past, although combinations of cytotoxic drugs with newer biological agents may prove useful. Whatever treatment approach is followed, good supportive care is essential. It is also important to consider the need to maintain quality of life, and to select and adapt treatment for the individual patient.

KEY POINTS

- Melphalan with or without prednisone remains the most appropriate initial treatment for elderly patients.
- Younger patients should receive a VAD-type regimen or high-dose dexamethasone as initial treatment prior to stem cell transplant.
- Treatment should not be continued beyond plateau phase in (or maximal response in the case of patients proceeding to transplant).
- Maintenance therapy with interferon prolongs remission by about 6 months with a smaller effect on survival, but is hampered by side effects, precluding a generalized recommendation for its use.

- Maintenance prednisone or dexamethasone appears promising.
- There are a wide variety of options for relapsed and refractory disease, including chemotherapy, transplant, thalidomide, and other new approaches.
- Good supportive care and attention to quality of life issues are important, whatever specific chemotherapy is chosen.

REFERENCES

- ● = Key primary paper
- ◆ = Major review article
- ∗ = Paper that represents the first formal publication of a management guideline

1. Bergsagel D. Phase II trials of mitomycin C, AB-100[2], NSC 1026[3], L-sarcolysin and meta sarcolysin in the treatment of multiple myeloma. *Cancer Cemother Rep* 1962; **16**:261–6.
- ●2. Alexanian R, Haut A, Khan A, Lane M, McKelvey E, Migliore P, *et al.* Treatment for multiple myeloma: combination chemotherapy with different melphalan dose regimes. *J Am Med Assoc* 1969; **208**:1680–5.
3. Dorr RT, von Hoff DD. *Cancer chemotherapy handbook*, 2nd edn. Norwalk, CT: Appleton and Lange, 1994.
4. Fischer DS, Knobf MT, Durivage HJ. *The cancer chemotherapy handbook*, 5th edn. St Louis: Mosby, 1999.
5. Arthur JR, Athens JW, Wintrobe MM, Cartwright GE. Melphalan and myeloma. Experience with a low dose continuous regimen. *Ann Intern Med* 1970; **72**:665–70.
6. Mellstedt H, Bjorkholm M, Holm G. Intermittent melphalan and prednisolone therapy in plasma cell myeloma. *Acta Med Scand* 1977; **202**:5–9.
7. Fernberg JG, Johansson B, Lewensohn R, Mellstedt H. Oral dosage of melphalan and response to treatment in multiple myeloma. *Eur J Cancer* 1990; **26**:393–6.
8. Bergsagel DE. The role of chemotherapy in the treatment of multiple myeloma. *Baillieres Clin Haematol* 1995; **8**:783–94.
9. Bergsagel DE, Bailey AJ, Langley GR, MacDonald RN, White DF, Miller AB. The chemotherapy on plasma-cell myeloma and the incidence of acute leukemia. *N Engl J Med* 1979; **301**:743–8.
10. Leone G, Voso MT, Sica S, Morosetti R, Pagano L. Therapy related leukemias: susceptibility, prevention and treatment. *Leuk Lymphoma* 2001; **41**:255–76.
- ●11. Belch A, Shelley W, Bergsagel D, Wilson K, Klimo P, White D, Willan A. A randomised trial of maintenance versus no maintenance melphalan and prednisone in responding multiple myeloma patients. *Br J Cancer* 1988; **57**:94–9.
12. Tricot G, Jagannath S, Vesole D, Nelson J, Tindle S, Miller L, *et al.* Peripheral blood stem cell transplants for multiple myeloma: identification of favorable variables for rapid engraftment in 225 patients. *Blood* 1995; **85**:588–96.
13. Demirer T, Buckner CD, Gooley T, Appelbaum FR, Rowley S, Chauncey T, *et al.* Factors influencing collection of peripheral blood stem cells in patients with multiple myeloma. *Bone Marrow Transplant* 1996; **17**:937–41.
14. Clark RE, Brammer CG. Previous treatment predicts the efficiency of blood progenitor cell mobilization: validation of a chemotherapy scoring system. *Bone Marrow Transplant* 1998; **22**:859–63.
- ◆15. Myeloma Trialists' Collaborative Group. Combination chemotherapy versus melphalan plus prednisone as treatment for multiple myeloma: an overview of 6,633 patients from 27 randomized trials. *J Clin Oncol* 1998; **16**:3832–42.
16. Osterborg A, Ahre A, Bjorkholm M, Bjoreman M, Brenning G, Gahrton G, *et al.* Oral versus intravenous melphalan and prednisone treatment in multiple myeloma stage II. A randomised study from the Myeloma Group of Central Sweden. *Acta Oncol* 1990; **29**:727–31.
17. Reece PA, Hill HS, Green RM, Morris R, Dale B, Kotasek D, *et al.* Renal clearance and protein binding of melphalan in patients with cancer. *Cancer Chemother Pharmacol* 1988; **22**:348–52.
18. Adair CG, Bridges JM, Desai ZR. Renal function in the elimination of oral melphalan in patients with multiple myeloma. *Cancer Chemother Pharmacol* 1986; **17**:185–8.
19. Cornwell GG 3rd, Pajak TF, McIntyre OR, Kochwa S, Dosik H. Influence of renal failure on myelosuppressive effects of melphalan: Cancer and Leukemia Group B experience. *Cancer Treatment Rep* 1982; **66**:475–81.
20. Osterborg A, Ehrsson H, Eksborg S, Wallin I, Mellstedt H. Pharmacokinetics of oral melphalan in relation to renal function in multiple myeloma patients. *Eur J Clin Oncol* 1989; **25**:899–903.
- ∗21. UK Myeloma Forum. Diagnosis and management of multiple myeloma *Br J Haematol* 2001; **115**:522–40.
23. MRC Working Party on Leukaemia in Adults. Report on the second myelomatosis trial after 5 years of follow-up. *Br J Cancer* 1980; **42**:813–22.
24. Palva IP, Ala-Harja K, Almquist A, *et al.* Corticosteroid therapy is not beneficial in multiple-drug combination chemotherapy for multiple myeloma. Finnish Leukaemia Group. *Eur J Haematol* 1993; **52**:98–101.
25. MacLennan ICM, Chapman C, Dunn J, Kelly K, for the MRC Working Party on Leukaemia in Adults. Combined chemotherapy with ABCM versus melphalan for treatment of myelomatosis. *Lancet* 1992; **339**:200–5.
26. MRC Working Party on Leukaemia in Adults. Treatment comparisons in the third MRC myelomatosis trial. *Br J Cancer* 1980; **42**:823–30.
27. Olojohungbe AB, Dunn JA, Drayson MT, MacLennan IM. Prednisolone added to the ABCM as treatment for multiple myeloma increases serological responses but not overall survival or the number of stable clinical responses. *Br J Haematol* 1996; **9**(Suppl 1):77.
28. Selby PJ, McElwain TJ, Nandi AC, Perren T, Powles R, Tillyer C, *et al.* Multiple myeloma treated with high-dose intravenous mephalan. *Br J Haematol* 1987; **66**:55–62.
29. Barlogie B, Jagannath S, Dixon DO, Cheson B, Smallwood L, Hendrickson A, *et al.* High-dose melphalan and granulocyte-macrophage colony-stimulating factor for refractory multiple myeloma. *Blood* 1990; **76**:677–80.

30. Tsakanikas S, Papanastasiou K, Stamatelou M, Maniatis A. intermediate dose of intravenous melphalan in advanced multiple myeloma. *Oncology* 1991; **48**:369–71.

31. Petrucci M, Avvisati G, Tribalto M, Czntonetti M, Giovangrossi P, Mandelli F. Intermediate-dose (25 mg/m^2) intravenous melphalan for patients with multiple myeloma in relapse or refractory to standard treatment. *Eur J Haematol* 1989; **42**:233–7.

32. Back H, Lindblad R , Rodjer S, Westin J. Single-dose intravenous melphalan in advanced multiple myeloma. *Acta Haematol* 1990; **83**:183–6.

33. Schey SA, Kazmi M, Ireland R, Lakhani A. The use of intravenous intermediate dose melphalan and dexamethasone as induction treatment in the management of de novo multiple myeloma. *Eur J Haematol* 1998; **61**:306–10.

34. Rivers SL, Whittington RM, Patno ME. Comparison of effect of cyclophosphamide and a placebo intreatment of multiple myeloma. *Cancer Chemother Rep* 1963; **29**:115–19.

35. Korst DR, Clifford GO, Fowler WM, Louis J, Will J, Wilson HE. Multiple myeloma: II. Analysis of cyclophosphamide therapy in 165 patients. *J Am Med Assoc* 1964; **189**:758–62.

36. Bergsagel DE, Cowan DH, Hasselback R. Plasma cell myeloma: response of melphalan-resistant patients to high-dose intermittent cyclophosphamide. *J Can Med Assoc* 1972; **107**:851–5.

37. Rivers SL, Patno ME. Cyclophosphamide vs melphalan in the treatment of plasma cell myeloma. *J Am Med Assoc* 1969; **207**:1328–34.

38. MRC Working Party on Leukaemia in Adults. Myelomatosis: comparison of melphalan and cyclophosphamide therapy. *Br Med J* 1971; **1**:640–1.

39. Brandes LJ, Israels LG. Treatment of advanced plasma cell myeloma with weekly cyclophosphamide and alternate-day prednisone. *Cancer Treat Rep* 1982; **66**:1413–15.

40. Brandes LJ, Israels LG. Weekly low-dose cyclophosphamide and alternate-day prednisone: an effective low-toxicity regimen for multiple myeloma. *Eur J Haematol* 1987; **39**:362–8.

41. Juma FD, Rogers HJ, Trounce JR. Effect of renal insufficiency on the pharacokinetics of cyclophosphamide and some of its metabolites. *Eur J Clin Pharacol* 1981; **19**:443–51.

●42. Alexanian R, Salmon S, Bonnet J, Gehan E, Haut A, Weick J. Combination therapy for multiple myeloma. *Cancer* 1977; **40**:2675–771.

43. Salmon SE. Expansion of the growth fraction in multiple myeloma with alkylating agents. *Blood* 1975; **45**:119–29.

44. Cornwell GG, Pajak TF, Kochwa S, McIntyre O, Glowienka L, Brunner K, *et al.* Comparison of oral melphalan, CCNU, and BCNU with and without vincristine in the treatment of multiple myeloma. Cancer and Leukaemia Group B experisnce. *Cancer* 1982; **50**:1669–75.

45. Alberts DS, Durie BGM, Salmon SE. Doxorubicin/BCNU chemotherapy for multiple myeloma in relapse. *Lancet* 1975; **1**:926–8.

46. Alberts DS, Salmon SE. Adriamycin in the treatment of alkylator-resistant multiple myeloma. A pilot study. *Cancer Chemother Rep* 1975; **59**:345–50.

47. MRC Working Party on Leukaemia in Adults. Objective evaluation of the role of vincristine in induction and maintenance therapy for myelomatosis. *Br J Cancer* 1985; **52**:52–158.

48. Case DCJ, Lee BJ, Clarkson BD. Improved survival times in multiple myeloma treated with melphalan, prednisolone, vincristine, cyclophosphamide and BCNU–M2 protocol. *Am J Med* 1977; **63**:897–903.

49. Oken MM, Tsiatis A, Abramson N, Glick J. Evaluation of intensive (VBMCP) vs standard (MP) therapy for multiple myeloma. *Proc Am Soc Clin Oncol* 1987; **6**:A 802.

50. Oken MM. Standard primary treatment of multiple myeloma: recent ECOG studies. *Abstracts of the IVth International Workshop on Multiple Myeloma*, Rochester, 1993: 70–1.

51. Palva IP, Ahrenberg P, Ala-Harja K, Almqvist A, Elonen E, Hallman H, *et al.* Intensive chemotherapy with combinations containing anthracyclines for refractory and relapsing multiple myeloma. *Eur J Haematol* 1990; **44**:121–4.

52. Finnish Leukaemia Group. Combination chemotherapy MOCCA in resistant and relapsing multiple myeloma. *Eur J Haematol* 1992; **48**:37–40.

53. Alexanian R, Dreicer R. Chemotherapy for multiple myeloma. *Cancer* 1984; **53**:583–8.

◆54. Maclennan ICM, Kelly K, Crockson RA, Cooper E, Cuzick J, Chapman C. Results of the MRC myelomatosis trials for patients entered since 1980. *Hematol Oncol* 1988; **6**:145–58.

55. Kelly K, Durie B, Maclennan ICM. Prognostic factors and staging system for multiple myeloma: comparisons between the MRC studies in the United Kingdom and the Southwest Oncology Group studies in the United States. *Hematol Oncol* 1988; **6**:131–40.

56. Peest D, Deicher H, Coldewey R, Leo R, Bartl R, Bartels H, *et al.* Melphalan and prednisone (MP) versus vincristine, BCNU, adriamycin, melphalan and dexamethasone (VBAMDex) induction chemotherapy and maintenance treatment in multiple myeloma; current results of a multicenter trial. *Onkologie* 1990; **13**:458–60.

57. Blade J, San Miguel J, Sanz-Sanz MA, *et al.* Treatment of melphalan-resistant multiple myeloma witn vincristine, BCNU, doxorubicin and high-dose dexamethasone. *Eur J Cancer* 1993; **29A**:57–60.

58. Salmon SE, Haut A, Bonnet JD, *et al.* Alternating combination chemotherapy and levamisole improves survival in multiple myeloma: a Southwest Oncology Group study. *J Clin Oncol* 1983; **1**:453–61.

59. Durie BGM, Dixon DO, Carter S, Stephens R, Rivkin S, Bonnet J, *et al.* Improved survival with combination chemotherapy induction for multiple myeloma: a Southwestern Oncology Group Study. *J Clin Oncol* 1986; **4**:1227–37.

60. Osterborg A, Ahre A, Bjorkholm M, Bjoreman M, Brenning G, Gahrton G, *et al.* Alternating combination chemotherapy (VMCP/VBAP) is not superior to melphalan/prednisone in the treatment of multiple myeloma patients stage III – A randomised study from the MGCS. *Eur J Haematol* 1989; **43**:54–62.

61. Boccadoro M, Marmont F, Tribalto M, Avvisati G, Andriani A, Barbui T, *et al.* Multiple myeloma: VMCP/VBAP alternating combination chemotherapy is not superior to melphalan and prednisolone even in high-risk patients. *J Clin Oncol* 1991; **9**:444–8.

62. Cuzick J, Galton DAG, Peto R, for the MRC Working Party on Leukaemia in Adults. Prognostic factors in the third MEC myelomatosis trial. *Br J Cancer* 1980; **43**:831–40.

◆63. Gregory WM, Richards MA, Malpas JS. Combination chemotherapy versus melphalan and prednisolone in the treatment of multiple myeloma: an overview of published trials. *J Clin Oncol* 1992; **10**:334–42.

64. Blade J, San Miguel JF, Fontanillas M, Esteve J, Maldonado J, Alcala A, *et al*. Increased conventional chemotherapy does not improve survival in multiple myeloma: long-term results of two PETHEMA trials including 914 patients. *Hematol J.* 2001; **2**:272–8.

65. Boccadoro M, Palumbo A, Argentino C, Dominietto A, Frieri R, Avvisati G, *et al*. Conventional induction treatments do not influence overall survival in multiple myeloma. *Br J Haematol* 1997; **96**:333–7.

66. Zervas K, Pouli A, Gregoraki B, Anagnostopoulos N, Dimopoulos MA, Bourantas K, *et al*. Comparison of vincristine, carmustine, melphalan, cyclophosphamide, prednisone (VBMCP) and interferon-alpha with melphalan and prednisone (MP) and interferon-alpha (IFN-alpha) in patients with good-prognosis multiple myeloma: a prospective randomized study. Greek Myeloma Study Group. *Eur J Haematol* 2001; **66**:18–23.

●67. Barlogie B, Smith L, Alexanian R. Effective treatment of advanced multiple myeloma resistant to alkylating agents. *N Engl J Med* 1984; **310**:1353–6.

68. Scheithauer W, Cortelezzi A, Kutzmits R, Baldini L, Ludwig H. VAD protocol for treatment of advanced refractory multiple myeloma. *Blut* 1987; **55**:245–52.

69. Anderson H, Scarffe JH, Lambert M, *et al*. VAD chemotherapy – toxicity and efficacy – in patients with multiple myeloma and other lymphoid malignancies. *Hematol Oncol* 1987; **5**:213–22.

70. Lokhorst HM, Meuwissen OJAT, Bast EJEG, Dekker AW. VAD chemotherapy for refractory multiple myeloma. *Br J Haematol* 1989; **71**:25–30.

71. Stenzinger W, Blomker A, Hiddeman W, van de Loo J. Treatment of refractory multiple myeloma with the vincristine–Adriamycin–dexamethasone (VAD) regimen. *Blut* 1990; **61**:55–9.

●72. Samson D, Gaminara E, Newland AC, Van de Pette J, Kearney J, McCarthey D, *et al*. Infusion of vincristine and doxorubicin with oral dexamethasone as first-line therapy for multiple myeloma. *Lancet* 1989; **2**:882–5.

73. Alexanian R, Barlogie B, Tucker S. VAD-based regimens as primary treatment for multiple myeloma. *Am J Hematol* 1990; **33**:86–9.

74. Abrahamson GM, Bird JM, Newland AC, Gaminara E, Giles C, Joyner M, *et al*. A randomised study of VAD therapy with either concurrent or maintenance interferon in patients with newly diagnosed multiple myeloma. *Br J Haematol* 1996; **94**:659–64.

75. Lejeune C, Sotto JJ, Fuzibet JG, Rossi JF, Lepeu G, Bataille R. Alternating combinations of alkylating agents and vincristine, doxorubicin and dexamethasone in multiple myeloma (letter). *J Clin Oncol* 1991; **9**:1090–1.

76. Kars A, Celik I, Kansu E, Tekuzman G, Ozisik Y, Guler N, *et al*. Maintenance therapy with alpha-interferon following first-line VAD in multiple myeloma. *Eur J Haematol* 1997; **59**:100–4.

77. Monconduit M, Menard JF, Michaux JL, Le Loet X, Bernard J, Grosbois B, *et al*. VAD or VBMCP in severe multiple myeloma. *Br J Haematol* 1992; **80**:199–204.

78. Aitchison RG, Reilly IA, Morgan AG, Russell NH. Vincristine, adriamycin and high-dose steroids in myeloma complicated by renal failure. *Br J Cancer* 1990; **61**:765–6.

79. Lieverse RJ, Ossenkoppele GJ. Prevention of doxorubicin-induced congestive cardiac failure by continuous intravenous infusion in multiple myeloma; a case report and review of the literature. *Netherlands J Med* 1991; **38**:33–4.

80. Browman GP, Belch A, Skillings J, Wilson K, Bergsagel D, Johnston D, *et al*. Modified Adriamycin–vincristine–dexamethasone (m-VAD) in primary refractory and relapsed plasma cell myeloma: an NCI (Canada) pilot study. *Br J Haematol* 1992; **82**:555–9.

●81. Segeren CM, Sonneveld P, van der Holt B, Baars JW, Biesma DH, Cornellissen JJ, *et al*. Vincristine, doxorubicin and dexamethasone (VAD) administered as rapid intravenous infusion for first-line treatment in untreated multiple myeloma. *Br J Haematol* 1999; **105**:127–30.

82. Tsiara SN, Kapsali E, Christou L, Panteli A, Pritsivelis N, Bourantas KL. Administration of a modified chemotherapeutic regimen containing vincristine, liposomal doxorubicin and dexamethasone to multiple myeloma patients:preliminary data. *Eur J Haematol* 2000; **65**: 118–22.

●83. Gore ME, Selby PJ, Viner C, Clark P, Meldnum M, Millar B, *et al*. Intensive treatment of multiple myeloma and criteria for complete remission. *Lancet* 1989; **2**:879–82.

84. Raje N, Powles R, Kulkarni S, Milan S, Middleton G, Singhal S, *et al*. A comparison of vincristine and doxorubicin infusional chemotherapy with methylprednisolone (VAMP) with the addition of weekly cyclophosphamide (C-VAMP) as induction treatment followed by autografting in previously untreated myeloma. *Br J Haematol* 1997; **97**:153–60.

85. Phillips JK, Sherlaw-Johnson C, Pearce R, Davies JM, Reilly JT, Newland AC, *et al*. A randomized study of MOD versus VAD in the treatment of relapsed and resistant multiple myeloma. *Leuk Lymphoma* 1995; **17**:465–72.

86. Gimsing P, Bjerrrum O, Brandt E, *et al*. Refractory myelomatosis treated with mitoxantrone in combination with vincristine and prednisone (NOP-regimen): a phase II study. *Br J Haematol* 1991; **77**:73–9.

87. Wisloff F, Gimsing P, Hedenus M, Hippe E, Palva I, Talstad I, *et al*. Bolus therapy with mitoxantrone and vincristine in combination with high-dose prednisone (NOP-bolus) in resistant multiple myeloma. *Eur J Haematol* 1992; **48**:70–4.

88. Keldsen N, Bjerrum OW, Dahl IMS, Drivsholm A, Ellegaard J, Gadeberg O, *et al*. Multiple myeloma treated with mitoxantrone in combination with vincristine and prednisolone (NOP regimen) versus melphalan and prednisolon: a phase III study. *Eur J Haematol* 1993; **51**:80–5.

89. Chisesi T, Capnist G, De Dominicis E, Dini E. A phase II study of idarubicin (4-methoxydaunorubicin) in advanced myeloma. *Eur J Cancer Clin Oncol* 1988; **24**:681–4.

90. Alberts AS, Falkson G, Rapoport BL, Uys A. A phase II study of idarubicin and prednisone in multiple myeloma. *Tumori* 1990; **70**:465–6.

91. Eridani S, Slater NGP, Singh AK, Pearson TC. Intravenous and oral demethoxydaunorubicin (NSC 256-439) in the treatment of acute leukaemia and lymphoma: a pilot study. *Blut* 1985; **50**:369–72.

●92. Cook G, Sharp RA, Tansey P, Franklin IM. A phase I/II trial of Z-Dex (oral idarubicin and dexamethasone), an oral equivalent of VAD, as initial therapy at diagnosis or progression in multiple myeloma. *Br J Haematol* 1996; **93**:931–4.

93. Glasmacher A, Haferlach T, Gorschluter M, Mezger J, Maintz C, Clemens MR, *et al.* Oral idarubicin, dexamethasone and vincristine (VID) in the treatment of multiple myeloma. *Leukemia* 1997; **11**(Suppl 5):S22–6.

94. Clark AD, Douglas KW, Mitchell LD, McQuaker IG, Parker AN, Tansey PJ, *et al.* Dose escalation therapy in previously untreated patients with multiple myeloma following Z-Dex induction treatment. *Br J Haematol* 2002; **117**:605–12.

95. Parameswaran R, Giles C, Boots M, Littlewood TJ, Mills MJ, Kelsey SM, *et al.* CCNU (lomustine), idarubicin and dexamethasone (CIDEX): an effective oral regimen for the treatment of refractory or relapsed myeloma. *Br J Haematol* 2000; **109**:571–5.

96. Dodwell DJ, McGill IG. The treatment of poor-prognosis myelomatosis with a cytosine arabinoside containing regimen. *Hematol Oncol* 1989; **7**:295–6.

97. Barlogie B, Velasquez WS, Alexanian R, Cabanillas F. Etoposide, dexamethasone, cytarabine and cisplatin in vincristine, doxorubicin and dexamethasone – refractory multiple myeloma. *J Clin Oncol* 1989; **7**:1514–17.

98. Ikeda K, Abe N, Morioka A, Inoo M, Nagai M, Kubota Y, *et al.* Etoposide and ifosfamide for MP (melphalan and prednisolone) and VAD (vincristine, adriamycin and dexamethasone)-resistant plasma-cell myeloma: a case report. *Jap J Med* 1990; **29**:516–18.

99. Ohrling M, Bjorkholm M, Osterborg A, Juliusson G, Bjoreman M, Brenning G, *et al.* Etoposide, doxorubicin, cyclophosphamide and high-dose betamethasone as outpatient salvage therapy for multiple myeloma. *Eur J Haematol* 1993; **51**:45–9.

100. Dimopoulos MA, Delasalle KB, Champlin R, Alexanian R. Cyclophosphamide and etoposide therapy with GM-CSF for VAD-resistant multiple myeloma. *Br J Haematol* 1993; **83**:240–4.

101. Giles FJ, Wickham NR, Rapoport BL, Somlo G, Lim SW, Shan J, *et al.* Cyclophosphamide, etoposide, vincristine, adriamycin, and dexamethasone (CEVAD) regimen in refractory multiple myeloma: an International Oncology Study Group (IOSG) phase II protocol. *Am J Hematol* 2000; **63**:125–30.

102. Ballester OF, Moscinski LC, Fields KK, Hiemenz JW, Zorsky PE, Goldstein SC, *et al.* Dexamethasone, cyclophosphamide, idarubicin and etoposide (DC-IE): a novel, intensive induction chemotherapy regimen for patients with high-risk multiple myeloma. *Br J Haematol* 1997; **96**:746–8.

103. Leoni F, Ciolli S, Salti F, Teodori P, Ferrini PR. Teniposide, dexamethasone and continuous infusion cyclophosphamide in advanced refractory multiple myeloma. *Br J Haematol* 1991; **77**:180–4.

104. Fossa A, Muer M, Kasper C, Welt A, Seeber S, Nowrousian MR. Bolus vincristine and epirubicin with cyclophosphamide and dexamethasone (VECD) as induction and salvage treatment in multiple myeloma. *Leukemia* 1998; **12**:422–6.

105. Munshi NC, Desikan KR, Jagannath S, *et al.* Dexamethasone, cyclophosphamide, etoposide and cis-platinum (DCEP), an

effective regimen for relapse after high-dose chemotherapy and autologous transplantation (AT). *Blood* 1996; **88**(Suppl 1): 586a.

106. Lichtman SM, Mittelman A, Budman DR, *et al.* Phase II trial of fludarabine phosphate in multiple myeloma using a loading dose and continuous infusion schedule. *Leuk Lymphoma* 1991; **6**:61–3.

107. Belch AR, Henderson JF, Brox LW. Treatment of multiple myeloma with deoxycoformycin. *Cancer Chemother Pharmacol* 1985; **14**:49–52.

108. Grever MR, Crowley J, Salmon S, McGee R, Kraut E, Buys S, *et al.* Phase II investigation of pentostatin in multiple myeloma: a Southwest Oncology Group study. *J Natl Cancer Inst* 1990; **82**:1778–9.

109. Hussein MA, Mason J, Ravandi F, Rifkin RM. A phase Ii clinical study of arsenic trioxide (ATO) in patients (Pts) with relapsed or refractory multiple myeloma (MM): a preliminary report. *Blood* 2001; **98**:378a.

110. Bahlis MJ, Jordan McMurry I, Grad JM, Reis I, Neel J, Kharfan-Dabaja MA, *et al.* Phase I results from a phase I/II study of arsenic trioxide (As_2O_3) and ascorbic acid (AA) in relapsed and chemorefractory multiple myeloma. *Blood* 2001; **98**:375a.

111. Dimopoulos MA, Arbuck S, Huber M, Weber D, Luckett R, Delasalle K, *et al.* Primary therapy of multiple myeloma with paclitaxel. *Ann Oncol* 1994; **5**:757–9.

112. Kraut EH, Crowley JJ, Wade JL, Laufman L, Alsina M, Taylor S, *et al.* Evaluation of topotecan in resistant and relapsing multiple myeloma: a Southwest Oncology Group study. *J Clin Oncol* 1998; **16**:589–92.

113. Weber DM, Bseiso A, Wood A, *et al.* All-trans-retinoic acid for multiple myaloma. *Blood* 1997; **90**(Suppl 1):375a.

114. Niesvizky R, Siegel DS, Busquets X, Nichols G, Muindi J, Warrell RP Jr, *et al.* Hypercalcaemia and increased serum interleukin-6 levels induced by all-trans retinoic acid in patients with multiple myeloma. *Br J Haematol* 1995; **89**:217–18.

115. Salmon SE, Crowley JJ, Grogan TM, *et al.* Combination chemotherapy, glucocorticoids and interferon alfa in the treatment of multiple myeloma: a Southwest oncology Group study. *J Clin Oncol* 1994; **12**:1405–14.

116. Alexanian R, Yap BS, Bodey CP. Predisone pulse therapy for refractory myeloma. *Blood* 1983; **62**:572–7.

117. Alexanian R, Barlogie B, Dixon D. High-dose glucocorticoid treatment of resistant myeloma. *Ann Intern Med* 1986; **105**:8–11.

●118. Alexanian R, Dimopoulos MA, Delasalle K, Barlogie B. Primary dexamethasone treatment of multiple myeloma. *Blood* 1992; **80**:887–90.

119. Friedenberg WR, Kyle RA, Knospe WH, Bennett JM, Tsiatis AA, Oken MM. High-dose dexamethasone for refractory relapsing multiple myeloma. *Am J Hematol* 1991; **36**: 171–5.

120. Norfolk DR, Child JA. Pulsed high dose oral prednisolone in relapsed or refractory multiple myeloma. *Hematol Oncol* 1989; **7**:61–8.

121. Kumar S, Lacy MQ, Disperienzi A, Rajkumar SV, Fonseca R, Geyer S, *et al.* Single agent dexamethasone for induction in patients with multiple myeloma undergoing autologous stem cell transplants. *Blood* 2002; **100**:432a.

122. Peest D, Blade J, Harousseau JL. Cytokine therapy in multiple myeloma. *Br J Haematol* 1996; **94**:425–32.

123. Cooper RB, Dear K, McIntyre OR, Ozer H, Ellerton J, Canellos G, *et al.* A randomised trial comparing melphalan/prednisolone with or without interferon alfa-2b in newly diagnosed patients with myeloma: a Cancer and Leukaemia Group B study. *J Clin Oncol* 1993; **11**:151–60.

124. Avvisati G, Petrucci MT, Mandelli F. The role of biotherapies (interleukin, interferons and erythropoietin) in multiple myeloma. *Baillieres Clin Haematol* 1995; **8**:815–29.

◆125. Myeloma Trialists' Collaborative Group. Interferon as therapy for multiple myeloma: an individual patient data overview of 24 randomized trials and 4012 patients. *Br J Haematol* 2001; **113**:1020–34.

◆126. Fritz E, Ludwig H. Interferon-alpha treatment in multiple myeloma: meta-analysis of 30 randomised trials among 3948 patients. *Ann Oncol* 2000; **11**:1427–36.

127. Wisloff F, Gulbrandsen N, Nord E. Therapeutic options in multiple myeloma: pharmaco-economic considerations. *Pharmacoeconomics* 1999; **16**:329–41.

●128. Mandelli F, Avvisati G, Amadori S, Boccadoro M, Gernone A, Lauta VM, *et al.* Maintenance treatment with recombinant-alpha-2b interferon in patients with multiple myeloma responding to conventional induction chemotherapy. *N Engl J Med* 1990; **332**:1430–4.

129. Westin J, Rodjer S, Turesson I, Cortelezzi A, Hjorth M, Zador G. Interferon alpha-2b versus no maintenance therapy during the plateau phase in multiple myeloma: a randomised study. *Br J Haematol* 1995; **89**:561–8.

130. Browman GP, Bergsagel D, Sicheri D, O'Reilly S, Wilson KS, Rubin S, *et al.* Randomised trial of interferon maintenance in multiple myeloma: a study of the National Cancer Institute of Canada Clinical Trials Group. *J Clin Oncol* 1995; **13**:2354–60.

131. Joshua DE, Penny R, Matthews JP, Laidlaw CR, Gibson J, Bradstock K, *et al.* Australian Leukaemia Study Group Myeloma II: a randomised trial of intensive combination chemotherapy with or without interferon in patients with myeloma. *Br J Haematol* 1997; **97**:38–45.

132. Drayson MT, Chapman CE, Dunn JA, Olujohungbe AB, Maclennan IC. MRC trial of α2b-interferon maintenance therapy in first plateau phase of multiple myeloma. *Br J Haematol* 1998; **101**:195–202.

133. Salmon SE, Crowley JJ, Balcerzak SP, Roach RW, Taylor SA, Rivkin SE, *et al.* Interferon versus interferon plus prednisone remission maintenance therapy for multiple myeloma: a Southwest Oncology Group Study. *J Clin Oncol* 1998; **16**:890–6.

134. Cunningham D, Powles R, Malpas J, Raje N, Milan S, Viner C, *et al.* A randomised trial of maintenance interferon following high-dose chemotherapy in multiple myeloma: long-term follow-up results. *Br J Haematol* 1998; **102**:495–502.

135. Bjorkstrand B, Svensson H, Goldschmidt H, Ljungman P, Apperley J, Mandelli F, *et al.* Alpha-interferon maintenance treatment is associated with improved survival after high-dose treatment and autologous stem cell transplantation in patients with multiple myeloma: a retrospective registry study from the European Group for Blood and Marrow Transplantation (EBMT). *Bone Marrow Transplant* 2001; **27**:511–15.

136. Ludwig H, Fritz E, Neuda J, Durie BG. Patient preferences for interferon alfa in multiple myeloma. *J Clin Oncol* 1997; **15**:1672–9.

137. SWOG Southwest Oncology Group. Remission maintenance therapy for mutliple myeloma. *Arch Intern Med* 1975; **135**:147–52.

138. Kildahl-Anderson O, Bjark P, Bondevik A, Bull O, Dehli O, Kvambe V, *et al.* Multiple myeloma in central Norway 1981–1982: a randomised clinicl trial of 5-drug combination therapy versus standard therapy. *Scand J Haematol* 1986; **35**:518–24.

139. Blade J, Esteve J. Viewpoint on the impact of interferon in the treatment of multiple myeloma: benefit for a small proportion of patients? *Med Oncol* 2000; **17**:77–84.

140. Zee B, Cole B, Li T, Browman G, James K, Johnston D, *et al.* Quality-adjusted time without symptoms or toxicity analysis of interferon maintenance in multiple myeloma. *J Clin Oncol.* 1998; **16**:2834–9.

141. Wisloff F, Hjorth M, Kaasa S, Westin J. Effect of interferon on the health-related quality of life of multiple myeloma patients: results of a Nordic randomised trial comparing melphalan-prednisolone to melphalan–prednisolone + alpha–interferon. The Nordic Myeloma Study Group. *Br J Haematol* 1996; **94**:324–32.

142. Berenson JR, Crowley JJ, Grogan TM, *et al.* Maintenance therapy with alternate-day prednisone improves survival in multiple myeloma patients. *Blood* 2002; **99**:3163–8.

143. Salmon SE, Crowley JJ, Balcerzak SP, Roach RW, Taylor SA, Rivkin SE, *et al.* Amlowski W. Interferon versus interferon plus prednisone remission maintenace therapy for multiple myeloma: a Southwest Oncology Group Study. *J Clin Oncol* 1998; **16**:890–6.

●144. Alexanian R, Weber D, Dimopoulos M, Delasalle K, Smith TL. Randomized trial of alpha-interferon or dexamethasone as maintenance treatment for multiple myeloma. *Am J Hematol* 2000; **65**: 204–9.

145. Sumpter K, Powles RL, Raje N, Ramiah V, Kulkarni S, Treleaven J, *et al.* Oral idarubicin as a single agent therapy in patients with relapsed or resistant multiple myeloma. *Leuk Lymphoma* 1999; **35**:593–7.

146. Tosi P, Cavo M. Thalidomide in multiple myeloma: state of art. *Haematologica* 2002; **87**:233–4.

147. Rajkumar SV, Fonseca R, Lacy MQ, Witzig TE, Lust JA, Greipp PR, *et al.* Autologous stem cell transplantation for relapsed and primary refractory myeloma. *Bone Marrow Transplant* 1999; **23**:1267–72.

148. Vesole DH, Crowley JJ, Catchatourian R, Stiff PJ, Johnson DB, Cromer J, *et al.* High-dose melphalan with autotransplantation for refractory multiple myeloma: results of a Southwest Oncology Group phase II trial. *J Clin Oncol* 1999; **17**:2173–9.

149. Sidra GM, Byrne JL, Myers B, Mitchell DC, Russell NH. Combination therapy with thalidomide, cyclophosphamide, and dexamethasone (C-ThaD) for relapsed and primary refractory multiple myeloma. *Br J Haematol* **117**(Suppl 1):64.

150. Tricot G, Jagannath S, Vesole DH, Crowley J, Barlogie B. (b) Relapse of multiple myeloma after autologous

transplantation: survival after salvage therapy. *Bone Marrow Transplant* 1995; **16**:7–11.

151. Mehta J, Tricot G, Jagannath S, Ayers D, Singhal S, Siegel D, *et al.* Salvage autologous or allogeneic transplantation refractory to or relapsing after a first line autograft. *Bone Marrow Transplant* 1998; **21**:887–98.

152. Lokhorst HM, Sonneveld P, Verdonck LF. Intensive treatment for multiple myeloma: where do we stand? *Br J Haematol* 1999; **106**:18–27.

153. Singer CR, Tobias JS, Giles F, Rudd GN, Blackman GM, Richards JD. Hemibody irradiation. An effective second-line therapy in drug-resistant multiple myeloma. *Cancer* 1989; **15**:2446–51.

154. Epstein J, Xiao H, Koba B. P-glycoprotein expression in myeloma is associated with resistance to VAD. *Blood* 1989; **74**:913–17.

155. Dalton WS, Grogan TM, Meltzer PS, Scheper R, Durie B, Taylor C, *et al.* Drug-resistance in multiple myeloma and non-Hodgkin's lymphoma: detection of p-glycoprotein and potential circumvention by addition of verapamil to chemotherapy. *J Clin Oncol* 1989; **7**:415–24.

156. Grogan TM, Spier CM, Salmon SE, *et al.* p-Glycoprotein expression in human plasma cell myeloma: correlation with prior chemotherapy. *Blood* 1993; **81**:490–5.

157. Salmon SE, Dalton WS, Grogan TM, *et al.* Multi-drug resistant myeloma: laboratory and clinical effects of verapamil as a senstitiser. *Blood* 1991; **78**:44–50.

158. Sonneveld P, Suciu S, Weijermans P, Beksac M, Neuwirtova R, Solbu G, *et al.* Cyclosporin A combined with vincristine, doxorubicin and dexamethasone (VAD) compared with VAD alone in patients with advanced refractory multiple myeloma: an EORTC–HOVON randomized phase III study (06914). *Br J Haematol* 2001; **115**:895–902.

15

Radiotherapy

DEBORAH A. FRASSICA AND MARIA C. JACOBS

INTRODUCTION

Radiotherapy has been utilized in the management of patients with plasma cell malignancies for much of the twentieth century and continues today. It has been estimated that radiotherapy will be required for up to 70% of patients with multiple myeloma at some point in the course of their disease,[1] and it is the primary treatment modality for patients with solitary extramedullary or bone plasmacytomas (see Chapter 25). The radiosensitivity of myeloma has been well established through clinical experience and in laboratory studies. Using a mouse plasma cell tumor model, Bergsagel estimated the D_0 (dose required to produce one natural log of cell kill) to be 1.1 Gray (Gy).[2] This chapter will review the current roles of radiotherapy in the palliative management of multiple myeloma and as part of the conditioning regimens for bone marrow transplant for multiple myeloma. In addition, the role of radioimmunotherapy will be discussed.

LOCAL RADIOTHERAPY

The primary indications for the use of radiotherapy in multiple myeloma are palliation of pain, prevention of bone destruction leading to pathologic fracture, prevention or treatment of neurologic complications of disease, such as nerve-root or spinal cord compression, and relief of symptoms caused by soft-tissue involvement. External beam treatment has been the mainstay of radiotherapeutic management. Both wide-field (total body or hemi-body) and localized field treatment have been utilized. Localized fields are most commonly used today owing to the low

risk of acute and late side effects, reduced effect on bone marrow activity, and ease of administration compared with wide-field therapy.

The total dose and fractionation (size and number of daily treatments) utilized for patients with multiple myeloma will vary based on the intent of treatment and the patient's prognosis and performance status. Patients with limited life expectancies and who require treatment for pain relief may achieve the therapeutic goal with a shorter course of therapy and a lower total dose. If the goal of treatment is long-term control of a localized area of myelomatous involvement, more aggressive therapy should be used, with doses similar to those for patients with solitary plasmacytomas (40–50 Gy). The potential side effects of radiotherapy are related to the total dose, fraction size, volume of treatment, and the area of the body treated. Organ tolerances are based on the use of 'standard fractionation', 1.8–2.0 Gy per fraction administered once daily, five times per week. When altered fractionation schemes are utilized, the total dose must be adjusted in order to avoid a higher risk of complications. Generally accepted normal tissue tolerances, measured as the total dose in standard fractionation that is associated with a 5% risk of a given complication at 5 years, are shown in Table 15.1.

Palliative treatment for pain relief

Relatively low doses of radiation have been associated with effective symptom control in patients with multiple myeloma, but controversy exists as to the optimal dose for palliative treatment. Numerous groups have reported on their dose–response experiences and rates of pain relief. Investigators at the Mallinckrodt Institute of Radiology[3] recorded the dose at which subjective pain relief was first

Table 15.1 *Commonly accepted normal tissue tolerances using fractionated ionizing irradiation (1.8–2.0 Gy/day)*

Organ (volume)	Complication	Dose (Gy)
Spinal cord	Myelopathy	45–50
Brain (partial volume)	Necrosis	60
Small bowel (large volume)	Chronic enteritis; small bowel	45
Small bowel (limited volume)	obstruction	54
Kidney (whole organ)	Renal failure	20–25
Liver (whole organ)	Hepatic failure	35
Esophagus	Stricture, ulcer	60–65
Lung	Fibrosis	20
Bone	Necrosis	60
Bone marrow (partial)	Fibrosis	20

reported by patients receiving localized radiotherapy. The median dose range was between 10 and 15 Gy, with 29 of 34 patients reporting pain relief with a dose of 20 Gy. In the same report, complete relief of pain by completion of therapy was obtained in 21% and partial relief in 70% of 116 patients. The authors commented that many of the patients with partial relief at completion of therapy subsequently went on to achieve complete pain relief within the next few weeks. The total dose most frequently prescribed was between 15 and 20 Gy. Six percent of the fields treated required retreatment for recurrence of pain. Leigh *et al.*[4] reviewed the experience at the University of Arizona. Ninety-seven percent of patients achieved pain relief with a median dose of 25 Gy. Complete relief was observed in 26% and partial relief in 71%. No differences in pain relief outcome were noted with doses less than or greater than 10 Gy (range 3–60 Gy), concurrent use of chemotherapy, or site of treatment. As in Mill's report,[3] 6% of patients had a local relapse after initial treatment. Retreatment of areas treated with lower doses of radiotherapy is generally considered feasible with respect to normal tissue toxicity. The effectiveness of retreatment has, however, been questioned by Adamietz and co-workers.[5] They found that the rate of complete pain relief decreased with subsequent courses of treatment, with no responses by the third course.

In distinction to the lack of benefit with concurrent chemotherapy noted by Leigh *et al.*,[4] the Hanover group[5] found an 80% local response rate in patients treated with melphalan, prednisone, and radiotherapy compared with a 40% response rate in patients managed with irradiation alone for local symptoms. The duration of response was also greater in the combined therapy group. Rates of prior use of chemotherapy differed in these studies, with nearly half of the Hanover patients being chemotherapy-naive and nearly all of the Arizona patients being heavily pre-treated. One might expect a better response to initial therapy in chemotherapy-naive compared with treatment of patients whose disease has become chemoresistant.

The issue of appropriate field size for localized treatment to long bones was addressed in a study by Catell *et al.*[6] They reviewed the experience at the New York University Medical Center using fields encompassing the symptomatic lesion plus a 1–2 cm margin. No attempts were made to cover the entire bone, as has been occasionally advocated. The average dose was 27.8 Gy. Even though the whole bone was not targeted, the length of the field relative to the bone length was 42% for the femurs treated and 68% for the humeri. Evidence of symptomatic progressive disease within the same bone was found in four of 41 long bones treated. In three of the four cases, the progressive disease was both adjacent to and within the previously irradiated volume. Symptomatic disease developed exclusively outside the original treatment volume in only one patient. This suggests that treatment to the symptomatic sites with an appropriate margin is not associated with a high rate of in-bone failure. Limiting the field sizes may help to limit marrow toxicity and other side effects of treatment.

Radiotherapeutic management of spinal cord compression

Neurologic compromise, such as nerve-root or cord compression, is an important problem that may occur in patients with myeloma. Six to twenty-four percent of patients with myeloma have been reported to require treatment for spinal cord compression.[3,7–10] Two of the more recent studies[7,8] have shown a risk of 10–15%. Treatment options include non-operative therapy with radiation, surgical treatment, and combined modality therapy. Patients with spinal instability or bone fragments from a compression fracture causing cord compression are generally offered surgery followed by radiotherapy. Wallington *et al.*[7] reviewed a series of 48 cases of spinal cord compression from myeloma (24 patients) and lymphoma (24 patients) treated with radiotherapy. Eleven of the 24 patients with myeloma had surgical decompression prior to initiation of radiotherapy. They evaluated factors leading to the endpoint of local control, defined as maintenance of or improvement to a grade 1 neurologic deficit or better without deterioration for 3 months from the start of radiotherapy. Sixty-three percent of the patients with myeloma achieved local control. Characteristics associated with a significantly improved chance of achieving local control on chi-squared analysis included age 65 or less, grade 1 or 2 neurologic deficit at presentation (ambulatory with or without assistance), and biologically equivalent radiation dose of 40 Gy or more. Benson *et al.*'s 1979 report[9] also showed an advantage to doses of 40 Gy compared with lower doses for myeloma patients with cord compression. Surgical decompression prior to radiotherapy was not associated with improvement in local control. Multivariate analysis showed grade 3 neurological deficit to be independently significant for duration of local control. Other studies[11–13] of treatment for spinal cord compression from all primary tumor types confirm that ambulatory status at presentation is predictive of outcome. Pain control can be achieved in patients with cord compression regardless of grade of neurologic deficit at presentation.[11]

The long-term effectiveness of spinal radiotherapy for patients presenting with neurologic symptoms (cord or nerve-root compression) was evaluated in an interesting report from Belgium.[14] Twelve patients were assessed with serial magnetic resonance imaging (MRI) scans prior to and following radiotherapy. Fifty-seven vertebral segments were included in the radiotherapy portals and were compared with 147 vertebrae outside the fields. All patients received between 30 and 40 Gy in standard fractionation (2 Gy/day) for neurological symptoms and pain. All of the patients also received chemotherapy for systemic management. With a mean follow-up of 35 months, new compression fractures were documented by MRI in 5% of irradiated and 20% of untreated vertebrae. New focal lesions were found in 4% of irradiated and 27% of untreated vertebrae. Management of vertebral disease with surgery or cement vertebroplasty alone may, therefore, be associated with a greater risk of subsequent disease, requiring additional procedures or radiotherapy. Whether this type of beneficial long-term effect would be achieved with lower doses of radiation is unknown but worthy of study. Treating a greater number of vertebral segments at the time of radiotherapy for symptomatic disease in order to reduce subsequent disease must be balanced with the effect of treating larger amounts of bone marrow, which could exacerbate hematologic toxicity.

Myelomatous involvement of the spine, ribs, or base of skull may cause neurological dysfunction owing to irritation or compression of nerves or nerve roots. Patients are more likely to have compressive symptoms when there is a soft-tissue component of disease. In some situations, progressive bone disease may be treated prior to development of significant symptoms, if the lesion is in a critical location, such as base of skull, clivus, or orbit (Fig. 15.1). In order to provide the greatest chance of long-term local control, doses in the range of 40–45 Gy would be recommended.

Local radiotherapy for bone lesions

Most patients with multiple myeloma and who are referred for radiotherapy have pain secondary to bone involvement. Alleviation of pain is a major endpoint of therapy but prevention of further destruction of bone and restitution of bone are also important goals, especially if the patient is expected to live more than 3–6 months. When life expectancy is very limited, the short-term control of pain, avoidance of treatment-related side effects, and ease of administration of therapy for the patient are the utmost concerns. However, when it is anticipated that survival may

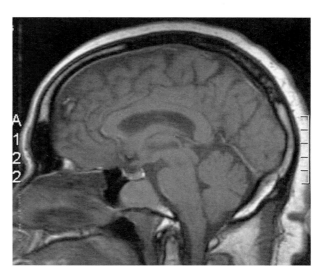

Figure 15.1 *Example of myeloma involving the clivus. Growth of a lesion in this location could result in significant neurologic impairment.*

be more extended, long-term local control or eradication of local tumor is of importance. Patients should be assessed for the risk of impending fracture when weight-bearing bones are involved. If the risk is felt to be high, patients will be offered surgical intervention prior to radiotherapy. If surgical intervention were not required, radiotherapy to the area of involvement would proceed. Fields encompassing the radiographic abnormality plus a margin of 3–5 cm are generally used. MRI may be helpful in delineating the extent of marrow involvement adjacent to the lesion visualized on standard films. When long-term local control is desired, the total dose should be higher (approximately 40–45 Gy or its equivalent) than if pain control is the only concern. If it is anticipated that a large amount of normal tissue will lie within the treatment fields, computed tomography (CT) planning could be utilized in order to devise a plan that would limit normal tissue exposure and reduce the potential for side effects. Radiographic evidence of healing may take many months following radiotherapy. Patients should be warned that the bone strength will not be improved in the short term after radiotherapy and care should be taken to avoid high stresses in the treated site. Higher doses of radiation may be associated with a greater late risk of fracture as noted in the study of fractionation patterns used for patients with metastatic bone disease by the Radiation Therapy Oncology Group (RTOG).[15] The rate of fracture was 17.5% in patients treated with 40.5 Gy in 15 fractions compared with 4% in patients receiving 20 Gy in five fractions ($P = 0.02$).

Post–operative radiotherapy

Radiotherapy following surgical fixation for pathologic fractures, impending fractures, or spinal instability is commonly recommended. In most situations, surgery for metastatic bone disease or myeloma is not designed to provide complete oncologic resection of disease. Post-operative radiotherapy has been associated with a decrease in the incidence of reoperation for tumor progression or failure of fixation.[16] In addition, the probability of achieving normal use of the extremity in one study was found to be 53% with post-operative radiotherapy versus 11.5% with surgery alone.[16] In patients with newly diagnosed myeloma, chemotherapy may be able to provide control of disease at surgical sites, eliminating the need for radiotherapy. Chen has indicated that chemotherapy has been used in lieu of radiotherapy in this situation at the Mayo Clinic[17] in recent years. Patients with chemorefractory disease or in whom chemotherapy will not be utilized should receive radiotherapy post-operatively. Doses similar to those used for primary palliative treatment are utilized for patients with widespread chemorefractory disease, but higher doses may be indicated for patients with more favorable prognoses. The field size is generally designed to encompass the entire prosthesis. Care should be taken to ensure adequate coverage of soft-tissue extension of disease. Review of all available pre-operative cross-sectional imaging may be helpful in defining the extent of soft tissue involvement. MRI and CT scans generally have limited usefulness as well, owing to the significant artifact produced by the rods or plates. In our experience, most patients will show evidence of radiographic healing; however, evidence of complete union of a fracture is not necessary to achieve the goals of stability, pain relief, and maintenance of fixation.

Osteosclerotic myeloma

An uncommon form of myeloma is the osteosclerotic variant. Lesions are often solitary or few in number. Approximately 50% of these cases are associated with peripheral neuropathy with or without the full POEMS syndrome (polyneuropathy, organomegaly, endocrinopathy, M-protein, and skin changes).[18–20] Treatment of the bone lesion in solitary cases has been associated with improvement in the neuropathy,[20,21] but reports of

significant improvement when multiple bone lesions are present have been uncommon. Rotta and Bradley[22] reported on a patient with three sclerotic bone lesions, features of POEMS syndrome, and a negative bone marrow and who had a marked improvement in the polyneuropathy that had left him non-ambulatory, with combined modality therapy, including excision of the largest bone lesion (for diagnosis), radiotherapy to the other skeletal lesions, plasmapheresis, and chemotherapy. This suggests that even patients with greater skeletal involvement and severe neuropathies may benefit from aggressive therapy.

Palliative wide–field radiotherapy

Wide-field (total body or hemi-body) irradiation has a long history of use in multiple myeloma. Total body irradiation (TBI) was utilized as initial management in the pre-chemotherapy era.[23,24] With the advent of chemotherapy, wide-field therapy was generally reserved for patients with refractory or recurrent myeloma, or for pain relief. Holder[24] as early as 1965 found that significant pain relief could be achieved with TBI. Hemi-body irradiation (HBI), which could be performed sequentially to the upper and lower hemi-body regions, largely replaced total body irradiation due to better tolerance. Numerous groups[25–34] have reported their results using single fraction HBI or sequential (double) HBI for palliation of pain and for treatment of refractory disease. Table 15.2 reviews the pain control results and hematologic toxicity from a number of studies.

Palliative hemi-body therapy is generally administered in a single fraction. Doses have ranged from 3 Gy[32] to 10 Gy.[26] Generally, the upper hemi-body dose is limited to 6–7.5 Gy[27,31,32,34] in order to reduce the risk of pneumonitis. Treating hemi-body regions sequentially with a rest between each portion allows for improved marrow tolerance compared with total body irradiation. The unirradiated marrow serves as a reserve for hematologic function and may allow reseeding of the irradiated marrow.[17,35] Hemi-body or sequential hemi-body therapy will lead to the need for red blood cell transfusion in

Table 15.2 *Results of palliative single or double hemi-body irradiation for chemotherapy refractory myeloma*

Study	Hemi-body radiation	Hematologic toxicity	Pain relief (%)
Bosch[27]	Single	Minimal	94
McSweeney[31]	Double	60% recovered sufficiently to receive α-interferon	95
Thomas[32]	Double	Severe; 1/7 fatal	All patients improved
Plesnicar[33]	Double	Full recovery by 6 weeks	83
Rostom[34]	12 double, 7 single	50% recovered fully after DHBI; 89.5% recovered after single HBI	89.5

DHBI, double hemi-body irradiation; HBI, hemi-body irradiation.

half to two-thirds of patients and approximately one-quarter will require platelet support.[29,31]

In chemorefractory patients, approximately 25–40% of patients will have a 50% or greater reduction in M-protein levels.[25,28,31] However, in a study from the Southwest Oncology Group,[36] only 5% of chemotherapy non-responders were converted to remission status. Plesnicar and colleagues treated six patients whose responses to chemotherapy had plateaued with sequential HBI but saw only one objective response.[33] HBI has also been shown to be inferior to chemotherapy when administered for remission consolidation following induction chemotherapy.[36] Therefore, the use of HBI for chemotherapy responders or non-responders is not generally recommended except for palliation of pain.[33,36,37]

TOTAL BODY IRRADIATION IN MULTIPLE MYELOMA

Over the past decade, bone marrow transplantation (BMT) has become an effective treatment for patients with various hematologic malignancies, particularly leukemias and lymphomas. More recently, autologous and allogeneic BMT has been introduced in the systemic treatment of multiple myeloma (see Chapters 16 and 17). Total body irradiation has played a significant role in the development of BMT clinical trials because it provided an effective cytoreductive conditioning regimen prior to high-dose chemotherapy and BMT. The use of autologous BMT is now accepted as primary treatment for younger patients with myeloma, but conditioning regimens, including melphalan–TBI, have been found to be inferior to melphalan alone.[38] Allogeneic transplant remains controversial because of the high mortality rate secondary to treatment-related complications, but TBI continues to be part of the standard conditioning regimens because it produces immunosuppression to allow engraftment of the donor marrow.[39–41] Recently, non-myeloablative doses of TBI (200 cGy) have been used with or without fludarabine, in an attempt to reduce the toxicities associated with allogeneic transplants, with promising results.[42]

Technical aspects of TBI

Radiation delivery in TBI should be as accurate as possible, keeping in mind that the dosimetry of this technique is most challenging, requiring the participation of the clinical physicist, dosimetrist, and the radiation therapist. In view of the irregular contour of the human body, to assure homogeneity in dose distribution most centers in the USA use linear accelerators with photon beam energies of 6–10 MeV. Patient position and immobilization must be considered during treatment planning to assure

reproducibility. Shank[43] has described a variety of positions, but today the most common positions are either standing up with anterior and posterior fields, or lying supine and/or prone with anterior and posterior fields, lateral fields, or a combination of both. Many centers have developed some form of TBI technique, attempting to provide patient comfort, since each treatment is significantly longer than the time required for delivery of standard-dose, localized treatments. For instance, at Memorial Sloan Kettering Cancer Center (MSKCC), a stand was developed to provide support and immobilization, which utilized a bicycle seat and handgrips for security.[44] At the University of Maryland Medical Center, a team of physicists and radiation oncologists developed a 'translational' couch, which facilitates reproducibility.[45] Beam spoilers are recommended to ensure adequate surface dose. At some institutions, compensators have been used at the neck, feet, and other thinner areas to increase homogeneity.[43] It is also important to consider the dose per fraction as well as the dose rate at which the treatment is delivered, since these factors relate to normal tissue toxicity, particularly interstitial pneumonitis (IP). Generally, treatment is administered with a dose rate of between 0.05 and 0.15 Gy/minute, significantly lower than the dose rates used for localized therapy of 2.0–3.0 Gy/minute.

The optimal schedule of TBI remains controversial. Most schedules have been based on either empiric or radiobiologic calculations. Vriesendorp[46,47] concluded that highly fractionated TBI with twice or three times daily regimen and total doses of 15 Gy produced effective immunosuppression and impressive sparing of the normal tissues, such as lung. Clinically, a variety of TBI regimens have been used, varying from single-dose treatment, to a regimen with a few fractions and higher doses per fraction, to highly fractionated daily regimens with multiple lower dose fractions per day. Ideally, when using twice-daily treatments, a 6-hour interval should be allowed between the fractions. This interval should be sufficient to allow maximal repair of sublethal damage of normal tissues prior to the next fraction. Fractionation has been shown to play a prominent role in the prevention of delayed toxicity of BMT. One of the major complications has been interstitial pneumonitis. Most recent studies support the use of hyperfractionated TBI to prevent this lethal complication. A randomized series from Seattle compared daily fractionation of 2 Gy for six fractions for a total dose of 12 Gy with a single dose of 10 Gy. In that study, IP was reported in 15% of the fractionated group compared with 26% of the single-dose group.[48] In a non-randomized comparative study, Cosset et al.[49] demonstrated a reduction in IP from 45% to 13% with single-dose TBI (10 Gy) versus fractionated TBI (13.2 Gy in 11 fractions over 4 days). A single dose of 10 Gy (lungs limited to 8 Gy) was compared with 14.85 Gy delivered in 11 fractions over 5 days in a prospective, randomized trial.[50] Cause-specific survival of patients receiving an allogeneic transplant was not significantly different based on the treatment schema. The incidence of veno-occlusive disease of the liver was significantly greater in the single dose group (14%) compared with the fractionated group (4%), but no differences were seen in the risk of IP. At the Mount Sinai Medical Center, a regimen consisting of a total dose of 15 Gy in ten fractions (1.5 Gy per fraction) over 5 days appeared as effective in achieving immunosuppression as 15 Gy in 12 fractions (1.25 Gy per fraction given three times daily) over 4 days used extensively at MSKCC.[44] While a variety of treatment schema have been used, the optimal fractionated regimen (total dose, number, and size of daily fractions) has not been established (see Table 15.3).

Toxicity of TBI

Common acute side effects of TBI are nausea and vomiting, usually occurring a few hours after the first fraction and improving over the course of hyperfractionated radiotherapy. Acute parotiditis with transient xerostomia[44] and oral mucositis are also common events in patients undergoing TBI. Fatigue, skin erythema, and hyperpigmentation are almost the rule. Late toxicities include graft versus host disease, interstitial pneumonitis, cataracts, liver and kidney dysfunction, hypothyroidism, and decreased gonadal function. The incidence of alterations of cognitive function and secondary malignancy is not well defined in the multiple myeloma population.

One of the most challenging problems associated with TBI is the potential development of interstitial pneumonitis, which has been reported to be fatal in the large majority of patients who develop this complication.[44] Radiobiology studies in animals have shown that increasing the number of fractions greatly decreases the incidence of IP.[44] Two TBI fractionation regimen were compared by Gopal et al.[51] to evaluate the incidence of acute and late pulmonary toxicity. Regimen A consisted of twice-daily fractions of 1.7 Gy over 3 days for a total dose of 10.2 Gy with no lung shielding. Regimen B consisted of 3.0 Gy daily over 4 days for a total dose of 12 Gy with lung shielding during the third dose. Patients were evaluated with pulmonary function tests (PFTs) and, after a median follow-up of 48 months, there was no significant difference in the PFTs or in late toxicity in either group. Della Volpe et al.[52] analyzed the effect of median lung dose on development of lethal pulmonary complications in patients treated with TBI in the conditioning regimen for BMT for hematologic malignancies. A regimen of fractionated TBI (10 Gy total dose in three fractions, one fraction/day, 0.055 Gy/minute) was utilized and individual lung doses were measured via in vivo dosimetry. They found that the risk of lethal pulmonary complications was 14.3% in patients with a median lung dose of greater than 9.4 Gy compared with 3.8% in patients with a lung dose of 9.4 Gy or less.

The lens is one of the most sensitive organs to ionizing radiation. Cataract formation has been considered nearly inevitable following TBI for BMT. Benyunes et al.[53] found that fractionated TBI regimens were associated with a reduction in cataract formation. Eighty-five percent of patients treated with a single 10 Gy dose exhibited cataract formation by 11 years compared with 34% of patients receiving 12 Gy fractionated TBI. Belkacemi et al.[54] evaluated treatment factors associated with cataract

Table 15.3 *Examples of total body irradiation techniques used for hematologic malignancies*

Study	Total dose (Gy)	Number of fractions	Instantaneous dose rate (IDR) (Gy/minute)	Toxicity (%) IP	Cataracts	VOD	Comments
Cosset[49]	10	1	0.125	45	–	13	Survival similar
	13.2	11	–	13		0	
Girinsky[50]	10	1	0.125	19	–	14	Survival similar
	14.85	11	0.25	14		4	
Gopal[51]	10.2	6	–	Same	–	–	OS 66%; FFP 31%
	12	4					OS 67% ; FFP: 82%
Della Volpe[52]	10	3	0.55	9	–	–	Lethal IP 14.3% vs. 3.8% for median lung dose > or ≤9.4 Gy
Benyunes[53]	10	1	–	–	85 (11 years)	–	Cataract risk in patients not receiving TBI – 19%
	12–15.75	6–7			>12 Gy: 50		
					12 Gy: 34		
Belkacemi[54]	10	1	0.03–0.15	–	11.3 (5 years)	–	High IDR and lack of heparin for VOD independently associated with increased frequency of cataracts
	12	6	0.03–0.089		4.4 (5 years)		
Feinstein[42]	2	1	–	–	–	–	Non-relapse mortality – 0%

FFP, freedom from progression; OS, overall survival; TBI, total body irradiation; VOD, veno-occlusive disease of the liver.

formation in patients treated with single-dose (10 Gy) or fractionated (12 Gy – 3 fractions – 3 days) TBI for allogeneic or autologous transplant for a variety of hematologic malignancies. For all patients, the estimated 5-year incidence of cataract formation was 23%. The risk was lower in patients receiving fractionated TBI than single-dose TBI(11% vs. 34%). Dose rate was also analyzed and was found to influence the risk of cataract formation. The 5-year risk was estimated to be 54%, 30%, and 3.5% for patients in the high-dose-rate group ($\geq$0.09 Gy/minute), the medium group ($\geq$0.048 Gy/minute but <0.09 Gy/minute), and low-dose-rate group (<0.048 Gy/minute), respectively. In addition to the radiation-related factors, Belkacemi et al.[54] also found that the use of heparin for prophylaxis against veno-occlusive liver disease was associated with a reduction in cataract formation (16% with heparin vs. 28% without). In multivariate analysis, only dose rate and heparin use were independently associated with the risk of cataract formation. These complications of TBI, as well as thyroid and gonadal dysfunction and decrease in cognitive abilities, are not life-threatening; however, they must be closely evaluated when assessing quality of life issues after high-dose chemotherapy and stem-cell rescue with TBI as part of the conditioning regimen. Many of these problems will be significantly reduced if the non-myeloablative TBI techniques become standard.

RADIOIMMUNOTHERAPY

Radioimmunotherapy (RIT) has been shown to be a useful technique for tumors such as the non-Hodgkin's lymphomas. Its use in multiple myeloma would potentially allow delivery of radiation to tumor cells while minimizing dose to normal tissue. A multitude of factors must be considered in the design of RIT techniques, including target-cell radiosensitivity, proliferation rate, ability to repair sublethal damage, tumor size, affinity and avidity of the antibody, target–non-target distribution ratios, etc.[55,56] As with external beam irradiation, currently available evidence does suggest a direct relationship between the administered dose of radiolabeled antibody and efficacy, as well as toxicity. The dosimetry of RIT, however, is less well defined and continues to be studied.[57]

In the myeloma model, where large, solid tumor masses are often not present, the choice of an α-emitting radioisotope with a very short range of action may be appropriate in order to maximize the target–non-target dose ratio. Another choice would be iodine-131 (^{131}I), a β-emitter with a relatively short range of action.[58,59] The efficacy of an α-emitter to produce cell mortality was demonstrated for myeloma cells with bismuth-213 (^{213}Bi) in an *ex vivo* model by Couturier et al.[59] Superiority of the α-emitter was validated in an *in vitro* study comparing ^{213}Bi and ^{131}I recently published by Supiot et al.[58]

The choice of an appropriate monoclonal antibody (MAb) is critical to RIT (see Chapter 20). Antibody distribution depends on multiple factors such as specificity, valency, and tumor-related conditions such as hypoxia.[55] Antibodies to epithelial mucin-1 glycoprotein (MUC-1), such as the MA5 anti-MUC1 monoclonal antibody, were found to be strongly reactive with human myeloma cell lines.[60] Supiot et al.[58] evaluated MA5 anti-MUC1 and B-B4, a monoclonal antibody that recognizes syndecan-1 (CD138). Treatment of myeloma cell lines with [^{213}Bi]B-B4 induced myeloma cell mortality and caused cell arrest in G2/M. The concentration required to create the same effect was fivefold higher with [^{213}Bi]MA5 than the B-B4 MAb. They also tested both MAbs with ^{131}I. Following treatment with [^{131}I]B-B4 MAb the percentage of cells arrested in the G2/M phase was nil and the effect on cell mortality was very limited. These results suggested that B-B4 was the more effective MAb and that use of an α-emitter was better than the use of ^{131}I. Targeting of normal tissues was seen with both MAbs. MA5 stained renal and pulmonary, tissues whereas B-B4 stained hepatic, pulmonary and duodenal tissue. Another approach that is being studied is the use of radioimmunoconjugates in the conditioning regimen for stem-cell transplantation. The use of a radiolabeled monoclonal antibody to an antigen, such as CD45 (common leukocyte antigen), may allow more specific targeting of the marrow and delivery of additional dose without unacceptable normal tissue exposure.[61] Clinical trials will be necessary to further test the effectiveness of various types of RIT for patients with multiple myeloma and assess for potential toxicities, but this type of targeted therapy holds promise for the future.

KEY POINTS

- Palliative external beam irradiation with doses in the range of 20–25 Gy is capable of providing the majority of patients with excellent pain control.
- Spinal cord compression and other symptoms of local disease can be treated effectively with radiotherapy. Slightly higher doses (30–40 Gy) may improve the likelihood of improving neurologic function and maintaining long-term local control.
- For long-term control of localized bone and soft-tissue lesions, doses of 40–45 Gy are generally recommended.
- Post-operative radiotherapy following fixation of pathologic or impending pathologic fractures is generally recommended to decrease the risk of further bone destruction and the need for additional surgery.

- Total body irradiation (TBI) is commonly used in the preparative regimen for allogeneic bone marrow transplantation. The use of fractionated TBI has significantly decreased the risk of interstitial pneumonitis. Low-dose, non-myeloablative TBI is being studied and appears to be associated with reduced toxicity.
- Radioimmunotherapy is currently being investigated and may become an important part of the armamentarium for the treatment of patients with multiple myeloma.

REFERENCES

● = Key primary paper

◆ = Major review article

1. Berenson JR, Lichtenstein A, Porter L, Dimopoulus M, Bordone R, Lipton A, et al. Efficacy of pamidronate in reducing skeletal events in patients with advanced multiple myeloma: Myeloma Aredia Sturdy Group. N Engl J Med 1996; **334**:488–93.

2. Bergsagel D. Total body irradiation for myelomatosis. Br Med J 1971; **2**:325.

3. Mill WB, Griffith R. The role of radiation therapy in the management of plasma cell tumors. Cancer 1980; **45**:647–52.

●4. Leigh B, Kurtts T, Mack C, Matzner M, Shimm D. Radiation therapy for the palliation of multiple myeloma. Int J Radiat Oncol Biol Phys 1993; **25**:801–4.

5. Adamietz IA, Schober C, Schulte RW, Peest D, Renner K. Palliative radiotherapy in plasma cell myeloma. Radiother Oncol 1991; **20**:111–16.

6. Catell D, Kogen Z, Donahue B, Steinfeld A. Multiple myeloma of an extremity: must the entire bone be treated? Int J Radiat Oncol Biol Phys 1998; **40**:117–19.

●7. Wallington M, Mendis S, Premawardhana U, Sanders P, Shahsavar-Haghighi K. Local control and survival in spinal cord compression from lymphoma and myeloma. Radiother Oncol 1997; **42**:43–7.

8. Plowman, PN. Radiotherapy of myeloma. In: Malpas JS, Bergsagel DE, Kyle RA (eds) Myeloma: biology and management. New York: Oxford University Press, 1995:314–21.

9. Benson WJ, Scarffe JH, Todd ID, Palmer M, Crowther D. Spinal cord compression in myeloma: an occasional review. Br Med J 1979; **18**:1541–4.

10. Woo E, Yu YL, Ng M, Haung CY, Todd D. Spinal cord compression in multiple myeloma: who gets it? Aust N Z Med 1986; **16**:671–5.

11. Turner S, Marosszeky B, Timms I, Boyages J. Malignant spinal cord compression: a prospective evaluation. Int J Radiat Oncol Biol Phys 1993; **26**:141–6.

12. Findlay GF. Adverse effects of the management of malignant spinal cord compression. J Neurol Neurosurg Psych 1984; **47**:761–8.

13. Gilbert RW, Kim JH, Posner JB. Epidural spinal cord compression from metastatic tumour: diagnosis and treatment. Ann Neurol 1978; **3**:40–51.

●14. Lecouvet F, Richard F, Vande Berg B, Malghem J, Maldague B, Jamart J, et al. Long-term effects of localized spinal radiation therapy on vertebral fractures and focal lesions appearance in patients with multiple myeloma. Br J Haematol 1997; **96**:743–5.

15. Blitzer P. Reanalysis of the RTOG study of palliation of symptomatic osseous metastases. Cancer 1985; **55**:1468–72.

16. Townsend PW, Rosenthal HG, Smalley SR, Cozad S, Hassanein R. Impact of postoperative radiation therapy and other factors on outcome after orthopedic stabilization of impending or pathologic fractures due to metastatic disease. J Clin Oncol 1995; **13**:2140–1.

17. Chen MG, Gertz MA. Multiple myeloma and other plasma cell neoplasms. In: Gunderson LL, Tepper J (eds) Clinical radiation oncology. Philadelphia: Churchill Livingstone, 2000:1189–202.

18. Bosch EP, Smith VE. Peripheral neuropathies associated with monoclonal proteins. Med Clin North Am 1993; **1**:125–39.

19. Miralles GD, O'Fallon JR, Talley NJ. Plasma-cell dyscrasia with polyneuropathy. The spectrum of POEMS syndrome. N Engl J Med 1992; **327**:1919–23.

◆20. Soubrier MJ, Dubost JJ, Sauvezie BJ. POEMS syndrome: a study of 25 cases and review of literature. Am J Med 1994; **97**:543–53.

21. Kelly JJ, Kyle RA, Miles JM, Dyck PJ. Osteosclerotic myeloma and peripheral neuropathy. Neurology 1983; **33**:202–10.

22. Rotta FT, Bradley WG. Marked improvement of severe polyneuropathy associated with multifocal osteosclerotic myeloma following surgery, radiation, and chemotherapy. Muscle Nerve 1997; **20**:1035–7.

23. Medinger FG, Craver LF. Total body irradiation, with review of cases. Am J Roentgenol 1942; **48**:651.

24. Holder DL. Total-body irradiation in multiple myeloma. Radiology 1965; **84**:83.

25. Jaffe JP, Bosch A, Raich PC. Sequential hemi-body radiotherapy in advanced multiple myeloma. Cancer 1979; **43**:124–8.

26. Rowland C, Garrett M, Crowley F. Half body radiation in plasma cell myeloma. Clin Radiol 1983; **34**:507–10.

27. Bosch A, Frias Z. Radiotherapy in the treatment of multiple myeloma. Int J Radiat Oncol Biol Phys 1988; **15**:1363–9.

28. Jacobs P, le Roux I, King HS. Sequential half-body irradiation as salvage therapy in chemotherapy-resistant multiple myeloma. Am J Clin Oncol 1988; **11**:104–9.

29. Singer C, Tobias J, Giles F, Rudd G, Blackman G, Richards J. Hemi-body irradiation. An effective second-line therapy in drug-resistant multiple myeloma. Cancer 1989; **63**:2446–51.

30. Giles FJ, McSweeney EN, Richards JD, Tobias J, Gaminora I, Grant I, et al. Prospective randomized study of double hemi-body irradiation with and without subsequent maintenance recombinant alpha 2b interferon on survival in patients with relapsed multiple myeloma. Eur J Cancer 1992; **28A**:1392–5.

31. McSweeney E, Tobias J, Blackman G, Goldstone A, Richards J. Double hemibody irradiation (DHBI) in the management of relapsed and primary chemoresistant multiple myeloma. Clin Oncol 1993; **5**:378–83.

32. Thomas PJ, Daban A, Bontoux D. Double hemibody irradiation in chemotherapy-resistant multiple myeloma. Cancer Treat Rep 1984; **68**:1173–5.

33. Plesnicar A, Jereb B, Zaletel-Kragelj L. Half-body irradiation in the treatment of multiple myeloma: a report of nine cases. Tumori 1996; **82**:588–91.

34. Rostom AY, O'Cathail SM, Folkes A. Systemic irradiation in multiple myeloma: a report on nineteen cases. *Br J Haematol* 1984; **58**:423–31.

◆35. Hu K, Yahalom J. Radiotherapy in the management of plasma cell tumors. *Oncology* 2000; **14**:101–11.

36. Salmon S, Tesh D, Crowley J, Saeed S, Finley P, Milder M, *et al.* Chemotherapy is superior to sequential hemibody irradiation for remission consolidation in multiple myeloma: a Southwest oncology Group study. *J Clin Oncol* 1990; **8**:1575–84.

37. MacKenzie MR, Wold H, George C, Gandara D, Ray G, Schiff S, *et al.* Consolidation hemibody radiotherapy following induction combination chemotherapy in high tumor burden multiple myeloma. *J Clin Oncol* 1992; **10**:1769–74.

38. Desikan KR, Tricot G, Dhodapkar M, Fassas A, Siegel D, Vesole D, *et al.* Melphalan plus total body irradiation (MEL-TBI) or cyclophosphamide (MEL-CY) as a conditioning regimen with second autotransplant in responding patients with myeloma is inferior compared to historical controls receiving tandem transplants with melphalan alone. *Bone Marrow Transplant* 2000; **25**:483–7.

39. Russell N, Bessell E, Stainer C, Haynes A, Das-Gupta E, Byrne J. Allogeneic haemopoietic stem cell transplantation for multiple myeloma or plasma cell leukaemia using fractionated total body radiation and high-dose melphalan conditioning. *Acta Oncol* 2000; **39**:837–41.

40. Gahrton G, Svensson H, Cavo M, Apperly J, Bacigulupo A, Bjorkstrand B, *et al.* Progress in allogenic bone marrow and peripheral blood stem cell transplantation for multiple myeloma: a comparison between transplants performed 1983–93 and 1994–8 at European Group for Blood and Marrow Transplantation centers. *Br J Haematol* 2001; **113**:209–16.

41. Bensinger W, Buckner D, Gahrton G. Allogeneic stem cell transplantation for multiple myeloma. *Hematol Oncol Clin North Am* 1997; **11**:147–57.

42. Feinstein L, Sandmaier B, Hegenbart U, McSweeney P, Maloney D, Gooley T, *et al.* Non-myeloablative allografting from human leucocyte antigen-identical sibling donors for treatment of acute myeloid leukaemia in first complete remission. *Br J Haematol* 2003; **120**:281–8.

◆43. Shank B. Techniques of magna-field irradiation. *Int J Radiat Oncol Biol Phys* 1983; **9**:1925.

44. Shank B. Total body irradiation. In: Leibel SA, Phillips TL (eds) *Textbook of radiation oncology.* Philadelphia: WB Saunders Company, 1998:253–75.

45. Sarfaraz M. Personal communication. April 20, 2001.

46. Vriesendorp HM, Chu H, Ochran TG, *et al.* Radiobiology of total body radiation. *Bone Marrow Transplant* 1994; **14**:54–8.

47. Vriesendrop HM, Chu H, Ochran TG, *et al.* Total body irradiation and the therapeutic ratio of bone marrow transplantation. *Bone Marrow Transplant* 1995; **15**:193–8.

48. Thomas ED, Clift RA, Hersman J. Marrow transplantation for acute nonlymphoblastic leukemia during first complete remission using fractionated or single-dose irradiation. *Int J Radiat Oncol Biol Phys* 1982; **8**:817–21.

49. Cosset JM, Baume D, Pico JL, Shank B, Girinski T, Benhamou E, *et al.* Single dose versus hyperfractionated total body irradiation before allogeneic bone marrow transplantation: a non-randomized comparative study of 54 patients at the Institut Gustave-Roussy. *Radiother Oncol* 1989; **15**:151–60.

50. Girinsky T, Benhamou E, Bourhis J-H, Dhermain F, Guillot-Vals D, Ganansia V, *et al.* Prospective randomized comparison of single-dose versus hyperfractionated total-body irradiation in patients with hematologic malignancies. *J Clin Oncol* 2000; **18**:981–6.

51. Gopal R, Ha CS, Tucker SL, Khouri I, Giratt S, Gajewski J, *et al.* Comparison of two total body irradiation fractionation regimens with respect to acute and late pulmonary toxicity. *Cancer* 2001; **92**:1949–58.

●52. Della Volpe A, Ferreri AJ, Annaloro C, Mangili P, Rosso A, Calandrino R, *et al.* Lethal pulmonary complications significantly correlate with individually assessed mean lung dose in patients with hematologic malignancies treated with total body irradiation. *Int J Radiat Oncol Biol Phys* 2002; **52**:284–8.

53. Benyunes M, Sullivan K, Deeg H, Mori M, Meyer W, Fisher L, *et al.* Cataracts after bone marrow transplantation: long-term follow-up of adults treated with fractionated total body irradiation. *Int J Radiat Oncol Biol Phys* 1995; **32**:661–70.

54. Belkacemi Y, Ozashin M, Pene F, Rio B, Laporte J, Lebland V, *et al.* Cataractogenesis after total body irradiation. *Int J Radiat Oncol Biol Phys* 1996; **35**:53–60.

55. Flynn AA, Green AJ, Pedley RB, Boxer G, Dearling J, Watson R, *et al.* A model-based approach for the optimization of radioimmunotherapy through antibody design and radionuclide selection. *Cancer* 2002; **94**:1249–57.

56. Goldenberg DM. Targeted therapy of cancer with radiolabeled antibodies. *J Nucl Med* 2002; **43**:693–713.

57. DeNardo SJ, Williams LE, Leigh BR, Wahl RL. Choosing an optimal radioimmunotherapy dose for clinical response. *Cancer* 2002; **94**:1275–86.

●58. Supiot S, Faivre-Chauvet A, Couturier O, Heymann M, Robillard N, Kraeber-Bordere F, *et al.* Comparison of the biologic effects of MA5 and B-B4 monoclonal antibody labeled with iodine-131 and bismuth-213 on multiple myeloma. *Cancer* 2002; **94**:1202–9.

59. Couturier O, Faivre-Chauvet A, Filippovich IV, Thedrez P, Sai-Maurel C, Bardies M, *et al.* Validation of 213Bi-alpha radioimmunotherapy for multiple myeloma. *Clin Cancer Res* 1999; **5**:3165s–70s.

60. Burton J, Mishina D, Cardillo T, Lew K, Rubin A, Goldenberg D, *et al.* Epithelial mucin-1 (MUC1) expression and MA5 anti-MUC1 monoclonal antibody targeting in multiple myeloma. *Clin Cancer Res* 1999; **5**:3065s–72s.

61. Pagel J, Matthews D, Appelbaum F, Bernstein I, Press O. The use of radioimmunoconjugates in stem cell transplantation. *Bone Marrow Transplant* 2002; **29**:807–16.

16

Autologous stem cell transplantation

JEAN-LUC HAROUSSEAU AND MICHEL ATTAL

THE ROLE OF AUTOLOGOUS STEM CELL TRANSPLANTATION IN MULTIPLE MYELOMA

In the absence of significant improvements in conventional chemotherapy (CC), high-dose therapy (HDT) with autologous stem cell transplantation (ASCT) has been increasingly used in the past 15 years in multiple myeloma (MM).[1] Non-randomized studies have shown that for patients responding to initial induction chemotherapy, ASCT is a safe (less than 5% toxic deaths) and effective consolidation therapy.[2] Notably, some of these studies have suggested that 30–50% complete remissions (CRs) could be achieved with this approach in newly diagnosed MM and, more importantly, tumor burden reduction could be converted into a prolongation of remission and of survival.[2] However, these pilot studies are difficult to analyze because the recruitment of patients is subject to selection bias regarding age, performance status, renal function, and response to initial chemotherapy. Blade et al.[3]

studied the outcome of a subgroup of patients who were potential candidates for HDT, but who were treated with CC in a randomized prospective trial comparing MP and combination chemotherapy. Out of 487 patients, 77 fulfilled the eligibility criteria for HDT (<65 years of age, stage II or III disease, performance status <3, and objective response following initial CC). Their median survival was 60 months and 52 months from the time when HDT would have been considered. They therefore stated that for these patients, survival duration was similar to that reported in selected series of patients given early HDT.

However, in three historical comparisons, HDT appeared superior to CC (Table 16.1). Barlogie et al.[4] compared the results achieved in 123 patients receiving tandem ASCT with the outcome of 116 matched pairs selected from 1123 patients treated with CC according to SWOG trials. Lenhoff et al.[5] compared the results achieved in 274 patients prospectively treated with ASCT prepared with melphalan 200 mg/m^2 with the outcome of 274 patients

Table 16.1 *Historical comparisons of conventional chemotherapy (CC) and high-dose therapy (HDT)*

| Study | Number of patients | | Type of HDT | Age (years) | Median survival (months) | | P value |
	HDT	CC			CC	HDT	
Barlogie et al.[4]	123	116[a]	Tandem transplantation	<70	48	62+	0.01
Lenhoff et al.[5]	274	274[b]	HDM 200 mg/m^2 + ASCT	<60	44	Not reached	0.001
Palumbo et al.[6]	71	71[c]	HDM 100 mg/m^2 + ASCT (2–3 courses)	55–75	48	56+	<0.01

[a] Matched for age, β_2-microglobulin, and creatinine.
[b] Fulfilling eligibility criteria for HDT.
[c] Matched for age and β_2-microglobulin.
ASCT, autologous stem cell transplantation; HDM, high-dose melphalan.

fulfilling the eligibility criteria for HDT and treated with conventional chemotherapy protocols in five previous studies. Palumbo et al.[6] compared the results achieved in older patients (55–75 years, median 64) with two to three courses of melphalan 100 mg/m^2 followed by ASCT with the outcome of 71 matched pairs matched for age and β_2-microglobulin and treated with melphalan prednisone (MP). All these comparisons showed a significant benefit for HDT as compared with CC (see Table 16.1)

The Intergroupe Français du Myelome (IFM) was the first to conduct a randomized trial showing the superiority of HDT with autologous bone marrow transplantation (ABMT) as compared with CC.[7] In this trial, at the time of diagnosis, patients under 65 years of age and with Durie–Salmon stage II or III MM were randomly assigned to receive either CC or HDT. CC consisted of alternating cycles of vincristine, melphalan, cyclophosphamide, and prednisone (VMCP) and of vincristine, carmustine, doxorubicin, and prednisone (VBAP) administered at 3-week intervals for 12 months, with a total of 18 cycles. In the HDT arm, HDT was administered after four to six cycles of VMCP/BVAP to all patients with World Health Organization (WHO) performance status of 2 or less, a serum creatinine level less than 150 μmol/L, and more than 2×10^8 nucleated cells/kg in the marrow harvest, which was unpurged. Patients were prepared with high-dose melphalan (HDM) (140 mg/m^2) and total body irradiation (TBI) (8 Gy delivered in four fractions over 4 days, without lung shielding). Interferon-α (IFNα) was administered at a dose of 3×10^6 U/m^2 three times a week until relapse in both arms. The criteria for response were the following: CR was defined as the absence of paraprotein on serum and urine electrophoresis (negative immunofixation was not required), and 5% or fewer plasma cells in the marrow. Very good partial response (VGPR) was defined as a decrease of 90% in the serum paraprotein level, partial remission (PR) as a decrease of 50% in the serum paraprotein level and/or a decrease of 90% in the urine Bence Jones protein, and minimal response as a decrease of 25% in the serum paraprotein level.

The 100 patients enrolled in the conventional chemotherapy arm received a median of 18 cycles (range 2–18). Seventy-four of 100 patients assigned to HDT actually underwent transplantation. The comparison of the two therapeutic modalities was made on an intention to treat basis, with all patients studied in their assigned treatment groups. None of the initial characteristics differed significantly between treatment groups. The response to initial chemotherapy and the compliance with interferon treatment were also comparable. In this IFM 90 trial, HDT significantly improved the response rate because 38% of patients enrolled in the HDT arm achieved a CR or VGPR versus 14% of patients enrolled in the CC arm ($P < 0.001$). An updated analysis of this study confirms that, with a median follow-up of 7 years, HDT significantly improves event-free survival (EFS; median 28 months vs. 18 months, 7-year EFS 16% vs. 8%; $P = 0.01$) and overall survival (OS; median 57 months vs. 44 months, 7-year OS 43% vs. 25%; $P = 0.03$).

Other randomized studies have also compared CC and HDT with autologous transplantation (Table 16.2). In the MAG91 trial performed by the French MAG group, 190 patients aged 55–65 years were randomized to receive CC or HDT.[8] In the CC arm, patients were treated with VMCP combination regimen. In the HDT arm, the conditioning regimen was HDM 200 mg/m^2 or HDM 140 mg/m^2, and busulfan 16 mg/kg. Although the results of HDT appeared comparable to those achieved in the IFM 90 trial (median survival 55 months), there was no significant difference in OS between the two arms, owing to an unexpectedly good survival in the CC arm (median 50 months). It should be noted that in the CC arm, 17 patients received ASCT at the time of relapse.

The design of the Spanish trial was different since only patients responding to initial CC were randomized.[9] In this trial, 216 patients under 65 years of age were initially treated with four cycles of the VMCP/VBAP combination. Of the 185 achieving at least minimal response, 164 were randomized either to further CC (83) or to HDT (HDM 140 mg/m^2 and TBI 12 Gy or HDM 200 mg/m^2) followed by autologous peripheral blood progenitor cell

Table 16.2 *Results of randomized studies for conventional chemotherapy (CC) and high-dose therapy (HDT)*

Trial	Number of patients	Age (years)	Median follow-up	CR rate (%) CC	CR rate (%) HDT	Median EFS (months) CC	Median EFS (months) HDT	Median OS (months) CC	Median OS (months) HDT
IFM 90[7]	200	<65	7 years	5[a]	22[a]	18[a]	28[a]	44[a]	57[a]
MAG 91[8]	190	55–65	56 months	NE	NE	19[a]	24[a]	50	55
Pethema[9]	164	Median 56	42 months	11[a]	30[a]	33	42	64	72
Italian MMSG[10]	195	<70	2 years	6[a]	28[a]	21[a]	34[a]	NR	NR
MRC7[11]	401	<65	–	8[a]	44[a]	20[a]	32[a]	42[a]	54[a]

[a] significant *P* value.

CR, complete remission; EFS, event-free survival; IFM, Intergroupe Français du Myelome; MAG, Myelome Auto Greffe; MMSG, Multiple Myeloma Study Group; MRC, Medical Research Council; NE, not evaluable; NR, not reached; OS, overall survival.

transplantation (PBPCT). Maintenance therapy consisted of IFNα and dexamethasone in both arms. In this trial, the CR rate was significantly higher in the HDT arm (30% vs. 11%). Although the median EFS and OS were longer in the HDT arm (42 months vs. 33 months, 72 months vs. 64 months), the differences were not significant.

The Italian study compared the classical MP combination with two courses of intermediate-dose melphalan (100 mg/m^2) followed by ASCT in patients up to the age of 70.[10] The CR rate and median EFS were significantly better with HDT. With a short median follow-up of 2 years, there was no significant difference in OS between the two arms but many patients received ASCT as salvage therapy in the CC arm.

Finally, the recent results of the British MRC Myeloma VII trial are also in favor of ASCT.[11] In this trial, 401 patients up to the age of 65 were randomly allocated to receive either ABCM or C-VAMP to maximum response followed by HDM 200 mg/m^2 with ASCT. Patients in both arms received maintenance with IFNα. The CR rate was 44% in the HDT arm versus 8% in the ABCM arm ($P < 0.001$). Intention to treat analysis showed a significant prolongation of progression-free survival (PFS) and of OS in the intensive-therapy arm (median PFS 31.6 months vs. 42.3 months; $P = 0.04$). These results confirm those observed 7 years earlier in the French IFM 90 trial.

Therefore, HDT improves the CR rate and the median EFS. The fact that OS is not always significantly increased may be explained by the results of another randomized trial conducted by the French MAG Group comparing early and late ASCT.[12] In this trial, although early transplantation significantly improved PFS, OS was not significantly different. These results confirm that ASCT is an effective salvage therapy when CC fails. In recently conducted randomized trials, a significant number of patients randomized to CC have received HDT following relapse, which will, therefore, tend to minimize any difference in OS between the two arms.

HOW TO IMPROVE THE RESULTS OF AUTOLOGOUS STEM CELL TRANSPLANTATION

In the IFM90 trial, the 7-year EFS was only 16% for patients enrolled in the HDT arm and there was no plateau of the survival curves. Therefore, strategies to improve these results were clearly warranted. Since, in this trial, achievement of CR or VGPR was significantly associated with a prolongation of survival (Fig. 16.1), the aim of subsequent studies has been to increase the CR rate.

Conditioning regimen

Improving the conditioning regimen could be one way to attain this objective. The optimal conditioning regimen

for ASCT in MM has not yet been determined. Since its introduction in 1987,[13] TBI has been used in multiple non-randomized studies. The combination of TBI plus HDM 140 mg/m^2 yields CR rates ranging from 20% to 50% according to the disease status at transplantation and to criteria used to define CR (see Chapter 13). This conditioning regimen was used in the IFM90 trial and, therefore, could be considered as the standard one. However, in newly diagnosed patients, the Royal Marsden Group reported an impressive 70% CR rate with HDM 200 mg/m^2 alone, with a low extramedullary toxicity.[14]

In 1995, the IFM initiated a randomized study comparing HDM 200 mg/m^2 and HDM 140 mg/m^2 plus TBI in 282 patients with newly diagnosed MM.[15] In this study, HDM 200 mg/m^2 was significantly less toxic (shorter duration of neutropenia and thrombocytopenia, lower incidence of grade ≥3 mucositis, no toxic death vs. 5 in the TBI group). Although the response rate and the EFS were identical (Fig. 16.2), OS was superior in the HDM 200 mg/m^2 apparently because of a better salvage after

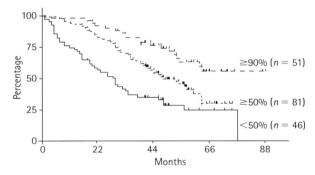

Figure 16.1 *IFM90 trial. The impact of complete remission achievement on survival.*

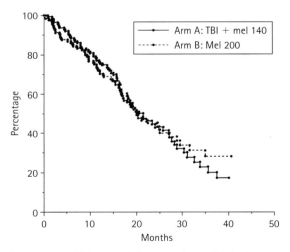

Figure 16.2 *IFM95-02 trial. Comparison of high-dose melphalan 140 mg/m^2 plus total body irradiation (TBI + mel 140) and melphalan 200 mg/m^2 (Mel 200). Event-free survival ($P = 0.6$).*

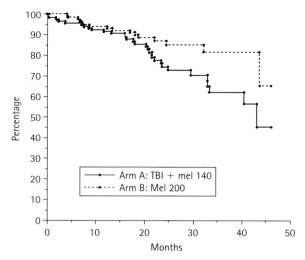

Figure 16.3 *IFM95-02 trial. Comparison of high-dose melphalan 140 mg/m² plus total body irradiation (TBI + mel 140) and melphalan 200 mg/m² (Mel 200). Overall survival (P = 0.05).*

Table 16.3 *Single versus double autologous stem cell transplantation (ASCT). Results of the IFM 94 trial*

	Single ASCT (n = 199)	Double ASCT (n = 200)	P value
CR rate (%)	34	35	
CR + VGPR rate (%)	42	50	
Median EFS (months)	25	30	0.03[a]
7 years EFS (%)	10	20	
Median OS (months)	48	58	0.01[a]
7 years OS (%)	21	42	

[a]Log-rank test.
CR, complete remission; EFS, event-free survival; OS, overall survival; VGPR, very good partial response.

relapse (Fig. 16.3). Two other non-randomized studies also failed to show a survival benefit for TBI-containing regimens.[16,17] In fact, the European Group for Blood and Marrow Transplantation (EBMT) registry data showed a worse outcome for TBI. Therefore, HDM 200 mg/m² should be preferred to HDM 140 mg/m² plus TBI as the conditioning regimen for ASCT in MM. Knowing the good tolerance of HDM 200 mg/m², higher doses of melphalan alone or in combination with an anti-interleukin-6 (IL-6) antibody have been explored with encouraging results.[18,19] In order to further improve the efficacy of conditioning regimens, studies are ongoing with agents that localize preferentially in the bone and that are coupled with radioelements (Holmium, Samarium). Other combinations have been explored, including busulfan plus cyclophosphamide or busulfan-melphalan. A recent retrospective analysis of 821 patients from the Spanish Registry showed that busulfan–melphalan combination yielded significantly better response rates compared with other regimens and suggested that EFS and OS could be longer as well.[20] However, since this was not a randomized study, HDM 200 mg/m² is still considered as the standard conditioning regimen with which all others should prospectively be compared.

Impact of tandem transplants

Another way to increase the CR rate could be to repeat intensive treatments. The IFM group was the first to explore this strategy but the hematopoietic toxicity of the first course of HDT was severe in the absence of any hematopoietic support.[21] Thanks to autologous transplantation of PBPCs and to hematopoietic growth factors,

the sequential use of two courses of HDT has become more feasible and appears to increase the CR rate,[22,23] and even to induce molecular remission.[24] The largest experience in this setting comes from the Little Rock group.[25] Of 495 patients enrolled to undergo two transplants, including 315 pre-treated patients, 95% completed the first course of HDM 200 mg/m² with PBPC transplantation and 73% completed two transplants. The CR rate increased from 24% after the first transplant to 43% after two transplants. This experience has now been extended to more than 1000 patients.[26] However, the actual impact of tandem transplantations on EFS and OS needed comparison with less aggressive strategies. While a case–control study has suggested that this approach is superior to CC,[4] the Little Rock group has not carried out a randomized study comparing tandem ASCT with single ASCT.

In 1994, the IFM initiated such a randomized trial (IFM94)[27] and, from October 1994 to March 1997, 403 untreated patients under the age of 60 years were enrolled by 45 centers. At diagnosis they were randomized to receive initial cytoreduction with VAD followed by either a single ASCT prepared with HDM (140 mg/m²) and TBI (8 Gy) or a double ASCT: the first one prepared with HDM (140 mg/m²), and the second one prepared with HDM (140 mg/m²) and TBI (8 Gy). After the initial cytoreduction, 343 patients eligible for transplantation underwent a second randomization (PBPCs vs. bone marrow) to support the HDT with HDM 140 mg/m² plus TBI.

Overall, 399 patients were evaluable. Of 199 patients assigned to the single ASCT arm, 177 (85%) actually received the planned transplant and there were three toxic deaths. Of 200 patients randomized in the double transplant arm, 156 (78%) actually received two transplants and there were five toxic deaths. The results are shown in Table 16.3. There is no significant difference in the CR rate between single and double transplantation. However, with a median follow-up of 6 years, the median EFS and the OS are superior in the double ASCT arm (Figs 16.4 and 16.5).

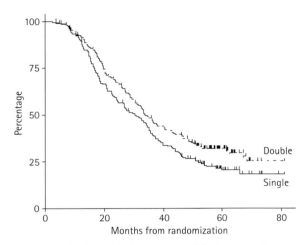

Figure 16.4 *IFM 94 trial. Comparison of single versus double autotransplantations (intention to treat analysis). Event-free survival (P = 0.03).*

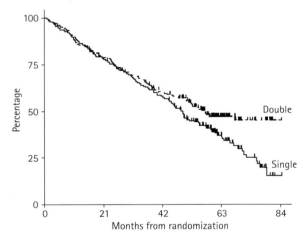

Figure 16.5 *IFM 94 trial. Comparison of single versus double autotransplantations (intention to treat analysis). Overall survival (P = 0.02).*

Three other studies have also addressed the issue of further intensification but with different intensity of the overall treatment (Table 16.4). Currently, two of these studies show a significant advantage for the more intensive treatment arm as regards EFS but none as regards survival.[28–30] However, it should be noted that in the IFM 94 trial, the OS curves separate after only 4 years. As the median follow-up time of these three studies is still relatively short, a longer observation period is needed before drawing any definite conclusions.

Source of stem cells

As in other malignancies, PBPCs have almost completely replaced bone marrow as the source of stem cells in ASCT for MM. The main reasons for this choice are easier

Table 16.4 *Single versus double autologous stem cell transplantation. Results of multicenter randomized studies*

Study	Number of patients	Median follow-up (months)	Results
IFM 94[25]	399	75	Better EFS and OS[a]
Hovon[26] [b]	255	40	Higher CR rate[a]
			Higher 4-year EFS rate
Bologna[27] [c]	220	38	Better median EFS
MAG 95[28] [d]	227	53	No difference

[a] In favor of the more intensive treatment arm.
[b] 2 × 70 mg/m² melphalan ± CTX-TBI/PBSCT.
[c] 200 mg/m² melphalan/PBSCT ± Bu-Mel/PBSCT.
[d] VAD + HD chemo + TBI/PBSCT vs. 140 mg/m² Mel/PBSCT + HD chemo + TBI/PBSCT.
Bu, busulfan; CR, complete remission; CTX, cyclophosphamide; EFS, event-free survival; IFM, Intergroupe Français du Myélome; HD chemo; high-dose chemotherapy; MAG, Myelome Auto Greffe; Mel, melphalan; OS, overall survival; PBSCT, peripheral blood stem cell transplantation; TBI, total body irradiation; VAD, vincristine, Adriamycin, and dexamethasone.

accessibility and availability, faster hematopoietic recovery, and possibly lower tumor contamination. However, several issues remain regarding the use of PBPCs. Although tumor cell contamination is lower in PBPC harvests than in bone marrow, the superiority of PBPC autologous transplantation as regards the clinical outcome has not yet been demonstrated. Sensitive immunofluorescence studies or polymerase chain reaction (PCR)-based techniques have demonstrated that virtually all PBPC harvests are contaminated with malignant cells. Although the prognostic significance of detecting malignant cells with such sensitive methods is still unknown, attempts to reduce tumor cell contamination of the grafts has been a great concern.

Purging marrow with cyclophosphamide derivatives or with monoclonal antibodies has proven feasible, although it induces prolonged mylosuppression. Selection of CD34+ progenitors appears to be a promising alternative with a 2.5–4.5 log-depletion of plasma cells.[31,32] Several pilot studies have confirmed the feasibility of autologous transplants with CD34+ selected PBPCs in MM. In a multicenter randomized phase III trial comparing selected and unselected PBPCs in 131 myeloma patients, successful neutrophil engraftement was achieved in all patients by day 15 and there was no significant difference between the two groups as regards platelet engraftment.[33] However, a recent analysis of this trial failed to show EFS or OS prolongation with CD34+ cell selection.[34] Two other randomized studies have not been published yet, but preliminary results do not show any benefit of CD34+ selected PBPCs. Moreover, in both studies, the incidence of opportunistic infections appears to be higher in the CD34+ selected PBPC arm.[30,35]

Sensitive PCR techniques using patient-specific oligonucleotide primers show the persistence of myeloma cells in the CD34+ cell fractions, but highly purified CD34+ Lin-thy 1+ stem cells do not apparently contain clonal myeloma cells.[36] Thus, an additional purging step might be necessary to obtain tumor-free grafts. The clinical impact of these cumbersome and expensive procedures is unknown. In a pilot study on ten patients, neutrophil and platelet engraftment was substantially delayed as compared with unmanipulated PBPC grafts.[37] Currently, unselected PBPCs appear to be the best source of stem cells for ASCT in MM.

Variables affecting PBPC mobilization and speed of engraftment have been analyzed.[38] There is a significant correlation between the number of CD34+ cells infused and hematopoietic reconstitution, and 2×10^6/kg CD34+ cells is the minimal dose to ensure a safe engraftment. Prior exposure to chemotherapy, especially to alkylating agents, significantly affects stem-cell collection and hemopoietic recovery. Thus, PBSCs should be collected before using alkylating agents and VAD-derived regimens are preferable prior to ASCT. The optimal regimen for mobilizing PBPCs is unclear. While some investigators use cyclophosphamide ($2–4 \, g/m^2$) plus granulocyte colony-stimulating factor (G-CSF) to increase the number of PBPCs, and possibly to reduce graft contamination and tumor cell mass, others use G-CSF alone to reduce morbidity and cost.[39] The combination of stem cell factor (SCF) and G-CSF is an attractive alternative[40] and could be used in poor mobilizers.

Maintenance therapy

As there is no plateau of the survival curves in published series with adequate follow-up, some form of maintenance therapy appears necessary. Several randomized studies have shown that in patients responding to CC, IFNα maintenance prolongs remission duration by 5–12 months as compared to observation. IFNα has also been used after HDT with the hypothesis that it could be more effective in patients with minimal residual disease. In a retrospective analysis of the EBMT registry, IFNα maintenance was associated with improved PFS and OS in patients responding to HDT.[41] However, it is important to note that in this study, the patients on IFNα had better prognostic factors and the authors could not conclude that the better survival was in fact due to IFNα. Only one randomized study has so far been completed.[42] This trial compared IFNα (3×10^6 UI/kg, three times weekly) following recovery from HDT and no further therapy. With a median follow-up of 77 months, the median PFS was longer (42 months vs. 27 months for the control arm), but the PFS and OS curves were not significantly different. This means that although IFNα delayed relapse, most if not all the patients ultimately relapsed. However, since this study

involved only 85 patients, these results should be interpreted cautiously. Further studies are needed and a large randomized trial is ongoing in the USA. It should be noted that in the IFM90 trial, although IFNα was to be administered to all patients after HDT, there is no plateau on the EFS curve.[7] Therefore, a single course of HDT followed by IFNα is unlikely to provide a cure for patients with MM. New strategies to control minimal residual disease after ASCT are necessary. They include the use of maintenance chemotherapy, thalidomide, bisphosphonates, and immunotherapy (idiotypic or DNA vaccination, vaccination with idiotype-pulsed dendritic cells). These strategies are currently being evaluated (see Chapters 19 and 20).

CURRENT ISSUES IN ASCT FOR MM

Prognostic factors

Barlogie et al.[43] recently published the results of an intensive program, including tandem transplants in 231 patients with newly diagnosed MM. In multivariate analysis, superior EFS and OS were observed in the absence of unfavorable karyotypes (11q breakpoints, and/or partial or complete deletion of chromosome 13) and with low β_2-microglobulin level at diagnosis ($\leq 4 \, mg/L$). When combining these factors, a subgroup of patients with a very poor prognosis was identified: patients with unfavorable cytogenetics and β_2-microglobulin level $>4 \, mg/L$ had a median survival of only 2.1 years, compared with 7 years for the remaining patients. New therapeutic approaches are clearly needed for these patients.

Using a larger cohort of 1000 consecutive patients including previously treated patients, the same authors confirmed that the most important independent favorable features were absence of chromosome 13 deletion and low β_2-microglobulin level, plus low C-reactive protein (CRP) level and less than 12 months of prior CC.[25] Plateaus on the EFS and OS curves were noted in 45% and 60% of patients with all these favorable characteristics. Thus, durable remissions and possibly cures can be achieved in a high proportion of good-risk patients with an intensive strategy, including tandem ASCT.

In a recent retrospective analysis of 110 patients treated with HDT in two IFM centers, the detection of chromosome 13 abnormalities (-13, 13 q$-$) by fluorescence *in situ* hybridization (FISH) was the most powerful adverse prognostic factor.[44] The combination of FISH analysis, β_2-microglobulin, and IgA isotype produced a very powerful staging system in the context of HDT. Again, patients with a high β_2-microglobulin level and chromosome 13 abnormalities had a very poor prognosis (Fig. 16.6).

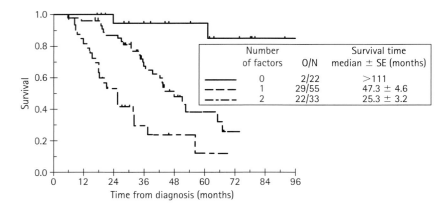

Figure 16.6 *Prognostic impact of β₂-microglobulin level and chromosome 13 abnormalities (detected by fluorescence in situ hybridization analysis). Overall survival. High β₂-microglobulin (>2.5 mg/L) and chromosome 13 deletions each score as one adverse factor.*

In addition to pre-HDT features, achievement of a CR defined by immunofixation[26,45,46] and timely administration[26] of the second ASCT are associated with better outcome.

Selection of patients

AGE

Usually, ASCT is limited to patients up to 65 years of age, with a performance status of 0–2 and with a normal renal function. The issue of age limits was emphasized by the IFM 90 trial, since ASCT was actually performed in 82% of patients 60 years of age or less, versus only 58% in patients aged 60–65.[7] As a consequence, in the intention-to-treat analysis, ASCT was significantly superior to CC only in younger patients. However, the introduction of hematopoietic growth factors has profoundly modified the practice of ASCT. With PBPCs collected after priming with G-CSF or granulocyte–macrophage colony-stimulating factor (GM-CSF), ASCT has become safer and could be offered to older patients. Recently, the Little Rock group has compared the outcome of 49 patients aged 65 years and older with 49 younger matched pairs selected in a cohort of 550 patients treated with HDT.[47] The CR rate was higher in younger patients (43% vs. 20%; $P = 0.02$) and the transplant related mortality appeared to be higher in older patients (8% vs. 2%). However, since the EFS and OS were comparable, the authors concluded that age is not a biologically adverse parameter for patients treated with HDT and PBPC support, and should not constitute an exclusion criterion for participation in what appears to be superior therapy in MM.

The same group recently published the results of ASCT in 70 patients over the age of 70 years. Although ASCT appeared feasible in this age subgroup, the use of a higher dose of melphalan (200 mg/m²) was too toxic (16% toxic deaths).[48] Palumbo *et al.*[6] reported that two to three courses of melphalan 100 mg/m² supported by PBPC support are feasible on an outpatient basis in patients up to 75 years of age. They compared 71 patients treated with this approach to 71 matched pairs treated with CC, and

concluded that intensive therapy was superior in terms of CR rate, EFS, and OS. However, the issue of selection bias should be raised in all studies on HDT in elderly patients. The benefit of ASCT in this patient population needs further evaluation by randomized trials.

Renal failure

Autologous stem cell transplantation is not usually offered to patients with renal failure (creatinine clearance <40 mL/minute) because of concerns regarding excessive toxicity of HDT and pharmacokinetics of melphalan in patients with renal dysfunction.[49] Therefore, a group of patients with a poor prognosis is excluded from the potential benefits of this procedure. However, several reports suggest that at least some patients may benefit from HDT in this context.[50–52] A recent retrospective study of the Spanish Registry showed a high transplant-related mortality (29%) in patients with renal failure at the time of transplant.[53] In multivariate analysis, transplant-related mortality was influence by performance status (Eastern Cooperative Oncology Group score >3), anemia (<9.5 g/dL), and severity of renal failure (creatinine >5 mg/dL). In a large study on 81 MM patients with renal failure at the time of ASCT, Badros *et al.*[49] stated that renal failure had no impact on the quality of stem cell collection and did not effect engraftment. ASCT was feasible even in patients on dialysis. However, extra-hematologic toxicities were more severe than in patients with normal renal function. The first 60 patients received melphalan 200 mg/m² but the authors observed a high incidence of mucositis (97%), and pulmonary complications (57%) as well as unusual cardiac and neurologic complications. Because of this excessive toxicity, the dose of melphalan was subsequently reduced to 140 mg/m², but 27% of patients still developed neurological complications.

It is, therefore, clear that treatment-related morbidity and mortality are increased in patients with renal failure, and the role of ASCT in such patients requires further evaluation.

CONCLUSION

Currently available results of multicenter randomized studies clearly show that ASCT is superior to CC in terms of response rate and event-free survival in patients up to the age of 65. The results are less clear cut in terms of overall survival, probably because many patients relapsing after CC can be salvaged by late ASCT. For older patients, uncontrolled studies are possibly biased by selection of patients fit enough to undergo ASCT. Randomized studies comparing CC and two courses of intermediate-dose melphalan plus ASCT are ongoing.

High-dose melphalan $200\,mg/m^2$ appears to be less toxic than HDM $140\,mg/m^2$ plus TBI, and should be considered as the standard conditioning regimen prior to ASCT. Although there is no convincing evidence that PBSCs are superior to bone marrow in terms of immediate and long-term outcome, PBSCs are preferred because of easier accessibility and faster hematopoietic reconstitution. CD34+ selection offers no significant advantage. The IFM94 trial is in favor of tandem ASCT compared with single ASCT. However, three other less mature trials do not confirm these results. Maintenance therapy with alpha interferon is currently widely used but other approaches, including thalidomide, are being evaluated.

Finally, a high β_2-microglobulin level and the presence of chromosome 13 abnormalities (by conventional cytogenetics or by FISH analysis) are associated with a poorer outcome. While patients with none of these adverse prognostic factors have a high probability of prolonged survival after ASCT, patients with both parameters have a very poor outcome even after double ASCT. For these patients, new approaches are clearly needed.

KEY POINTS

- Autologous stem cell transplantation (ASCT) prolongs remission duration and overall survival, although all patients ultimately relapse.
- The addition of total body irradiation to the conditioning regimen does not improve outcome.
- CD34 selection of stem cells reduces tumor contamination but does not reduce the risk of relapse.
- It is not clear at present whether double transplant programmes offer a definite survival advantage over a single procedure.
- Selected patients over 60 years of age may be suitable candidates for ASCT, but at present ASCT is not generally recommended for patients with severe renal failure.

REFERENCES

● = Key primary paper
◆ = Major review article

◆1. Bataille R, Harousseau JL. Multiple myeloma (review article). N Engl J Med 1997; **36**:1657–64.

◆2. Harousseau JL, Attal M. The role of autologous hematopoietic stem cell transplantation in multiplemyeloma. Semin Hematol 1997; **34**(Suppl 1):61–6.

3. Blade J, San Miguel JF, Montserrat F, Alcala A, Maldonado J, Garcia-Conde J, et al. Survival of multiple myeloma patients who are potential candidates for early high-dose therapy intensification/autotransplantation and who were conventionally treated. J Clin Oncol 1996; **14**:2167–73.

4. Barlogie B, Jagannath S, Vesole D, Naucke S, Cheson B, Mattox S, et al. Superiority of tandem autologous transplantation over standard therapy for previously untreated multiple myeloma. Blood 1997; **89**:789–93.

5. Lenhoff S, Hjorth M, Holmberg E, Turesson I, Westin J, Nielsen JL, et al. Impact of survival of high-dose therapy with autologous stem cell support in patients younger than 60 years with newly diagnosed multiple myeloma. Blood 2000; **95**:7–11.

6. Palumbo A, Triolo S, Argentino C, Bringhen S, Dominietto A, Rus C, et al. Dose intensive melphalan with stem-cell support is superior to standard treatment in elderly myeloma patients. Blood 1999; **94**:1248–53.

◆7. Attal M, Harousseau JL, Stoppa AM, Sotto JJ, Fuzibet JG, Rossi JF, et al. A prospective, randomized trial of autologous bone marrow transplantation and chemotherapy in multiple myeloma. N Engl J Med 1996; **335**:91–7.

8. Fermand JP, Ravaud P, Katsahian S, Divine M, Leblond V, Belanger C, et al. High dose therapy and autologous blood stem cell transplantation versus conventional treatment in multiple myeloma: results of a randomized trial in 190 patients 55 to 65 years of age. Blood 1999; **94**(Suppl 1):396a (abstract).

9. Blade J, Sureda A, Ribera JM, Diaz-Mediavilla J, Palomera L, Fernandez-Calvo J, et al. High-dose therapy autotransplantation/intensification vs. continued conventional chemotherapy in multiple myeloma in patients responding to initial treatment chemotherapy. Results of a prospective randomized trial from the Spanish Cooperative Group PETHEMA. Blood 2001; **98**:815a (abstract).

10. Palumbo A, Bringhen S, Rus C, Petrucci M, Mandelli F, Musto P, et al. A prospective randomized trial of intermediate dose melphalan (100 mg/m²) vs. oral melphalan/prednisone: an interim analysis. Blood 2001; **98**:849a (abstract).

11. Child JA, Morgan GJ, Davies FC, et al. High-dose chemotherapy with hematopoietic stem-cell rescue for multiple myeloma. N Engl J Med 2003; **348**:1875–83.

12. Fermand JP, Ravaud P, Chevret S, Divine M, Leblond V, Belanger C, et al. High-dose therapy and autologous peripheral blood stem cell transplantation in multiple myeloma: up-front or resume treatment? Results of a multicenter sequential randomized clinical trial. Blood 1998; **92**:3131–6.

13. Barlogie B, Alexanian R, Dicke K, Zagars G, Spitzer G, Jagannath S, et al. High dose chemoradiotherapy and autologous bone marrow transplantation for resistant multiple myeloma. Blood 1987; **70**:869–72.

14. Cunningham D, Paz-Ares L, Milan S, Powles R, Nicolson M, Hickish T, et al. High dose melphalan and autologous bone marrow transplantation as consolidation in previously untreated myeloma. J Clin Oncol 1994; 12:759–63.

15. Moreau P, Facon T, Attal M, Hulin C, Michallet M, Maloisel F, et al. Comparison of 200 mg/m^2 melphalan and 8 Gy total body irradiation plus 140 mg/m^2 as conditioning regimens for peripheral blood stem cell transplantation in patients with newly diagnosed multiple myeloma. Final analysis of the IFM 95-02 randomized trial. Blood 2002; 99:731–5.

16. Goldschmidt H, Hegenbart U, Wallmeier M, Hohaus S, Engenhart R, Wannenmacher M, et al. High-dose therapy with peripheral blood progenitor cell transplantation in multiple myeloma. Ann Oncol 1997; 8:243–6.

17. Bjorkstrand B, Svensson H, Goldschmidt H, Ljungman PT, Apperley J, Remes K, Ljungman PT, Apperley J, Remes K, et al. 5489 autotransplants in multiple myeloma: a registry from the EBMT. Blood 1999; 94(Suppl 1):714a (abstract).

18. Moreau P, Milpied N, Mahé B, Juge-Morineau N, Rapp MJ, Bataille R, et al. Melphalan 220 mg/m^2 followed by peripheral blood stem cell transplantation in 27 patients with advanced multiple myeloma. Bone Marrow Transplant 1999; 23:1000–6.

19. Moreau P, Harousseau JL, Wijdenes J, Morineau N, Milpied N, Bataille R. A combination of anti-interleukin 6 murine monoclonal antibody with dexamethasone and high-dose Melphalan induces high complete response rate in advanced multiple myeloma. Br J Haematol 2000; 109:661–4.

20. Lahuerta JJ, Grande C, Blade J, Martinez-Lopez J, Alegre A, Garcia-Conde J, et al. Myeloablative treatments for multiple myeloma: update of comparative study of different regimens used in patients from the Spanish Registry for Transplantation in Multiple Myeloma. Leuk Lymphoma 2002; 43:67–74.

21. Harousseau JL, Milpied N, Laporte JP, Collombat P, Facon T, Tigaud JD, et al. Double intensive therapy in high-risk multiple myeloma. Blood 1992; 79:2827–33.

22. Vesole D, Barlogie B, Jagannath S, Cheson B, Tricot G, Alexanian R, et al. High-dose therapy for refractory multiple myeloma: improved prognosis with better supportive care and double transplants. Blood 1994; 84:950–6.

23. Weaver CH, Zhen B, Schwartzberg LS, Leff R, Magee M, Geier L, et al. Phase I-II evaluation of rapid sequence tandem high-dose melphalan with peripheral blood stem cell support in patients with multiple myeloma. Bone Marrow Transplant 1998; 22:245–51.

24. Bjorkstrand B, Ljungman P, Bird JM, Samson D, Gahrton G. Double high-dose chemoradiotherapy with autologous stem cell transplantation can induce molecular remission in multiple myeloma. Bone Marrow Transplant 1995; 15:367–71.

25. Vesole D, Tricot G, Jagannath S, Desikan KR, Siegel D, Bracy D, et al. Autotransplant in multiple myeloma: what have we learned? Blood 1996; 88:838–47.

26. Desikan R, Barlogie B, Sawyer J, Ayers D, Tricot G, Badros A, et al. Results of high dose therapy for 1000 patients with multiple myeloma: durable complete remission and superior survival in the absence of chromosome 13 abnormalities. Blood 2000; 95:4008–10.

27. Attal M, Harousseau JL, Facon T, et al. for the IFM. Single versus double transplant in myeloma: a randomized trial of the IFM. Proceeding of the VIIIth International Myeloma Workshop 2001, S15 p 28 (abstract).

28. Sonneveld P, Van Der Holt P, Sergeren CM, et al. Intensive versus double intensive therapy in untreated multiple myeloma: updated results of the prospective Phase III study Hovon 24 MM. Proceedings of the IXth Myeloma Workshop. Hematol J 2003; 4(Suppl 1):S59.

29. Cavo M, Zamagni E, Cellini C, et al. Single versus tandem autologous transplants in Multiple Myeloma: Italian experience. Proceedings of the IXth Myeloma Workshop. Hematol J 2003; 4(Suppl 1):S60.

30. Fermand JP, Marolleau JP, Alberti C, Divine M, Leblond V, Macro M, et al. Single versus tandem high dose therapy supported with autologous stem cell transplantation using unselected or CD 34 enriched ABSC: preliminary results of a two by two designed randomized trial in 23 young patients with multiple myeloma. Blood 2001; 98:815a (abstract).

31. Schiller G, Vescio R, Freytes C, Spitzer G, Sahebi F, Lee M, et al. Transplantation of CD 34+ peripheral blood progenitor cell after high-dose chemotherapy for patients with advanced multiple myeloma. Blood 1995; 86:390–7.

32. Lemoli RM, Fortuna A, Motta MR, Rizzi S, Giudice V, Nannetti A, et al. Concomittant mobilization of plasma cells and hematopoietic progenitors into peripheral blood of multiple myeloma patients: positive selection and transplantation of enriched CD 34+ cells to remove circulating tumor cells. Blood 1996; 87:1625–34.

33. Vescio RA, Schiller G, Stewart K, Ballester O, Noga S, Rugo H, et al. Multicenter Phase III trial to evaluate CD 34+ selected versus unselected autologous peripheral blood progenitor cell transplantation in multiple myeloma. Blood 1999; 93:1858–68.

34. Stewart AK, Vescio K, Schiller G, Ballester O, Noga S, Rugo H, et al. Purging of autologous peripheral blood stem cells using CD34 selection does not improve overall or progression free survival after high-dose therapy for multiple myelome: results of a multicenter randomized controlle trial. J Clin Oncol 2001; 198:3771–9.

35. Goldschmidt H, Bouko Y, Bourhis JH, Greinix H, Salles G, Derigs G, et al. CD 34+ selected PBPCT results in an increased infective risk without prolongation of event free survival in newly diagnosed myeloma: a randomised study from the EBMT. Blood 2000; 96:558a (abstract).

36. Gazitt Y, Reading CC, Hoffman R, Wickrema A, Vesole DH, Jagannath S, et al. Purified CD 34+ Lin-thy + stem cells do not contain clonal myeloma cells. Blood 1995; 86:381–9.

37. Tricot G, Gazitt Y, Leemhuis S, Jagannath S, Desikan KR, Siegel D, et al. Collection, tumor contamination and engraftment kinetics of highly purified hematopoietic progenitor cells to support high dose therapy in multiple myeloma. Blood 1998; 91:4489–95.

38. Tricot G, Jagannath S, Vesole D, Nelson J, Trindle S, Miller L, et al. Peripheral blood stem cell transplants for multiple myeloma: identification of favorable variables for rapid engraftment in 225 patients. Blood 1995; 85:588–96.

39. Harousseau JL. Optimizing peripheral blood progenitor cell autologous transplantation in multiple myeloma. Haematologica 1999; 84:548–53.

40. Facon T, Harousseau JL, Maloisel F, Attal M, Odriozola J, Alegre A, et al. Stem cell factor in combination with filgrastim after chemotherapy improves peripheral blood progenitor cell yield and reduces apheresis requirements in multiple myeloma: a randomized, controlled trial. Blood 1999; 94:1218–25.

41. Bjorkstrand B, Svensson H, Goldschmidt H, Ljungman P, Apperley JF, Mandelli F, et al. Alpha-interferon maintenance treatment is associated with improved survival after high-dose treatment and autologous stem cell transplantation in patients with multiple myeloma: a retrospective registry study from the EBMT. Bone Marrow Transplant 2001; 27:511–15.

42. Cunningham D, Powles R, Malpas J, Raje N, Milan S, Viner C, et al. A randomized trial of maintenance interferon following high-dose chemotherapy in multiple myeloma: long term follow-up results. Br J Haematol 1998; 102:195–202.

43. Barlogie B, Jagannath S, Desikan KR, Mattox S, Vesole D, Siegel D, et al. Total therapy with tandem transplants for newly diagnosed multiple myeloma. Blood 1999; 93:66–75.

44. Facon T, Avet-Loiseau H, Guillerm G, Moreau P, Genevieve F, Zan M, et al. Chromosome 13 abnormalities identified by Fish analysis and serum β2 microglobulin produce powerful myeloma staging system for patients receiving high-dose therapy. Blood 2001; 97:1566–71.

45. Lahuerta JJ, Martinez-Lopez J, de la Serna J, Blade J, Grande C, Alegre A, et al. Remission status defined by immunofixation vs. electrophoresis after autologous transplantation has a major impact on the outcome of multiple myeloma patients. Br J Haematol 2000; 109:438–46.

46. Davies FE, Forsyth PD, Rawstron AC, Owen RG, Pratt G, Evans PA, et al. The impact of attaining a minimal disease state after high-dose melphalan and autologous transplantation for multiple myeloma. Br J Haematol 2001; 112:814–19.

47. Siegel DS, Desikan KR, Mehta J, Singhal S, Fassas A, Munshi N, et al. Age is not a prognostic variable with autotransplants for multiple myeloma. Blood 1999; 93:51–4.

48. Badros A, Barlogie B, Siegel E, Morris C, Desikan R, Zangari M, et al. Autologous stem cell transplantation in elderly multiple myeloma patients over the age of 70 years. Br J Haematol 2001; 114:600–7.

49. Badros A, Barlogie B, Siegel E, Roberts J, Langmaid C, Zangari M, et al. Results of autologous stem cell transplant in multiple myeloma patients with renal failure. Br J Haematol 2001; 114:822–9.

50. Tricot G, Alberts DS, Johnson C, Roe DJ, Dorr RT, Bracy D, et al. Safety of autotransplants with high-dose melphalan in renal failure: a pharmacokinetic and toxicity study. Clin Cancer Res 1996; 2:947–52.

51. Ballester B, Tummala R, Janssen WE, Fields KK, Hiemenz JW, Goldstein SC, et al. High dose therapy and autologous peripheral blood stem cell transplantation in patients with multiple myeloma and renal failure. Bone Marrow Transplant 1997; 20:653–6.

52. Tosi P, Zamagni E, Ronconi S, Benni M, Motta MR, Rizzi S, et al. Safety of autologous hematopoietic stem cell transplantation in patients with multiple myeloma and chronic renal failure. Leukemia 2000; 14:1310–13.

53. San Miguel J, Lahuerta JJ, Garcia-Sanz R, Alegre A, Blade J, Martinez R, et al. Are myeloma patients with renal failure candidate for autologous stem cell transplantation. Hematol J 2000; 1:28–36.

17

Allogeneic transplantation and treatment with donor lymphocytes

GÖSTA GAHRTON AND PER LJUNGMAN

INTRODUCTION

Allogeneic bone marrow transplantation became an established method for treatment of hematological malignancies in the early 1970s.[1,2] The rationale for allogeneic transplantation is firstly that the bone marrow ablative therapy may have the potential to eradicate the malignant disease. The patient is thereafter saved from the consequences of ablating the marrow by infusion of normal cells from a donor. Secondly, the donor cells *per se* have a graft-versus-tumor effect.[3,4] The exact nature of this effect is not known. However, it is well documented for chronic myelocytic leukemia,[4,5] acute leukemia,[4,5] and multiple myeloma.[6–8] The graft-versus-tumor effect may be different from, but is associated with, graft-versus-host disease.

Most allogeneic transplants in multiple myeloma have been performed with bone marrow from human leukocyte antigen (HLA) identical sibling donors.[9–12] Originally, the source of cells was bone marrow but, since the mid-1990s, peripheral blood stem cells have been used increasingly.[13] Until recently, conditioning treatment has been myeloablative (high-dose) but there is currently considerable interest in the use of non-myeloablative (low-dose) regimens (Table 17.1).

Only a small number of transplants have been performed with syngeneic[14,15] or HLA-matched unrelated donors.[10,16–18] So far, results have been rather poor using unrelated donors; however, most of these patients have received high-dose myeloablative conditioning before the transplant.

In general, allogeneic bone marrow transplantation in myeloma is associated with a relatively high transplant-related mortality compared with other hematological malignancies, and relapse also remains a major problem. The long-term transplant-related mortality (TRM) is at least 30%, while disease progression or relapse occurs in most of those that survive the transplant. Nevertheless, a proportion of patients enter long-term complete remission, and it is possible that some of these patients may be cured, although very late relapses have been reported.

TRANSPLANTATION USING HLA-MATCHED SIBLING DONORS

Early transplants and present frequency

The first attempts to perform allogeneic transplantation with sibling donor marrow in multiple myeloma were made in the early 1980s.[9,19–22] Out of three patients reported from our group at Huddinge University Hospital,[21] one patient who was resistant to melphalan + prednisolone treatment went into complete remission following transplantation. She remained without signs of multiple myeloma for 4 years but then relapsed. Similar results were reported by the Bologna group.[22] Subsequently, the number of reported transplants for myeloma increased

Table 17.1 *Myeloablative and non-myeloablative conditioning regimens in multiple myeloma*

Total body irradiation (Gy)	Fractions	Cyclophosphamide (mg/kg)	Busulfan (mg/kg)	Other drugs	Reference
Myeloablative					
10	1	60 × 2			Gahrton *et al.* (1986)[21]
8	1	50 × 2			Ozer *et al.* (1984)[20]
10	1	60 × 2		BCNU 5 mg/kg × 1 and/or oral melphalan 1 mg/kg × 5	Tura *et al.* (1986)[22]
7.5–10.5	5–7	60 × 2	3.5 × 4		Bensinger *et al.* (1996)[12]
		50 × 4	4 × 4		Tura *et al.* (1989)[114]
		60 × 2	3.5–4 × 4		Bensinger *et al.* (1996)[12]
Non–myeloablative					
0.2	1				McSweeney *et al.* (2001)[45]
0.2	1			Fludarabine 30 mg/m²	Storb *et al.* (2001);[95] Bensinger *et al.* (2001)[30]
		30 × 2		Thiotepa 5 mg/kg × 2; fludarabine 30 mg/m² × 2	Corradini *et al.* (2002)[115]
				Melphalan 100 mg/m² × 1 (sibling donors)	Badros *et al.* (2002)[116]
0.25	2			Melphalan 100 mg/m² × 1; fludarabine 30 mg/m² × 2 (unrelated donors)	Badros *et al.* (2002)[116]

steadily. However, in comparison to acute leukemia and chronic myelocytic leukemia, the number of allogeneic transplants performed in multiple myeloma remains relatively small. The Myeloma Registry of the European Group for Blood and Marrow Transplantation (EBMT) has reports of more than 1500 allogeneic transplants, and the International Bone Marrow Transplant Registry (IBMTR) has reports of 2216 allogeneic transplants performed up to the year 2000 (M. Horowitz, unpublished communication). However, a proportion of these patients are also reported to the EBMT registry. The Seattle group has performed about 180 transplants that are not reported to EBMT or IBMTR (W. Bensinger, unpublished communication). Considering both some double reporting to EBMT and IBMTR and an uncertain number of unreported patients, the estimated number of myeloma allotransplants that have been performed worldwide is about 4000–5000. This relatively small number of transplants in myeloma in comparison to transplants in many other hematological malignancies is probably due to the fact that only about 7% of patients with myeloma are below the age of 55 years.[23] Also, because of the high treatment-related mortality of allogeneic BMT, many centers prefer to use autologous transplantation (Chapter 16), although this is not a curative approach.

The results presented in this chapter are mainly based on data from the EBMT registry, but reports from Seattle and other centers are also discussed.

Myeloablative conditioning treatment

The aim of myeloablative conditioning treatment (Table 17.1) is to eradicate the malignant cell population. The myeloma cell is highly sensitive to both irradiation and cytotoxic drugs, particularly the alkylating agents melphalan and cyclophosphamide. Most myeloablative allogeneic transplants in patients with multiple myeloma have been performed with conditioning regimens, including total body irradiation (TBI). The irradiation has been combined with cyclophosphamide (mainly according to the original Seattle protocol), or melphalan, or other drugs in combination.

In a recent updated report from EBMT, TBI + cyclophosphamide was the most common conditioning regime.[13] It was used in 37% of patients who were transplanted before 1994, 39% of patients who received bone marrow transplants 1994–1998, and 27% of those who received peripheral blood stem cells during this later time period (see later). In later years, melphalan-containing regimens have been increasingly used in combination with TBI. Busulfan + cyclophosphamide was used in about 10% of patients, while melphalan alone has rarely been used as a conditioning regimen for allogeneic transplantation. In EBMT studies, it has not been possible to detect differences in outcome owing to the conditioning method used. However, the great variation in dosages and schedules, etc., makes comparison difficult.

Busulfan combined with cyclophosphamide was originally used by Tutschka *et al.*[24] and later in multiple myeloma by the Seattle group.[12,25] In leukemia, one randomized study comparing busulfan + cyclophosphamide with the classical Seattle regimen, TBI + cyclophosphamide, indicated that busulfan + cyclophosphamide might be associated with more complications, such as hemorrhagic cystitis and veno-occlusive disease.[26] Also, for some patient groups, busulfan + cyclophosphamide seemed to be inferior to TBI.[26] Later studies found a tendency for poorer survival with busulfan + cyclophosphamide in acute myeloid leukemia (although not in chronic myeloid leukemia) and a greater incidence of cataract was observed with TBI-containing regimens.[27] The Seattle group used busulfan + cyclophosphamide in 20 patients with multiple myeloma, most of whom had refractory disease, and considered the regimen promising.[25] However, the series was small and the transplant-related mortality high. Later, the busulfan + cyclophosphamide regimen ($n = 57$ patients) was compared with 'modified' (7.5–10.5 Gy) TBI + busulfan + cyclophosphamide ($n = 23$ patients) in mainly refractory or relapsed myeloma patients.[12] No obvious difference in outcome was seen. The transplant-related mortality at 100 days was high in both groups of patients, i.e. 44% and 43%, respectively.

Thus, there are no data available that could clearly tell which myeloablative regimen might be the best one. So far, no myeloablative regimen appears to be superior to the classical Seattle combination of TBI + cyclophosphamide.

Engraftment

The number of CD34-positive cells infused is probably of importance for engraftment, as it is for other hematological malignancies.[28,29] However, the issue has not been well investigated for allotransplants in multiple myeloma. With current techniques, practically all patients engraft, and the median time to neutrophils $>0.5 \times 10^9$/L is around 20 days with bone marrow and 14 days with peripheral blood stem cells following ablative conditioning.[13] The time to platelets $>50 \times 10^9$/L is at a median of 27 days with bone marrow and 18 days with peripheral blood stem cell.[13] Thus, the rate of engraftment is more rapid with peripheral blood stem cells, as has also been documented for other hematological malignancies.[30]

Response

The complete response–remission (CR) rate is highly dependent on many factors, such as stage of disease at diagnosis, number of pre-transplant treatment regimens, and the response to pre-transplant treatment (Tables 17.2–17.4).[11] Among the patients who have been reported to the EBMT registry, the prognosis has in many

Table 17.2 *Bone marrow transplantation (BMT) in multiple myeloma: complete remission (CR) by stage of disease at diagnosis*

Stage at diagnosis	Number of patients	CR following BMT	
		Number of patients	%
I	22	15	68
II	30	11	37
III	109	45	41

Table 17.3 *Bone marrow transplantation (BMT) in multiple myeloma: complete remission (CR) following BMT by number of lines of treatment*

Number of lines before BMT	Number of patients	CR following BMT	
		Number of patients	%
One	64	36	56
Two	50	19	38
Three	46	16	35

Table 17.4 *Bone marrow transplantation (BMT) in multiple myeloma: complete remission (CR) by response status at conditioning*

Response status at conditioning	Number of patients	CR following BMT	
		Number of patients	%
CR	18	15	83
Partial remission	66	28	42
Stable disease	22	11	50
Primary refractory	14	5	36
Progressive disease	25	6	24
Relapse	14	6	43

cases been considered poor. Many patients have received transplants after resistance to conventional chemotherapy or relapse following autologous transplantation. Nevertheless, in the EBMT material, a complete hematological response was seen in more than 50% of the patients at 6 months and about 60% of the patients at 2 years following transplantation.[13]

The highest CR rate is obtained in patients who are diagnosed in stage I irrespective of the stage at the time of the transplant (Table 17.2), and those who receive fewer treatment regimens (Table 17.3) or are in a responsive state at the time of transplantation (Table 17.4). Thus, in the EBMT studies, patients who had received several lines of treatment had a CR rate of 35%, and those who were in a progressive state of disease at the time of transplantation had a CR rate of 24%. However, patients who were in stage I at diagnosis, irrespective of the stage at transplantation, were responsive at the time of transplantation, and had received only one treatment regimen before the transplant had CR rates of 68%, 51% and 56%, respectively. The CR rate was similar whether transplantation was performed with bone marrow or peripheral blood stem cells.

The CR rate is also dependent on the criteria used to define response. Until recently, the EBMT has required only disappearance of immunoglobulins or light chains in the urine following either conventional electrophoresis *or* immunofixation, and less than 5% plasma cells in the marrow or absence of myeloma cells.[10,11] Recently, more strict criteria to define response and relapse have been adopted.[31] Complete remission requires absence of detectable paraprotein on immunofixation and $\leq 4\%$ plasma cells in the marrow as well as no progression of bone lesions on X-ray, if X-ray has been performed. However, these criteria have not been required by EBMT until recently and, therefore, CR rates still rely on the earlier definition. In comparison to CR rates in smaller series of patients reported by other groups that have required absence of detectable paraprotein by immunofixation,[12,17,25] it appears that the reduction in CR rate with the new criteria should be relatively small.

Molecular remissions are frequent following allogeneic transplantation in contrast to autologous transplantation, where persistent polymerase chain reaction (PCR) negativity is rarely observed. About 50% of those patients who enter a complete hematological remission after allogeneic transplantation also appear to enter a molecular remission.[32–35] Recent studies indicate that those patients who enter a molecular remission have a better chance of long-term survival and long-term relapse-free survival than patients who do not enter molecular remission.[35]

Survival, and progression-free and relapse-free survival

The results of bone marrow transplantation with sibling donors have improved dramatically from 1994 as compared with results of bone marrow transplants during the time period 1983–1993.[13] The overall 4-year survival was only 32% before 1994, but 50% from 1994 to 2000 (Fig. 17.1). This dramatic improvement over time was not due to the use of peripheral blood stem cells, since results of peripheral blood stem cell transplantation and bone marrow transplantation were similar (Fig. 17.2). Instead there seem to be several other reasons for the improvement. During the later time period, patients have been transplanted earlier in the course of their disease. They have received fewer treatment regimens before the transplant, and more effective antibacterial and antiviral drugs have been used both for treatment and

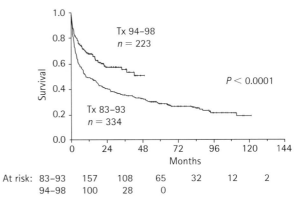

Figure 17.1 *Overall actuarial survival after bone marrow transplantation according to the time of transplantation. The Kaplan–Meier curves show a significantly better survival among patients who received the transplant (Tx) 1994–98 than among those who received the transplant 1983–93. (Reproduced with permission from Gahrton et al., Br J Haematol 2001; 113:209–16.[13])*

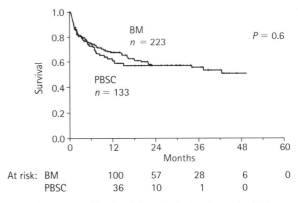

Figure 17.2 *Overall actuarial survival after transplantation performed 1994–98 according to the type of graft. The Kaplan–Meier curves show a similar survival among patients who received bone marrow (BM) cells and those who received peripheral blood stem cells (PBSC). (Reproduced with permission from Gahrton et al., Br J Haematol 2001; 113:209–16.[13])*

prevention of transplant-related complications. This, in turn, has decreased transplant-related mortality (Fig. 17.3) and resulted in the improvement in overall survival.

Several non-procedural prognostic factors for survival have been delineated. Females do better than males (Fig. 17.4) and younger patients do better than older patients.[16] Patients who are diagnosed in stage I appear to have a better survival than other patients irrespective of the stage in which they are transplanted. Those with low β_2-microglobulin have better survival than those with high β_2-microglobulin. IgA myelomas seem to do better than other types of myelomas.[11] Recently, it has been shown that patients with IgD myeloma do less well following both

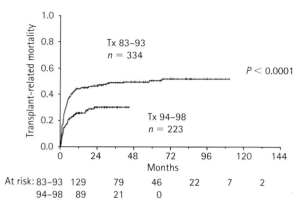

Figure 17.3 *Transplant-related mortality (TRM) according to the time of bone marrow transplantation. The Kaplan–Meier curves shown significantly less TRM among patients who received the transplant 1994–98 than those who received the transplant 1983–93. (Reproduced with permission from Gahrton et al., Br J Haematol 2001; 113:209–16.[13])*

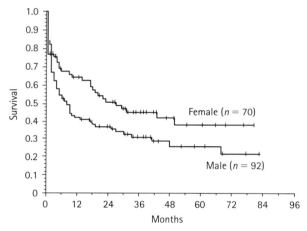

Figure 17.4 *Actuarial survival after bone marrow transplantation according to the sex of the patient. The Kaplan–Meier curves show significantly better survival among females than among males. (Reproduced withpermission from Gahrton et al. J Clin Oncol 1995; 13:1312–22.[11])*

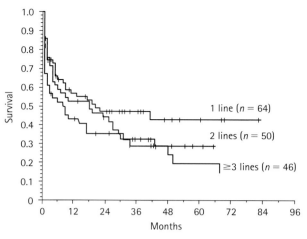

Figure 17.5 *Actuarial survival after bone marrow transplantation according to the number of lines of treatment regimens used before transplantation. The Kaplan–Meier curves show significantly better survival among patients who had received only one line of treatment as compared with those who had received three ore more line of treatment (Reproduced with permission from Gahrton et al. J Clin Oncol 1995; 13:1312–22.[11])*

An interesting observation is that there seems to be an adverse effect of female-to-male[38] as well as male-to-female[12] transplantation as compared with transplantation with donors of the same gender. An influence of donor gender has also been shown for leukemia.[39,40] Differences in minor transplantation antigens dependent on loci on the Y chromosome may play a role.[41,42]

Because of the reduction in TRM in recent years, the progression-free survival and relapse-free survival of patients in complete remission have also improved with time.[13] However, the relapse rate of patients who enter a complete remission has not changed significantly (Fig. 17.6). The relapse rate is between 20% and 25% at 2 years following transplantation. Although there seems to be no clear plateau in relapse rate or relapse-free survival, it is of interest that about 20% of patients survive more than 10 years from transplantation, some of them in complete remission. Furthermore, in some patients, clonal cells could not be detected with PCR-based techniques using patient-specific primers.[32–35] Thus, it may be possible that the myeloma cell clone can be eradicated completely in some patients.

The rate of disappearance of the myeloma cell clone varies considerably between patients. In EBMT studies, the median time for disappearance of monoclonal immunoglobulins was 4 months following conditioning, although some patients did not lose their monoclonal component until 2 years post-transplant.[10,11] To enter a complete remission is an important factor for survival following transplantation.[10] Patients who did engraft but did not enter a complete remission had a survival that was significantly poorer than the survival for those who entered a

autotransplantation and allotransplantation than those with other isotypes.[36] In contrast, non-secretory myelomas do not have a significantly worse outlook.[36] Plasma-cell leukemia is associated with a very poor prognosis.[37]

Patients who are on first-line treatment at the time of transplantation do better than those who are on second- or third-line treatment (Fig. 17.5). Those who are in complete remission already before transplantation do better than those who have more advanced disease or who are unresponsive to conventional chemotherapy. However, most importantly, a small fraction of patients who are considered unresponsive to treatment before transplantation become long-term survivors.[11]

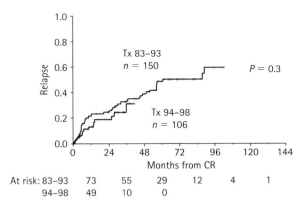

Figure 17.6 *Relapse rate according to the time of bone marrow transplantation. The Kaplan–Meier curves show no significant difference in relapse rate among patients who received the transplant (Tx) 1983–93 and those who received the transplant 1994–98. (Reproduced with permission from Gahrton et al., Br J Haematol 2001; 113:209–16.[13])*

CR. However, it has to be noted that 20% of patients who did not enter CR survived more than 3 years following transplantation. Thus, although CR post-transplant is the most important factor for survival, patients who do not enter CR can survive for a significant period of time. Some of these patients have stable disease for many years with only a small monoclonal component in serum or minimal amounts of light chains in the urine. Thus, high-dose therapy followed by allogeneic transplantation does improve survival for a fraction of patients who are non-responsive to other types of treatment or who do not enter CR following transplantation.

Treatment–related complications and mortality

Treatment-related mortality using myeloablative conditioning regimens is significant and until 1994 was close to 40% at 6 months, and between 40% and 50% at 2 years.[10,11] Since1994, there has been a significant reduction in TRM to 21% at 6 months and 30% at 2 years. This is not due to increasing use of peripheral blood stem cells, and there is no significant difference in TRM between transplants with bone marrow or peripheral blood stem cells.[13] Although the transplant-related mortality is still high, it is now similar to that seen in many other hematologic disorders.

GRAFT–VERSUS–HOST DISEASE

Acute graft-versus-host disease (GVHD) is an important cause of death in allogeneic transplantation. In the EBMT study, 11% of patients transplanted with bone marrow and 18% of those transplanted with peripheral blood stem cells between 1994 and 1998 had GVHD grades III–IV cells.[13] GVHD was considered either the main cause or a contributing cause of death in 11% of patients transplanted with bone marrow and in 22% of those who were transplanted with peripheral blood stem cells. However, there was no statistically significant difference between the incidence of GVHD with bone marrow or peripheral blood stem cells.

Other centers have also found a high incidence of severe GVHD in myeloma transplants.[12] In one study,[17] 20 out of 26 patients (78%) had grade II–IV acute GVHD, including 68% of those who had received matched sibling donor transplants. GVHD was the cause of death in 11% of the patients.

There are several possible ways of reducing the incidence and severity of GVHD by prophylactic treatment. The most common treatment modality is the one originally used by the Seattle group with methotrexate + cyclosporin.[43] The rationale for this treatment is that these drugs inhibit the T-cell-dependent graft-versus-host reaction. Another regimen that has recently been used, particularly in association with non-myeloablative treatment, is the combination of cyclosporin and mycophenylate mofetil.[44–46]

T-cell depletion may be the most effective method of preventing severe GVHD, but the EBMT data do not indicate a survival advantage for patients who received T-cell-depleted grafts. In one recent study,[47] selective CD6 T-cell depletion appeared promising; in 24 reported patients, GVHD grade III was seen in only one patient (4%) and grade II in four patients (17%). However, T-cell depletion may increase the risk of relapse and should, therefore, probably be combined with donor lymphocyte infusion given either prophylactically or as early treatment at signs of recurrence of monoclonal protein in serum or light chains in urine. So far, there is no proof that T-cell depletion will improve survival.

When GVHD appears despite prevention, treatment should be initiated with prednisolone and, if possible, increased dosages of cyclosporin.

Chronic GVHD is seen in a frequency that seems similar to that seen in other hematological disorders. In the EBMT study, it was seen in 11% of patients transplanted after 1994 who received bone marrow and in 27% of those receiving peripheral blood stem cells.[13] However, there may be some under-reporting of chronic GVHD in EBMT studies. In the Seattle experience, acute and chronic GVHD contributed to death in 14% of patients[12] and, in the study by Reece et al.,[17] three of 26 patients died of chronic GVHD.[17]

INFECTIONS AND OTHER TRANSPLANT–RELATED COMPLICATIONS AND SIDE EFFECTS

During the aplastic phase following stem cell transplantation, bacterial and fungal infections are common,[48] while viral infections predominate during the later post-transplant period.[49] Early instigation of broad-spectrum antimicrobial therapy has decreased the mortality from bacterial infections.[50]

Prophylaxis with fluconazole reduces the mortality from fungal infections[51,52] and has resulted in improved long-term survival.[53] However, fungal infections, in particular with aspergillus, remain a major problem.[54] In contrast to yeast infections, most aspergillus infections occur during the phase of acute GVHD and not during the aplastic phase.[54] Treatment of aspergillus infections has remained unsatisfactory.[55] The use of liposomal amphotericin has reduced the toxicity of antifungal therapy and possibly improved the efficacy.[56,57] New antifungal drugs, such as voriconazole[58] and caspofungin, show promising results in the treatment of invasive aspergillosis.

The most frequent serious viral infection is caused by cytomegalovirus (CMV). During the past few years, major advances have been made in the prophylaxis and therapy of CMV infections.[59] High-dose aciclovir prophylaxis can reduce CMV viremia and infectious mortality.[60] Prophylaxis with ganciclovir reduces the frequency of CMV disease.[61-63] New diagnostic techniques, such as detection of pp65 antigenemia[64,65] or detection of CMV DNA by PCR, allow very early instigation of antiviral therapy (pre-emptive therapy) and is effective in reducing the risk for CMV disease.[59,66,67] The outcome of patients with CMV pneumonia is still poor despite use of ganciclovir and immune globulin, the combination of ganciclovir and foscarnet, or cidofovir.[68,69]

The pattern of CMV disease has changed in recent years, with more disease occurring late after transplantation[70] and new forms of disease, such as retinitis, becoming more frequent.[71,72] CMV disease also remains an important complication after non-myeloablative stem cell transplantation, occurring most frequently after day 100.[73] The most important risk factors for development of CMV infection and disease are pre-existing exposure to CMV infection (recipient seropositive) and delayed specific immune reconstitution. Therefore, strategies such as monitoring of the immune response to select high-risk patients for late CMV disease, thereby allowing directed interventions,[74-76] and the development of adoptive immunotherapy with CMV-specific cytotoxic T-cells are currently being investigated.[75,77,78]

Other viral infections that can cause fatal infections in bone marrow transplant recipients include adenovirus, respiratory syncytial virus, parainfluenza viruses, and human herpesvirus 6.[49] Important late infections are *Pneumocystis* pneumonias, Herpes zoster, and infections caused by pneumococci and *H. influenzae*. The risk is increased in patients with chronic GVHD and prophylactic measures to prevent infections are indicated. These include antibiotic prophylaxis against bacterial infections and *P. carinii*, possibly long-term prophylaxis with aciclovir against Varicella zoster virus,[79,80] and revaccinations against several infections agents, such as pneumococci, *H. influenzae*, influenza, tetanus, diphtheria, and poliovirus.[79-81]

CAUSE OF DEATH

Although the transplant-related mortality in multiple myeloma has improved dramatically since 1994, it is still significant. At the time of follow-up of patients reported to the EBMT registry in 2000, 250 out of 344 patients who were transplanted between 1983 and 1993 had died.[13] Of those who were transplanted with bone marrow between 1994 and 1998, 84 out of 233 (36%) had died, and, of those who had received peripheral blood stem cells, 44 out of 133 (33%) had died. The causes of death were similar in both groups, i.e. bacterial and fungal infections, viral infections, interstitial pneumonitis, acute and chronic GVHD, adult respiratory distress syndrome, capillary leak syndrome, rejection or poor graft function, organ failure, disseminated intravascular coagulation, veno-occlusive disease, hemorrhage, and cardiac toxicity. However, the frequencies of some causes of death were different before and after 1994. Interstitial pneumonitis was the cause of death in 37 patients (15%) during the earlier time period, while only seven patients died of this complication thereafter (5%). The causes of death were bacterial and fungal infections in 43 patients (17%) before 1994, but in only 11 patients (9%) after this time. There were no apparent differences between the causes of death with bone marrow or peripheral blood stem cells during the time period 1994–2000. The improvement with time in overall survival appeared to be due mainly to fewer deaths from bacterial and fungal infections and interstitial pneumonitis. This, in turn, was probably due to earlier transplantation, as well as better treatment with new and more effective antibacterial and antifungal drugs and new antiviral drug treatment. Death due to progressive disease was still the most important cause of death.

Conclusions – sibling donor transplantation

- The results of allogeneic transplantation have improved dramatically since the mid-1990s.
- Transplant-related mortality is still high with a long-term transplant related mortality of about 30%.
- About 50% of the patients enter a complete hematologic remission and about 50% of these patients enter a molecular remission.
- Although the relapse rate is significant, it is lower than with autologous transplantation.
- The best candidate for an allogeneic transplantation is a responsive female patient who has received only one line of treatment and with a female sibling donor.

TRANSPLANTATION USING HLA–MATCHED NON–RELATED VOLUNTEER DONORS

Only about 25% of patients are expected to have an HLA-matched sibling donor. Thus, about 75% of patients who otherwise would have had an indication for allogeneic transplantation cannot be transplanted unless a suitable alternative donor can be found.

Because of the lack of sibling or other related donors, and the increasing need for allogeneic transplantation, several countries have established registries of volunteer HLA-typed donors. More than seven million donors are now registered at about 50 registries throughout the world. Of these HLA-A and HLA-B-typed donors, about half have also been typed for HLA-DR. In the year 2000, close to 4000 transplants were performed with unrelated donor marrow or peripheral blood stem cells as reported to the World Marrow Donor Association (WMDA).[82] This organization consists of representatives for registries of volunteer donors throughout the world. It collects annual information about the use of volunteer donors. Its main aim is to facilitate hematopoietic stem cell transplantation using volunteer donors. It also provides guidelines on issues relating to donors, such as ethical guidelines and guidelines on logistics. It has recently started a project of accrediting registries to enhance quality. Another organization is Bone Marrow Donors Worldwide, which collects information on the results of HLA typing on volunteer donors and allows worldwide searching for a donor.

Although the results of transplantation using volunteer unrelated donors are poorer than results of sibling donor transplantation,[16] recent studies suggest that if a well-matched volunteer donor is selected, the results seem to approach those of sibling donor transplantation.[83]

Cord blood transplantation is another possibility for patients who do not have a sibling donor.[84,85] Cord blood cells appear to be as effective for transplantation as stem cells from bone marrow or peripheral blood. However, the problem is that the number of cells that can be recovered from the cord is frequently insufficient for transplantation to adult patients.[86] More than 30 cord blood banks have collected more than 100 000 units of cord blood that are available for transplantation. In the year 2001, more than 500 transplants were performed with cord blood throughout the world according to reports to the WMDA.[82]

In multiple myeloma, unrelated donors have been used in only a relatively small number of patients and transplants with cord blood have not yet been reported. Since unrelated donor transplants appear to be associated with higher transplant-related mortality than transplants that uses sibling donors, unrelated donors should preferentially be used in combination with non-myeloablative conditioning (see later).

SYNGENEIC TRANSPLANTATION

Syngeneic transplantation lacks the graft-versus-tumor effect but has the advantage in comparison with allogeneic transplantation that it also lacks GVHD (with some possible exceptions).[14,15] The first results of syngeneic transplantation in myeloma were published in the early 1980s. Fefer et al.[87] and Osserman et al.[88] each reported one patient at this time. More recently, the EBMT reported a case-matched analysis comparing 25 syngeneic transplants with 125 autologous and 125 allogeneic transplants. The results of syngeneic transplants were superior to both the other transplant modalities. Most striking was the significantly lower relapse rate as compared with autologous transplantation, while the transplant-related mortality was not higher than with an autologous transplant. The results of syngeneic transplants previously published by the Seattle group appear poorer but may be due to different conditioning regimens or selection of patients with poorer prognostic factors. The EBMT data indicate that younger patients with a twin donor should receive a transplant when there is an indication for treatment.

NON–MYELOABLATIVE TRANSPLANTATION

The idea of non-myeloablative low-dose conditioning in allogeneic transplantation for hematological malignancies is that reduced myelosuppression may reduce transplant-related mortality and still allow engraftment.[89,90] Furthermore, the most important reason for killing the tumor cells may not be total body irradiation or cytotoxic drugs, but the graft-versus-tumor effect.[89] Although it cannot be expected that the antitumor effect *per se* should be more pronounced with non-myeloablative treatment, the predicted gain in transplant-related mortality could result in improved survival. Also, since there is a graft-versus-tumor effect,[3,4] donor-lymphocyte transfusion (see later) following the transplant could further improve results by preventing recurrence of the disease. Donor lymphocytes could also be used to treat recurrence.[5,91] Hopefully, the overall outcome with these procedures should be better than with myeloablative allogeneic transplantation.

Non-myeloablative regimens (Table 17.1) have been increasingly used during the last few years.[89,90] In studies on transplantation in dogs, Storb and co-workers found that conditioning with 200 cGy total body irradiation was enough to promote engraftment.[92] However, in humans a significant number of rejections were seen. It was later shown that combining 200 cGy total body irradiation with fludarabine 30 mg/m^2 for 3–5 days preceding total body irradiation promoted engraftment and only occasional rejections were seen in patients who had previously been treated with autologous stem cell transplantation.[83] Other so-called non-myeloablative regimens have included melphalan 100–140 mg/m^2 combined with fludarabine in different schedules.[93] Low-dose busulfan + cyclophosphamide has also been used. These and other phase II-studies show that engraftment as well as remissions can be obtained with non-myeloablative low-dose conditioning in both previously untreated and refractory patients.[94,95]

One of the most promising regimen seems to be the combination of total body irradiation 200 cGy and fludarabine 30 mg/m^2 × 3–5 days preceding the irradiation.[45,83] The best results seem to be obtained if this procedure follows 2–4 months after autologous transplantation.[44,46] Irradiation alone in this dosage (200 cGy), combined with post-transplant immunosuppression with mycophenolate mofetil for 28 days, combined with cyclosporin for at least 56 days was recently used to treat 32 patients with previously treated stage II–III myeloma. A total of 43% of the previously autotransplanted patients were refractory or in relapse.[46] All patients engrafted. The transplant-related toxicity was very low. More than half of the patients did not have to be hospitalized and had no neutropenia or thrombocytopenia. The response rate was 84% and the complete hematologic remission rate was 53%. It usually takes between 6 months and 1 year for the paraprotein to disappear,[83] i.e. longer than following myeloablative conditioning. With a median follow-up time of 423 days after the autologous transplantation and 328 days after non-myeloablative transplantation, the overall survival was 81%. However, 45% of the patients developed grade II–IV GVHD and 55% developed chronic GVHD. Six patients had died at the time of follow-up owing to progression, infections or GVHD.

Other studies have used 100–140 mg melphalan,[96] low-dose melphalan plus fludarabine,[93] melphalan plus Campath IH, or low-dose busulfan plus fludarabine[97] for conditioning. Overall, engraftment has been high, but addition of fludarabine to irradiation or an alkylating agent seems to be advisable in order to secure engraftment.

A survey of EBMT centers collected results of non-myeloablative transplantation in 54 myeloma patients.[94] Many different low-dose regimens were used. Eighteen patients were refractory to other treatment at the time of conditioning, 28 were in partial remission, and only one was in complete remission. After the transplant with non-myeloablative conditioning, 19 patients were in complete remission and 21 in partial remission. Of the good-risk patients (those in remission at the time of transplant), 83% were alive at 1 year, but only 25% of the poor-risk patients (refractory at transplant) were alive. The transplant related mortality was only 11% at 1 year

in good-risk patients but 68% in poor-risk ones. Donor lymphocytes were given to four patients in partial remission and to three who were refractory. Two of them entered complete remission.

Although non-myeloablative transplantation appears promising, owing to the seemingly decreased transplant-related mortality as compared with myeloablative conditioning, the long-term results are not yet known. It is possible that the relapse rate will be higher and that progression may occur earlier than following myeloablative treatment. In comparison to autologous transplantation alone, the procedure-related mortality is higher. Thus, it is now important that this new procedure is properly evaluated in prospective comparative studies. Within the Myeloma Subcommittee of the EBMT such a study is in progress, comparing autologous transplantation alone with the tandem procedure, i.e. non-myeloablative allogeneic transplantation following autologous transplantation. Patients with an HLA-matched sibling donor will be offered the tandem procedure, while other patients will receive autologous transplantation alone. The conditioning regimen for the autologous transplant will be melphalan 200 mg/m^2. Similar studies, but with different non-myeloablative conditioning regimens, are planned or ongoing at other centers. Hopefully, this will eventually clarify the role of non-myeloablative transplantation in multiple myeloma. In the mean time, this type of procedure should only be offered to patients in the context of an approved research protocol.

RELAPSE AND DONOR LYMPHOCYTE TRANSFUSIONS

Relapse is still the most important cause of failure following bone marrow transplantation of patients with multiple myeloma.[11,98] Patients seemingly in complete remission relapse as late as 9 years following transplantation.

Post-transplant drug treatment has been used with the aim of preventing or delaying relapse. Interferon has been used in a dose-finding study by the EBMT[99] and is included in current phase II studies.[100,101] However, it was associated with a risk of provoking GVHD and its role in preventing relapse after allogeneic transplantation is debated. Thalidomide treatment has been most successful in inducing response in patients relapsing after autologous transplantation,[102] and has recently also been shown to induce response and complete remission in patients who have relapsed following allogeneic transplantation.[102–104]

Most encouraging has been the use of donor lymphocytes in the treatment of relapse following allogeneic transplantation. Donor lymphocyte infusions have been used both following myeloablative[6,8,105–109] and non-myeloablative conditioning regimens.[46] In one study,[108] 14 responses were achieved in 27 patients (52%) and in six of them (22%) the remission was complete. The dose ranged from 1×10^6 lymphocytes/kg to more than 1×10^8/kg. The best results were obtained with doses more than 1×10^8 lymphocytes/kg. However, donor lymphocyte transfusions are not without complications. Severe acute graft-versus-host disease occurred in 26% of the patients and chronic graft-versus-host disease in 55%. Two patients who responded died of bone marrow aplasia. Five patients remained in complete remission more than 30 months following donor lymphocyte transfusion.

In another recent study,[47] selected CD4-positive lymphocytes were used in an attempt to induce remission following T-cell-depleted allogeneic transplantation. Donor lymphocyte infusions were administered 6–9 months after transplantation in 24 patients who had received allogeneic transplants from matched sibling donors. The transplants were performed with CD6 T-cell-depleted donor marrow, and this was the only graft-versus-host prevention. Fourteen of the patients received donor lymphocyte infusion, three of whom were in complete remission and 11 of whom had persistent disease after the transplant. Significant graft-versus-myeloma responses were noted after donor lymphocyte infusion in 10 of the 11 patients with persistent disease. Six entered complete remission and four partial remission. Fifty percent of the patients developed grade II–IV acute GVHD or extensive chronic GVHD. The 2-year overall survival of all the patients was 55% and progression-free survival 42%, while those who had received donor lymphocyte infusions had a 2-year progression-free survival of 65%.

In current attempts to use non-myeloablative transplantation, donor lymphocyte infusion may be the method of choice to prevent or treat early relapse. In the current study organized by the EBMT (see earlier), donor lymphocyte infusions are used following non-myeloablative treatment. Low initial doses, i.e. 1×10^6 CD3-positive cells/kg, are used in patients with asymptomatic persistence of monoclonal protein detected by immunofixation. In progression or symptomatic relapse after complete remission, higher initial doses of donor lymphocytes are used (5×10^7 CD3-positive cells/kg) following two cycles of vincristine + doxorubicin + dexamethasone (VAD). In both situations, escalating dosages will be used.

Relapse following allogeneic transplantation is still the most serious problem. It is too early to know whether donor lymphocyte transfusion or thalidomide will decrease the frequency of relapses when used as a preventive measure, or whether it will significantly improve survival after treatment of relapsed disease.

INDICATIONS FOR ALLOGENEIC TRANSPLANTATION – PROSPECTS FOR THE FUTURE

Myeloablative allogeneic transplantation is hampered by high transplant-related mortality. Therefore, patients over 55 years of age should not be considered for such allogeneic transplantation. Among the younger patient group, it remains difficult to decide which patients should be offered myeloablative allogeneic transplantation. The competing treatment modalities are conventional chemotherapy, autologous stem cell transplantation, and non-myeloablative allogeneic transplantation, perhaps in combination with previous autologous transplantation. For patients with stage III disease and many with stage II disease, it seems clear that intensification of treatment followed by autologous transplantation is superior to conventional low-dose chemotherapy.[110] Conventional chemotherapy does not have the potential to cure multiple myeloma. It results in a median survival of only 3–4 years. Nor does high-dose myeloablative chemotherapy followed by autologous stem cell transplantation have the potential to cure the disease. Eradication of the malignant cells is more difficult than with allogeneic transplantation. Molecular analysis has clearly shown that the multiple myeloma clone only rarely disappears with autologous transplantation but disappears in about half of patients in hematologic remission after allogeneic transplantation.[32,33] There is also the risk of reinfusion of malignant cells, which may cause relapse following autologous transplantation. Tandem autologous transplantation may induce molecular remission in some patients,[111] but the principal argument that autologous transplantation does not cure the disease is the same for double as for single transplantation. The arguments in favor of autologous transplantation are a lower transplant-related mortality, and perhaps that tandem autologous transplantation in combination with a later drug treatment, for example with thalidomide, may be curative . However, the chance for this outcome seems to be less than for allogeneic transplantation.

The arguments in favor of allogeneic transplantation are the potential of eradicating the disease without infusion of malignant cells during transplantation, and the possible help by a graft-versus-myeloma effect[6,8] and later donor-lymphocyte infusions.[47,105,108] However, the transplant-related mortality remains high. For most patients, it is, therefore, difficult today to recommend myeloablative allogeneic transplantation as an upfront treatment method.

Non-myeloablative allogeneic transplantation may radically reduce transplant-related mortality in comparison to myeloablative allogeneic transplantation. The recent preliminary results of non-myeloablative transplantation following autologous transplantation indicate that this might be the method of choice.[43,46] This approach is now being evaluated in a number of different protocols. The EBMT has started a trial comparing autologous transplantation alone with autologous transplantation followed by non-myeloablative transplantation, provided that the patient has an HLA-matched sibling donor. The approach is feasible but it will take many years to prove its possible superiority.

New approaches, such as proteosome inhibitors, selected donor-lymphocyte infusions or antibodies to specific targets on myeloma cells, might change the indications for allogeneic transplantation. It is also likely that new technologies such as gene transfer of immune-enhancing genes to myeloma cells will result in more efficient induction of antitumor immunity in the post-transplant period. It has been shown that genes can be transferred to multiple myeloma cells,[112,113] and in experimental systems transfer of genes can enhance immunogenicity of malignant cells. Hopefully, these new methods added to a less toxic allogeneic transplantation modality may eventually cure a growing number of patients with multiple myeloma.

KEY POINTS

- Allogeneic hematopoietic stem cell transplantation induces sustained molecular remission in about 25% of myeloma patients and may, therefore, have the potential to cure some patients.
- Allogeneic transplantation is still associated with significantly higher transplant-related mortality than autologous transplantation, which, therefore, is the method of choice for most myeloma patients.
- Subgroups of patients with an ideal donor (e.g. a young female stage III with an identical female sibling donor) may profit from an allogeneic transplant, while others (e.g. a male with a female donor) may do better with an autologous transplant.
- Non-myeloablative conditioning and allogeneic transplantation is still an experimental method, but indications are that transplant-related mortality is reduced considerably compared with myeloablative conditioning, particularly if the patient receives the allotransplant after a previous response to an autologous transplant.
- Most patients who are progressive or primary refractory to other treatment modalities also do poorly with an allogeneic transplant; however, a few do well and, therefore, allogeneic transplantation may be a last possibility for some patients.

- Donor lymphocyte transfusions may be used to prevent or to treat relapse following allogeneic transplantation.

REFERENCES

● = Key primary paper
◆ = Major review article
∗ = Paper that represents the first formal publication of a management guideline

◆1. Thomas E, Storb R, Clift RA, Fefer A, Johnson FL, Neiman PE, et al. Bone-marrow transplantation (first of two parts). N Engl J Med 1975; **292**:832–43.

◆2. Thomas ED, Storb R, Clift RA, Fefer A, Johnson L, Neiman PE, et al. Bone-marrow transplantation (second of two parts). N Engl J Med 1975; **292**:895–902.

●3. Weiden PL, Sullivan KM, Flournoy N, Storb R, Thomas ED. Antileukemic effect of chronic graft-versus-host disease: contribution to improved survival after allogeneic marrow transplantation. N Engl J Med 1981; **304**:1529–33.

4. Horowitz MM, Gale RP, Sondel PM, Goldman JM, Kersey J, Kolb HJ, et al. Graft-versus-leukemia reactions after bone marrow transplantation. Blood 1990; **75**:555–62.

●5. Kolb HJ, Schattenberg A, Goldman JM, Hertenstein B, Jacobsen N, Arcese W, et al. Graft-versus-leukemia effect of donor lymphocyte transfusions in marrow grafted patients. European Group for Blood and Marrow Transplantation Working Party Chronic Leukemia. Blood 1995; **86**:2041–50.

●6. Tricot G, Vesole DH, Jagannath S, Hilton J, Munshi N, Barlogie B. Graft-versus-myeloma effect: proof of principle. Blood 1996; **87**:1196–8.

7. Verdonck LF, Lokhorst HM, Dekker AW, Nieuwenhuis HK, Petersen EJ. Graft-versus-myeloma effect in two cases. Lancet 1996; **347**:800–1.

8. Aschan J, Lonnqvist B, Ringden O, Kumlien G, Gahrton G. Graft-versus-myeloma effect [letter; comment]. Lancet 1996; **348**:346.

●9. Gahrton G, Tura S, Flesch M, Gratwohl A, Gravett P, Lucarelli G, et al. Bone marrow transplantation in multiple myeloma: report from the European Cooperative Group for Bone Marrow Transplantation. Blood 1987; **69**:1262–4.

●10. Gahrton G, Tura S, Ljungman P, Belanger C, Brandt L, Cavo M, et al. Allogeneic bone marrow transplantation in multiple myeloma. European Group for Bone Marrow Transplantation. N Engl J Med 1991; **325**:1267–73.

11. Gahrton G, Tura S, Ljungman P, Blade J, Brandt L, Cavo M, et al. Prognostic factors in allogeneic bone marrow transplantation for multiple myeloma. J Clin Oncol 1995; **13**:1312–22.

12. Bensinger WI, Buckner CD, Anasetti C, Clift R, Storb R, Barnett T, et al. Allogeneic marrow transplantation for multiple myeloma: an analysis of risk factors on outcome. Blood 1996; **88**:2787–93.

●13. Gahrton G, Svensson H, Cavo M, Apperly J, Bacigalupo A, Björkstrand B, et al. Progress in allogenic bone marrow and peripheral blood stem cell transplantation for multiple myeloma: a comparison between transplants performed 1983–93 and 1994–8 at European Group for Blood and Marrow Transplantation centres. *Br J Haematol* 2001; **113**:209–16.

14. Bensinger WI, Demirer T, Buckner CD, Appelbaum FR, Storb R, Lilleby K, et al. Syngeneic marrow transplantation in patients with multiple myeloma. *Bone Marrow Transplant* 1996; **18**:527–31.

15. Gahrton G, Svensson H, Björkstrand B, Apperley J, Carlson K, Cavo M, et al. Syngeneic transplantation in multiple myeloma – a case-matched comparison with autologous and allogeneic transplantation. *Bone Marrow Transplant* 1999; **24**:741–5.

16. Gahrton G, Tura S, Ljungman P, Blade J, Cavo M, De Laurenzi A, et al. An update of prognostic factors for allogeneic bone marrow transplantation in multiple myeloma using matched sibling donors. European Group for Blood and Marrow Transplantation. *Stem Cells* 1995; **13**(Suppl 2):122–5.

17. Reece DE, Shepherd JD, Klingemann HG, Sutherland HJ, Nantel SH, Barnett MJ, et al. Treatment of myeloma using intensive therapy and allogeneic bone marrow transplantation. *Bone Marrow Transplant* 1995; **15**:117–23.

◆18. Bensinger WI, Gahrton G. Allogeneic hematopoietic cell transplantation for multiple myeloma. In: Forman SJ, Blume KG, Thomas ED (eds) *Hematopoietic cell transplantation.* Oxford: Blackwell Science; 1999:887–91.

19. Higby DBC, Fitzpatrick J, Henderson ES. Bone marrow transplantation in multiple myeloma: a case report with protein studies. *ASCO Proceedings* 1982; C747.

20. Ozer H, Han T, Nussbaum-Blumenson A, Henderson ES, Fitzpatrick J, Higby DJ. Allogeneic BMT and idiotypic monitoring in multiple myeloma. *AACR* abstract; 1984; 161.

21. Gahrton G, Ringden O, Lönnqvist B, Lindquist R, Ljungman P. Bone marrow transplantation in three patients with multiple myeloma. *Acta Med Scand* 1986; **219**:523–7.

22. Tura S, Cavo M, Baccarani M, Ricci P, Gobbi M. Bone marrow transplantation in multiple myeloma. *Scand J Haematol* 1986; **36**:176–9.

23. Registry NBoHaWTC. *Cancer incidence in Sweden 1989.* Stockholm: Kommentus Förlag, 1992.

24. Tutschka PJ, Copelan EA, Klein JP. Bone marrow transplantation for leukemia following a new busulfan and cyclophosphamide regimen. *Blood* 1987; **70**:1382–8.

25. Bensinger WI, Buckner CD, Clift RA, Petersen FB, Bianco JA, Singer JW, et al. Phase I study of busulfan and cyclophosphamide in preparation for allogeneic marrow transplant for patients with multiple myeloma. *J Clin Oncol* 1992; **10**:1492–7.

26. Ringden O, Ruutu T, Remberger M, Nikoskelainen J, Volin L, Vindelov L, et al. A randomized trial comparing busulfan vs total body irradiation in allogeneic marrow transplant recipients with hematological malignancies. *Transplant Proc* 1994; **26**:1831–2.

27. Socie G, Clift RA, Blaise D, Devergie A, Ringden O, Martin PJ, et al. Busulfan plus cyclophosphamide compared with total-body irradiation plus cyclophosphamide before marrow transplantation for myeloid leukemia: long-term follow-up of 4 randomized studies. *Blood* 2001; **98**:3569–74.

28. Demirer T, Gooley T, Buckner CD, Petersen FB, Lilleby K, Rowley S, et al. Influence of total nucleated cell dose from

marrow harvests on outcome in patients with acute myelogenous leukemia undergoing autologous transplantation. *Bone Marrow Transplant* 1995; **15**:907–13.

29. Zaucha JM, Gooley T, Bensinger WI, Heimfeld S, Chauncey TR, Zaucha R, et al. CD34 cell dose in granulocyte colony-stimulating factor-mobilized peripheral blood mononuclear cell grafts affects engraftment kinetics and development of extensive chronic graft-versus-host disease after human leukocyte antigen-identical sibling transplantation. *Blood* 2001; **98**:3221–7.

30. Bensinger WI, Storer B, Clift R, Forman SJ, Negrin R, Kashyap A, et al. Transplantation of bone marrow as compared with peripheral blood cells from HLA-identical relatives in patients with hematologic cancers. *N Engl J Med* 2001; **344**:175–81.

∗31. Blade J, Samson D, Reece D, Apperley J, Bjorkstrand B, Gahrton G, et al. Criteria for evaluating disease response and progression in patients with multiple myeloma treated by high-dose therapy and haemopoietic stem cell transplantation. Myeloma Subcommittee of the EBMT. European Group for Blood and Marrow Transplant. *Br J Haematol* 1998; **102**:1115–23.

●32. Corradini P, Voena C, Tarella C, Astolfi M, Ladetto M, Palumbo A, et al. Molecular and clinical remissions in multiple myeloma: role of autologous and allogeneic transplantation of hematopoietic cells. *J Clin Oncol* 1999; **17**:208–15.

33. Cavo M, Terragna C, Martinelli G, Ronconi S, Zamagni E, Tosi P, et al. Molecular monitoring of minimal residual disease in patients in long-term complete remission after allogeneic stem cell transplantation for multiple myeloma. *Blood* 2000; **96**:355–7.

34. Martinelli G, Terragna C, Zamagni E, Ronconi S, Tosi P, Lemoli RM, et al. Molecular remission after allogeneic or autologous transplantation of hematopoietic stem cells for multiple myeloma. *J Clin Oncol* 2000; **18**:2273–81.

35. Corradini P, Lokhorst H, Martinelli G, Russel N, Majolini M, Boccadoro M, et al. Molecular remissions are frequently achieved in myeloma patients undergoing allografting with peripheral blood stem cells. *Bone Marrow Transplant* 2001; **27**(Suppl 1):S39.

36. Morris TCM, Björkstrand B, Gahrton G. Transplantation outcome in rare myelomas. *Bone Marrow Transplant* 2002; **29**(Suppl 2):S11.

37. Drake M, Hagman A, Björkstrand B, Gahrton G, Apperley J. Transplantation in plasma cell leukemia. *Bone Marrow Transplant* 2002; **29**(Suppl 2):S11.

◆38. Gahrton G, Ljungman P. Bone marrow transplantation with syngeneic or allogeneic marrow in multiple myeloma. In: Gahrton G, Durie B (eds) *Multiple myeloma.* London: Arnold, 1996:194–204.

39. Zwaan FE, Hermans J, Barrett AJ, Speck B. Bone marrow transplantation for acute nonlymphoblastic leukaemia: a survey of the European Group for Bone Marrow Transplantation (E.G.B.M.T.). *Br J Haematol* 1984; **56**:645–53.

40. Gratwohl A, Niederwieser D, van Biezen A, van Houwelingen H, Apperley J. Female donors influence transplant-related mortality and relapse incidence in male recipients of sibling blood and marrow transplants. *Hematol J* 2001; **2**:363–70.

41. Den Haan JM, Sherman NE, Blokland E, Huczko E, Koning F, Drijfhout JW, et al. Identification of a graft versus host disease-associated human minor histocompatibility antigen. Science 1995; 268:1476–80.

42. Vogt MH, de Paus RA, Voogt PJ, Willemze R, Falkenburg JH. DFFRY codes for a new human male-specific minor transplantation antigen involved in bone marrow graft rejection. Blood 2000; 95:1100–5.

●43. Storb R, Deeg HJ, Pepe M, Appelbaum F, Anasetti C, Beatty P, et al. Methotrexate and cyclosporine versus cyclosporine alone for prophylaxis of graft-versus-host disease in patients given HLA-identical marrow grafts for leukemia: long-term follow-up of a controlled trial. Blood 1989; 73:1729–34.

44. Molina A, McSweeney P, Maloney DG, Sanmaier B, Bensinger W, Nash R, et al. Non myeloablative peripheral blood stem cell (PBSC) allografts following cytoreductive autotransplants for treatment of multiple myeloma (MM). Blood 1999; 94(10, Suppl 1):347a (Abstract 1551).

45. McSweeney PA, Niederwieser D, Shizuru JA, Sandmaier BM, Molina AJ, Maloney DG, et al. Hematopoietic cell transplantation in older patients with hematologic malignancies: replacing high-dose cytotoxic therapy with graft-versus-tumor effects. Blood 2001; 97:3390–400.

46. Maloney D, Sahebi F, Stockerl-Goldstein K, Molina A, Bensinger W, McSweeney P, et al. Combining an allogeneic graft-vs-myeloma effect with high-dose autologous stem cell rescue in the treatment of multiple myeloma. Blood 2001; 98(11)(Part 1):434a.

47. Alyea E, Weller E, Schlossman R, Canning C, Webb I, Doss D, et al. T-cell-depleted allogeneic bone marrow transplantation followed by donor lymphocyte infusion in patients with multiple myeloma: induction of graft-versus-myeloma effect. Blood 2001; 98:934–9.

48. Sparrelid E, Hägglund H, Remberger M, Ringden O, Lönnqvist B, Ljungman P, et al. Bacteraemia during the aplastic phase after allogeneic bone marrow transplantation is associated with early death from invasive fungal infection. Bone Marrow Transplant 1998; 22:795–800.

49. Ljungman P. Prevention and treatment of viral infections in stem cell transplant recipients. Br J Haematol 2002; 118:44–57.

50. Wingard JR, Leather HL. Bacterial infections. In: Blume KG, Forman SJ, Appelbaum FR (eds) Thomas' hematopoietic cell transplantation, 3rd edn. Oxford: Blackwell Science, 2003;665–82.

51. Goodman JL, Winston DJ, Greenfield RA, Chandrasekar PH, Fox B, Kaizer H, et al. A controlled trial of fluconazole to prevent fungal infections in patients undergoing bone marrow transplantation. N Engl J Med 1992; 326:845–51.

52. Slavin MA, Osborne B, Adams R, Levenstein MJ, Schoch HG, Feldman AR, et al. Efficacy and safety of fluconazole prophylaxis for fungal infections after marrow transplantation – a prospective, randomized, double-blind study. J Infect Dis 1995; 171:1545–52.

53. Marr KA, Seidel K, Slavin MA, Bowden RA, Schoch HG, Flowers ME, et al. Prolonged fluconazole prophylaxis is associated with persistent protection against candidiasis-related death in allogeneic marrow transplant recipients: long-term follow-up of a randomized, placebo-controlled trial. Blood 2000; 96:2055–61.

54. Wald A, Leisenring W, van Burik JA, Bowden RA. Epidemiology of Aspergillus infections in a large cohort of patients undergoing bone marrow transplantation. J Infect Dis 1997; 175:1459–66.

55. Denning DW. Invasive aspergillosis. Clin Infect Dis 1998; 26:781–803; quiz 804–5.

56. Leenders A, Daenen S, Jansen R, Hop W, Löwenberg B, Wijermans P, et al. Liposomal amphotericin B compared with amphotericin B deoxycholate in the treatment of documented and suspected neutropenia-associated invasive fungal infections. Br J Haematol 1998; 103:205–12.

57. Tollemar J, Klingspor L, Ringden O. Liposomal amphotericin B (AmBisome) for fungal infections in immunocompromised adults and children. Clin Microbiol Infect 2001; 7(Suppl 2): 68–79.

58. Denning DW, Ribaud P, Milpied N, Caillot D, Herbrecht R, Thiel E, et al. Efficacy and safety of voriconazole in the treatment of acute invasive aspergillosis. Clin Infect Dis 2002; 34:563–71.

59. Ljungman P, Aschan J, Lewensohn-Fuchs I, Carlens S, Larsson K, Lönnqvist B, et al. Results of different strategies for reducing cytomegalovirus-associated mortality in allogeneic stem cell transplant recipients. Transplantation 1998; 66:1330–4.

60. Prentice HG, Gluckman E, Powles RL, Ljungman P, Milpied N, Fernandez Ranada JM, et al. Impact of long-term acyclovir on cytomegalovirus infection and survival after allogeneic bone marrow transplantation. European Acyclovir for CMV Prophylaxis Study Group. Lancet 1994; 343:749–53.

61. Winston DJ, Ho WG, Bartoni K, Du Mond C, Ebeling DF, Buhles WC, et al. Ganciclovir prophylaxis of cytomegalovirus infection and disease in allogeneic bone marrow transplant recipients. Results of a placebo-controlled, double-blind trial. Ann Intern Med 1993; 118:179–84.

62. Goodrich JM, Bowden RA, Fisher L, Keller C, Schoch G, Meyers JD. Ganciclovir prophylaxis to prevent cytomegalovirus disease after allogeneic marrow transplant. Ann Intern Med 1993; 118:173–8.

63. Zaia JA. Cytomegalovirus infection. In: Blume KG, Forman SJ, Appelbaum FR (eds) Thomas' hematopoietic cell transplantation, 3rd edn. Oxford: Blackwell Science, 2003;701–26.

64. Boeckh M, Gooley TA, Myerson D, Cunningham T, Schoch G, Bowden RA. Cytomegalovirus pp65 antigenemia-guided early treatment with ganciclovir versus ganciclovir at engraftment after allogeneic marrow transplantation: a randomized double-blind study. Blood 1996; 88:4063–71.

65. Boeckh M, Bowden RA, Gooley T, Myerson D, Corey L. Successful modification of a pp65 antigenemia-based early treatment strategy for prevention of cytomegalovirus disease in allogeneic marrow transplant recipients [letter]. Blood 1999; 93:1781–2.

66. Einsele H, Ehninger G, Hebart H, Wittkowski KM, Schuler U, Jahn G, et al. Polymerase chain reaction monitoring reduces the incidence of cytomegalovirus disease and the duration and side effects of antiviral therapy after bone marrow transplantation. Blood 1995; 86:2815–20.

67. Reusser P, Einsele H, Lee J, Volin L, Rovira M, Engelhard D, et al. Randomized multicenter trial of foscarnet versus ganciclovir for preemptive therapy of cytomegalovirus infection after allogeneic stem cell transplantation. Blood 2002; 99:1159–64.

68. Nguyen Q, Champlin R, Giralt S, Rolston K, Raad I, Jacobson K, et al. Late cytomegalovirus pneumonia in adult allogeneic blood and marrow transplant recipients. Clin Infect Dis 1999; 28:618–23.

69. Ljungman P, Deliliers GL, Platzbecker U, Matthes-Martin S, Bacigalupo A, Einsele H, et al. Cidofovir for cytomegalovirus infection and disease in allogeneic stem cell transplant recipients. The Infectious Diseases Working Party of the European Group for Blood and Marrow Transplantation. Blood 2001; 97:388–92.

70. Einsele H, Hebart H, Kauffmann-Schneider C, Sinzger C, Jahn G, Bader P, et al. Risk factors for treatment failures in patients receiving PCR-based preemptive therapy for CMV infection. Bone Marrow Transplant 2000; 25:757–63.

71. Crippa F, Corey L, Chuang EL, Sale G, Boeckh M. Virological, clinical, and ophthalmologic features of cytomegalovirus retinitis after hematopoietic stem cell transplantation. Clin Infect Dis 2001; 32:214–19.

72. Larsson K, Lönnqvist B, Ringdén O, Hedquist B, Ljungman P. CMV retinitis after allogeneic bone marrow transplantation: a report of five cases. Transplant Infect Dis 2002; 4:75–9.

73. Junghanss C, Boeckh M, Carter RA, Sandmaier BM, Maris MB, Maloney DG, et al. Incidence and outcome of cytomegalovirus infections following nonmyeloablative compared with myeloablative allogeneic stem cell transplantation, a matched control study. Blood 2002; 99:1978–85.

74. Keenan RD, Ainsworth J, Khan N, Bruton R, Cobbold M, Assenmacher M, et al. Purification of cytomegalovirus-specific CD8 T cells from peripheral blood using HLA-peptide tetramers. Br J Haematol 2001; 115:428–34.

75. Kleihauer A, Grigoleit U, Hebart H, Moris A, Brossart P, Muhm A, et al. Ex vivo generation of human cytomegalovirus-specific cytotoxic T cells by peptide-pulsed dendritic cells. Br J Haematol 2001; 113:231–9.

76. Krause H, Hebart H, Jahn G, Muller CA, Einsele H. Screening for CMV-specific T cell proliferation to identify patients at risk of developing late onset CMV disease. Bone Marrow Transplant 1997; 19:1111–16.

77. Szmania S, Galloway A, Bruorton M, Musk P, Aubert G, Arthur A, et al. Isolation and expansion of cytomegalovirus-specific cytotoxic T lymphocytes to clinical scale from a single blood draw using dendritic cells and HLA-tetramers. Blood 2001; 98:505–12.

78. Walter EA, Greenberg PD, Gilbert MJ, Finch RJ, Watanabe KS, Thomas ED, et al. Reconstitution of cellular immunity against cytomegalovirus in recipients of allogeneic bone marrow by transfer of T-cell clones from the donor. N Engl J Med 1995; 333:1038–44.

79. Ljungman P, Cordonnier C, de Bock R, Einsele H, Engelhard D, Grundy J, et al. Immunisations after bone marrow transplantation: results of a European survey and recommendations from the infectious diseases working party of the European Group for Blood and Marrow Transplantation. Bone Marrow Transplant 1995; 15:455–60.

*80. CDC. Guidelines for preventing opportunistic infections among hematopoietic stem cell transplant recipients. Recommendations of CDC, the Infectious Disease Society of America, and the American Society of Blood and Marrow Transplantation. MMWR Morb Mortal Wkly Rep 2000; 49(RR-10):1–125.

81. Ljungman P. Immunization of transplant recipients. Bone Marrow Transplant 1999; 23:635–6.

82. WMDA. Donor registries annual report, 4th edn. Leiden: World Marrow Donor Association (WMDA); 2000 November 5 2001. Report no. 4.

83. Bensinger WI, Maloney D, Storb R, Allogeneic hematopoietic stem cell transplantation for multiple myeloma. Semin Hematol 2001; 38:243–9.

84. Gluckman E, Rocha V, Chevret S. Results of unrelated umbilical cord blood hematopoietic stem cell transplant. Transfus Clin Biol 2001; 8:146–54.

85. Rubinstein P, Carrier C, Scaradavou A, Kurtzberg J, Adamson J, Migliaccio AR, et al. Outcomes among 562 recipients of placental-blood transplants from unrelated donors. N Engl J Med 1998; 339:1565–77.

86. Laughlin MJ, Barker J, Bambach B, Koc ON, Rizzieri DA, Wagner JE, et al. Hematopoietic engraftment and survival in adult recipients of umbilical-cord blood from unrelated donors. N Engl J Med 2001; 344:1815–22.

87. Fefer A, Cheever MA, Greenberg PD. Identical-twin (syngeneic) marrow transplantation for hematologic cancers. J Natl Cancer Inst 1986; 76:1269–73.

88. Osserman EF, DiRe LB, DiRe J, Sherman WH, Hersman JA, Storb R. Identical twin marrow transplantation in multiple myeloma. Acta Haematol 1982; 68:215–23.

89. Slavin S, Nagler A, Naparstek E, Kapelushnik Y, Aker M, Cividalli G, et al. Nonmyeloablative stem cell transplantation and cell therapy as an alternative to conventional bone marrow transplantation with lethal cytoreduction for the treatment of malignant and nonmalignant hematologic diseases. Blood 1998; 91:756–63.

◆90. Sandmaier BM, McSweeney P, Yu C, Storb R. Nonmyeloablative transplants: preclinical and clinical results. Semin Oncol 2000; 27(2 Suppl 5):78–81.

91. Kolb HJ. Donor leukocyte transfusions for treatment of leukemic relapse after bone marrow transplantation. EBMT Immunology and Chronic Leukemia Working Parties. Vox Sang 1998; 74(Suppl 2):321–9.

92. Zaucha JM, Yu C, Zellmer E, Takatu A, Junghanss C, Little MT, et al. Effects of extending the duration of postgrafting immunosuppression and substituting granulocyte-colony-stimulating factor-mobilized peripheral blood mononuclear cells for marrow in allogeneic engraftment in a nonmyeloablative canine transplantation model. Biol Blood Marrow Transplant 2001; 7:513–16.

93. Giralt S, Weber D, Aleman A, Anagnastopoulos A, Anderlini P, Braunschweig I, et al. Non Myeloablative conditioning with Fludarabine/Melphalan (FM) for patients with multiple myeloma (MM). Blood 1999; 94(10 Suppl 1):347a (Abstract 1549).

94. Lalancette M, Rezvani K, Szydlo R, Mackinnon S, Juliusson G, Michallet M, et al. Excellent outcome of non-myeloablative stem cell transplant (NMSCT) for good risk myeloma: the EBMT experience. Blood 2000; 96:204a.

◆95. Storb RF, Champlin R, Riddell SR, Murata M, Bryant S, Warren EH. Non-myeloablative transplants for malignant disease. Hematology (Am Soc Hematol Educ Program) 2001; 375–91.

96. Mehta J, Singhal S. Graft-versus-myeloma. Bone Marrow Transplant 1998; 22:835–43.

97. Garban F, Attal M, Rossi JF, Payen C, Fegueux N, Sotto JJ. Immunotherapy by non-myeloablative allogeneic stem cell transplantation in multiple myeloma: results of a pilot study as salvage therapy after autologous transplantation. *Leukemia* 2001; **15**:642–6.

98. Gahrton G, Tura S, Ljungman P, Belanger B, Brandt L, Cavo M, *et al.* Allogeneic bone marrow transplantation in multiple myeloma using HLA-compatible sibling donors – an EBMT Registry Study. *Bone Marrow Transplant* 1991; **7**(Suppl 2):32.

99. Samson D, Volin L, Schanz U, Bosi A, Gahrton G. Feasibility and toxicity of interferon maintenance therapy after allogeneic BMT for multiple myeloma: a pilot study of the EBMT. *Bone Marrow Transplant* 1996; **17**:759–62.

100. Russell NH, Miflin G, Stainer C, McQuaker JG, Bienz N, Haynes AP, *et al.* Allogeneic bone marrow transplant for multiple myeloma [letter]. *Blood* 1997; **89**:2610–1.

101. Russell N, Bessell E, Stainer C, Haynes A, Das-Gupta E, Byrne J. Allogeneic haemopoietic stem cell transplantation for multiple myeloma or plasma cell leukaemia using fractionated total body radiation and high-dose melphalan conditioning. *Acta Oncol* 2000; **39**:837–41.

●102. Singhal S, Mehta J, Desikan R, Ayers D, Roberson P, Eddlemon P, *et al.* Antitumor activity of thalidomide in refractory multiple myeloma. *N Engl J Med* 1999; **341**:1565–71.

103. Barlogie B, Desikan R, Eddlemon P, Spencer T, Zeldis J, Munshi N, *et al.* Extended survival in advanced and refractory multiple myeloma after single-agent thalidomide: identification of prognostic factors in a phase 2 study of 169 patients. *Blood* 2001; **98**:492–4.

104. Biagi JJ, Prince HM. Thalidomide is effective for extramedullary relapse of multiple myeloma post-allogeneic bone marrow transplantation. *Br J Haematol* 2001; **115**:484–5.

105. Lokhorst HM, Schattenberg A, Cornelissen JJ, Thomas LL, Verdonck LF. Donor leukocyte infusions are effective in relapsed multiple myeloma after allogeneic bone marrow transplantation. *Blood* 1997; **90**:4206–11.

106. Verdonck LF, Petersen EJ, Lokhorst HM, Nieuwenhuis HK, Dekker AW, Tilanus MG, *et al.* Donor leukocyte infusions for recurrent hematologic malignancies after allogeneic bone marrow transplantation: impact of infused and residual donor T cells. *Bone Marrow Transplant* 1998; **22**:1057–63.

107. Van der Griend R, Verdonck LF, Petersen EJ, Veenhuizen P, Bloem AC, Lokhorst HM. Donor leukocyte infusions inducing remissions repeatedly in a patient with recurrent multiple myeloma after allogeneic bone marrow transplantation. *Bone Marrow Transplant* 1999; **23**:195–7.

108. Lokhorst HM, Schattenberg A, Cornelissen JJ, van Oers MH, Fibbe W, Russell I, *et al.* Donor lymphocyte infusions for relapsed multiple myeloma after allogeneic stem-cell transplantation: predictive factors for response and long-term outcome. *J Clin Oncol* 2000; **18**:3031–7.

109. Salama M, Nevill T, Marcellus D, Parker P, Johnson M, Kirk A, *et al.* Donor leukocyte infusions for multiple myeloma. *Bone Marrow Transplant* 2000; **26**:1179–84.

●110. Attal M, Harousseau JL, Stoppa AM, Sotto JJ, Fuzibet JG, Rossi JF, *et al.* A prospective, randomized trial of autologous bone marrow transplantation and chemotherapy in multiple myeloma. Intergroupe Francais du Myelome. *N Engl J Med* 1996; **335**:91–7.

111. Björkstrand B, Bird JM, Samson D, Gahrton G. Double high-dose chemoradiotherapy with autologous stem cell transplantation can induce molecular remission in multiple myeloma. *Bone Marrow Transplant* 1995; **15**:367–71.

112. Stewart AK, Prince HM, Cappe D, Chu P, Lutzko C, Sutherland DR, *et al.* In vitro maintenance and retroviral transduction of human myeloma cells in long-term marrow cultures. *Cancer Gene Ther* 1997; **4**:148–56.

◆113. Gahrton G, Björkstrand B, Dilber MS, Sundman-Engberg B, Ljungman P, Smith CI. Gene marking and gene therapy in multiple myeloma. *Adv Exp Med Biol* 1998; **451**:493–7.

114. Tura S, Cavo M, Gobbi M, Rosti G, Bandini G, Miggiano C, *et al.* High-dose chemoradiotherapy and allogenic bone marrow transplantation in multiple myeloma. *Eur J Haematol Suppl* 1989; **51**:191–5.

115. Corradini P, Tarella C, Olivieri A, Gianni AM, Voena C, Zallio F, *et al.* Reduced-intensity conditioning followed by allografting of hematopoietic cells can produce clinical and molecular remissions in patients with poor-risk hematologic malignancies. *Blood* 2002; **99**:75–82.

116. Badros A, Barlogie B, Siegel E, Cottler-Fox M, Zangari M, Fassas A, *et al.* Improved outcome of allogeneic transplantation in high-risk multiple myeloma patients after nonmyeloablative conditioning. *J Clin Oncol* 2002; **20**:1295–303.

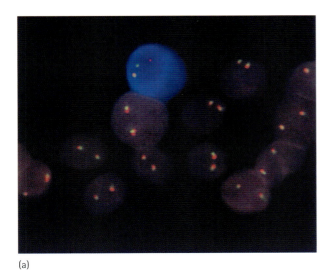

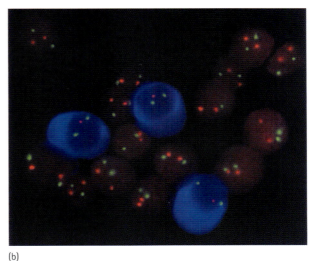

(a)

(b)

Plate 1 *Interphase fluorescence* in situ *hybridization of myelomatous plasma cells. (a) Detection of a translocation involving the* IgH *locus at 14q32. Two probes flanking the breakpoints are used; thus, presence of a red/green fusion signal indicates a normal pattern, whereas separation of the red and green signals indicates presence of a translocation. The plasma cell is identified after staining for cytoplasmic immunoglobulin light-chain expression and shows evidence for a* IgH *translocation, whereas a normal pattern of 14q32 is observed in the surrounding bone marrow cells. (b) Detection of a deletion of 13q14. The red signals are derived from a retinoblastoma-1 (rb-1) gene specific probe (13q14) and green signals represent a reference probe hybridizing to the centromeric region of chromosome 11. Note loss of a* rb-1 *signal in all plasma cells.*

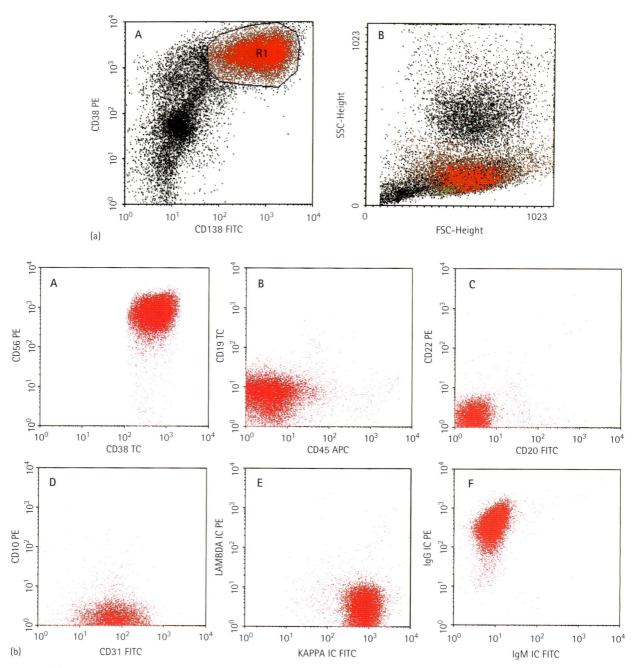

Plate 2 *(a) Typical co-expression of CD38 at high fluorescence intensity and CD138 in multiple myeloma plasma cells (red, A) and their physical distribution compared with lymphocytes (green, B) in a bone marrow sample. (b) Immunophenotype of multiple myeloma plasma cells. Usually CD56 is expressed at high density (A); CD19 CD45 (B), CD20 and CD22 (C) are negative; CD31 is expressed on the majority of cases; CD10, usually negative on myeloma, can be positive on plasma cell leukemias (D); monoclonal immunoglobulin light and heavy chains are detectable in the cytoplasm (E and F).*

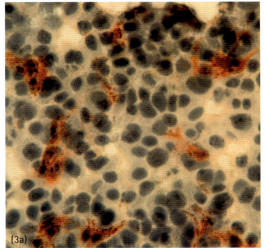

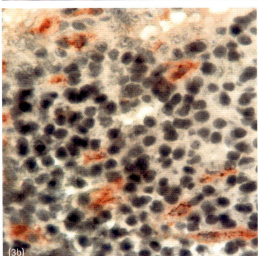

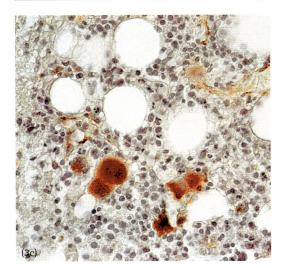

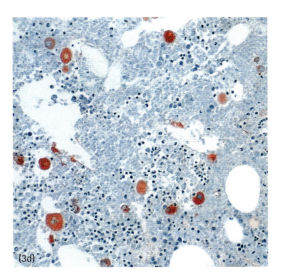

Plate 3 *Neo-angiogenesis is markedly prominent in the bone marrow (BM) of patients with progressive myeloma (a) as compared with the BM of patients who undergo disease remission (b) and patients with monoclonal gammopathy of undetermined significance (MGUS) (c). Anti-factor VIII immunostaining (d) (megakaryocyte positivity provides the internal positive control). (Courtesy of Professor A. Vacca, University of Bari, Italy.)*

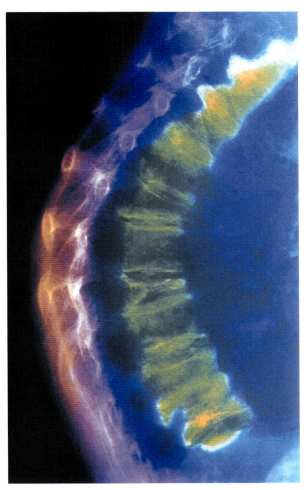

Plate 4 *Standard X-rays of (a) skull, showing lytic lesions, and (b) spine, showing osteoporosis and vertebral collapse.*

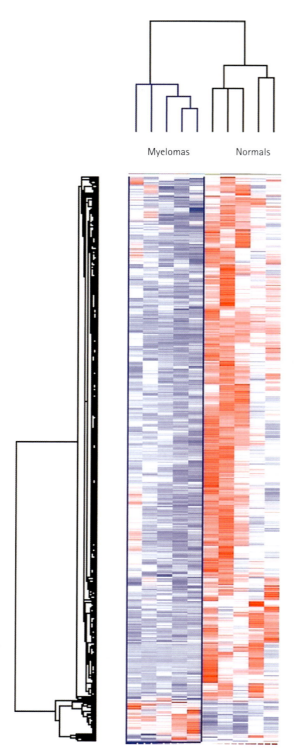

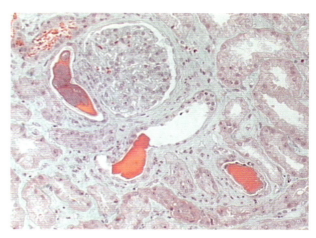

Plate 6 *Myeloma kidney (cast nephropathy). Typical intratubular lesions consisting of large, dense, proteinaceous casts composed of immunoglobulin light chains (Masson's Trichrome, × 100).*

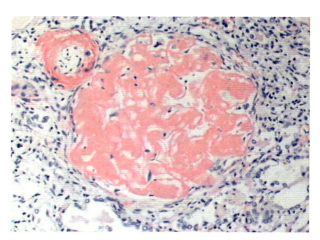

Plate 7 *Extensive glomerular involvement by amyloid deposition (Congo red, × 200).*

Plate 5 *Hierarchical clustering of normal and myeloma samples. Samples are initially clustered on the horizontal axis with the samples being most similar next to each other. In a similar fashion, genes are clustered on the vertical axis. A dendrogram is generated and drawn on each axis, and represents the similarities and differences between samples/genes and splits the samples into different subgroups. Traditionally, red squares represent an upregulated gene and blue squares represent a downregulated gene. In this example, normal and myeloma samples clearly have a different gene expression pattern.*

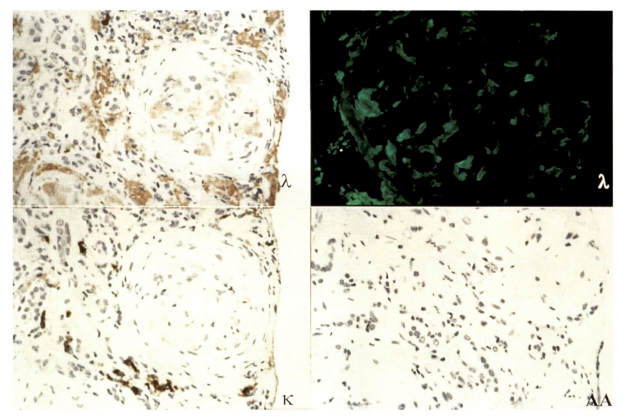

Plate 8 *Characterization of amyloid deposits in a patient with nephrotic syndrome and primary amyloidosis. λ light-chain positivity by immunohistochemical and immunofluorescence studies, and negativity for κ light chain and amyloid A (original × 200).*

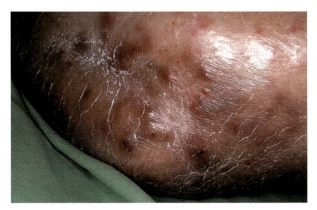

Plate 9 *Diffuse skin infiltrates from plasma cells.*

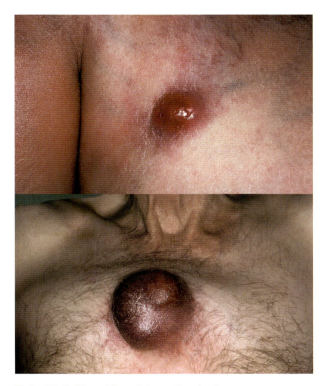

Plate 10 *Solitary skin nodules on the chest.*

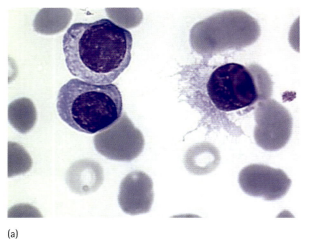

(a)

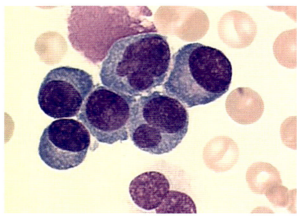

(b)

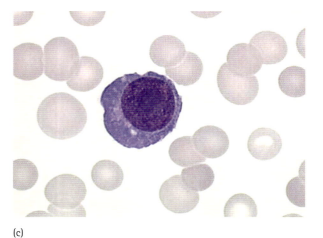

(c)

Plate 11 *Plasma cell leukemia (PCL): peripheral blood findings. (a) Plasma cells from a IgA κ primary PCL demonstrating coarse nuclear chromatin and moderately abundant cytoplasm. (b) Some cells from IgG λ secondary PCL sustain classical morphology, whereas others demonstrate irregular nuclear shape. (c) This plasma cell (secondary IgA λ PCL) shows dispersed chromatin and prominent nucleolus.*

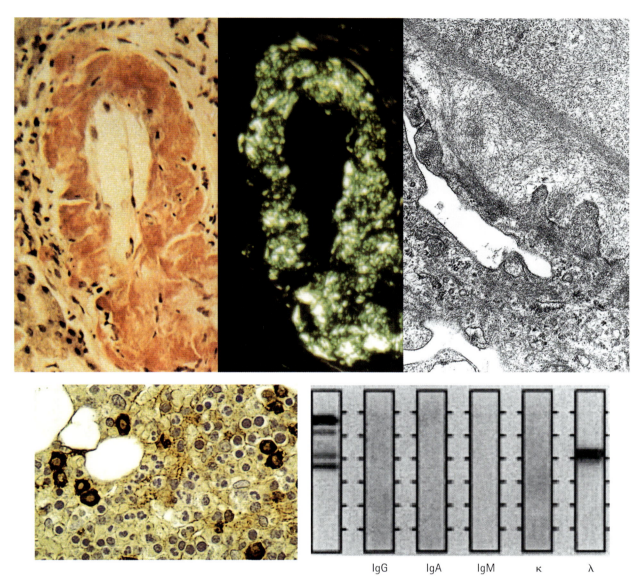

| IgG | IgA | IgM | κ | λ |

Plate 12 *Top: images of a Congo red-stained section of liver tissue in non-polarized light (left), the same tissue viewed in polarized light showing apple-green refringence (center) and an electron microscopy view of amyloid fibrils. Bottom: a section of bone marrow biopsy showing immunostained λ -restricted plasma cells (left, brown cells) and a urine immunofixation showing free monoclonal λ light chains (right). These findings are typical images of AL amyloidosis.*

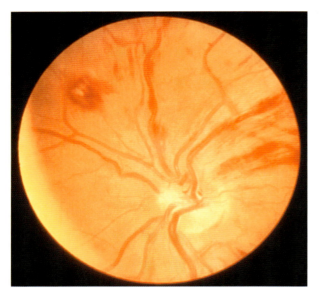

Plate 13 *The circulatory disturbances caused by blood hyperviscosity are best appreciated by ophthalmoscopy, which shows distended and tortuous retinal veins, hemorrhages, and papilledema.*

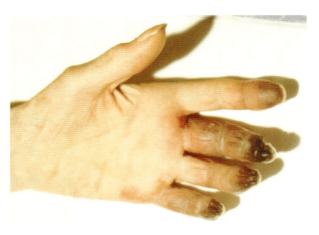

Plate 14 *Necrosis of the tips of the fingers in a patient with Waldenström's macroglobulinemia and type I cryoglobulinemia.*

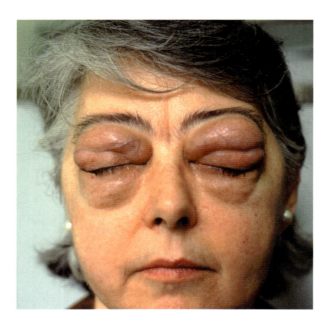

Plate 15 *Involvement of the periorbital structures by neoplastic cells in a patient with Waldenström's macroglobulinemia.*

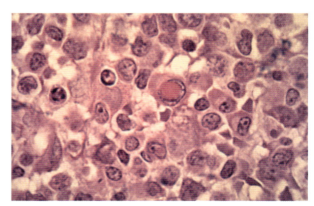

Plate 16 *Lymphoplasmacytic population with abundant plasma cell component and presence of a Dutcher–Fahey body in a lymph node. (Courtesy of Professor Umberto Magrini, Department of Human Pathology, University of Pavia, Italy.)*

18

Supportive care

HEINZ LUDWIG AND JOHANNES DRACH

INTRODUCTION

Patients with multiple myeloma often suffer from complications that stem from characteristic features of the disease, such as bone destruction, renal failure, and immunological impairment. Therefore, in addition to chemotherapy of the underlying plasma cell dyscrasia, prophylaxis and supportive treatment of bone destruction, pain, anemia, fatigue, infections, hypercalcemia, and emotional distress are an essential part of the therapeutic management of myeloma patients. Even in progressive disease, adequate supportive care can considerably improve the patient's quality of life.

BONE DESTRUCTION

Skeletal involvement is a characteristic feature of multiple myeloma. At diagnosis, almost all patients present with osteoporosis in the vertebral spine: 70% show osteolytic lesions and 30% have fractures. Initially, some patients show both increased bone degradation and elevated osteogenesis but, as the disease progresses, bone degradation by far outweighs bone formation.[1]

Mechanisms of bone disease

In myeloma, as discussed in Chapter 6, several cytokines contribute to the increased formation, differentiation, and stimulation of osteoclasts. These cytokines are mainly secreted by bone marrow stroma cells and often are induced by direct myeloma–stroma cell contact. Interleukin-1b (IL-1b), tumor necrosis factor α (TNFα), TNFβ, IL-6, macrophage colony-stimulating factor (M-CSF), vascular endothelial growth factor (VEGF), and other cellular growth hormones have all been implicated as major osteoclast activators.[2,3] Recently, a probably more important mechanism of osteoclast stimulation has been discovered: receptor activator of nuclear factor-kappa B ligand (RANKL),[4] which is produced by bone marrow stromal cells. This induces differentiation of osteoclast progenitors and activates mature osteoclasts by binding to its receptors (RANK) on the respective cell types. In normal homeostasis, RANKL and its natural decoy receptor osteoprotegerin (OPG) are carefully balanced. In myeloma, an imbalance between OPG and RANKL is frequently observed (see Chapter 6), with impaired OPG production and part of the available OPG binding to syndecan-1 (CD138), which results in an excess of RANKL. Macrophage inflammatory protein-1α (MIP-1α) is another inflammatory cytokine that has recently been shown to enhance RANKL- and IL-6-induced osteoclast formation.[5] Restoring the balance between RANKL and OPG not only stops myeloma-induced bone resorption[6,7] but also inhibits growth and survival of myeloma cells. The latter effect occurs only when the disease process is restricted to the bone marrow, whereas extramedullary myeloma cell clones seem to have a different growth pattern.[8] The clinical symptoms of excessive bone resorption are bone pain, hypercalcemia, and fractures. Compression fractures of the vertebrae may lead to neurological symptoms from spinal cord compression.

Table 18.1 *Recommended regimens for long-term bisphosphonate therapy in myeloma*

	Substance		
	Pamidronate	**Zoledronic acid**	**Clodronate**
Dose (mg)	90	4	1600
Administration	90-minute infusion	15-minute infusion	Oral
Treatment interval	Monthly	Monthly	Daily
Treatment duration	Indefinitely, even in patients with progressive bone disease		

Bisphosphonates

Symptomatic myeloma-associated bone resorption should be treated with: (1) effective myeloma therapy; (2) local radiotherapy, if appropriate; and (3) the administration of bisphosphonates. Bisphosphonates are derived from pyrophosphates by substitution of an oxygen atom with a carbon atom, and modifying one or both lateral chains of the molecule. Bisphosphonates inhibit the recruitment of osteoclasts from their precursor cells and suppress their subsequent cellular proliferation and differentiation. They also bind to bone surfaces, thus protecting them from destruction,[9] inhibit the production of IL-6, the most important growth hormone for myeloma cells, and stimulate apoptosis of osteoclasts and myeloma cells.[10–13] The efficacy of the bisphosphonates clodronate and pamidronate in preventing bone lesions has been investigated in several randomized trials, as discussed in detail in Chapter 21. A multicenter Finnish study, in which 2.4 g clodronate was used daily for 2 years, reported a 50% reduction in the progression of osteolytic lesions, an increase in the proportion of patients feeling no pain, and greater decreases in serum and urinary calcium in the clodronate arm as compared with placebo-treated controls.[14] A German trial reported significant reductions of bone pain and a trend towards decreased progression of bone lesions.[15] The most extensive trial of clodronate was carried out by the Medical Research Council.[16] This involved 536 patients who were randomized to receive orally, in addition to chemotherapy, either 1600 mg clodronate daily or placebo. Treatment with clodronate was associated with a 50% reduction in non-vertebral fractures and a 50% decrease in the proportion of patients with severe hypercalcemia. In the clodronate arm, significantly fewer patients experienced vertebral fractures and back pain; performance status after 24 months was better and loss of body height during 3 years was significantly less as compared with patients in the placebo arm. Even patients without overt skeletal disease at enrolment benefited from clodronate. However, survival time was comparable in the two treatment arms.[16]

A Danish–Swedish, multicenter, randomized trial of oral pamidronate (300 mg/day) versus placebo showed significant reductions in bone pain and loss of body height in the treatment arm, but found no significant differences regarding hypercalcemia, pathologic fractures, or progression of osteolytic lesions.[17]

The parenteral application of pamidronate (90 mg, as intravenous 4-hour infusion, monthly for 21 months) resulted in significant reductions in bone pain, episodes of hypercalcemia, and skeletal complications.[18] In patients starting pamidronate treatment during second-line or subsequent chemotherapy regimens, a prolongation of survival was also observed.[19] Parenteral pamidronate treatment proved to be safe and was tolerated well.[18,19] In a dose-escalation study evaluating tolerability and effectiveness of repeated pamidronate infusions, a close correlation was found between dose intensity and treatment effects. Dose intensities of 25–45 mg/week resulted in a significant palliative effect, whereas the best results were obtained with high doses of 60 or 90 mg pamidronate per week.[20] The currently recommended dose of pamidronate is 90 mg monthly, given as an infusion over at least 90 minutes (Table 18.1).

Newer, more potent substances, such as zoledronic acid,[21] ibandronate,[22] and incadronate,[12] might further improve treatment outcomes and/or convenience of administration. Zoledronic acid, given as 5-minute infusions at doses of 2 or 4 mg, was reported to be as effective as 2-hour infusions of 90 mg pamidronate.[21] Because higher doses of zoledronic acid (e.g. 8 mg) were occasionally associated with renal impairment, the recommended dose is 4 mg, administered by a 15-minute infusion, at monthly intervals. Caution is required when zoledronic acid is combined with thalidomide, because this combination possibly impairs renal function. In contrast to the bisphosphonates listed above, monthly treatment with ibandronate (2 mg intravenously) failed to render any benefits so far,[21] probably due to inadequate dosages. Table 18.2 shows a synopsis of the main randomized, placebo-controlled trials on bisphosphonate treatment in myeloma patients.[14–19,21,24–28]

Risedronate, which is also a new bisphosphonate, was used orally in 11 myeloma patients at a daily dose of 30 mg for 6 months, with monitoring of these patients for an additional 6 months. Serum calcium levels decreased from day 4 onwards. At the end of the treatment period, pyridinoline and deoxypyridinoline, established markers of bone resorption, had decreased to 50% of their initial values. In addition, significant reductions were observed

Table 18.2 *Main placebo-controlled clinical trials on bisphosphonates*

Study	Number of patients	Patient population	Dose and regimen	Treatment duration	Benefits	No influence on
Clodronate						
Lathinen (1992)[14]	350	Multiple myeloma	2.4 g, orally, daily	24 months	Sig. ↓ progression of bone lesions, ↓ progression of vertebral fractures, sig. ↑ painless, ↓ hypercalcemia	Nothing reported
Clemens (1993)[23]	26	Multiple myeloma or metastatic bone disease	1600 mg, orally, daily	At least 1 year	Sig. ↓ lytic bone lesions, ↓ hypercalcemia, ↓ vertebral fractures	Nothing reported
Heim (1995)[15]					Sig. ↓ bone pain, ↓ progression of bone lesions	
McCloskey (1998)[16]	536	Multiple myeloma	1600 mg, orally, daily		Sig. ↓ vertebral fractures, sig. ↓ height loss, sig. ↓ back pain, sig. ↓ poor PS, ↓ hypercalcemia	Survival
McCloskey (2001)[24]	535	Multiple myeloma	1600 mg, orally, daily	8.6 years (median)	Previously reported	Survival
Pamidronate						
Harvey (1996)[25]	377	Multiple myeloma	90 mg, IV, every 4 weeks		Sig. ↓ bone pain, sig. ↓ incidence and time to skeleton-related events	Nothing reported
Berenson (1996)[18]	392	Stage III myeloma with ≥1 lytic lesion	90 mg, 4-hour infusion, every 4 weeks	9 cycles	Sig. ↓ skeletal events, sig. ↓ bone pain no deterioration in PS and QoL pain, no deterioration in PS and QoL	Nothing reported
Berenson (1998)[19]	392	Stage III myeloma with ≥1 lytic lesion	90 mg, 4-hour infusion, every 4 weeks	21 cycles	Sig. ↓ skeletal events, sig. ↑ survival on second-line therapy	Survival in patients on first-line therapy
Brincker (1998)[17]	300	Multiple myeloma requiring chemotherapy	300 mg, orally, daily	550 days (mean)	Sig. ↓ severe pain, sig. ↓ reduction of body height	Skeletal-related morbidity, frequency of hypercalcemia, survival
Kraj (2000)[26]	46	Stage III myeloma with osteolytic lesions	60 mg, IV, 4-hour infusion, monthly	1 year	Sig. ↓ skeletal events, ↓ progression of osteolysis	Nothing reported
Ibandronate						
Menssen (2002)[27]	198	Stage II or III myeloma	2 mg, IV, monthly	12–24 months	None	Number of skeletal-related events, bone pain, analgesic drug use, QoL, survival
Zoledronic acid vs. pamidronate						
Berenson (2001)[21]	280	Multiple myeloma or metastatic breast cancer	Zoledronic acid 0.4, 2.0, or 4.0 mg, 5-minute infusion; pamidronate 90 mg, 2-hour infusion		2.0 or 4.0 mg zoledronic acid or pamidronate: sig. ↓ need for radiation therapy to bone, ↓ skeletal-related events, ↓ hypercalcemia	No benefits from 0.4 mg zoledronic acid
Meta-analysis						
Djulbegovic (2001)[28]	2183 (11 trials)	Multiple myeloma			Sig. prevention of pathological vertebral fractures, sig. amelioration of pain	Mortality, reduction of non-vertebral fractures, incidence of hypercalcemia

IV, intravenously; PS, performance status; QoL, quality of life; Sig, significant; ↓, decrease in; ↑, increase in.

in the number of osteoclasts, their activation frequencies, and their erosion depths.[29]

Apart from the gastrointestinal adverse effects caused by some oral preparations, tolerance of intravenous bisphosphonates is usually good. Shortly after their infusion, amino-bisphosphonates may induce an inflammatory reaction, which usually persists no longer than 24 hours and only seldom requires symptomatic treatment with non-steroidal anti-inflammatory drugs. The most likely cause of this reaction is stimulation of inflammatory cytokines. In addition, a transient reduction of IL-6 levels may be seen as a result of infusion therapy. Tolerance of oral treatment is limited by the gastrointestinal adverse effects of bisphosphonates, with nausea, emesis, and diarrhea being the most frequent symptoms. Because intestinal resorption of oral bisphosphonates is poor (only approximately 3%), patients are required to fast for at least 1 hour prior to and after ingesting the medication.

Bisphosphonates have been used prophylactically to prevent or delay the progression of monoclonal gammopathy of undetermined significance (MGUS) or asymptomatic early-stage myeloma. Even though only few data are available on this issue in humans, ibandronate has been shown to have some effect on the development of bone lesions in a murine myeloma model.[30] Experimental data strongly suggest an inhibitory influence of bisphosphonates on myeloma-promoting cytokines,[10,11] as well as direct cytotoxic effects, particularly of third-generation bisphosphonates.[13,21,31] An *in vitro* study of ibandronate-induced apoptosis of human myeloma cells confirmed that inhibition of the mevalonate pathway played a role in the observed antitumor effect.[12]

In conclusion, treatment with bisphosphonates is presently recommended in myeloma patients, in order to reduce the progression of osteolytic lesions and, thereby, reduce bone pain, fractures, and the need for palliative pain treatment. Pamidronate at a dose of 90 mg, given over at least 90 minutes, or 4 mg zoledronic acid, given as a 15-minute infusion, are presently the most commonly used regimes, but oral clodronate, 1600 mg, taken orally once daily, is an effective alternative to infusion therapies. The definite duration of bisphosphonate therapy has not been addressed in clinical trials but it is currently recommended to continue treatment indefinitely, even when progression of bone disease is evident, with the hope of reducing the rate of progression, and thus reducing bone pain and the risk of hypercalcemia.

PAIN

Characteristics and causes of pain

Many myeloma patients suffer from moderate to severe pain in the skeleton, particularly in the lumbar spine.

Table 18.3 *Main causes of pain in multiple myeloma*

Bone pain
  Pathological fractures
  Microfractures
  Bone lesions
  Irritation of sensory nerves in the bone marrow
Neurological damage
  Nerve root and spinal cord compression
  Post-herpetic neuralgia
Lesions in skin and mucosal tissue
  Herpes virus infections
  Mucosal ulceration

This type of pain is not only frequently the predominant symptom of myeloma at diagnosis but also a common indicator of relapse or progressive disease. Microfractures and pathological fractures of vertebral bodies, ribs, pelvis, or long bones cause severe pain, which is characterized by its sudden onset. In addition, pain results from irritation of sensory nerves in the bone marrow by inflammatory cytokines and prostaglandins.

Other important causes of pain in myeloma are nerve root and spinal cord compression caused by extraosseous extension of myeloma deposits or by compression fractures. These neurological impairments require rapid diagnosis and treatment, in order to prevent possible monoplegia or paraplegia. Post-herpetic neuralgia, active herpetic virus infections, and mucosal ulcerations, common complications of high-dose chemotherapy, also cause considerable pain. A synopsis of the main causes of pain in myeloma patients is shown in Table 18.3.

Even though myeloma-associated pain usually subsides during effective chemotherapy and/or local irradiation, specific treatment for pain relief is required in most patients, particularly in those who respond poorly to myeloma treatment. It is noteworthy that the degree of pain, a subjective experience, is often estimated differently by patients, doctors, and nurses,[32] resulting in inadequate analgesia.[33] In order to maintain a satisfactory quality of life, the causes of pain should be carefully assessed and analgesia needs to be sufficient.

Medical pain treatment

In almost all myeloma patients, effective analgesia can be achieved by regular administration of oral medication. A three-step treatment plan, the so-called 'World Health Organization (WHO) pain treatment ladder' (Fig. 18.1)[35] has been widely accepted for the treatment of tumor-related pain. The first step, non-opioid drugs, may suffice even in patients suffering from severe pain. In case of persisting or increasing pain, treatment should readily be escalated according to the second step, which covers weak opioid drugs. Strong opioids and specific adjuvant

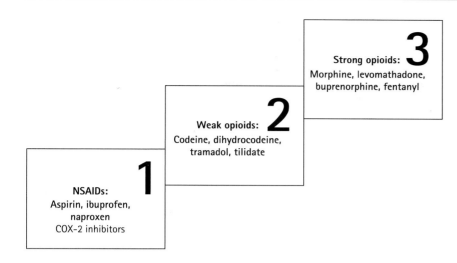

Figure 18.1 *World Health Organization (WHO) pain treatment ladder. A three-step treatment plan, which starts with non-opioid drugs and, if necessary, proceeds first to weak and, finally, to strong opioids, has been recommended by the WHO for the treatment of cancer-related pain. NSAIDs, non-steroidal anti-inflammatory drugs; COX-2, cyclo-oxygenase 2.*

analgesic drugs, the third step, are necessary if pain is still persisting or increasing.

Non-steroidal anti-inflammatory drugs (NSAIDs) have analgesic as well as anti-inflammatory effects and may, in addition, retard prostaglandin-induced bone resorption. NSAIDs are useful in myeloma but should be used with caution in patients with renal impairment. However, common NSAIDs are being widely replaced or supplemented by the more recently developed cyclo-oxygenase 2 (COX-2) inhibitors, which have milder adverse effects, particularly less gastrointestinal and possibly less renal toxicity.[35] Because the analgesic effects of the first-step drugs are limited and dose escalations beyond a certain level do not result in enhanced analgesia, insufficient pain control at the first step of the WHO pain treatment ladder requires the addition or sole application of weak opioids as soon as possible.

Typical opioids recommended by the WHO for the second step of pain treatment are codeine, dihydrocodeine, tramadol, and tilidine. These weak opioids exert their analgesic effect by binding to microreceptors on brain cells. Both affinity to these receptors and activation of the intrinsic receptor activity are important characteristics of opioids but only the latter is responsible for the analgesic effect. Substances with a high potential for triggering intrinsic activity (morphine and pethidine) are agonists, whereas substances with high receptor affinity but lack of triggering intrinsic activity (naloxone and naltrexone) are antagonists. Agonists/antagonists (buprenorphine and pentazocine) both trigger relatively high intrinsic activity and have receptor affinity, thus potentially competing with agonists for receptor binding site. Therefore, agonist and agonist/antagonist opioids must not be mixed or alternated. In several European countries, buprenorhine is also available as a patch, which may be particularly helpful in patients who have difficulty in swallowing medication.

Typical opioids for the third step of pain treatment are morphine, levomethadone, and buprenorphine, as well as transdermal fentanyl, which has the advantages of

Table 18.4 *Recommended doses and intervals of opioid analgesics*

	Dose	Treatment interval (hours)
Oral application		
Codeine	180–200 mg	3–4
Hydrocodone	30 mg	3–4
Morphine	10–30 mg	3–4
Buprenorphine	0.2 mg	6–8
Morphine, controlled release	90–120 mg	6–12
Levomethadone	2.5–5 mg	6–12
Transdermal application		
Fentanyl patch	25–100 μg/hour	72
Buprenorphine patch	35–70 μg/hour	72

long-term activity and better tolerance, particularly less gastrointestinal toxicity, but is more expensive. Buprenorphine is more potent than morphine but, when administered orally, it is subject to the first-pass effect of the liver. Its bioavailability is, therefore, low, unless it is administered sublingually or systemically. The latter application mode is facilitated by the recent introduction of a transdermal buprenorhine patch.

A strict classification of opioids into second- and third-step drugs is not always possible. Dosage plays an important role, and opioids vary widely in the duration of their analgesic effect and partly also in their adverse effects. Table 18.4 lists recommended doses and treatment intervals for various opioids.

The adverse effects of opioids can frequently be well controlled by supportive measures[36] but, in some patients, they can become problematic. At the start of treatment, nausea and emesis may prevail, requiring antiemetics, and dryness of mouth is a common complaint. Impairment of vigilance and temporary confusion may require transient dose reduction. Initial nausea and sedation often subside or lessen during the course of treatment. Impairment of visceral motor function may manifest as inadequate colonic motility or bladder distension. As prophylaxis against constipation, a fiber-rich diet and adequate hydration should be recommended; treatment with laxatives may be necessary. In addition, patients should be aware of the fact that urinary retention, caused by opioid-induced bladder atony, is a possible complication of pain treatment with opioids. Respiratory depression, another possible adverse effect of opioids, however, occurs only rarely during pain treatment.

Sufficient dosing and adequate scheduling of pain treatment are essential in order to ascertain sufficient and continuous pain control, rather than dosing on demand. Combinations of opioids and NSAIDs may increase the efficacy of pain control and curb toxicities. Additional benefits may be achieved by adding glucocorticosteroids, antidepressants, or neuroleptics to pain treatment according to the WHO pain treatment ladder. In some patients, however, pain cannot be sufficiently controlled by these conventional forms of pain therapy. In these cases, sufficient pain control is often achieved by continuous intravenous infusion of morphines with portable pump systems or intrathecal application of morphines with or without potentiating drugs, such as calcium antagonists.

ANEMIA

Pathogenesis of anemia

Anemia is a common complication of myeloma and its treatment. Twenty percent to 60% of patients already have mild or moderate anemia at the time of diagnosis, and almost all patients with uncontrolled long-standing disease become anemic. Myeloma-associated anemia is induced by one or several of a variety of factors, namely erythropoietin deficiency,[37] which occurs in practically all patients with impaired kidney function and in about 25% of patients with normal creatinine levels,[38] decreased responsiveness of the erythron to proliferative signals of erythropoietin, insufficient numbers of erythroid precursor cells, a direct proapoptotic effect on erythroid precursor cells by FAS-ligand- and/or TRAIL-positive myeloma cells, a shortened life span of red blood cells, impaired iron utilization, and paraprotein-induced expansion of the plasma volume leading to dilutional anemia. In addition, myeloma therapy, chemotherapy, and radiotherapy may cause anemia or aggravate an already existing anemic state.

The blunted erythropoietin response to the anemic condition seen in the majority of anemic myeloma patients is mediated by inflammatory cytokines (IL-1, TNFα, and interferon-γ) that suppress both erythropoietin synthesis[39] and proliferation of erythroid precursor cells.[40,41] Another contributing factor to blunted erythropoietin response is increased plasma viscosity caused by high

paraprotein levels.[42] Functional iron deficiency is a result of inadequate iron release from macrophages, even when iron stores are normal or overloaded. Activated macrophages also remove slightly damaged red blood cells from circulation, thus shortening their life span.

Clinical symptoms of anemia

Anemic myeloma patients may present with various symptoms. Almost all of them suffer from fatigue,[43] which is often associated with depression, emotional disturbance, or impaired cognitive function. The peripheral hypoxia of moderate to severe anemia induces vasodilation, which may lead to compensatory tachycardia, left ventricular hypertrophy, and, in cases with severe anemia, congestive heart failure and pulmonary edema (Table 18.5). As myeloma patients are typically elderly and often have other morbid conditions, the symptoms of anemia may be pronounced, even at relatively high hemoglobin levels. It is evident that symptomatic anemia diminishes the patient's quality of life, but even asymptomatic anemia is a negative prognostic factor and possibly reduces the efficacy of myeloma therapy.[44]

Treatment of anemia

Anemia in myeloma patients should be adequately treated. It has been clearly demonstrated that treatment of mild to moderate anemia significantly improves the patient's quality of life (Fig. 18.2).[45,46] Blood transfusion may be used as needed but the benefit is transient. A number of clinical studies have shown that treatment with recombinant human erythropoietin (rhEPO)[47] improves or normalizes myeloma-associated anemia in the majority of patients. A pilot study,[48] published in 1990, reported increases of hemoglobin levels by at least 2 g/dL in 85% of myeloma patients who had received

Table 18.5 *Symptoms of anemia in multiple myeloma*

Cardiovascular system	Reduced physical capacity Dyspnea Pulmonary edema Tachycardia Left ventricular hypertrophy Congestive heart failure
Central nervous system	Fatigue Depression Emotional disturbance Impairment of cognitive function
Immune system	Impaired immune reactions
Skin	Pallor Low temperature
Sexual function	Menstrual disturbances Decreased libido Impotence

150–300 units/kg rhEPO. The symptoms of anemia subsided and no adverse effects occurred. These results were confirmed in a series of subsequent phase II trials, in which response rates between 71% and 78% were observed.[49–51] However, poor-prognosis myeloma patients who were refractory to chemotherapy showed a lower response rate (35%).[52] Several prospective, randomized trials comparing the results of rhEPO treatment with those of an untreated control group confirmed the highly significant beneficial effects of rhEPO treatment, with typical response rates of 60% vs. 0%[53] or 75% vs. 21%[54] in myeloma patients and controls, respectively. Two trials that also included patients with non-Hodgkin's lymphoma (NHL) reported respective response rates of 60% vs. 24%[55] and 62% vs. 7%.[56] In both trials, superior results were observed in myeloma patients as compared with patients with NHL. A recent randomized, placebo-controlled trial confirmed that, regardless of the patients' transfusion history, transfusion requirements were significantly reduced in the rhEPO arm.[44] The best response to erythropoietin treatment is achieved by patients with absolute or relative deficiencies in endogenous erythropoietin (O/P, i.e. ratio of observed by expected hemoglobin level, <0.9).[56] Table 18.6 lists the major placebo-controlled clinical trials on rhEPO in myeloma patients.[44,53–59]

A dose-escalation study[56] identified as optimal initial rhEPO dose 5000 units/day seven times/week, which is approximately equivalent to 150 units/kg three times a week. Thus, it is recommended to start erythropoietin treatment in patients with hemoglobin levels below 12 g/dL or with symptomatic anemia at a dose of 10 000 units subcutaneously three times a week, or at a dose of 40 000 U subcutaneously once a week.[60] Hemoglobin values should be monitored weekly and, if necessary, the dosage should be tapered, in order to prevent overshooting of hemoglobin levels. In patients who fail to respond within 6 weeks, the initial dose may be doubled. Additional benefits can be expected from iron supplementation during the phases of high iron demands from enhanced erythropoiesis. In patients with renal anemia, intravenous iron supplementation reduced the required weekly rhEPO dose by 30–70%.[61] Parenteral iron should be administered in cancer patients with overt iron deficiency, as indicated by low transferrin saturation (<20%) and/or high numbers (>10%) of hypochromic red cells. Dosing of parenteral iron will depend on the patient's hemoglobin, serum ferritin, and transferrin saturation levels. Oral iron treatment is often beneficial during the early phase of erythropoietin therapy but scientific data substantiating this recommendation are still missing.

Adverse effects of erythropoietin treatment are negligible. They are usually limited to slight pain or mild erythema at the injection site, which occurs in about 15% of treated patients. Patients who respond to rhEPO therapy are able to benefit from this treatment for long periods of time. Transient loss of responsiveness to erythropoietin treatment has to be expected during episodes of severe complications of multiple myeloma, such as intermittent infections, or after surgery. Progression of myeloma is usually mirrored by rhEPO unresponsiveness, which lasts until the disease can be controlled again.

A more recent development in the treatment of cancer-associated anemia is the so-called 'novel erythropoiesis

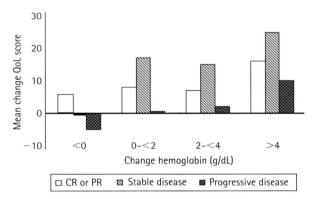

Figure 18.2 *Quality of life (QoL) score increases with increasing hemoglobin (Hb) level. Comparisons of changes in QoL scores with various degrees of gains in Hb level, stratified according to response to chemotherapy. If Hb increases substantially, QoL improves even in patients with progressive disease. (Adapted from Demetri et al.[45])*

Table 18.6 *Main placebo-controlled clinical trials on erythropoietin*

Study	Number of patients	Erythropoietin dose	Regimen	Response criterion	Response rate
Silvestris (1995)[57]	54	150–300 U/kg	s.c., TIW	Hemoglobin increase	78%
Garton (1995)[53]	25	150–300 U/kg	s.c., TIW	+ ≥ 6% hematocrit	60% vs. 0%
Cazzola (1995)[56]	84	1000–10 000 U	s.c., daily	+ ≥ 2 g/dL hemoglobin	62% vs. 7%
Österborg (1996)[55]	121 MM or NHL	10 000 U or 2000 U, escalated	s.c., daily	+ ≥ 2 g/dL hemoglobin	60% vs. 24%
Dammacco (1998)[54]	71	150–300 U/kg	s.c., TIW	Hemoglobin increase	75% vs. 21%
Dammacco (2001)[44]	145	150–300 U/kg	s.c., TIW	Transfusion incidence	28% vs. 47%
Österborg (2002)[58]	117	150–300 U/kg	s.c., TIW	+ ≥ 2 g/dL hemoglobin	67% vs. 27%
Hedenus (2002)[59]	88	Darbepoetin 1.0, 2.25, 4.5 μg/kg	s.c., weekly	+ ≥ 2 g/dL hemoglobin	45/55/62% vs. 10%

s.c., subcutaneous; TIW, three times per week.

stimulating protein' (NESP or darbepoetin). This stimulates erythropoiesis by the same mechanisms as rhEPO, but has a two- to three-fold longer serum half-life. Therefore, it is likely that darbepoetin can be administered at less frequent intervals. Darbepoetin has already been shown to be efficient and safe in cancer patients on chemotherapy[62] and also in anemic patients with multiple myeloma or other lymphoproliferative malignancies.[59]

The financial costs of erythropoietin treatment can be reduced by selecting patients who are most likely to respond, namely those who show low endogenous erythropoietin levels and lack concomitant complications, such as infections, surgery, or rapidly progressive disease. In addition to these basic principles, more sophisticated models for predictions of response to rhEPO treatment have been developed. These prediction models are based either on an observed blunted EPO response[56] or on objective indications of therapeutic benefits during the early treatment phase.[63] The most precise prediction models combine these two criteria, evaluating baseline erythropoietin levels and the serum concentration of soluble transferrin receptor,[64] blunted erythropoietin response, and changes in hemoglobin levels,[65] or baseline erythropoietin levels and changes in hemoglobin levels.[66] In principle, these models propose to select patients with inadequate endogeneous erythropoietin levels and to monitor indications of early response to rhEPO treatment. If hemoglobin levels fail to increase within 2 weeks, the initial erythropoietin dose of 30 000–40 000 U/week (which may be administered as 10 000 U three times per week or as 30 000–40 000 U once weekly) or of 2.25 μg/kg darbepoetin per week should be increased by 50–100%. Treatment should be discontinued if this dose elevation fails to induce a rapid therapeutic response.

Treatment of myeloma-associated anemia with erythropoietin is primarily a supportive therapy that aims to improve the patient's quality of life. Patients who respond to erythropoietin treatment experience an increased sense of well-being, better exercise capacity, less fatigue, and improvements in several other parameters that contribute to quality of life.[45,46] It is noteworthy that the largest gain in quality of life from incremental increases of 1 g/dL hemoglobin occurs when the hemoglobin increases from 11 to 12 g/dL, and quality of life keeps improving with further increases of hemoglobin levels.[67]

In addition, recent investigations suggest that adequate treatment of anemia might also have a beneficial effect on the outcome of cancer therapy. It had previously been shown that low hemoglobin levels have a negative influence on the outcome of radiotherapy,[68–70] and that rhEPO treatment prolonged survival and reduced mortality in murine myeloma models.[71] A recent randomized, placebo-controlled trial, involving 375 patients with solid tumors or hematological malignancies on concurrent non-platinum-based chemotherapy, demonstrated a tendency towards increased survival in the rhEPO arm as compared with the placebo arm (median: 17 vs. 11 months).[72] Several trials are in progress that aim to confirm these preliminary data, suggesting that erythropoietin treatment of anemic cancer patients, particularly those with multiple myeloma, might improve the outcome of cancer therapy and prolong survival.

FATIGUE

Prevalence and consequences of fatigue

Most myeloma patients suffer from fatigue, a debilitating symptom that can impair the patient's quality of life to a considerable degree (Table 18.7). Fatigue is mainly caused by progressive disease, anemia, cachexia, infections, adverse effects of chemotherapy and/or opioid analgesia, depression, hypercalcemia, and impaired organ function due to secondary amyloidosis. The majority of cancer patients on chemotherapy experience fatigue at least for a few days during each cycle; 30% suffers from fatigue on a daily basis.[73]

Physicians tend to underestimate the impact of fatigue on quality of life, particularly when compared with the impairment of quality of life that they attribute to pain (Fig. 18.3).[74] In a large survey, approximately 90% of the cancer patients who experienced fatigue reported that this symptom prevented a 'normal' life, required alterations in their daily routine, and made participation in social activities and performance of typical cognitive tasks difficult. Seventy-five percent of the patients who were employed had changed their employment status as a result of fatigue.[73] In spite of these partly severe fatigue-related impairments of their quality of life, only approximately 30% of these patients reported fatigue to their oncologists.[74] The outcomes of this and similar surveys[73,75] emphasize the importance of asking explicit questions

Table 18.7 Impact of fatigue on quality of life

Physical	Weakness, exhaustion
	Heaviness of the limbs
	Lack of energy
	Post-exertional malaise
	Decreased tolerance of pain
Functional	Insomnia or hypersomnia
	Reduced capability to work
	Difficulties in performing daily chores
Psychological	Concentration problems
	Impaired short-term memory
	Lack of motivation and interest
	Depression
	Emotional instability
	Reduced tolerance of frustration
Social	Limited capacity for social activities
	Withdrawal from social contacts

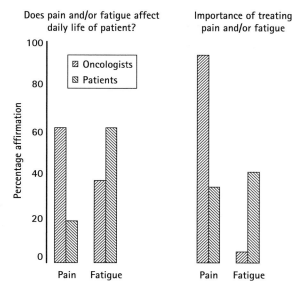

Figure18.3 *Perceptions of cancer-related fatigue by oncologists and patients. When asked to rate the influence of cancer-related pain and fatigue on the patients' daily life and the importance of treating these symptoms, oncologists place much more emphasis on pain, whereas patients rate fatigue much higher. (Adapted from Vogelzang et al.[74])*

about fatigue and, if appropriate, initiating adequate treatment.

Treatment of fatigue

Whenever possible, treatment should aim to eliminate the causes of fatigue, i.e. effective myeloma therapy, treatment of underlying infections with antibiotics, antifungals, or antivirals, and treatment of anemia with eyrthropoietin should be applied, if necessary. If these treatment modes are not indicated or if treatment response is insufficient, psychological support, physical exercise programs, nutrition counseling, and even treatment with antidepressants and/or psychostimulating drugs, such as methylphenidat, phentermine, or modafinil, should be considered.

INFECTIONS

Causes of infections

Infections, particularly those of bacterial origin, are frequent complications of multiple myeloma and are among the most common causes of death in myeloma patients.[76] The susceptibility of myeloma patients to infections results mainly from granulocytopenia and deficiencies in humoral and/or cellular immunity (Table 18.8).[77–80]

During active disease, the risk of infections is about four times higher than during remission;[81] during the first

Table 18.8 *Main causes of infections in multiple myeloma*

Neutropenia – disease and/or treatment
Steroid therapy
Immunosuppression
- Reduced proliferative T-cell response to antigenic stimulation
- Suppressed production of polyclonal B-cell response
- Decreased natural killer cell activity
- Reduced level of polyclonal immunoglobulins
Damage to mucosal or skin barriers
- Chemotherapy- or radiation-induced mucositis
- Catheter-induced bacteremia

2 months of induction chemotherapy, bacterial infections occur twice as frequently as during the rest of the course of the disease. Some of these early infections are fatal; others can prevent adequate doses of chemotherapy.[82] After reaching the plateau phase of their disease, only patients who show poor IgG responses to exogenous antigens, such as pneumococcal capsular polysaccharides, or tetanus and diphtheria toxoids, have an increased risk of serious infections.[81] Mortality from infections is particularly high in immunosuppressed patients who have received allografts from unrelated donors.[83] Patients on high-dose glucocorticoids are particularly prone to newly acquired or reactivated viral and fungal infections, with the latter frequently manifesting as oral or oroesophageal candidiasis.

The spectrum of microorganisms that patients are susceptible to changes during the course of the disease. In early-stage myeloma, the most common infections involve the respiratory tract, manifesting as bronchitis and pneumonia. These infections are predominantly caused by *Haemophilus influenzae* or *Streptococcus pneumoniae*. In patients with advanced myeloma and during the neutropenic phases of intensive chemotherapy, *Staphylococcus aureus* and Gram-negative bacteria are more common. However, Gram-positive bacteria have recently become more frequent in neutropenic myeloma patients. They were the predominant source of infection in the episodes of sepsis observed in 20–40% of patients after high-dose therapy and autologous stem cell transplantation.[84,85] Patients with advanced myeloma also tend to suffer from infections of the urinary tract and septicemia. Table 18.9 lists microorganisms frequently involved in myeloma-associated infections.

Early diagnosis and treatment of infections are particularly important in myeloma patients. Diagnostic measures should include differential blood counts, urine tests, bacterial cultures from blood, urine, and other specimens, chest X-rays, serum electrophoresis, and quantitative assessment of immunoglobulins. Neutropenic patients may fail to show fever as a symptom of sepsis; suddenly emerging fatigue and weakness can be the only obvious symptoms of severe infections in these patients. In these cases, immediate treatment with adequate doses of broad-spectrum antibiotics is essential.

Table 18.9 *Microorganisms frequently involved in myeloma-associated infections*

Class	Organism	Predominant source
Gram-negative bacteria	*Escherichia coli, Klebsiella pneumoniae, Pseudomonas aeruginosa*	Gastrointestinal tract
Gram-positive bacteria	*Staphylococcus aureus*	Oropharynx, skin, catheter locations
	Staphylococcus pneumoniae, Haemophilus influenzae	Respiratory tract
Fungi	*Candida* spp.	Skin, mucosal surfaces
	Aspergillus spp.	Respiratory tract
Viruses	*Adenovirus*	Respiratory tract
	Herpes simplex, Varicella zoster, Cytomegalovirus	Latent infections

Prophylaxis of infections

Infections can be prevented to some degree in myeloma patients by the administration of immunoglobulin preparations. A randomized placebo-controlled study in plateau-phase patients using monthly immunoglobulin infusions (0.4 g/kg) for a period of 1 year showed significant reductions in frequency and severity of infections, with patients who responded poorly to pneumococcal immunization benefiting most from immunoglobulin infusions.[86] Another randomized trial in patients with lymphoproliferative syndromes or myeloma showed significant effects of nebulizations with IgA (every 12 hours for 3 months) in preventing respiratory infections or at least delaying their onset.[87] Therefore, regular immunoglobulin substitution should be considered in all myeloma patients who suffer from recurrent infections but not in those without any history infectious complications.

Effective infection prophylaxis in patients undergoing induction chemotherapy can also be achieved by the administration of trimethoprim/sulfamethoxazole (co-trimoxazole, 160 mg/800 mg, twice daily, orally). In a randomized trial, the use of this regimen during the first 2 months of conventional induction chemotherapy resulted in significantly decreased frequencies and severities of bacterial infections.[82] However, solid scientific data on prophylactic antimicrobial therapy in myeloma are scarce. Experience in several centers suggests prophylactic intervention based on the individual patient's risk profile. This depends on the patient's previous history of infections and, particularly, on the type and dose of myeloma therapy. Patients on VAD or dexamethasone monotherapy are at a high risk of reactivation or new acquisition of herpetic infections and of acquiring fungal infections, in particular oral and upper gastrointestinal tract candidiasis.

For antiherpetic prophylaxis or treatment, oral aciclovir, 800 mg, four times daily, or one of the newer antiviral drugs, such as famciclovir or valaciclovir, may be used. Dose adaptation according to renal function is required for aciclovir but not for the newer azoles. Oral amphotericin suspension, swallowed four times daily, may be used for prophylaxis of oro-oesophageal candidiasis; oral fluconazole, 50 mg daily, may be considered for antifungal prophylaxis.

Treatment of infections

Patients who undergo high-dose chemotherapy and autologous or allogeneic transplantation are prone to additional infectious complications. Ganciclovir or foscarnet are the treatments of choice for cytomegalovirus infections; ribavirin is indicated for severe pulmonary infections by respiratory syncytial virus (RSV). Dosing of these antiviral drugs should be adjusted in patients with renal impairment.

Invasive aspergillosis and infections with other filamentous fungi, which may occur in neutropenic patients, particularly after allogeneic transplantation, have a high mortality rate.[88,89] Patients who develop cerebral abscesses and/or aspergillosis lesions in the vicinity of the pulmonary artery require emergency surgery in addition to antifungal drugs.[90] For the treatment of invasive fungal infections, amphotericin B is still the established standard drug, and the degree of resistance of the invading aspergillus species to *in vitro* cultivation with amphotericin B is a reliable predictor of the clinical outcome of this anitfungal treatment.[88] Amphotericin B or imidazoles also serve as prophylaxis against fungal infections in neutropenic patients, where, in cases of severe neutropenia, a combination with granulocyte colony-stimulating factor (G-CSF) is recommended.[88] Caspofungin acetate and voraconazole are new antifungal agents with even higher activity against aspergillosis and better tolerance than amphothericin.

G-CSF is routinely used to speed up the neutrophil recovery after autologous or allogeneic transplantation. It has also been shown to enhance the efficacy of antibiotic treatment of infections in severely granulocytopenic patients after high-dose chemotherapy. A randomized trial in myeloma patients showed that the addition of G-CSF (5 μg/kg per day) to broad-spectrum antibiotics improved the outcome of antibiotic treatment. In addition, it decreased the mortality rate, shortened the length of hospital stay, curbed superinfections, and prevented fungal infections.[91] However, in other cancer patients who were febrile and neutropenic, two similar placebo-controlled randomized trials failed to confirm these results fully.[92,93] Patients who received antibiotic treatment in combination with G-CSF had significantly reduced periods of febrile neutropenia but did not differ from controls with regard to days of fever and days of hospitalization.[92] The addition of granulocyte–macrophage colony-stimulating factor (GM-CSF) to antibiotics significantly increased response rates but failed to prolong survival.[93] Even though the growth factors G-CSF and GM-CSF have been reported to stimulate proliferation of myeloma cells *in vitro*,[94] this effect has not been observed *in vivo*,[95] and their use for prophylaxis and treatment of infections in neutropenic myeloma patients is considered safe.

HYPERCALCEMIA

Diagnosis and symptoms

Hypercalcemia, the most frequent metabolic complication of multiple myeloma, is predominantly caused by tumor-induced bone resorption. In myeloma patients with impaired kidney function, hypercalcemia can be aggravated by their decreased renal calcium excretion. Bone resorption in myeloma is mediated by various osteoclast-activating factors, i.e. various cytokines and prostaglandins, and, particularly, by the potent stimulators of osteoclast formation, RANKL and MIP-1α.

Diagnosis of hypercalcemia based solely on increased serum calcium levels is unreliable, because the binding of albumin to circulating calcium tends to lead to underestimations of biologically active calcium. For more accurate results, the concentration of ionized calcium should be determined. Alternatively, the calcium level should be corrected as follows:[96]

Corrected serum calcium (mmol/L) = Measured serum calcium (mmol/L) − [0.025 × albumin (g/L)] + 1

The frequency and intensity of the symptoms of hypercalcemia depend on its severity. Patients with slightly increased calcium levels (<3 mmol/L) are often asymptomatic, whereas more pronounced hypercalcemia (3–4 mmol/L) is associated with symptoms, such as dry mouth, nausea, vomiting, anorexia, constipation, polydipsia, polyuria, fatigue, depression, confusion, impairment of cognitive function, and, rarely, even coma (Table 18.10). Beyond levels of 4 mmol/L, the patient may develop a hypercalcemic crisis, which can be fatal if not immediately treated.

Table 18.10 *Symptoms of hypercalcemia*

Gastrointestinal	Nausea
	Vomiting
	Anorexia
	Constipation
Cardiac	Tachycardia
	Increased myocardial contractility
	Shortened ventricular systole
	Shortened QT interval
	Increased diastolic blood pressure
Renal	Polyuria
	Polydipsia
	Dryness of mouth
	Nocturia
Neurologic	Fatigue
	Confusion
	Depression
	Drowsiness
	Lethargy
	Coma

Treatment of hypercalcemia

Successful myeloma treatment is the best therapy for myeloma-associated hypercalcemia. However, symptomatic hypercalcemia requires immediate supportive therapy. It should start with intravenous saline (3–6 L/day), in order to restore extracellular fluid and induce calcium diuresis. By this treatment measure alone, serum calcium levels may be reduced by 0.3–0.5 mmol within 48 hours.

Forced saline diuresis with the addition of high doses of loop diuretics (furosemide 80–100 mg/day) can be used to induce sodium-linked calcium diuresis, but this requires careful monitoring of central venous pressure and frequent evaluations of serum electrolytes, with electrolyte replacements if appropriate. Under intensive clinical observation, the load of intravenous fluid may be increased to 500–750 mL/hour. However, if the patient receives only moderate amounts of saline under routine monitoring conditions, diuretics may aggravate volume depletion and, therefore, are only recommended when fluid balance can be carefully monitored (Table 18.11).

Within the past few years, saline replenishment in combination with bisphosphonates, such as pamidronate or clodronate, has become the standard treatment of myeloma-associated hypercalcemia.[97–99] Clodronate is given either as a single infusion over 6 hours at a dose of 1200 mg or repeatedly at daily doses of 300–600 mg. Pamidronate may be given at a dose of 60–90 mg as a single 3-hour infusion. However, the manifestation of the effect of bisphosphonates is delayed, so that 2–3 days may elapse before decreases in calcium levels occur, and full treatment effect may take 10–14 days for clodronate and 20–30 days for pamidronate. Bisphosphonate

Table 18.11 *Recommended treatment of hypercalcemia*

	Dose	Comments
Hydration		
Normal saline	3–6 L/day	Monitor fluid balance
Bisphosphonates		
Pamidronate	60–90 mg in 1 L saline over 4 hours	Start after replacement of fluid deficit, effect after 24–48 hours
Ibandronate	4–8 mg as slow intravenous injection	
Zoledronic acid	4 mg as 15-minute infusion	
Calcitonin	5–10 U/kg in 500 mL saline over 6 hours, followed by the same dose, s.c., once or twice daily	Causes a rapid drop of calcium, but tachyphylaxis sets in soon
Forced saline diuresis		
Normal saline	500 mL/h	Start furosemide after replacement of fluid deficit; monitor and replace electrolytes (especially potassium and magnesium)
Furosemide	80–100 mg/day	

s.c., subcutaneous.

treatment should be continued with oral clodronate (400 mg three times a day) or intermittent monthly clodronate (600–1200 mg) or pamidronate (60–90 mg). Pamidronate treatment may induce transient pyrexia as an adverse effect.

Ibandronate and zoledronic acid, third-generation bisphosphonates, are more potent than pamidronate;[100] in addition, they require shorter infusion periods. Ibandronate can even be applied as a slow intravenous injection. At a dose of 4–8 mg, it reduces serum calcium levels sufficiently within 3–4 days and maintains this reduction for up to 30 days.[101] Zoledronic acid, given as a 15-minute infusion at a dose of 4 mg, induced calcium normalization in a larger number of patients and prevented relapses for longer time periods than pamidronate, while still showing a good safety profile.[101,102]

Additional treatment with calcitonin is particularly important in patients who are at risk of developing a hypercalcemic crisis. Calcitonin, which effectively suppresses osteoclastic bone resorption and inhibits renal tubular calcium reabsorption, can reduce serum calcium levels within 2 hours. Because osteoclasts receptors are being downregulated, the effect of calcitonin on bone resorption is transient, whereas its effect on renal calcium excretion persists and is responsible for long-term control of hypercalcemia.[97]

Today, bisphosphonates have replaced previous recommendation for the treatment of hypercalcemia, such as intravenous phosphate infusions, mithramycin, and gallium nitrate, which have become obsolete. Corticosteroids, which are routinely included in many chemotherapy regimens for the treatment of myeloma, can also inhibit bone resorption to some degree and curb intestinal calcium absorption. Therefore, they are often included in combination therapies for hypercalcemia.

EMOTIONAL DISTRESS

The knowledge that multiple myeloma is incurable can be an enormous psychological burden to patients, particularly the elderly, who may lack adequate social networks and hence emotional support. Doctors and nurses should consider the patient's emotional vulnerability in all their interactions with them.

It is common practice now that physicians disclose cancer diagnoses to their patients. This is a positive development because the majority of patients in all age groups prefer frank communication about their disease and, after overcoming the initial shock, have high hopes about the outcome of their disease.[103] However, individuals vary in their need to know details about their disease, its treatment options, and prognosis. Therefore, doctors should carefully assess their patients' desire for information and tell them as much or as little as they want to know. In general, younger patients are more likely to want to be well informed, whereas older patients tend to expect and prefer a less active, less participatory patient role.[103] There are many exceptions to this rule, however, because educational, socio-economic, and ethnic backgrounds have a strong influence on the amount of medical information a patient seeks and on his/her desired extent of involvement in therapeutic decision-making.

Bad news about poor prognosis, a relapse, and the necessity of surgery or chemotherapy are difficult to accept. In this situation, the patient deserves secluded surroundings and the full attention of his or her physician. The first reaction may be denial, a natural protective mechanism, or even hostility, which should never be taken personally by doctors or other caregivers. Most patients need ample time to accept such information and to adjust their lives to the changed situation. Nevertheless, empathetically presented realistic information about the patient's current situation neither diminishes hope nor increases anxiety.[103]

Patients who prefer to be involved in treatment decisions show significantly more hope than those who reject participation in therapeutic mangement.[103] Being allowed to participate in medical decision-making indicates a certain degree of control over one's own fate, rather than feeling completely dependent on an oncological expert. Having a choice might even play a role in the popularity of unproven cancer treatments, and a confirmed experience of actively fighting the disease might partially explain the possible life-prolonging effect claimed by reports of some psychosocial therapies.[104]

A severe stressor in myeloma patients is uncertainty about the outcome of their disease, an anxiety that does not diminish during remission, when the threat of relapse remains. Physicians and some of their myeloma patients face the dilemma of having or wanting to approach treatment with high hopes for cure, while they know that the natural course of myeloma will eventually lead to death. Even though it might be difficult, doctors, nurses, and other caregivers should resist the temptation to offer false hope and superficial reassurance. The long-term effects of this approach may be loss of confidence and trust, which can be detrimental to the patient. Nurses should be reminded that their efforts to improve the patient's quality of life and their emotional support are as important to the patient as the physician's medical skills.

An important psychological support that medical staff can provide is listening to the patients. Listening communicates interest in the person and shows that his/her problems are being taken seriously. It relieves anxiety and, thus, has a therapeutic effect. However, in order to be able to listen constructively, doctors, nurses, and other caregivers of myeloma patients have to be aware of their own anxieties about incurable cancer, and must have come to terms with them. This is one of the reasons why all medical staff should ideally be professionally supervised in their dealings with cancer patients.

It is also very important for the emotional well-being of patients that they can trust their physicians that they will never be given up as hopeless cases. In fact, there is always something a doctor can do to make the patient feel more comfortable; and focusing on improved quality of life not only benefits the patient but also diminishes frustration in doctors, when they are unable to aim for cure. If the doctor feels genuinely sad about a patient's poor situation, there is nothing wrong about showing it. On the contrary, this expression of empathy will strengthen the bond between doctor and patient, and might motivate the patient to become more engaged in the therapeutic alliance with his or her doctor.

Many cancer patients have an increased need for physical contact.[105] Being tenderly handled by nurses and a

Table 18.12 *How to decrease emotional distress*

Communication
Listen actively to the patient
Show empathy
Adjust information about disease and treatment to the patient's need
Avoid giving false hope and superficial reassurance
Instead, offer realistic hope

Patient–doctor relationship
Offer participation in therapeutic decision-making
Allow enough time for adjustment to changed situations
Aim to improve the patient's quality of life

Attitude
Perceive the patient as a person
Never give up the patient as a hopeless case
Arrange professional supervision for all medical staff

Environment
Make the patient feel secure
Provide for visits with the same physician or a small team of physicians
If possible, admit the patient to a familiar hospital ward

doctor's firm handshake will help the patient to feel more comfortable. In addition, continuity of care is important for the patient's feeling of security. Therefore, he or she should be seen regularly by the same physician or a small team of physicians, and, if possible, should be admitted to a familiar hospital ward.

Myeloma and its treatment can be associated with psychological problems, such as depression, impaired cognitive function, and delirium, which may require psychiatric consultation[106] and specific medication. Depression also aggravates fatigue, one of the most common symptoms of myeloma. For severe depression, treatment with antidepressant medication and psychotherapy are recommended.

Even though psychological parameters have no influence on response to myeloma therapy and survival,[107] mood disturbances, which are more severe in patients with multiple myeloma than in other cancer patients,[108] do decrease the patient's quality of life.[108] Therefore, optimal psychological support (Table 18.12) by all members of the medical staff is important for the patient's emotional well-being, and will help to improve his or her quality of life.

KEY POINTS

- Supportive treatment is an essential part of the therapeutic management of myeloma patients.
- Bone destruction should be curbed by treatment with bisphosphonates.

- Pain treatment should follow the three-step plan of the World Health Organization pain treatment ladder (non-steroidal anti-inflammatory drugs, weak and strong opioids).
- Anemia below 12 g/dL hemoglobin decreases the patient's quality of life; it can successfully be treated with erythropoietin.
- Fatigue, weakness, and exhaustion can severely impair the patient's quality of life, but are often neglected by oncologists.
- Myeloma patients are susceptible to bacterial, fungal, and viral infections.
- Hypercalcemia in myeloma patients should be promptly diagnosed and treated without delay.
- Emotional distress of the patient should be met with consideration and empathy.

ACKNOWLEDGMENT

Supported by the Wilhelminen Cancer Institute of the Austrian Forum Against Cancer.

REFERENCES

● = Key primary paper
◆ = Major review article
* = Paper that represents the first formal publication of a management guideline

1. Taube T, Beneton MN, McCloskey EV, Rogers S, Greaves M, Kanis JA, et al. Abnormal bone remodelling in patients with myelomatosis and normal biochemical indices of bone resorption. Eur J Haematol 1992; 49:192–8.
2. Bataille R, Manolagas SC, Berenson JR. Pathogenesis and management of bone lesions in multiple myeloma. Hematol Oncol Clin North Am 1997; 11:349–61.
3. Podar K, Tai YT, Davies FE, Lentzsch S, Sattler M, Hideshima, T, et al. Vascular endothelial growth factor triggers signaling cascades mediating multiple myeloma cell growth and migration. Blood 2001; 98:428–35.
●4. Roux S, Meignin V, Quillard J, Meduri G, Guiochon-Mantel A, Fermand JP, et al. RANK (receptor activator of nuclear factor-kappaB) and RANKL expression in multiple myeloma. Br J Haematol 2002; 117:86–92.
5. Han JH, Choi SJ, Kurihara N, Koide M, Oba Y, Roodman G. Macrophage inflammatory protein-1alpha is an osteoclastogenic factor in myeloma that is independent of receptor activator of nuclear factor kappaB ligand. Blood 2001; 97:3349–53.
6. Croucher PI, Shipman CM, Lippitt J, Perry M, Asosingh K, Hijzen A, et al. Osteoprotegerin inhibits the development of osteolytic bone disease in multiple myeloma. Blood 2001; 98:3534–40.

7. Hofbauer LC, Neubauer A, Heufelder AE. Receptor activator of nuclear factor-kappaB ligand and osteoprotegerin: potential implications for the pathogenesis and treatment of malignant bone diseases. Cancer 2001; 92:460–70.
8. Yaccoby S, Pearse RN, Johnson CL, Barlogie B, Choi Y, Epstein J. Myeloma interacts with the bone marrow microenvironment to induce osteoclastogenesis and is dependent on osteoclast activity. Br J Haematol 2002; 116:278–90.
9. Siris ES. Breast cancer and osteolytic metastases: can bisphosphonates help? Nat Med 1997; 3:151–2.
10. Abildgaard N, Rungy J, Glerup H, Brixen K, Kassem M, Brincker H, et al. Long-term oral pamidronate treatment inhibits osteoclastic bone resorption and bone turnover without affecting osteoblastic function in multiple myeloma. Eur J Med 1998; 61:128–34.
11. Shipman CM, Rogers MJ, Apperely JF, Russell R, Croucher P. Bisphosphonates induce apoptosis in human myeloma cell lines: a novel anti-tumor activity. Br J Haematol 1997; 98:665–72.
12. Shipman CM, Croucher PI, Russell RG, Helfrich MH, Rogers MJ. The bisphosphonate incadronate (YM175) causes apoptosis of human myeloma cells in vitro by inhibiting the mevalonate pathway. Cancer Res 1998; 58:5294–7.
13. Takahashi R, Shimazaki C, Inaba T, Okano A, Hatsuse M, Okamoto A, et al. A newly developed bisphosphonate, YM529, is a potent apoptosis inducer of human myeloma cells. Leuk Res 2001; 25:77–83.
●14. Lathinen R, Laakso M, Palva I, Virkkunen P, Elomaa I. Randomised, placebo-controlled multicentre trial of clodronate in multiple myeloma. Lancet 1992; 340:1049–52.
15. Heim ME, Clemens MR, Queisser W, Pecherstorfer M, Boewer C, Herold M, et al. Prospektive randomized trial of dichloromethylene bisphosphonate (clodronate) in patients with multiple myeloma requiring treatment: a multicenter study. Onkologie 1995; 18:439–48.
●16. McCloskey EV, MacLennan IC, Drayson MT, Chapman C, Dunn J, Kanis JA. A randomized trial of the effect of clodronate on skeletal morbidity in multiple myeloma. MRC Working Party on Leukaemia in Adults. Br J Haematol 1998; 100:317–25.
17. Brincker H, Westin J, Abildgaard N, Gimsing P, Turesson I, Hedenus M, et al. Failure of oral pamidronate to reduce skeletal morbidity in multiple myeloma: a double-blind placebo-controlled trial. Danish-Swedish co-operative study group. Br J Haematol 1998; 101:280–6.
●18. Berenson JR, Lichtenstein A, Porter L, Dimopoulous M, Bordoni R, George S, et al. Efficacy of pamidronate in reducing skeletal events in patients with advanced multiple myeloma. N Engl J Med 1996; 334:488–93.
●19. Berenson JR, Lichtenstein A, Porter L, Dimopoulous M, Bordoni R, George S, et al. Long-term pamidronate treatment of advanced multiple myeloma patients reduces skeletal events. Myeloma Aredia Study Group. J Clin Oncol 1998; 16:593–602.
20. Thürlimann B, Morant R, Jungi WF, Radziwill A. Pamidronate for pain control in patients with malignant osteolytic bone disease: a prospective dose-effect study. Support Care Cancer 1994; 2:61–5.
21. Berenson JR, Rosen LS, Howell A, Porter L, Coleman R, Morley W, et al. Zoledronic acid reduces skeletal-related events in patients with osteolytic metastases. Cancer 2001; 91:1191–200.

22. Coleman RE, Purohit OP, Black C, Vinholes J, Schlosser K, Huss H, *et al.* Double-blind, randomised, placebo-controlled, dose-finding study of oral ibandronate in patients with metastatic bone disease. *Ann Oncol* 1999; **10**:311–16.

23. Clemens MR, Fessele K, Heim ME. Multiple myeloma: effect of daily dichloromethylene bisphosphonate on skeletal complications. *Ann Hematol* 1993; **66**:141–6.

●24. McCloskey EV, Dunn JA, Kanis JA, MacLennan IC, Drayson MT. Long-term follow-up of a prospective, double-blind, placebo-controlled randomized trial of clodronate in multiple myeloma. *Br J Haematol* 2001; **113**:1035–43.

25. Harvey HA, Lipton A. The role of bisphosphonates in the treatment of bone metastases – the U.S. experience. *Support Care Cancer* 1996; **4**:213–17.

26. Kraj M, Poglod R, Pawlikowski J, Maj S, Nasilowska B. Effect of pamidronate on skeletal morbidity in myelomatosis. Part 1. The results of the first 12 months of pamidronate therapy. *Acta Pol Pharm* 2000; **57**(Suppl):113–16.

●27. Menssen HD, Sakalova A, Fontana A, Herrmann Z, Boewer C, Facon T, *et al.* Effects of long-term intravenous ibandronate therapy on skeletal-related events, survival, and bone resorption markers in patients with advanced multiple myeloma. *J Clin Oncol* 2002; **20**:2353–9.

◆28. Djulbegovic B, Wheatley K, Ross J, Clark O, Bos G, Goldschmidt H, *et al.* Bisphosphonates in multiple myeloma. *Cochrane Database Syst Rev* 2001; CD003188.

29. Roux C, Ravaud P, Cohen-Solal M, de Vernejoul M, Guillemant S, Cherruau B, *et al.* Biologic, histologic and densitometric effects of oral risedronate on bone in patients with multiple myeloma. *Bone* 1994; **15**:41–9.

30. Cruz JC, Alsina M, Craig F, Yoneda T, Anderson J, Dallas M, *et al.* Ibandronate decreases bone disease development and osteoclast stimulatory activity in an in vivo model of human myeloma. *Exp Hematol* 2001; **29**:441–7.

31. Aparicio A, Gardner A, Tu Y, Savage A, Berenson J, Lichtenstein A. In vitro cytoreductive effects on multiple myeloma cells induced by bisphosphonates. *Leukemia* 1998; **12**:220–9.

●32. Grossman SA, Sheidler VR, Swedeen K, Mucenski J, Piantadosi S. Correlation of patient and caregiver ratings of cancer pain. *J Pain Symptom Manage* 1991; **6**:53–7.

33. Grossman SA. Undertreatment of cancer pain: barriers and remedies. *Support Care Cancer* 1993; **1**:74–8.

*34. World Health Organization. *Cancer pain relief and palliative care: report of a WHO Expert Panel.* WHO Technical Report 804. Geneva: WHO, 1990.

◆35. Michalowski J. COX-2 inhibitors: cancer trials test new uses for pain drug. *J Natl Cancer Inst* 2002; **94**:248–9.

36. Cherny NI, Portenoy RK. The management of cancer pain. *CA Cancer J Clin* 1994; **44**:263–303.

37. Musto P. The role of recombinant erythropoietin for the treatment of anemia in multiple myeloma. *Leuk Lymphoma* 1998; **29**:283–91.

●38. Beguin Y, Yerna M, Loo M, Weber M, Fillet G. Erythropoiesis in multiple myeloma: defective red cell production due to inappropriate erythropoietin production. *Br J Haematol* 1992; **82**:648–53.

39. Faquin WC, Schneider TJ, Goldberg MA. Effect of inflammatory cytokines on hypoxia-induced erythropoietin production. *Blood* 1992; **79**:1987–94.

40. Balkwill F, Osborne R, Burke F, Naylor S, Talbot D, Durbin H, *et al.* Evidence for tumor necrosis factor/cachectin production in cancer. *Lancet* 1987; **ii**:1229–32.

41. Denz H, Fuchs D, Huber H, Nachbaur D, Reibnegger G, Thaler J, *et al.* Correlation between neopterin, interferon-gamma and haemoglobin in patients with haematological disorders. *Eur J Haematol* 1990; **44**:186–9.

42. Singh A, Eckardt KU, Zimmermann A, Gotz K, Hamann M, Ratcliffe P, *et al.* Increased plasma viscosity as a reason for inappropriate erythropoietin formation. *J Clin Invest* 1993; **91**:251–6.

43. Maxwell MB. When the cancer patient becomes anemic. *Cancer Nurs* 1984; **7**:321–6.

●44. Dammacco F, Castoldi G, Rodjer S. Efficacy of epoetin alfa in the treatment of anaemia of multiple myeloma. *Br J Haematol* 2001; **113**:172–9.

●45. Demetri GD, Kris M, Wade J, Degos L, Cella D. Quality-of-life benefit in chemotherapy patients treated with epoetin alfa is independent of disease response or tumor type: results from a prospective community oncology study. *J Clin Oncol* 1998; **16**:3412–25.

46. Leitgeb C, Pecherstorfer M, Fritz E, Ludwig H. Quality of life in chronic anemia of cancer during treatment with recombinant human erythropoietin. *Cancer* 1994; **73**:2535–42.

●47. Means RT, Krantz SB. Inhibition of human erythroid colony-forming units by gamma interferon can be corrected by recombinant human erythropoietin. *Blood* 1991; **78**:2564–7.

●48. Ludwig H, Fritz E, Kotzmann H, Hocker P, Gisslinger H, Bamas U. Erythropoietin treatment of anemia associated with multiple myeloma. *N Engl J Med* 1990; **322**:1693–9.

49. Ludwig H, Leitgeb C, Fritz E, Krainer M, Kuhrer I, Kornek G, *et al.* Erythropoietin treatment of chronic anemia of cancer. *Eur J Cancer* 1993; **29A**(Suppl 2):8–12.

50. Barlogie B, Beck T. Recombinant human erythropoietin and the anemia of multiple myeloma. *Stem Cells* 1993; **11**:88–94.

51. Mittelman M, Zeidman A, Fradin Z, Magazanik A, Lewinski U, Cohen A. Recombinant human erythropoietin in the treatment multiple myeloma-associated anemia. *Acta Haematol* 1997; **98**:204–10.

52. Musto P, Falcone A, D'Arena G, Scalzulli P, Matera R, Minervini M, *et al.* Clinical results of recombinant erythropoietin in transfusion-dependent patients with refractory multiple myeloma; role of cytokines and monitoring of erythropoiesis. *Eur J Haematol* 1997; **58**:314–19.

53. Garton JP, Gerz MA, Witzig TE, Greipp P, Lust J, Schroeder G, *et al.* Epoetin alfa for the treatment of the anemia of multiple myeloma. A prospective, randomized, placebo-controlled, double-blind trial. *Arch Intern Med* 1995; **155**:2069–74.

54. Dammacco F, Silvestris F, Castoldi GL, Grassi B, Bernasconi C, Nadali G, *et al.* The effectiveness and tolerability of epoetin alfa in patients with multiple myeloma refractory to chemotherapy. *Int J Clin Lab Res* 1998; **28**:127–34.

●55. Österborg A, Boogaerts MA, Cimino R, Essers U, Holowiecki J, Juliusson G, *et al.* Recombinant human erythropoietin in transfusion-dependent anemic patients with multiple myeloma and non-Hodgkin's lymphoma – a randomized multicenter study. The European Study Group of Erythropoietin (Epoetin Beta) Treatment in Multiple Myeloma and Non-Hodgkin's Lymphoma. *Blood* 1996; **87**:2675–82.

●56. Cazzola M, Messinger D, Battistel V, Bron D, Cimino R, Enller-Ziegler L, *et al.* Recombinant human erythropoietin in the anemia associated with multiple myeloma or non-Hodgkin's lymphoma: dose finding and identification of predictors of response. *Blood* 1995; **86**:4446–53.

57. Silvestris F, Romito A, Fanelli P, Vacca A, Dammacco F. Long-term therapy with recombinant human erythropoietin (rHu-EPO) in progressing multiple myeloma. *Ann Hematol* 1995; **70**:313–18.

58. Österborg A, Brandberg Y, Molostova V, Iosava G, Abdulkadyrov K, Hedenus M, *et al.* Randomized, double-blind, placebo-controlled trial of recombinant human erythropoietin, epoetin Beta, in hematologic malignancies. *J Clin Oncol* 2002; **20**:2486–94.

●59. Hedenus M, Hansen S, Taylor K, Arthur C, Emmerich B, Dewey C, *et al.* Randomized, dose-finding study of darbepoetin alfa in anaemic patients with lymphoproliferative malignancies. *Br J Haematol* 2002; **119**:79–86.

●60. Gabrilove JL, Cleeland CS, Livingston RB, Sarokhan B, Winer E, Einhorn L. Clinical evaluation of once-weekly dosing of epoetin alfa in chemotherapy patients: improvements in hemoglobin and quality of life are similar to three-times-weekly dosing. *J Clin Oncol* 2001; **19**:2875–82.

61. Sunder-Plassmann G, Hörl WH. Importance of iron supply for erythropoietin therapy. *Nephrol Dial Transplant* 1995; **10**:2070–6.

●62. Glaspy J, Jadeja JS, Justice G, Kessler J, Richards D, Schwartzberg L, *et al.* A dose-finding and safety study of novel erythropoiesis stimulating protein (NESP) for the treatment of anaemia in patients receiving multicycle chemotherapy. *Br J Cancer* 2001; **84**(Suppl 1): 17–23.

●63. Henry D, Abels R, Larholt K. Prediction of response to recombinant human erythropoietin (r-HuEPO/epoetin-alpha) therapy in cancer patients. *Blood* 1995; **85**:1676–8.

●64. Cazzola M, Ponchio L, Pedrotti C, Farina G, Cerani P, Lucotti C, *et al.* Prediction of response to recombinant human erythropoietin (rHuEpo) in anemia of malignancy. *Haematologica* 1996; **81**:434–41.

●65. Henry D, Glaspy J. Predicting response to epoetin alfa in anemic cancer patients receiving chemorx. *J Clin Oncol* 1997; **16**:49a (abstract).

●66. Ludwig H, Fritz E, Leitgeb C, Pecherstorfer M, Samonigg H, Schuster J. Prediction of response to erythropoietin treatment in chronic anemia of cancer. *Blood* 1994; **84**:1056–63.

67. Cleeland C, Demetri G, Glaspy J, Cella D, Portenoy R, Cremieux P, *et al.* Identifying hemoglobin level for optimal quality of life: results of an incremental analysis. *Proc Am Soc Clin Oncol* 1999; **18**:574a (abstract).

68. Pedersen D, Sogaard H, Overgaard J, Bentzen SM. Prognostic value of pretreatment factors in patients with locally advanced carcinoma of the uterine cervix treated by radiotherapy alone. *Acta Oncol* 1995; **34**:787–95.

69. Dubray B, Mosseri V, Brunin F, Jaulerry C, Poncet P, Rodriguez J, *et al.* Anemia is associated with lower local-regional control and survival after radiation therapy for head and neck cancer: a prospective study. *Radiology* 1996; **201**:553–8.

70. Lee WR, Berkey B, Marcial V, Fu K, Cooper J, Vikram B, *et al.* Anemia is associated with decreased survival and increased locoregional failure in patients with locally advanced head and neck carcinoma: a secondary analysis of RTOG 85-27. *Int J Radiat Oncol Biol Phys* 1998; **42**:1069–75.

●71. Mittelman M, Neumann D, Peled A, Kanter P, Haran-Ghera N. Erythropoietin induces tumor regression and antitumor immune responses in murine myeloma models. *Proc Natl Acad Sci USA* 2001; **98**:5181–6.

●72. Littlewood TJ. Possible relationship of hemoglobin levels with survival in anemic cancer patients receiving chemotherapy. *Proc Am Soc Clin Oncol* 2000; **19**:605a (abstract).

●73. Curt GA, Breitbart W, Cella D, Groopman J, Horning S, Itri L, *et al.* Impact of cancer-related fatigue on the lives of patients: new findings from the Fatigue Coalition. *Oncologist* 2000; **5**:353–60.

●74. Vogelzang NJ, Breitbart W, Cella D, Curt G, Groopman J, Horning S, *et al.* Patient, caregiver, and oncologist perceptions of cancer-related fatigue: results of a tripart assessment survey. The Fatigue Coalition. *Semin Hematol* 1997; **34**(Suppl 2):4–12.

*75. Portenoy RK, Itri LM. Cancer-related fatigue: guidelines for evaluation and management. *Oncologist* 1999; **4**:1–10.

76. Peest D, Coldewey R, Deicher H. Overall vs. tumor-related survival in multiple myeloma. *Eur J Cancer* 1991; **27**:672.

77. Massaia M, Dianzani U, Bianchi A, Camponi A, Boccadoro M, Pileri A. Defective generation of alloreactive cytotoxic T lymphocytes (CTL) in human monoclonal gammopathies. *Clin Exp Immunol* 1988; **73**:214–18.

78. Osterborg A, Nilsson B, Bjorkholm M, Holm G, Mellstedt H. Natural killer cell activity in monoclonal gammopathies: relation to disease activity. *Eur J Haematol* 1990; **45**:153–7.

79. Peest D, Holscher R, Weber R, Leo R, Deicher H. Suppression of polyclonal B cell proliferation mediated by supernatants from human myeloma bone marrow cell cultures. *Clin Exp Immunol* 1989; **75**:252–7.

80. Jacobson DR, Zolla-Pazner S. Immunosuppression and infection in multiple myeloma. *Semin Oncol* 1986; **13**:282–90.

81. Hargreaves RM, Lea JR, Griffiths H, Faux J, Holt J, Reid C, *et al.* Immunological factors and risk of infection in plateau phase myeloma. *J Clin Pathol* 1995; **48**:260–6.

●82. Oken MM, Pomeroy C, Weisdorf D, Bennett JM. Prophylactic antibiotics for the prevention of early infection in multiple myeloma. *Am J Med* 1996; **100**:624–8.

●83. Mattsson J, Ringden O, Aschan J, Barkholt L, Dalianis T, Hagglund H, *et al.* A low incidence of grade II to IV acute GVHD, but high mortality from infection using HLA-A, -B, and -DR-identical unrelated donors and immunosuppression with ATG, cyclosporine, and methotrexate. *Transplant Proc* 1997; **29**:735–6.

84. Salutari P, Sica S, Laurenti L, Leone F, Chiusolo P, Piccirillo N, *et al.* Incidence of sepsis after peripheral blood progenitor cells transplantation: analysis of 86 consecutive hemato oncological patients. *Leuk Lymphoma* 1998; **30**:193–7.

85. Kolbe K, Domkin D, Derigs HG, Bhakdi S, Huber C, Aulitzky W. Infectious complications during neutropenia subsequent to peripheral blood stem cell transplantation. *Bone Marrow Transplant* 1997; **19**:143–7.

●86. Chapel HM, Lee M, Hargreaves R, Pamphilon D, Prentice A. Randomised trial of intravenous immunoglobulin as prophylaxis against infection in plateau-phase multiple myeloma. The UK Group for Immunoglobulin

Replacement Therapy in Multiple Myeloma. *Lancet* 1994; **343**:1059–63.

87. Bezares R, Murro H, Diaz A, Cavagnaro F, Caviglia G, Santome J. Prevention of infections in patients with lymphoproliferative syndromes and myeloma by nebulization of an IgA concentrate. [in Spanish]. *Sangre* 1997; **42**:219–22.

88. Florl C, Kofler G, Kropshofer G, Hermans J, Kreczy A, Dierich M, et al. In-vitro testing of susceptibility to amphotericin B is a reliable predictor of clinical outcome in invasive aspergillosis. *J Antimicrob Chemother* 1998; **42**:497–502.

●89. Pagano L, Girmenia C, Mele L, Ricci P, Tosti M, Nasari A, et al. Infections caused by filamentous fungi in patients with hematologic malignancies. A report of 391 cases by GIMEMA Infection Program. *Haematologica* 2001; **86**:862–70.

90. Bernard A, Caillot D, Couaillier JF, Casasnovas O, Guy H, Favre J. Surgical management of invasive pulmonary aspergillosis in neutropenic patients. *Ann Thorac Surg* 1997; **64**:1441–7.

●91. Aviles A, Guzman R, Garcia EL, Talavera A, Diaz-Maqueo J. Results of a randomized trial of granulocyte colony-stimulating factor in patients with infection and severe granulocytopenia. *Anticancer Drugs* 1996; **7**:392–7.

●92. Maher DW, Lieschke GJ, Green M, Bishop J, Stuart-Harris R, Wolf M, et al. Filgrastim in patients with chemotherapy-induced febrile neutropenia. A double-blind, placebo-controlled trial. *Ann Intern Med* 1994; **121**:492–501.

93. Anaissie EJ, Vartivarian S, Bodey GP, Legrand C, Kantarjian H, Abi-Said D, et al. Randomized comparison between antibiotics alone and antibiotics plus granulocyte–macrophage colony-stimulating factor (Escherichia coli-derived) in cancer patients with fever and neutropenia. *Am J Med* 1996; **100**:17–23.

94. Klein JB, Scherzer JA, McLeish KR. IFN-gamma enhances expression of formyl peptide receptors and guanine nucleotide-binding proteins by HL-60 granulocytes. *J Immunol* 1992; **148**:2483–8.

●95. Barlogie B, Jagannath S, Dixon DO, Cheson B, Smallwood L, Hendrickson A, et al. High-dose melphalan and granulocyte-macrophage colony-stimulating factor for refractory multiple myeloma. *Blood* 1990; **76**:677–80.

96. Payne RB, Carver ME, Morgan DB. Interpretation of serum total calcium: effects of adjustment for albumin concentration on frequency of abnormal values and on detection of change in the individual. *J Clin Pathol* 1979; **32**:56–60.

●97. Ralston SH, Gardner MD, Dryburgh FJ, Jenkins A, Cowan R, Boyle I. Comparison of aminohydroxypropylidene diphosphonate, mithramycin and corticosteroids/calcitonin in treatment of cancer-associated hypercalcaemia. *Lancet* 1985; **ii**:907–10.

●98. Body JJ, Bartl R, Burckhardt P, Delmas P, Diel I, Fleisch H, et al. Current use of bisphosphonates in oncology. International Bone and Cancer Study Group. *J Clin Oncol* 1998; **16**:3890–9.

●99. Carano A, Teitelbaum SI, Konsek JD, Schlesinger P, Blair H. Bisphosphonates directly inhibit the bone resorption activity of isolated avian osteoclasts in vitro. *J Clin Invest* 1990; **85**:456–61.

100. Pecherstorfer M, Steinhauer E-U, Pawsey SD. Ibandronic acid is more effective than pamidronate in lowering serum calcium in patients with severe hypercalcemia of malignancy (HCM), and has at least equal efficacy to pamidronate in HCM patients with lower baseline calcium levels. Results of a randomised, open label, comparative study. *Proc Am Soc Clin Oncol* 2001; **20**: A1535 (abstract).

◆101. Body JJ. Dosing regimens and main adverse events of bisphosphonates. *Semin Oncol* 2001; **28**(Suppl 11): 49–53.

102. Major PP, Coleman RE. Zoledronic acid in the treatment of hypercalcemia of malignancy: results of the International Clinical Development program. *Semin Oncol* 2001; **28**(Suppl 3):17–24.

●103. Cassileth BR, Zupkis RV, Sutton-Smith K, March V. Information and participation preferences among cancer patients. *Ann Intern Med* 1980; **92**:832–6.

104. Spiegel D, Bloom JR, Kraemer HC, Gottheil E. Effect of psychosocial treatment on survival of patients with metastatic breast cancer. *Lancet* 1989; **2**:888–91.

105. Leiber L, Plumb MM, Gerstenzang ML, Holland JC. The communication of affection between cancer patients and their spouses. *Psychosom Med* 1976; **9**:1–17.

106. Silberfarb PM, Bates GM Jr. Psychiatric complications of multiple myeloma. *Am J Psychiat* 1983; **140**:788–9.

●107. Silberfarb PM, Anderson KM, Rundle AC, Holland J, Cooper M, McIntyre O. Mood and clinical status in patients with multiple myeloma. *J Clin Oncol* 1991; **9**:2219–24.

●108. Poulos AR, Gertz MA, Pankratz VS, Post-White J. Pain, mood disturbance, and quality of life in patients with multiple myeloma. *Oncol Nurs Forum* 2001; **28**:1163–71.

19

Biological basis of therapy: new molecular targets

TERRY H. LANDOWSKI AND WILLIAM S. DALTON

INTRODUCTION

Traditionally, the design of cytotoxic agents used for the treatment of malignant disease has attempted to take advantage of unique biochemical characteristics of the tumor cell. For example, many of the most potent cytotoxic agents act at specific stages of the cell cycle and are most effective in tumors with a large growth fraction. Although the systemic toxicity of these agents is often quite high, this approach has produced treatment regimens with curative results in many tumor types. In contrast, multiple myeloma remains an incurable disease with a median survival of 30–40 months. The major obstacle to successful treatment of myeloma is the emergence of drug-resistant disease. Although 50–60% of patients initially respond to standard chemotherapeutic regimens, essentially all patients ultimately relapse with tumor that is refractory to further treatment. Recent advances in molecular genetics have provided the means to identify tumor-specific pathways that regulate myeloma cell growth and survival. Furthermore, in a revival of the 'seed and soil' hypothesis,[1] the contribution of the tumor microenvironment to the growth and survival of malignant cells has identified tumor-cell interactions with the microenvironment as a potential point of therapeutic intervention. Identification of the molecular mechanisms contributing to tumor cell survival and the pathways involved are providing fertile ground for the development of molecular inhibitors with high tumor specificity and low systemic toxicity.

The vast majority of molecular targeting agents currently under development are small molecules that block a critical pathway in the malignant cell with minimal impact on normal tissues. These pathways may be intrinsic to the myeloma cell or may involve an interaction between the tumor cells and the bone marrow microenvironment (Fig. 19.1). This chapter will describe some of the recently identified molecular targets and agents in development providing opportunities for therapeutic intervention in myeloma. Indeed, genetic analysis may ultimately allow the selection of specific treatment opportunities for individual patients based on molecular profiling and characterization of individual disease (see Chapter 11).

TYROSINE KINASE INHIBITORS

Basic principle

The vast majority of signal transduction pathways regulating the growth and proliferation of hematopoietic cells utilize proteins of the tyrosine kinase family, and a large number of proto-oncogenes have been identified with tyrosine kinase activity (reviewed in Kolibaba[2]). The enzymatic function of tyrosine kinases is to activate specific effector proteins by catalyzing the transfer of a gamma-phosphate from ATP to the hydroxyl group of a tyrosine residue. This phosphorylation-dependent

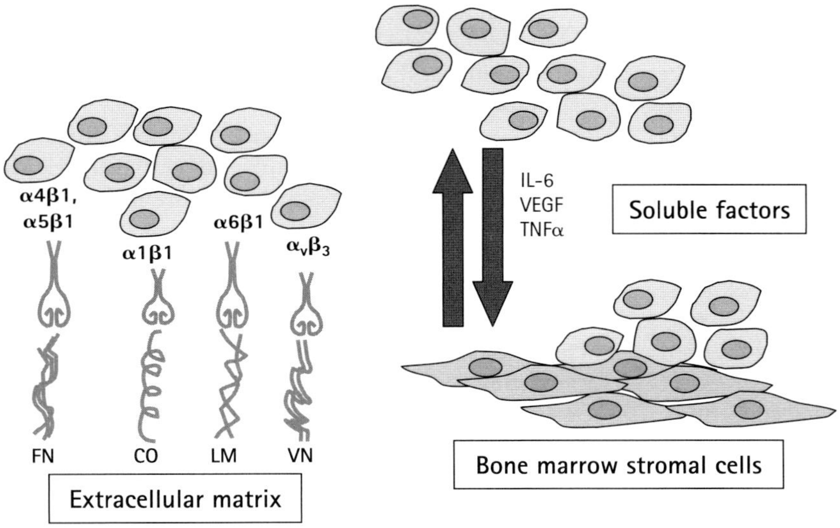

Figure 19.1 *Three primary components of the bone marrow microenvironment contribute to the enhanced survival of multiple myeloma cells: (1) ligation of receptors for extracellular matrix components, including fibronectin (FN), collagen (CO), laminin (LM), and vitronectin (VM); (2) soluble factors produced by both myeloma tumor cells and bone marrow resident cells, including stroma and other accessory cells; (3) direct physical contact with bone marrow stromal cells through integrin and non-integrin receptors. IL-6, interleukin-6; TNFα, tumor necrosis factor α; VEGF, vascular endothelial growth factor.*

activation frequently initiates protein–protein interactions and a phosphorylation cascade regulating gene expression and the resulting transformed phenotype. The c-*src* tyrosine kinase was the first viral oncogene identified, originally demonstrated by Peyton Rous in 1911, and identified as a cellular gene by Bishop and Varmus in 1976.[3] Since that time, over 100 tyrosine kinases have been identified, which can be generally divided into two groups: the receptor tyrosine kinases (RTKs) and the non-receptor tyrosine kinases (NRTKs). Common structural features of the RTKs include an extracellular ligand binding domain, a transmembrane sequence, and intracellular domains for substrate recognition and catalytic activity. These transmembrane proteins transduce a signal from the extracellular environment to cytoplasmic effectors, and ultimately to the nucleus, eliciting a response from the cell such as proliferation, differentiation, or enhanced survival. Initial demonstration of the role of RTKs in oncogenesis was provided by Schlessinger and Ullrich in the late 1980s, when they demonstrated the transforming potential of the epidermal growth factor receptor (EGFR) and the mechanism of activation by autophosphorylation in response to ligand binding.[4] Gene amplification and/or overexpression of RTK proteins, or functional alterations caused by mutations, can result in constitutive RTK signaling, ultimately leading to dysregulated cell growth and cancer. Thus, inhibition of RTK activity has been proposed as a means of selectively inhibiting the growth of transformed cells with minimal impact on normal cellular function. Similarly, NRTKs are cytoplasmic effector proteins that can be activated by a wide variety of initiating factors to transmit, and often amplify, a signal from the extracellular milieu, such as cytokines, hormones, and cellular adhesion receptors. The prototypical NRTK is the c-*src* family of proto-oncogenes, which function as second messengers for cell-surface receptors that lack intrinsic

kinase activity.[5] NRTK proteins are typically maintained in an inactive state, either through their secondary structure, as in the case of c-*src*, or in association with inhibitory factors, as in the case of Raf-1 interaction with the scaffold protein, 14-3-3.[6] As with the RTKs, constitutive activation of NRTKs, either by overexpression or mutation of the protein itself, or alterations in upstream effectors, can lead to unregulated growth and transformation.

Small molecules that inhibit the kinase activity of RTKs or NRTKs represent highly specific therapeutic agents that may restore growth control and sensitivity to programmed cell death. As such, they may potentially be developed as single-agent therapeutics, chemosensitizers, or immune modulators. Most tyrosine kinase inhibitors currently under development are small synthetic molecules that inhibit enzyme activity by blocking the ATP binding site or by interfering with the substrate recognition domain, thereby preventing signal transduction by the tyrosine kinase enzyme.[7,8] Several RTK and NRTK pathways have been identified as potential therapeutic targets in multiple myeloma.

Interleukin-6 signal transduction as a target for tyrosine kinase inhibitors

Interleukin-6 (IL-6) is generally considered to be the major growth factor for myeloma. Although many myeloma tumors are dependent on either exogenous or intrinsic production of IL-6 for growth and survival, the vast majority of transformed plasma cells have developed IL-6 independence through mutations that result in constitutive activation of the IL-6 receptor (IL-6R) signal-transduction pathway. The IL-6R is a heterodimer consisting of a p80 and a p130 subunit, which has intrinsic tyrosine kinase activity (reviewed in Heinrich[9] and

Hirano[10]). Upon binding by IL-6, the heterodimeric IL-6R oligomerizes to form a high-affinity quaternary receptor, resulting in autophosphorylation of tyrosine residues in the cytoplasmic domain of gp130, analogous to that originally described for the EGFR. This phosphorylation recruits and activates the NRTK Jak2, which, in turn, recruits and activates the signal transducer and transcriptional regulator (STAT) STAT3. Activated STAT3 dimers are then further modified by phosphorylation on serine and threonine, and translocated to the nucleus for induction of specific gene expression. Constitutive activation of STAT3 has been identified in the majority of myeloma patient plasma cells, and has been associated with overexpression of a number of proteins that contribute to the growth and survival of myeloma tumors, including Bcl-x_L, mcl-1, and cyclin D1.[11–13] Furthermore, in experimental tumor models, inhibition of STAT3-mediated gene expression by blocking the activation of the RTK IL-6R, or the NRTK Jak2, has been shown to enhance programmed cell death.[14–16] These pre-clinical studies suggest that inhibition of this cytokine signaling pathway may represent an opportunity for therapeutic intervention in myeloma patients.

The Jak2-selective tyrosine kinase inhibitor, AG490, has been shown to inhibit STAT3 in myeloma models, leading to reduced expression of the antiapoptotic molecules, bcl-x_L and mcl-1, and enhanced sensitivity to programmed cell death.[14,17] However, the cytotoxic response to standard chemotherapeutic drugs was found to be highly drug-dependent, suggesting the involvement of additional STAT3 responsive genes.[11] These findings support the use of JAK-Stat3 inhibitors after cytoreduction with chemotherapy to prolong *in vivo* responses and enhance immune surveillance; however, the data also demonstrate that a thorough understanding of how specific signal transduction pathways regulate downstream gene expression is necessary to design strategies for using targeted therapy to enhance the activity of cytotoxic agents.

Molecular analysis of myeloma patient cells has identified a second mechanism of constitutive STAT3 activation in many tumors that may provide additional targets for Jak/Stat inhibitors. Chesi *et al.*[18] reported that approximately 25% of myeloma patients harbor a t(4;14) translocation inserting the fibroblast growth factor receptor 3 into the IgH locus. This translocation results in the constitutive overexpression of FGFR3. Additionally, myeloma cells with the t(4;14) translocation frequently display activating mutations within the receptor, resulting in constitutive FGFR3 signaling in the absence of ligand stimulus. In animal models, FGFR3 expression has been shown to confer IL-6 independence through the activation of STAT3 in a Jak-independent manner.[19] Several FGFR inhibitors, including the quinazolines SU9902 and SU9803 and the pyridopyrimidines PD166285 and PD173074, have been reported to inhibit myeloma cell proliferation in

pre-clinical studies.[20] These data suggest that patients harboring the t(4;14) chromosomal abnormality may benefit from FGFR kinase inhibitors.[21]

Clinically, the most successful tyrosine kinase inhibitor to date has been the bcr-abl inhibitor, Imatinib (Gleevec/STI-571) for the treatment of chronic myelogenous leukemia.[22] Imatinib is an ATP analog that selectively inhibits the kinase activity of the abl kinase with a 50% inhibitory concentration (IC_{50}) of 0.1–0.3 μM. In contrast, the tyrosine kinases Flt-3, erbB2, v-src, and Jak2 are inhibited only at concentrations of 10–100 μM. Inhibition of c-kit, the natural receptor for stem cell factor, has been demonstrated at 0.1 μM, suggesting additional clinical applications for this agent.[23] Activation by ligand binding or function altering mutations in the c-Kit receptor has been shown to induce interactions with a network of effector kinases that result in diverse cellular responses, including differentiation, adhesion, and resistance to programmed cell death.[24] Because c-kit is a RTK that has been found to be overexpressed in 32% of myeloma patients, Imatinib may show antitumor activity in a subset of myeloma patients.[25,26] Additional kinase inhibitors such as AG957 and PD180970[27] that were initially identified as bcr-abl inhibitors may also be effective in myeloma tumors with overexpression or mutation of the c-kit RTK.

Targets of tyrosine kinase inhibitors associated with the microenvironment

Just as tyrosine kinase inhibitors may show activity against constitutively activated pathways in malignant plasma cells, activation of kinase-dependent signal transduction by interaction of the tumor cells with the bone marrow microenvironment may also represent an opportunity for therapeutic intervention. It has long been recognized that the tumor cell microenvironment may determine the phenotype of malignant cells, influencing diverse characteristics, such as growth and proliferation, metastatic potential, and response to therapy.[1] Within the past 5 years, these principles have been demonstrated in myeloma cells, and it is becoming increasingly clear that therapeutic agents that interfere with signal transduction events initiated by the microenvironment may enhance the initial response to therapy or alter the emergence of refractory disease.[28,29]

Kinase inhibitors of angiogenesis

Studies in solid tissues have demonstrated that tumor growth is highly dependent on the establishment of adequate vascularization to support increased tumor burden. Accumulating data support a central role for angiogenesis in the progression of hematologic malignancies as well. Targeting the tumor vasculature should produce minimal toxicity and prevent the development of acquired drug resistance, and has been proposed as a therapeutic strategy in multiple myeloma.

Neovascularization of the microenvironment surrounding malignant cells has been well characterized in numerous tumor models (reviewed in Liotta and Kohn[30]). Tumor cells stimulate quiescent endothelial cells to divide and form new blood vessels by releasing growth factors, which bind to resident endothelial cells. Binding of vascular endothelial growth factor (VEGF) to one of its receptors initiates the signaling cascade that regulates new blood vessel formation. A number of RTKs have been identified as endothelial cell receptors for VEGF, including the Flk-1 receptor, which is believed to play a critical role in angiogenesis. Binding of VEGF to the extracellular domain of FLK-1 activates the tyrosine kinase activity of the receptor, initiating a signaling cascade leading to endothelial cell proliferation. Recent reports have provided evidence that angiogenesis occurs in hematopoietic malignancies including multiple myeloma.[31] Vacca et al.[32] reported that angiogenesis was significantly associated with active myeloma as compared with non-active myeloma or patients with monoclonal gammopathy of unknown significance (MGUS). Myeloma patients who had the highest proliferative fraction also had the greatest bone marrow microvessel density.[33] Additionally, Bellamy et al.[34] reported that VEGF was overexpressed in all human myeloma cell lines studied and in myeloma cells from 12 of 16 patients. In contrast, plasma cells from normal subjects expressed minimally detectable levels of VEGF. These data support the possibility that agents that interfere with VEGF signal transduction may inhibit myeloma growth and progression.

The adenine analogs SU5416 and SU6668 have been shown to be potent and selective inhibitors of Flk-1 tyrosine kinase activity.[35,36] In vitro experiments have demonstrated the ability of SU5416 to inhibit endothelial cell proliferation and new blood vessel formation following stimulation by VEGF. Additionally, studies in animal models have demonstrated growth inhibition of a number of tumor types in xenobiotic transplants, suggesting that interference with neovascularization represents an effective therapeutic strategy. Phase I/II clinical trials of VEGF inhibitors have shown promising results in carcinomas and trials are under way in hematologic malignancies, including multiple myeloma.

NON-KINASE INHIBITORS OF ANGIOGENESIS: THALIDOMIDE AND IMMUNOMODULATORY DRUGS

Thalidomide was originally introduced as a sedative in Europe and Canada in the late 1950s, and was widely used to treat insomnia and nausea during pregnancy. Severe teratogenic effects led to its withdrawal in 1961. Subsequent investigation demonstrated that thalidomide is a potent antiangiogenic and immunomodulatory agent with anticancer activity.[37] Thalidomide was approved for use as an antiangiogenic agent in the USA in July 1998 under 21 CFR 314.520 Subpart H, restricting the distribution of drugs with special safety concerns, and has been investigated in a number of cancers, including multiple myeloma, myelodysplastic syndromes, gliomas, Kaposi's sarcoma, renal cell carcinoma, advanced breast cancer, and colon cancer. The mechanism by which thalidomide inhibits angiogenesis is unclear; however, its teratogenicity is believed to be due to intercalation into G-rich promoter regions of DNA and inhibition of growth factor transcription during limb bud outgrowth, suggesting regulation of specific gene expression as a potential action.[38,39] As an anti-inflammatory agent, thalidomide has been reported to block the production of tumor necrosis factor α (TNFα), IL-6, IL-10, and IL-12, while enhancing the production of IL-2, IL-4, and IL-5, and stimulating T-cell cytotoxicity (Fig. 19.2). The exact mechanism by which thalidomide acts in myeloma is unclear, but thalidomide and thalidomide analogs have been remarkably active in multiple myeloma, as both single agents and in combination.[40]

In 1999, Singhal et al.[41] reported a 32% response rate to thalidomide, with 20% of the responders demonstrating at least a 50% reduction in M-protein. Drowsiness, constipation, weakness, fatigue, tingling, and/or numbness in the hands and feet, dizziness, and rash were reported as the predominant adverse effects. However, most side effects were grade I or II, and only 10% of patients chose to discontinue the study.[41] These results were updated by Barlogie et al.[42] in a report of 169 patients. Major and partial responses were observed in 30% of patients, with 9% displaying >grade 3 neuropathy, which was resolved in most patients with dose reduction. The dose of thalidomide used in these studies was 400–800 mg/day, administered as a single oral dose. Based on the 6–7 hour reported half-life of the drug, the Swedish group of Juliusson et al.[43] examined the benefits of divided doses, starting at 200 mg/day and escalating to 400, 600, or 800 mg/day. Forty-three percent of patients in the divided dose group achieved partial response (PR), with the median time to PR at 31 days, compared with 70 or 116 days in the two responding patients receiving one dose per day. A retrospective analysis by Neben et al.,[44] examining the cumulative dose effect on progression-free survival and overall survival, further supports the use of a dose-intensive treatment schedule, at least for the first 3 months of therapy. However, this study additionally noted that dose intensity correlated with the incidence of serious adverse events, such as deep vein thrombosis. Durie and Stephen[45] noted that initial responses tended

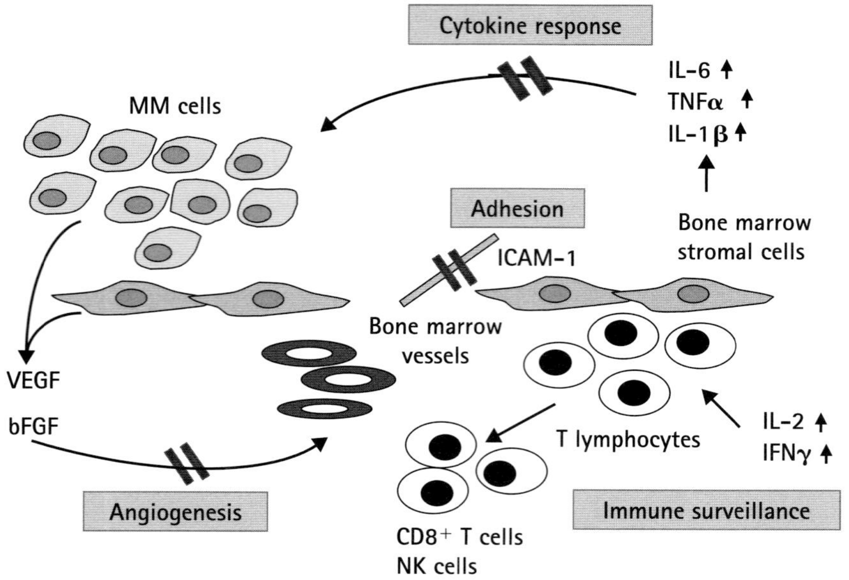

Figure 19.2 *Although the specific mechanism of thalidomide and the immunomodulatory drugs has not been fully identified, multiple activities have been demonstrated, including inhibition angiogenesis, inhibition of myeloma cell adhesion to stromal cells, enhanced immune surveillance by NK and CD8+ T cells, and reduced response to growth-promoting cytokines. bFGF, basic fibroblast growth factor; ICAM-1, intracellular adhesion molecule; IFNγ, interferon-γ; IL, interleukin; MM, multiple myeloma; NK, natural killer; TNFα, tumor necrosis factor α; VEGF, vascular endothelial growth factor.*

to occur early, and dose escalation significantly increased toxicity. In a trial designed to examine the efficacy of less toxic lower doses, patients with relapsing or progressive myeloma were treated with thalidomide at doses of between 50 and 400 mg/day. Dose escalation was based upon lack of response following an 8-week course. Overall response in this trial was 44%, highly comparable with the trials described above, with all responding patients remaining in remission at 6 months, 67% at 18 months, and 22% at 2 years. Interestingly, the two patients maintaining remission status at 30 months were those who received the lowest dose, 50 mg/day. However, progressive peripheral neuropathy appeared as a long-term toxicity. Thus, the optimum dose of thalidomide and the factors contributing to response and toxicity remain to be determined.[46]

Patients with multiple myeloma frequently display paraprotein-associated coagulopathies, including both hypercoagulability and anticoagulant syndromes. Recently, several studies have identified an increased risk of thrombo-embolism in myeloma patients receiving thalidomide, particularly when given with anthracycline therapy.[46–52] In the largest of these studies, Zangari et al.[47] reported an incidence of deep vein thrombosis (DVT) in 14 of 50 patients (28%) randomly assigned to receive thalidomide in addition to combination chemotherapy, but in only two of 50 patients (4%) who did not receive the agent. The mechanism of this phenomenon is unknown; however, in most cases, thromboses were successfully treated with anticoagulant therapy and patients were able to resume thalidomide treatment.

The thalidomide analogs SelCIDs (selective cytokine inhibitory drugs), which are phosphodiesterase 4 inhibitors, and ImiDs (immunomodulatory drugs), have recently entered phase I and I/II clinical trials, are well tolerated,

and have shown reduced toxicity compared with thalidomide. Richardson et al.[53] reported a phase I trial of the ImiD CC-5013 (Revimid) in 27 patients with relapsed and refractory multiple myeloma. Dose escalation identified the maximum tolerated dose (MTD) as 25 mg/day, with limiting toxicities appearing after 28 days of therapy. The most common serious adverse events included grade 3 thrombocytopenia and grades 3 and 4 neutropenia. Clinical response was noted in 17 of 24 evaluable patients (71%), primarily at 25 or 50 mg/day.

Thalidomide and other immunomodulatory agents may be best utilized as combination therapies in patients not responding to, or relapsing on, either thalidomide alone or standard cytotoxic therapies. Two combinations have been reported, DT-PACE (dexamethasone, thalidomide, cisplatin, doxorubicin, cyclophosphamide, etoposide) and BLT-D (clarithromycin, thalidomide, dexamethasone) with varied results. Additionally, thalidomide has been reported to overcome the resistance of myeloma cells to standard chemotherapy,[54] suggesting that this agent may be highly effective in relapsed or refractory disease.

More recently, thalidomide has been suggested as a first-line therapy, either as a single agent or in combination with dexamethasone. Two clinical trials have been reported in which thalidomide or thalidomide plus dexamethasone were administered to newly diagnosed or previously untreated myeloma patients.[55,56] This protocol was proposed as a less toxic alternative to VAD (vincristine, Adriamycin, and dexamethasone) as induction therapy in preparation for autologous stem cell transplant. In 28 patients treated with thalidomide alone, Weber et al.[56] reported ten patients (36%) with disease remission and a median time to remission of 4.2 months. Combination therapy of thalidomide plus dexamethasone resulted in a significantly higher response rate, 29 of 40 (72%), with five patients (16%) achieving a complete remission. Similarly, Rajkumar et al.[55] reported 32 of 50 patients (64%) demonstrating a response to thalidomide–dexamethasone, with an additional 14 patients (28%) categorized as stable disease. Dose-limiting toxicities were comparable to those reported when thalidomide is used as salvage therapy in advanced or refractory disease. In both studies, tumor burden was reduced as effectively as VAD induction; however, the long-term effects of thalidomide on stem-cell yield or engraftment are not known. Further studies are warranted to identify the most appropriate time of use in the course of the disease, and the long-term toxicities of thalidomide and thalidomide analogs.

FARNESYL TRANSFERASE INHIBITORS

Mutations of the *ras* gene are among the most commonly identified transforming events in multiple myeloma. Examination of myeloma patient tumor cells for oncogenic Ras mutations has revealed activating mutations in 30–47% of either K- or N-ras.[57–59] More importantly, however, the incidence of Ras mutations demonstrated a direct correlation with a number of critical clinical parameters. Median survival of patients with K-ras mutation was approximately 2.0 years, compared with 3.7 years for patients with no K-ras mutations. Based on these observations, agents that inhibit Ras function have been proposed as molecular agents in the treatment of myeloma. The Ras oncoprotein is a small G-protein signal transducer that requires a prenyl lipid modification and membrane association for signal transduction activity.[60,61] Two enzymes, farnesyltransferase (FTase) and geranylgeranyltransferase I (GGTase I), catalyze this prenyl post-translational modification by transferring farnesyl and geranylgeranyl to the cysteine of the carboxyl terminal CAAX (C = cysteine, A = aliphatic, X = any amino acid). H-, N-, and K-Ras are all farnesylated. Because prenylation is required for the oncogenic activity of Ras, FTase (FTIs) and GGTase inhibitors (GGTIs) have been developed as potential anticancer drugs (Fig. 19.3).[62,63] The first generation of FTIs were designed as peptidomimetics of the CVIM, the CAAX sequence of K-ras. These agents were highly efficient at selectively blocking FTase compared with the related enzyme GGTase I. Current-generation FTIs are largely non-peptide-, non-thiol-containing compounds with nanomolar potency. They represent a variety of different structures, including improved molecules based on the rationally designed CAAX peptidomimetics, farnesyl pyrophosphate analogs, and non-peptide compounds identified by screening of random libraries from combinatorial chemistry.

Phase I clinical trials using FTIs as single agents have demonstrated that it is possible to achieve plasma drug

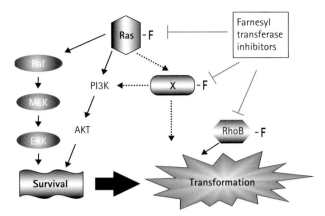

Figure 19.3 *Farnesyl transferase inhibitors inhibit the prenylation, and thus block the signal transduction function, of proteins including Ras, RhoB, and other as yet unidentified targets (X) that may contribute to myeloma cell growth and survival. AKT, protein kinase B; F-, farnesylation; PI3K, phosphoinositide-3 kinase.*

concentrations that inhibit FTase activity by both oral and intravenous administration. Alsina et al.[64] have reported a phase II clinical study with FTI (R11577/Zarnestra) in heavily pre-treated myeloma patients that demonstrated disease stabilization in 50% of patients, as defined by a reduction of the monoclonal protein of less than 25%. Treatment with R115777 suppressed FTase, but not GGTase I, activity in bone marrow and peripheral blood mononuclear cells of multiple myeloma patients. Similarly, R115777 inhibited the prenylation of the exclusively farnesylated protein, HDJ-2, in all patients. Inhibition of farnesylation did not correlate with clinical activity, supporting additional pre-clinical studies that suggest the specific prenylated target of the FTIs in myeloma tumors is not yet defined. A similar report by Cortes et al.[65] that included ten patients with refractory or relapsed myeloma demonstrated only one response. However, the dosing schedule utilized in this study, 600 mg twice daily, allowed median treatment of only 7 weeks before interruption due to toxicity. In contrast, the study by Alsina et al.[64] initiated treatment at 300 mg twice daily for 3 weeks, repeated every 4 weeks. At the time of publication, four of six responding patients had completed four cycles of therapy without significant toxicity. These data suggest that myeloma patients may benefit from prolonged treatment at lower doses; however, additional studies are needed to identify the optimum scheduling for FTI efficacy in myeloma.

Pre-clinical studies have demonstrated the greatest inhibition of growth in myeloma tumor cells with N-ras mutations, whereas myeloma cells with K-ras mutations are the most resistant to the cytotoxic effects of FTIs.[66,67] In these studies, cytotoxicity does not strictly correlate with inhibition of prenylation, and clinical studies in myeloma and other malignancies have shown no correlation of ras mutation status with response to FTIs. These studies suggest that ras may not be the primary target of these agents *in vivo*, and many laboratories are actively involved in attempts to define the molecular activity of FTIs. Other farnesylated targets that have been proposed include the ras-related family of Rho proteins, particularly RhoB (Fig. 19.3), and the mitotic spindle segregation proteins CENP-E and CENP-F; however, these targets have not been validated in all cell types.[68,69] More importantly, however, studies using myeloma cells with acquired mechanisms of resistance to standard chemotherapeutic drugs have demonstrated that FTIs are equally active in drug-sensitive and drug-resistant cells, supporting the use of these agents in refractory disease either as single agents or in combination therapy.

INHIBITION OF GENE EXPRESSION BY ANTISENSE

Biological targeted therapies that inhibit the activity of proto-oncogenes have generally been found to be most effective in malignancies that rely on those gene products for proliferation. However, multiple myeloma is largely a latent disease, and it has been suggested that the primary transforming events are those that dysregulate programmed cell death.[70] Therefore, strategies that block the expression of antiapoptotic molecules and pathways that promote extended cell survival may represent one of the most promising approaches for myeloma therapy.

Bcl-2 was one of the first genes identified as a proto-oncogene with antiapoptotic activity.[71,72] Originally isolated from follicular B-cell lymphoma, the *Bcl-2* gene has been found to be translocated into the IgH locus in over 80% of follicular B-cell malignancies, resulting in high constitutive expression of the protein product. The frequency of *Bcl-2* translocations is much lower in myeloma than in other B-cell malignancies; however, overexpression of Bcl-2 protein or other antiapoptotic *Bcl-2* family members has been demonstrated in 80–100% of myeloma patient specimens and cell lines examined.[73–76] Bcl-2 is a 25-kDa protein that has been proposed to function as an ion gate in the mitochondrial membrane. Overexpression of Bcl-2 allows it to form stable homodimers in the mitochondrial membrane, thereby preventing the release of cytochrome *c* and inhibiting the terminal steps of the apoptotic cascade. Additionally, high levels of Bcl-2 protein lead to the formation of heterodimers with pro-apoptotic members of the *Bcl-2* family, including *Bax* and *Bad*, thereby blocking their apoptotic function. Inhibition of Bcl-2 expression has been shown to increase the ratio of pro-apoptotic to antiapoptotic factors and promote programmed cell death. Strategies to inhibit the expression of antiapoptotic proteins include inhibition of translation

by antisense oligonucleotides and destruction of the mRNA by ribozymes or siRNA.

Antisense oligonucleotides (ODNs) are short segments of DNA that are complementary to a target mRNA. The ODNs selectively hybridize to their complementary RNA and prevent the translation of target RNA, thereby blocking gene expression. Two mechanisms of action have been described, one in which the complementary ODN physically inhibits the progression of splicing or the translational machinery, and one in which the ODN directs the activity of endogenous RNase H to degrade the RNA strand of the RNA/DNA duplex.[77,78] The majority of the antisense drugs currently being investigated in clinical trials function via an RNase H-dependent mechanism, although the precise mechanism by which RNase H recognizes the RNA/DNA hybrids is not well understood. Target sequences must be selected based on the accessibility of the mRNA for heteroduplex formation in the context of predicted mRNA secondary structure. Additionally, the development of ODN-based therapeutics requires chemical modification of the ODN to prevent degradation by exonucleases and endonucleases, both during delivery and following tumor uptake. One of the most common modifications used is the substitution of a sulfur atom for an oxygen in the phosphate backbone, forming a phosphorothioate.

Phase I clinical trials of ODN targeting the mRNA of Bcl-2 in non-Hodgkin's lymphoma demonstrated one complete response, two minor responses, nine patients with stable disease, and nine patients with progressive disease. No important systemic toxicity was identified at doses up to $147.2 \, \text{mg/m}^2$ daily, and phase II trials have been initiated.[79] The prevalence of Bcl-2 overexpression in multiple myeloma suggests that Bcl-2 ODNs may represent a therapeutic strategy in this disease. Additionally, the *Bcl-2* family members Bcl-x$_L$ and Mcl-1 have been identified as survival factors in multiple myeloma, and overexpression has been associated with drug-resistant tumors, further supporting the development of *Bcl-2* family ODNs for the treatment of myeloma.

INHIBITION OF THE UBIQUITIN–PROTEASOME SYSTEM OF PROTEIN DEGRADATION

One of the most novel molecular pathways emerging as a target for cancer therapy is the ubiquitin–proteasome system of protein degradation. The ubiquitin–proteasome system has been shown to regulate the cellular activity of a large number of proteins known to be involved in carcinogenesis, including transcription factors such as AP-1 and p53, signal transduction molecules such as Jak2 and cbl, the cell cycle regulator p27, and regulatory factors such as the nuclear factor κ B (NF-κB) inhibitors IκBα, β, ε, and p100. Based on these observations, proteasome inhibitors have been developed as anticancer agents.[80,81] One of the most potent, and least toxic, proteasome inhibitors currently in clinical trials is the dipeptide boronic acid, bortezomib (VELCADE™), formerly known as PS-341.[82] Bortezomib forms a covalent bond with the active site threonine in the core of the 20S proteasome and inhibits the chymotrypsin activity of the proteasome; however, its exact mechanism of cytotoxicity and selectivity for transformed cells is not known. Several studies have suggested NF-κB as a potential bortezomib target. Using 8226 myeloma cell lines selected for resistance to standard chemotherapeutic drugs,[83–85] Berenson et al.[86] demonstrated inhibition of NF-κB activity and enhanced cytotoxicity of chemotherapeutic drugs when combined with bortezomib. Additionally, Cusack et al.[87] demonstrated that combining bortezomib with CPT-11, an agent that activates NF-κB, significantly enhanced drug response in human colorectal cancer cells. However, in both studies, the dose of bortezomib required to inhibit NF-κB activity was far greater than the toxic dose, suggesting that NF-κB may not be the primary target of the agent.

Investigation into the role of p53 in bortezomib-mediated apoptosis demonstrated that, although inhibition of proteasome activity increased p53 protein levels, bortezomib-mediated apoptosis was not dependent on p53.[88] Using a number of cell lines with differing p53 status, An et al.[88] demonstrated that PS-341-mediated apoptosis occurred in cell lines lacking wild-type (wt) p53, and introduction of wt p53 into p53 null cell lines did not enhance the cytotoxicity of the proteasome inhibitors. These investigators further demonstrated an accumulation of p21 correlating with PARP cleavage; however, no differential effects were seen in cells lacking p21 compared with those that express the protein. Thus, the exact target and mechanism of cytotoxicity are not known (Fig. 19.4).

In addition to displaying a high degree of tumor specificity, bortezomib has been suggested to target the microenvironment in MCF-7 breast carcinoma,[81] and ovarian and prostate carcinomas grown in spheroid culture, which represents a model for solid tumor 'multicellular resistance.'[89] Using an ovarian cancer multicellular spheroid model, Frankel et al.[89] demonstrated greater cytoxicity in the SKOV3 cell line grown in spheroid culture than when cells were grown in monolayer culture. These data support the hypothesis that bortezomib molecular targets may be more active in cells following cell–cell or cell–matrix interactions such as would be encountered in the bone marrow microenvironment. In vivo studies using mouse mammary carcinoma and

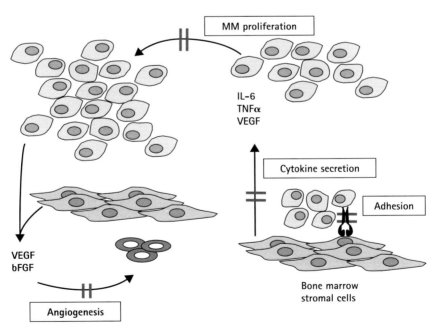

Figure 19.4 *Potential targets of the proteasome inhibitor bortezomib (VELCADE™) in multiple myeloma (MM). Bortezomib inhibits myeloma cell proliferation, angiogenesis, and cytokine response, suggesting that the in vivo activities may be even greater than those seen in pre-clinical models. Bortezomib may directly inhibit myeloma cell growth through: (1) altered stability of proteins that regulate cell-cycle progression; (2) inhibition of adhesion molecules, such as ICAM-1 and VCAM-1, thus disrupting the myeloma cell–bone marrow (BM) interactions; (3) inhibition of the antiapoptotic effects of BM-derived TNFα and VEGF on myeloma cells; and (4) inhibition of the angiogenic effects of VEGF and bFGF on BM microvessel formation. bFGF, basic fibroblast growth factor; ICAM-1, intracellular adhesion molecule; IL, interleukin; TNFα, tumor necrosis factor α; VCAM-1, vascular cellular adhesion molecule-1; VEGF, vascular endothelial growth factor.*

Lewis lung carcinoma demonstrated antitumor activity toward both primary and metastatic disease,[81] again supporting the role of the microenvironment in activation of molecular targets for proteosome inhibitors.

Pre-clinical studies in human myeloma cells have demonstrated that bortezomib acts directly on the tumor cells as well as the bone marrow microenvironment.[90] Hideshima *et al.*[91] reported that bortezomib inhibited the paracrine growth of multiple myeloma cells by decreasing the adhesion of myeloma cells to bone marrow stromal cells, reducing TNFα-stimulated NF-κB activation, and inhibiting the mitogen-activated protein kinase signaling pathway in both myeloma cell lines and freshly isolated myeloma cells from patient bone marrow aspirates.

In phase I clinical trials, bortezomib was well tolerated, with the MTD determined at $1–2\,mg/m^2$. Primary toxicities identified included low-grade fever and fatigue, thrombocytopenia, which was not dose-limiting, and low-grade diarrhea, all of which were manageable. Preliminary reports from a large phase II trial enrolling >200 patients at nine centers have demonstrated responses or stabilization of disease in 75% of the 54 patients currently analyzable.[90] Additional phase II studies are planned in mantle cell lymphoma, indolent non-Hodgkin's lymphoma, chronic myelogenous leukemia, diffuse large B-cell leukemia, and chronic lymphocytic leukemia. A phase III trial of bortezomib in multiple myeloma is in progress, which compares bortezomib alone or in combination with dexamethasone. Bortezomib perhaps represents the most promising of the new therapeutic agents.

SUMMARY

The treatment of myeloma has not improved substantially in the past three decades, and treatment continues to rely on cytotoxic drugs and glucocorticoids. Enhancing the efficacy of these drugs by preventing or overcoming drug resistance may improve the frequency of response and response duration; however, studies in myeloma cell models have demonstrated that when one mechanism of resistance, such as drug efflux, is inhibited, a second mechanism of resistance emerges.[92] Recent developments in molecular genetics now provide a unique opportunity to target biological aspects of myeloma for the design of novel therapeutic approaches. A major challenge to improving treatment outcome is not only discovering new therapeutic targets but also identifying the patients most likely to benefit from a given therapeutic approach, and utilizing biological endpoints to monitor safety and efficacy. Because many of the biological targets are most likely to be useful in preventing disease progression or enhancing the efficacy of standard chemotherapeutic agents, it will be essential to design clinical trials to

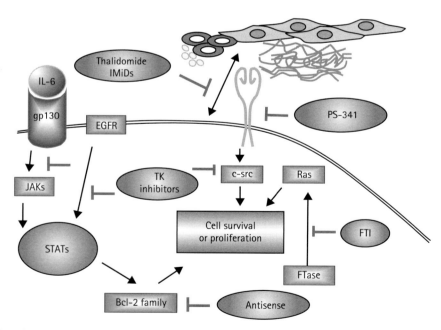

Figure 19.5 *The identification of pathways important to the growth and survival of myeloma cells has provided molecular targets for therapeutic intervention. These targets include inhibition of signal transduction by tyrosine kinase (TK) inhibitors, blocking the expression of antiapoptotic and survival genes by antisense oligonucleotides, prevention of second-messenger localization by prenylation inhibitors, and inhibition of microenvironmental survival mechanisms by bortezomib and thalidomide. EGFR, epidermal growth factor receptor; FTase, farnesyltransferase; FTI, farnesyltransferase inhibitor; IL-6, interleukin-6; ImiDs, immunomodulatory drugs; JAKs, janus kinases; STATs, signal transducers and activators of transcription.*

determine the specific activity of the investigational agent vs. combination therapy for the best clinical outcome.

A second major consideration in the identification of novel molecular targets in multiple myeloma is the influence of the bone marrow microenvironment on tumor cell response to therapy. Historically, pre-clinical studies have relied on tissue culture models in which transformed cells are examined independent of extracellular components. It is now well accepted that the tumor microenvironment supports the growth and survival of myeloma cells, and although extracellular matrix (ECM)-mediated signal transduction pathways may represent opportunities for therapeutic intervention, their antiapoptotic effects must be considered in therapeutic strategies (Fig. 19.5).

KEY POINTS

- Advances in genetics have provided molecular targets for the development of therapeutic agents, which are likely to be more effective and less toxic than standard cytotoxic agents.
- Interleukin 6 (IL-6) is the major growth factor associated with multiple myeloma proliferation and survival.
- Small-molecule tyrosine kinase inhibitors can be used to block the IL-6 signal transduction pathway in myeloma therapy.
- Thalidomide and thalidomide analogs demonstrate activity in myeloma patients, perhaps through inhibition of growth factor production or response.
- Antisense oligonucleotides that prevent the expression of pro-survival genes, such as *Bcl-2*, may be the most specific and least toxic of the new therapeutics.
- Proteasome inhibitors are highly selective antitumor agents with a unique mechanism of activity.
- Molecular target-based therapies must be integrated with existing therapies in both pre-clinical and clinical settings to determine optimal application strategies.
- Therapeutic considerations include both the tumor itself and the interactions of the tumor with the surrounding microenvironment.

REFERENCES

● = Key primary paper
◆ = Major review article

1. Paget S. The distribution of secondary growths in cancer of the breast. *Lancet* 1889; **1**:571–3.

◆2. Kolibaba KS, Druker BJ. Protein tyrosine kinases and cancer. *Biochim Biophys Acta* 1997; **1333**:F217–48.
3. Stehelin D, Varmus HE, Bishop JM, Vogt PK. DNA related to the transforming gene(s) of avian sarcoma viruses is present in normal avian DNA. *Nature* 1976; **260**:170–3.
4. Riedel H, Dull TJ, Schlessinger J, Ullrich A. A chimaeric receptor allows insulin to stimulate tyrosine kinase activity of epidermal growth factor receptor. *Nature* 1986; **324**:68–70.
◆5. Smithgall TE. Signal transduction pathways regulating hematopoietic differentiation. *Pharmacol Rev* 1998; **50**:1–19.
6. Li S, Janosch P, Tanji M, Rosenfeld GC, Waymire JC, Mischak H, et al. Regulation of Raf-1 kinase activity by the 14-3-3 family of proteins. *EMBO J* 1995; **14**:685–96.
7. Levitt ML, Koty PP. Tyrosine kinase inhibitors in preclinical development. *Invest New Drugs* 1999; **17**:213–26.
8. Showalter HD, Kraker AJ. Small molecule inhibitors of the platelet-derived growth factor receptor, the fibroblast growth factor receptor, and Src family tyrosine kinases. *Pharmacol Ther* 1997; **76**:55–71.
9. Heinrich PC, Behrmann I, Muller-Newen G, Schaper F, Graeve L. Interleukin-6-type cytokine signalling through the gp130/Jak/STAT pathway. *Biochem J* 1998; **334**:297–314.
◆10. Hirano T, Ishihara K, Hibi M. Roles of STAT3 in mediating the cell growth, differentiation and survival signals relayed through the IL-6 family of cytokine receptors. *Oncogene* 2000; **19**:2548–56.
11. Oshiro MM, Landowski TH, Catlett-Falcone R, Hazlehurst LA, Huang M, Jove R, et al. Inhibition of JAK kinase activity enhances Fas-mediated apoptosis but reduces cytotoxic activity of topoisomerase II inhibitors in U266 myeloma cells. *Clin Cancer Res* 2001; **7**:4262–71.
12. Epling-Burnette PK, Liu JH, Catlett-Falcone R, Turkson J, Oshiro M, Kothapalli R, et al. Inhibition of STAT3 signaling leads to apoptosis of leukemic large granular lymphocytes and decreased Mcl-1 expression. *J Clin Invest* 2001; **107**:351–62.
13. Sinibaldi D, Wharaton S, Turkson J, Bowman T, Pledger WJ, Jove R. Induction of p21waf/cip1 and cyclin D1 expression by the Src oncoprotein in mouse fibroblasts: role of activated STAT3 signaling. *Oncogene* 2000; **19**:5419–27.
●14. Catlett-Falcone R, Landowski TH, Oshiro MM, Turkson J, Levitzki A, Savino R, et al. Constitutive activation of Stat3 signaling confers resistance to apoptosis in human U266 myeloma cells. *Immunity* 1999; **10**:105–15.
15. Sporeno E, Savino R, Ciapponi L, Paonessa G, Cabibbo A, Lahm A, et al. Human interleukin-6 receptor super-antagonists with high potency and wide spectrum on multiple myeloma cells. *Blood* 1996; **87**:4510–19.
●16. Demartis A, Bernassola F, Savino R, Melino G, Ciliberto G. Interleukin 6 receptor superantagonists are potent inducers of human multiple myeloma cell death. *Cancer Res* 1996; **56**:4213–18.
●17. Puthier d, Derenne S, Barille S, Moreau P, Harousseau JL, Bataille R, et al. Mcl-1 and Bcl-xL are co-regulated by IL-6 in human myeloma cells. *Br J Haematol* 1999; **107**:392–5.
●18. Chesi M, Nardini E, Brents LA, Schrock E, Ried T, Kuehl WM, et al. Frequent translocation t(4;14)(p16.3;q32.3) in multiple myeloma is associated with increased expression and

activating mutations of fibroblast growth factor receptor 3. *Nat Genet* 1997; **16**:260–4.

19. Plowright EE, Li Z, Bergsagel PL, Chesi M, Barber DL, Branch DR, *et al.* Ectopic expression of fibroblast growth factor receptor 3 promotes myeloma cell proliferation and prevents apoptosis. *Blood* 2000; **95**:992–8.

20. Dimitroff CJ, Klohs W, Sharma A, Pera P, Driscoll D, Veith J, *et al.* Anti-angiogenic activity of selected receptor tyrosine kinase inhibitors, PD166285 and PD173074: implications for combination treatment with photodynamic therapy. *Invest New Drugs* 1999; **17**:121–35.

21. Panek RL, Lu GH, Klutchko SR, Batley BL, Dahring TK, Hamby JM, *et al.* In vitro pharmacological characterization of PD 166285, a new nanomolar potent and broadly active protein tyrosine kinase inhibitor. *J Pharmacol Exp Ther* 1997; **283**:1433–44.

22. Mauro MJ, O'Dwyer M, Heinrich MC, Druker BJ. STI571: a paradigm of new agents for cancer therapeutics. *J Clin Oncol* 2002; **20**:325–34.

♦23. Griffin J. The biology of signal transduction inhibition: basic science to novel therapies. *Semin Oncol* 2001; **28**(5 Suppl 17):3–8.

24. Zhao S, Zoller K, Masuko M, Rojnuckarin P, Yang XO, Parganas E, *et al.* JAK2, complemented by a second signal from c-kit or flt-3, triggers extensive self-renewal of primary multipotential hemopoietic cells. *EMBO J* 2002; **21**:2159–67.

25. Gooding RP, Bybee A, Cooke F, Little A, Marsh SG, Coelho E, *et al.* Phenotypic and molecular analysis of six human cell lines derived from patients with plasma cell dyscrasia. *Br J Haematol* 1999; **106**:669–81.

26. Lemoli RM, Fortuna A. C-kit ligand (SCF) in human multiple myeloma cells. *Leuk Lymphoma* 1996; **20**:457–64.

27. Dorsey JF, Jove R, Kraker AJ, Wu J. The pyrido[2,3-d]pyrimidine derivative PD180970 inhibits p210Bcr-Abl tyrosine kinase and induces apoptosis of K562 leukemic cells. *Cancer Res* 2000; **60**:3127–31.

●28. Damiano JS, Cress AE, Hazlehurst LA, Shtil AA, Dalton WS. Cell adhesion mediated drug resistance (CAM-DR): role of integrins and resistance to apoptosis in human myeloma cell lines. *Blood* 1999; **93**:1658–67.

29. Hazlehurst LA, Damiano JS, Buyuksal I, Pledger WJ, Dalton WS. Adhesion to fibronectin via beta1 integrins regulates p27kip1 levels and contributes to cell adhesion mediated drug resistance (CAM-DR). *Oncogene* 2000; **19**:4319–27.

♦30. Liotta LA, Kohn EC. The microenvironment of the tumour–host interface. *Nature* 2001; **411**:375–9.

♦31. Rajkumar SV, Kyle RA. Angiogenesis in multiple myeloma. *Semin Oncol* 2001; **28**:560–4.

32. Vacca A, Ribatti D, Roccaro AM, Frigeri A, Dammacco F. Bone marrow angiogenesis in patients with active multiple myeloma. *Semin Oncol* 2001, **28**:543–50.

33. Munshi NC, Wilson C. Increased bone marrow microvessel density in newly diagnosed multiple myeloma carries a poor prognosis. *Semin Oncol* 2001; **28**:565–9.

●34. Bellamy WT, Richter L, Frutiger Y, Grogan TM. Expression of vascular endothelial growth factor and its receptors in hematopoietic malignancies. *Cancer Res* 1999; **59**:728–33.

35. Fong TA, Shawver LK, Sun L, Tang C, App H, Powell TJ, *et al.* SU5416 is a potent and selective inhibitor of the vascular endothelial growth factor receptor (Flk-1/KDR) that inhibits tyrosine kinase catalysis, tumor vascularization, and growth of multiple tumor types. *Cancer Res* 1999; **59**:99–106.

36. Laird AD, Vajkoczy P, Shawver LK, Thurnher A, Liang C, Mohammadi M, *et al.* SU6668 is a potent antiangiogenic and antitumor agent that induces regression of established tumors. *Cancer Res* 2000; **60**:4152–60.

37. Singhal S, Mehta J. Thalidomide in cancer. *Biomed Pharmacother* 2002; **56**:4–12.

38. Stephens TD, Bunde CJ, Fillmore BJ. Mechanism of action in thalidomide teratogenesis. *Biochem Pharmacol* 2000; **59**:1489–99.

39. Stephens TD, Fillmore BJ. Hypothesis: thalidomide embryopathy-proposed mechanism of action. *Teratology* 2000; **61**:189–95.

40. Mitsiades N, Mitsiades CS, Poulaki V, Chauhan D, Richardson PG, Hideshima T, *et al.* Apoptotic signaling induced by immunomodulatory thalidomide analogs in human multiple myeloma cells: therapeutic implications. *Blood* 2002; **99**:4525–30.

●41. Singhal S, Mehta J, Desikan R, Ayers D, Roberson P, Eddlemon P, *et al.* Antitumor activity of thalidomide in refractory multiple myeloma. *N Engl J Med* 1999; **341**:1565–71.

●42. Barlogie B, Desikan R, Eddlemon P, Spencer T, Zeldis J, Munshi N, *et al.* Extended survival in advanced and refractory multiple myeloma after single-agent thalidomide: identification of prognostic factors in a phase 2 study of 169 patients. *Blood* 2001; **98**:492–4.

43. Juliusson G, Celsing F, Turesson I, Lenhoff S, Adriansson M, Malm C. Frequent good partial remissions from thalidomide including best response ever in patients with advanced refractory and relapsed myeloma. *Br J Haematol* 2000; **109**:89–96.

44. Neben K, Moehler T, Benner A, Kraemer A, Egerer G, Ho AD, *et al.* Dose-dependent effect of thalidomide on overall survival in relapsed multiple myeloma. *Clin Cancer Res* 2002; **8**:3377–82.

45. Durie BG, Stephen AG. Low dose thalidomide alone and in combination: Long term follow-up. *Blood* 2001; **98**:163a.

♦46. Cavenagh JD, Oakervee H. Guideline: thalidomide in multiple myeloma: current status and future prospects. *Br J Haematol* 2003; **120**:18–26.

●47. Zangari M, Anaissie E, Barlogie B, Badros A, Desikan R, Gopal AV, *et al.* Increased risk of deep-vein thrombosis in patients with multiple myeloma receiving thalidomide and chemotherapy. *Blood* 2001; **98**:1614–15.

48. Zangari M, Siegel E, Barlogie B, Anaissie E, Saghafifar F, Fassas A, *et al.* Thrombogenic activity of doxorubicin in myeloma patients receiving thalidomide: implications for therapy. *Blood* 2002; **100**:1168–71.

49. Camba L, Peccatori J, Pescarollo A, Tresoldi M, Corradini P, Bregni M. Thalidomide and thrombosis in patients with multiple myeloma. *Haematologica* 2001; **86**:1108–9.

50. Cavo M, Zamagni E, Cellini C, Tosi P, Cangini D, Cini M, *et al.* Deep-vein thrombosis in patients with multiple myeloma receiving first-line thalidomide-dexamethasone therapy. *Blood* 2002; **100**:2272–3.

51. Escudier B, Lassau N, Leborgne S, Angevin E, Laplanche A. Thalidomide and venous thrombosis. *Ann Intern Med* 2002; **136**:711.

●52. Osman K, Comenzo R, Rajkumar SV. Deep venous thrombosis and thalidomide therapy for multiple myeloma. *N Engl J Med* 2001; **344**:1951–52.

53. Richardson PG, Schlossman RL, Weller E, Hideshima T, Mitsiades C, Davies F, *et al.* Immunomodulatory drug CC-5013 overcomes drug resistance and is well tolerated in patients with relapsed multiple myeloma. *Blood* 2002; **100**:3063–7.

54. Hideshima T, Chauhan D, Shima Y, Raje N, Davies FE, Tai YT, *et al.* Thalidomide and its analogs overcome drug resistance of human multiple myeloma cells to conventional therapy. *Blood* 2000; **96**:2943–50.

55. Rajkumar SV, Hayman S, Gertz MA, Dispenzieri A, Lacy MQ, Greipp PR, *et al.* Combination therapy with thalidomide plus dexamethasone for newly diagnosed myeloma. *J Clin Oncol* 2002; **20**:4319–23.

56. Weber D, Rankin K, Gavino M, Delasalle K, Alexanian R. Thalidomide alone or with dexamethasone for previously untreated multiple myeloma. *J Clin Oncol* 2003; **21**:16–19.

57. Portier M, Moles J-P, Mazars G-R, Jeanteur P, Bataille R, Klein B, *et al.* p53 and RAS gene mutations in multiple myeloma. *Oncogene* 1992; **7**:2539–43.

58. Corradini P, Ladetto M, Inghirami G, Boccadoro M, Pileri A. N- and K-Ras oncogenes in plasma cell dyscrasias. *Leuk Lymphoma* 1994; **15**:17–20.

59. Liu P, Leong T, Quam L, Billadeau D, Kay NE, Greipp PR, *et al.* Activating mutations of N- and K-ras in multiple myeloma show different clinical associations: analysis of the Eastern Cooperative Oncology Group phase III trial. *Blood* 1996; **88**:2699–706.

60. Hancock JF, Magee AI, Childs JE, Marshall CJ. All ras proteins are polyisoprenylated but only some are palmitoylated. *Cell* 1989; **57**:1167–77.

61. Willumsen BM, Christensen A, Hubbert NL, Papageorge AG, Lowy DR. The p21 ras C-terminus is required for transformation and membrane association. *Nature* 1984; **310**:583–6.

62. Sebti S, Hamilton AD. Farnesyltransferase and geranylgeranyltransferase I inhibitors in cancer therapy: important mechanistic and bench to bedside issues. *Expert Opin Investig Drugs* 2000; **9**:2767–82.

63. Cox AD. Farnesyltransferase inhibitors: potential role in the treatment of cancer. *Drugs* 2001; **61**:723–32.

●64. Alsina M, Overton R, Belle N, Wilson EF, Sullivan DM, Djulbegovic B, *et al.* Farnesyl transferase inhibitor FTI-R115777 is well tolerated, induces stabilization of disease and inhibits farnesylation and oncogenic tumor survival pathways in patients with advanced multiple myeloma. *Proc AACR* 2002; **43**:1000.

65. Cortes JE, Albitar M, Thomas D, Giles F, Kurzrock R, Thibault A, *et al.* Efficacy of the farnesyl transferase inhibitor, ZARNESTRATM (R115777), in chronic myeloid leukemia and other hematological malignancies. *Blood* 2002; **101**:1692–7.

●66. Bolick SCE, Landowski TH, Boulware D, Oshiro MM, Ohkanda J, Hamilton AD, *et al.* The farnesyl transferase inhibitor, FTI-277, inhibits growth and induces apoptosis in drug resistant myeloma tumor cells. *Leukemia* 2003; **17**:451–7.

67. Lerner EC, Qian Y, Blaskovich MA, Fossum RD, Vogt A, Sun J, *et al.* Ras CAAX peptidomimetic FTI-277 selectively blocks oncogenic Ras signaling by inducing cytoplasmic accumulation of inactive Ras-Raf complexes. *J Biol Chem* 1995; **270**:26802–6.

68. Prendergast GC, Rane N. Farnesyltransferase inhibitors: mechanism and applications. *Expert Opin Investig Drugs* 2001; **10**:2105–16.

♦69. Sebti S, Hamilton AD. Inhibitors of prenyl transferases. *Curr Opin Oncol* 1997; **9**:557–61.

70. Hallek M, Bergsagel PL, Anderson KC. Multiple myeloma: Increasing evidence for a multistep transformation process. *Blood* 1998; **91**:3–21.

71. Reed JC. Bcl-2 family proteins: regulators of apoptosis and chemoresistance in hematologic malignancies. *Semin Hematol* 1997; **34**(4 Suppl 5):9–19.

♦72. Strasser A, Huang DCS, Vaux DL. The role of the bcl-2/ced-9 gene family in cancer and general implications of defects in cell death control for tumourigenesis and resistance to chemotherapy. *Biochim Biophys Acta* 1997; **1333**:F151–78.

73. Pettersson M, Jernberg-Wiklund H, Larsson LG, Sundstrom C, Givol I, Tsujimoto Y, *et al.* Expression of the bcl-2 gene in human multiple myeloma cell lines and normal plasma cells. *Blood* 1992; **79**:495–502.

74. Harada N, Hata H, Yoshida M, Soniki T, Nagasaki A, Kuribayashi N, *et al.* Expression of Bcl-2 family of proteins in fresh myeloma cells. *Leukemia* 1998; **12**:1817–20.

75. Hamilton MS, Barker HF, Ball J, Drew M, Abbot SD, Franklin IM. Normal and neoplastic human plasma cells express bcl-2 antigen. *Leukemia* 1999; **9**:768–71.

76. Nishida K, Taniwaki M, Misawa S, Abe T. Nonrandom rearrangement of chromosome 14 at band q32.33 in human lymphoid malignancies with mature B-cell phenotype. *Cancer Res* 1989; **49**:1275–81.

♦77. Galderisi U, Cascino A, Giordano A. Antisense oligonucleotides as therapeutic agents. *J Cell Physiol* 1999; **181**:251–7.

78. Tamm I, Dorken B, Hartmann G. Antisense therapy in oncology: new hope for an old idea? *Lancet* 2001; **358**:489–97.

79. Waters JS, Webb A, Cunningham D, Clarke PA, Raynaud F, di Stefano F, *et al.* Phase I clinical and pharmacokinetic study of bcl-2 antisense oligonucleotide therapy in patients with non-Hodgkin's lymphoma. *J Clin Oncol* 2000; **18**:1812–23.

♦80. Adams J. Proteasome inhibition in cancer: development of PS-341. *Semin Oncol* 2001; **28**:613–19.

●81. Teicher BA, Ara G, Herbst R, Palombella VJ, Adams J. The proteasome inhibitor PS-341 in cancer therapy. *Clin Cancer Res* 1999; **5**:2638–45.

82. Adams J, Behnke M, Chen S, Cruickshank AA, Dick LR, Grenier L, *et al.* Potent and selective inhibitors of the proteasome: dipeptidyl boronic acids. *Bioorg Med Chem Lett* 1998; **8**:333–8.

83. Dalton WS, Durie BGM, Alberts DS, Gerlach JH, Cress AE. Characterization of a new drug resistant human myeloma cell line that expresses P-glycoprotein. *Cancer Res* 1986; **46**:5125–30.

84. Bellamy WT, Dalton WS, Gleason MC, Grogan TM, Trent JM. Development and characterization of a melphalan resistant human multiple myeloma cell line. *Cancer Res* 1992; **51**:995–1002.

♦85. Damiano JS, Dalton WS. Integrin-mediated drug resistance in multiple myeloma. *Leuk Lymphoma* 2000; **38**:71–81.

86. Berenson JR, Ma HM, Vescio R. The role of nuclear factor-kappaB in the biology and treatment of multiple myeloma. *Semin Oncol* 2001; **28**:626–33.

87. Cusack JC Jr, Liu R, Houston M, Abendroth K, Elliott PJ, Adams J, *et al.* Enhanced chemosensitivity to CPT-11 with proteasome inhibitor PS-341: implications for systemic nuclear factor-kappaB inhibition. *Cancer Res* 2001; **61**:3535–40.

88. An WG, Hwang SG, Trepel JB, Blagosklonny MV. Protease inhibitor-induced apoptosis: accumulation of wt p53, p21WAF1/CIP1, and induction of apoptosis are independent markers of proteasome inhibition. *Leukemia* 2000; **14**:1276–83.

●89. Frankel A, Man S, Elliott PJ, Adams J, Kerbel RS. Lack of multicellular drug resistance observed in human ovarian and prostate carcinoma treated with the proteasome inhibitor PS-341. *Clin Cancer Res* 2000; **6**:3719–928.

90. Richardson PG, Barlogie B, Berenson J, Singhal S, Jagannath S, Irwin D, *et al.* A phase 2 study of bortezomib in relapsed, refractory myeloma. *N Engl J Med* 2003; **348**:2609–17.

91. Hideshima T, Richardson P, Chauhan D, Palombella VJ, Elliott PJ, Adams J, *et al.* The proteasome inhibitor PS-341 inhibits growth, induces apoptosis, and overcomes drug resistance in human multiple myeloma cells. *Cancer Res* 2001; **61**:3071–6.

92. Abbaszadegan MR, Cress AE, Futscher BW, Bellamy WT, Dalton WS. Evidence for cytoplasmic P-glycoprotein location associated with increased multidrug resistance and resistance to chemosensitizers. *Cancer Res* 1996; **56**:5435–42.

20

Immunotherapeutic approaches

HÅKAN MELLSTEDT

INTRODUCTION

Both active and passive immunotherapeutic approaches can be used for treatment of malignant diseases, including myeloma. Active immunotherapy might be effective in myeloma as evidenced by the graft versus myeloma (GvM) effect of allogeneic transplantation (see Chapter 17), and immunization has shown clinical benefit in hematological malignancies (e.g. non-Hodgkin's lymphoma, chronic lymphocytic leukemia) as well as in solid tumors (e.g. colorectal carcinoma, melanoma). Moreover, the patient's immune system might also spontaneously recognize myeloma cell-associated structures, such as the idiotypic protein and the cancer testis antigen sperm protein 17 (see later).

Tumor cells express tumor-associated protein antigen molecules on the cell surface as well as peptides of the protein presented in the groove of MHC complexes. Although the vast majority of tumor antigens are shared self-antigens, operationally these structures can be regarded as tumor-specific antigens and used as targets for immunotherapy.

The tumor clone in multiple myeloma consists of plasma cells and clonogenic B lymphocytoid precursors. Plasma cells usually express only MHC class I molecules on their surface, while B lymphocytes exhibit both MHC class I and class II antigens. In myeloma, clone-specific idiotypic immunoglobulin structures are expressed on the surface membrane of the malignant tumor cells and these structures might be an ideal antigen for targeting.[1] Idiotypic immunoglobulin molecules (Fig. 20.1) are

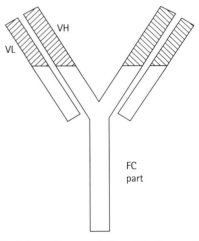

Figure 20.1 *Schematic presentation of the tumor-derived immunoglobulin molecule in myeloma. Hatched areas indicate the V-region, the idiotypic region. VL, variable region of the light chain; VH, variable region of the heavy chain; FC part, biological active part of the immunoglobulin molecule.*

unique antigens, which are normally involved in immune regulation. The protein is expressed as a complete molecule on the surface of B cells but also as peptides in the grooves of MHC class I and II molecules. Other surface antigens exhibited as membrane-bound molecules or as peptides in the context of MHC molecules in multiple myeloma may also be considered for targeting in an immunological therapeutic approach. These include MAGE-1, sperm-17, the interleukin-6 (IL-6) receptor, and B-cell-associated CD antigens.

PRINCIPLES OF IMMUNOTHERAPY

There are two major forms of immunotherapy, specific and non-specific. In the non-specific approach, immune effector cells, which specifically recognize tumor cells not via MHC restriction but through evolutionary conserved recognition receptors, could be activated to kill the tumor cells. These include natural killer (NK) cells, monocytes, and neutrophils, which act through various soluble factors released from activated cells. These cells may be activated by, for example, cytokines such as IL-2 and granulocyte–macrophage colony-stimulating factor (GM-CSF). The specific approach involves activation of immune effectors, which specifically recognize and bind to tumor-associated antigens on tumor cells, resulting in cell death. It is becoming clear that an effective antitumor immunity depends on activation of both arms of the immune system, humoral and cellular.

There are two major forms of specific immunotherapy: active immunotherapy (tumor vaccination) and passive immunotherapy (e.g. monoclonal antibodies). Unconjugated monoclonal antibodies induce tumor cell death by activating various immune functions, such as ADCC (antibody-dependent cellular cytotoxicity), CDC (complement-dependent cytotoxicity), and the induction of an idiotypic network response, resulting in a tumor-specific humoral and cellular immunity. Depending on the nature of the target, antibodies can also induce apoptosis, cell-cycle arrest, inhibition of proliferation, and bystander killing through a local inflammatory response with release of pro-inflammatory cytokines from activated cells, e.g. monocytes, neutrophils, and NK cells. Antibodies can also be used as carriers of cytotoxic substances.

When a tumor-derived antigen is used for vaccination of patients (Fig. 20.2), the antigen is taken up, processed, and presented on MHC molecules of antigen presenting cells (APCs) – dendritic cells (DCs), monocytes/macrophages, and B lymphocytes. The most effective are DCs. Immature DCs take up and process the antigen. DCs have then to be activated by cytokines, mainly GM-CSF, IL-4, tumor necrosis factor α (TNFα), and IL-12, to present the antigen and initiate an immune response. Exogenous antigens may use both the class II and class I antigen presentation pathways. After degradation in the endosomes, the peptides are bound to MHC class II molecule complexes and then transported to the cell surface. Exogenous antigens may, however, also enter proteasomes using the ubiquitin system. Processed peptides are transported to the endoplasmatic reticulum, where they bind to MHC class I complexes, which are then transported to the surface of APCs. This process seems to be facilitated by GM-CSF.[2] Thus, both MHC class II-restricted (CD4) helper T cells and MHC class I-restricted cytotoxic (CD8) T lymphocytes can be induced when tumor antigens are used for

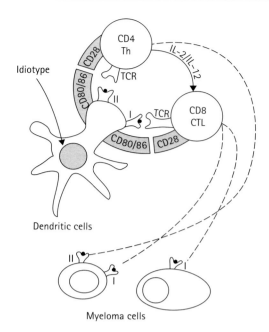

Figure 20.2 *Schematic presentation of the principle of idiotype vaccination. The idiotype is brought by various means to be taken up in vivo or ex vivo by dendritic cells (DCs). The idiotype is then presented on MHC class I and II molecules of DCs. Specific CD4 T cells interact with MHC class II molecules and start to produce cytokines, including interleukin (IL)-2 and IL-12. These cytokines activate CD8 cells that have specifically recognized idiotypes on MHC class I molecules on DCs. Idiotype-specific CD4 and CD8 cells can then bind specifically to myeloma cells expressing class II and class I molecules, respectively, and kill the myeloma cells. CTL, cytotoxic T lymphocytes; TCR, T-cell receptor; Th, T helper.*

vaccination. Both these types of T-cell population are mandatory for the induction of a fully competent and effective antitumor response. Consequently, the immunogen should contain T-helper (Th) epitopes as well as cytotoxic T lymphocytes (CTLs) epitopes. Th_1 cells are instrumental in inducing a CD8 CTL response and are also able to induce humoral immunity by switching to a Th_2 response. Helper T cells are essential to maintain a memory response. Furthermore, Th_1 and Th_2 cells might themselves also mediate tumor cell killing. Th_1 cells have been shown to lyze tumor cells directly and to produce interferon-γ, which activates monocytes to release nitrogen oxide and hydrogen superoxide, which are toxic to tumor cells. Upon antigen-specific activation, Th_2 cells secrete IL-5, which stimulates eosinophils to produce molecules toxic for the tumor cells.[3]

To induce an effective immune response, adjuvants have to be added. Several adjuvants for human use are available. These can be chemical compounds, products derived from various microorganisms, and cytokines. Low-dose

GM-CSF seems to be a key cytokine for the induction of an immune response.[4] GM-CSF activates APC, upregulates MHC complexes and co-stimulatory molecules, promotes migration to the local lymph nodes, where the immune response is initiated. Other important cytokines are IL-2 and IL-12. IL-2 expands T cells, and IL-12 promotes a type I T-cell response and amplifies the magnitude of the response. It is also becoming apparent that a more effective antigen-specific immunity can be elicited by targeting antigen to APCs via ligands for cell-surface receptors, such as mannose receptors, FcR, and chemokine receptors.[5–7] This might favor the use of complete idiotypic immunoglobulin molecules rather than the idiotypic region alone.

IDIOTYPE IMMUNIZATION IN ANIMAL MODELS

Eisen et al.[8–10] were the first to show that syngeneic BALB/c mice immunized with purified myeloma immunoglobulin proteins (obtained from mineral-oil-induced plasmacytomas (MOPCs) and coupled with complete Freund's adjuvant) developed a sustained humoral response specific for the idiotype used for immunization. Moreover, these animals were capable of specifically rejecting a tumor challenge with the parental neoplasm, but were not resistant to other MOPC tumors, thus demonstrating the specificity of this antitumor immunity for idiotype. A few years later, Jorgensen et al.[11] showed that immunization with MOPC-315 plamacytoma-derived light chains alone was sufficient to confer protection against subsequent tumor challenge. In this system, tumor resistance correlated with splenocyte proliferation in vitro, with no apparent antibody production.

Subsequently, the demonstration that immunoglobulin immunization can induce an idiotype-specific, protective antitumor immunity was reproduced in several myeloma, leukemia, and lymphoma animal models.[12–14] However, studies designed to elucidate cellular mechanisms of tumor resistance have yielded mixed results, as exemplified by the BCL-1 and 38C13 lymphomas, in which tumor protection could actually be transferred by mixing serum from immune mice with the tumor cells before challenge of naive mice, suggesting an essential role for antibodies.[13,15] Nevertheless, protection against a subsequent tumor challenge could also be reversed by treating immunized mice with depleting monoclonal antibodies against T cells.[15]

Additional insights into the role of T cells in the response against tumor idiotype have been achieved with experiments in which cloned, idiotype-specific T cells were used. Immunization of mice with light chains derived from MOPC-315 elicited MHC class II-restricted CD4+T-cell clones of both Th$_1$ and Th$_2$ subtypes.[16] When either of these clones was administered subcutaneously, together with a challenge of syngenic cells transfected with the cognate idiotype, each protected the mouse in an idiotypic-specific and dose-dependent manner. To mimic the in vivo situation more closely, wherein naive lymphocytes are able to interact with target tumor cells immediately following activation and in the complete absence of pre-formed antibodies, mice transgenic for the T-cell receptor (TCR) isolated from these T-cell clones were generated. Such transgenic mice were found to be resistant to challenge with immunoglobulin-secreting tumor.[17] Furthermore, in as much as the tumor was MHC class II-negative, an indirect mechanism of tumor cell neutralization was postulated.[18] Finally, the adoptive transfer of lymphocytes obtained from mice transgenic for the TCR into SCID mice, devoid of B cells, produced resistance to challenge with MOPC-315, thus demonstrating that such idiotype-specific T cells were sufficient for tumor resistance. Perhaps the best evidence for CD8+ idiotype-specific T cells has been provided by the unexpected finding of cross-reactivity of murine influenza virus hemagglutinin-specific T-cell clones against an epitope nine amino acids long and contained in the CDR-2 region of an immunoglobulin heavy-chain variable region of a myeloma.[19]

Kwak et al.[20] screened series of selected recombinant cytokines for their ability to enhance the protective effect of immunization with tumor-derived idiotypic immunoglobulin (Id) conjugated to keyhole limpet hemocyanin (KLH) in a murine model. It had been previously demonstrated that conjugation to an immunogenic carrier protein, such as KLH, was required to elicit protection against a subsequent tumor challenge in this model system.[14] For such studies, a single dose of Id-KLH was injected subcutaneously, followed by free recombinant murine GM-CSF, administered either locally as close as possible to the initial immunization site or systemically, i.e. intraperitoneally. GM-CSF was administered daily for 4 days, starting on the vaccination day. Fourteen days later, immunized mice were challenged with 10 000 tumor cells, i.e. 100-fold the minimum lethal dose, and followed for survival. All groups of mice receiving GM-CSF showed significantly prolonged median survival as well as an increased number of long-term survivors, compared with the groups of mice immunized with the Id-KLH conjugate alone. Moreover, GM-CSF injected locally, i.e. subcutaneously, was more effective than GM-CSF administered systemically, i.e. intraperitoneally, and a reproducible trend, approaching statistical significance, favoring lower doses was observed. The addition of human IL-2, murine interferon-γ, human IL-1α or IL-1β, or murine IL-12 by various routes, doses, and schedules of administration described by others failed to produce significantly augmented protection following tumor challenge, compared with a single subcutaneous immunization with Id-KLH alone in these studies.

The mechanism of the additive tumor protection conferred by GM-CSF was investigated further, and was found to be critically dependent upon effector CD4+ and CD8+ T cells, as demonstrated by the abrogation of protection in immunized mice after depleting either subset with monoclonal antibodies *in vivo*. This clear-cut requirement for T cells was not associated with any apparent increase in antibody response directed against idiotype, suggesting that the mechanism of augmented protective antitumor immunity by GM-CSF was dependent on the selective activation of the T-cell arm of the immune response.[20]

The prototypic Ig coupled with KLH does not induce efficient cell-mediated immune responses and antitumor immunity in every B-cell tumor model. New formulations of Id vaccines have been designed to streamline production of these individual vaccines and to optimally recruit appropriate effector cellular functions to elicit potent antitumor immunity.

The new generation of vaccines in animal models takes into account the fact that unique determinants of Ig are localized in two short regions designated as VH and VL (Fig. 20.1, p. 305). These fragments can be cloned from an individual myeloma cell and expressed as scFv (single-chain antibody, consisting of solely VH and VL fragments linked together in frame with a short peptide linker sequence), which usually retains all the unique features of the parenteral tumor-derived Ig. Recombinant scFv can be produced with a variety of fusion proteins in order to increase immunogenecity. An alternative and much simpler approach to produce Id vaccine is, however, vaccination with naked DNA.[21] Naked DNA vaccine requires only that the gene of interest is cloned under eukaryotic or viral regulatory elements into an expression cassette, which is then either injected in solution via intramuscular or intradermal routes, or delivered into the epidermis by particle-mediated bombardment of DNA-coated gold particles (gene gun approach). Animal studies have shown that DNA vaccines can induce both a humoral and a cellular response.

The first anti-idiotypic responses using DNA immunization were induced in mice by injection of human V genes from B-cell tumors.[22] However, scFv is usually only weakly immunogenic in syngeneic mice. The immunogenicity can be increased by fusion of cytokines, such as GM-CSF, IL-4, and IL-2.[23] Moreover, a growing number of reports support the hypothesis that activation of innate immunity through evolutionary conserved recognition receptors is essential for the initiation of adaptive immunity.[24] Furthermore, optimal recognition of self-antigens (idiotypes) and induction of pro-inflammatory rather than tolerogenic responses may require activation of innate immunity by a danger signal.[25] Engagement of

pattern-recognition receptors induces upregulation of CD80 and CD86 co-stimulatory molecules and production of various pro-inflammatory mediators, such as cytokines and chemokines. Bacterial components, CpG motifs, etc. are major activators of innate immunity. An alert signal, fragment C of tetanus toxin (FrC) was successfully used to elicit Id-specific immunity.[26] To increase the immunogenecity of DNA-vaccine scFv can also be fused to chemotactic factors, which attract immature DC and elicit effector CD4 and CD8 T cells. This approach can generate antitumor immunity and eradicate established B-cell tumors.[27]

From animal models, it seems clear that the idiotypic protein together with appropriate cytokines (preferentially GM-CSF) can elicit protective and therapeutic immunity. DNA immunization with fusion proteins may even enhance the effector anti-idiotypic cellular responses.

NATURAL ANTITUMOR IMMUNITY IN MONOCLONAL GAMMOPATHIES IN MAN

T cells in monoclonal gammopathies

Although some studies have reported a relatively low number of blood T cells in patients with multiple myeloma and monoclonal gammopathy of undetermined significance (MGUS),[28] the total number of T lymphocytes was within the normal range in most studies.[29] However, a consistent finding has been a low CD4/CD8 ratio, which is most pronounced in patients with advanced disease. An increase in the CD4+/CD45RO+ subset (suppressor/inducer T cells) in MGUS[30] and a reduced number of these cells in multiple myeloma[31] have also been described.

The presence of activated (HLA-DR+) T cells in myeloma patients has also been reported.[32] These T cells produced large amounts of IL-2 and interferon-γ and were shown to recognize myeloma plasma cells *in vitro* after stimulation with CD3. Moreover, clonal expansions of CD4+ as well as CD8+ T cells have been noted.[33,34] CD8+ clonal T-cell populations were more frequently seen in patients with low tumor burden as compared with those with advanced disease.[35] The relevance of such clonal T cells with regard to recognition of malignant B cells is not known. In one patient, two large expansions within the CD8+ subsets displayed no reactivity against the idiotype. Idiotype recognition was confined to a small non-expanded T-cell population but with a monoclonal restricted TCR usage (TCRBV22).[35] In addition, T lymphocytes cytotoxic for autologous plasma cells have been reported.[36]

The susceptibility of T cells to apoptosis in patients with multiple myeloma has been analyzed by determining the expression on the cell surface of the Fas antigen and the intracellular exhibition of the bcl-2 protein.[37] The number of Fas+ cells was significantly higher in patients than in controls. Spontaneous and triggered apoptosis was higher in multiple myeloma patients than in controls and mainly restricted to HLA-DR+ T cells. An increase in CD8+/CD57+ cells with a suppressive effect on T-cell function has also been observed in myeloma patients.[38] Thus, myeloma patients appear to have an increase in suppressor T-cell activity and susceptibility of T cells to apoptosis. These abnormalities may contribute to an impaired T-cell function in patients with monoclonal gammopathies. Moreover, we have also recently shown that signal transduction molecules involved in T-cell signaling from the T-cell receptor to the nucleus are downregulated. Cytokine production is impaired. These dysfunctions are probably of importance in idiotype vaccination, i.e. patients with an impaired T-cell dysfunction might have a lower capability to mount an idiotype-specific cellular response. Measures should be taken to restore T-cell functions in vaccination protocols. This might be achieved by adding cytokines, e.g. IL-2.

Tumor-specific immunity

The presence of idiotype-specific (tumor-derived) blood T cells in patients with multiple myeloma or MGUS has been studied by activating T cells with the autologous myeloma-derived idiotypic immunoglobulin. We have observed that naturally occurring idiotype-specific T cells are frequently detected in patients with indolent myeloma or MGUS.[39] An idiotype-specific type I T-cell response (characterized by interferon-γ and IL-2 secretion) predominated in MGUS and early-stage myeloma patients, whereas a type II response pattern (IL-4 production) was seen preferentially in patients with a high tumor load.[40] Idiotype reactivity was confined to both CD4+ and CD8+ T-cell subsets as well as to MHC class I- and II-restricted T cells.[41] The median total number of idiotype-specific blood T cells in patients was calculated to be about $20/10^5$ peripheral blood mononuclear cells (PBMCs), corresponding roughly to 1/5000 mononuclear cells. The fine specificity of idiotype-reactive T cells was mapped using peptides corresponding to the complete CDR1–3 regions of the heavy and light chains as well as to MHC-restricted sequences of the CDR2 and 3 heavy-chain regions. T cells specifically reacting with peptides corresponding to each of the three CDRs of the heavy-chain variable part of the idiotype were found. Peptides corresponding to the CDRs of the variable part of the light chain of the monoclonal immunoglobulin or unrelated immunoglobulin fragments were not efficient in eliciting an idiotype-specific immune response.[42–44] Taken together, these studies provide convincing support for the existence of MHC-restricted idiotype-specific T cells,

which may target immunogenic CDR peptides in monoclonal gammopathies. Such T cells might be an important part of a naturally occurring, antitumor-specific immune response.

In addition, evidence of humoral immunity has also been detected using an ELISPOT assay for anti-idiotypic antibodies, especially in patients with MGUS and multiple myeloma stage I.[45] Such antibodies are most likely to bind *in vivo* to the tremendous excess of free circulating monoclonal immunoglobulin and may not be of importance for an immune defense against the tumor.

Antigens expressed by myeloma cells other than the idiotype might also spontaneously be recognized by the patient's immune system. Sperm protein 17 (Sp-17), a cancer testis antigen, has been shown to elicit naturally a CTL response in myeloma patients. Sp-17 is expressed in tumor cells from about 30% of myeloma patients.[46] This induction of natural immunity against a tumor-associated antigen is considered to be an indication that the antigen might be a candidate to explore as a therapeutic vaccine.

IDIOTYPE IMMUNIZATION IN PATIENTS WITH MULTIPLE MYELOMA

As indicated above, tumor-derived idiotypic immunoglobulin may elicit a humoral and cellular anti-idiotypic response, which conferred resistance to tumor cell challenge in animal models. A rewarding therapeutic approach might thus be to immunize myeloma patients with the autologous idiotype. A schematic presentation for the principle of idiotype immunization in man is shown in Fig. 20.2.

One of the first studies of immunoglobulin immunization in patients with multiple myeloma actually provided proof of principle for a novel strategy of successful transfer of tumor antigen-specific T-cell immunity from an immunized healthy donor to a recipient with multiple myeloma undergoing bone marrow transplantation.[47] The patient was a 43-year-old woman with progressive myeloma, which was refractory to VAD chemotherapy, and who presented with considerable tumor burden. Myeloma immunoglobulin protein was isolated from the plasma of the recipient. Her 47-year-old HLA-matched male sibling bone marrow transplantation (BMT) donor received two subcutaneous immunizations of myeloma immunoglobulin-KLH. In the recipient, after transfer of unmanipulated donor marrow, significant lymphoproliferative responses against the idiotype were detectable. Additional support for the demonstration of T-cell immunity transfer was provided by the successful isolation of CD4+ T-cells. The patient experienced only grade II skin graft-versus-host disease, which required and was resolved by corticosteroid therapy. Bone marrow examination on day 90 revealed no residual myeloma, and by day 220 a greater than 90% serum M-protein level reduction was recorded, which persisted for three and a half years. These encouraging results have led to the opening of several clinical trials to confirm the potential of marrow donor immunization in multiple myeloma. Results from these trials are not yet available.

The idiotypic immunoglobulin isolated from serum can also be used to vaccinate patients. Several approaches have been used. Idiotypes have been given together with alum or KLH as well as with adjuvant cytokines. Idiotypes have been loaded *ex vivo* on to DCs, which have been fused back or given as subcutaneous injections.

In our first reported study, five patients with stage I multiple myeloma were immunized with the autologous serum M-protein alone precipitated in alum. An idiotype specific T-cell immunity was induced in two of the patients, but the T-cell response was of a modest magnitude and of short duration.[48]

GM-CSF is a potent stimulator for the induction of a specific antitumor immunity (see earlier).[4,20] In our second series, therefore, seven patients with indolent multiple myeloma were immunized with the autologous idiotypic immunoglobulin (precipitated in alum) at day 1 together with 75 μg/day of GM-CSF subcutaneously at days 1–4. GM-CSF was given at the same site as the idiotypic immunoglobulin. The immunization procedure was repeated at weeks 2, 4, 6, 8, and 14. An idiotype-specific T-cell immunity was induced in five of seven patients. In four of five patients, predominantly CD8+ MHC class I-restricted idiotype-specific T cells were noted but CD4+ MHC II-restricted T cells were also induced. Epitope mapping revealed a reactivity against peptides corresponding to the CDR 1, 2, and 3 regions of the heavy chains but not to CDR peptides from idiotypic proteins of other myeloma patients. The magnitude of the T-cell response was higher and the duration of the specific T-cell immunity was longer compared with the first series, where no GM-CSF was given. In one of the patients in the second series, the M-component concentration was reduced by 65%. No other treatment was given.[49]

In a subsequent series, the adjuvant cytokine GM-CSF and IL-12 were added. A much higher amplitude of the immune response was noted. A total of 90% of the patients in the GM-CSF/IL-12 group ($n = 13$) mounted an idiotype specific antimyeloma clone T-cell response and 45% ($n = 13$) in the IL-12 group. One major response has so far been noted. However, in four out of six analyzed patients, a decrease/disappearance of blood circulating tumor cells was noted. These data indicate that idiotype immunity might only be able to eradicate minimal residual disease and should, therefore, preferentially be applied after cytoreductive therapy in patients in

complete remission with the aim to prevent relapse. This is similar to the results seen in follicular lymphoma patients immunized with the idiotypic protein when entering complete remission. Eleven patients still had circulating tumor cells after clinical remission induction by chemotherapy. Idiotype vaccination eradicated this population in eight of the patients.[50]

Another vaccine strategy is to use DC. DCs are potent professional APCs capable of presenting antigen (idiotype) in the context of MHC class I and class II molecules as well as of co-stimulatory molecules mediating signals necessary for T-cell activation. Although present in low numbers in the blood, DCs can be reproducibly generated *ex vivo* from their precursors by culturing in the presence of GM-CSF and IL-4. When pulsed with the tumor antigen *in vitro*, DCs have attracted attention as a promising adjuvant for vaccination. DCs generated from the blood of myeloma patients have been shown to have a normal functional capacity[51] and induce a stronger *in vitro* idiotype-specific response than monocytes, involving mainly type I T cells.[44]

In the first report, autologous DCs from one patient with myeloma were cultured *ex vivo* with GM-CSF and IL-4, and thereafter incubated with the idiotypic immunoglobulin. The idiotype-loaded DCs were then infused intravenously. An idiotype-specific MHC class I- and II-restricted T-cell response was induced and classical tumor-recognizing CTLs could be expanded from the blood. A 20% reduction of the serum M-component was noted.[52] There are several ongoing studies using idiotype-loaded DCs in patients in clinical remission after high-dose chemotherapy and in refractory patients. All studies have shown the induction of idiotype-specific T cells. In some cases, classical CTLs were generated.[53–55] It is, however, too early to evaluate the clinical impact.

A number of phase I/II studies are ongoing using the idiotype as the target structure. About 200 patients have been included. Various protocols have been used, including idiotype protein vaccination and idiotype protein loaded on to DCs *ex vivo*. In common for all studies is the use of GM-CSF. Patients in different clinical settings have been recruited: stage I, advanced disease or in remission after high-dose therapy (HDT), and peripheral blood stem cell transplantation (PBSCT). In the majority of the studies, most of the patients mounted an idiotype-specific cellular response (proliferation and/or cytokine assay). In 3%, complete response/remission (CR) was reported, 2% achieved partial response/remission (PR), and 11% achieved a reduction of the M-component concentration to less than 50% (unpublished data).[49,56] The 5% major responses were seen in patients with early-stage disease (stage I) or in remission after HDT and PBSCT. It cannot be ruled out that the major responses seen after HDT and PBSCT were the result of the intensive chemotherapy regimen. This problem can only be solved by phase III studies and a phase III study is ongoing exploring DCs loaded with the idiotype given as immunization in the maintenance phase.

Taken together, the results indicate that an idiotype-specific T-cell response can be induced in patients at an early stage of the disease, at an advanced stage, and after intensive chemotherapy. Several issues remain to be addressed in future clinical studies of idiotype vaccination in patients with multiple myeloma. The potential effect of large amounts of circulating antigens or induction of tolerance to idiotype should be considered in the design of vaccination trials.[57] This obstacle may favor the goal of administering vaccination in a minimal residual disease setting or very early during the course of the disease. The problem of circulating antigen underscores the importance of focusing on the induction of a T-cell response rather than antibodies, which may simply be blocked by the M-protein. However, idiotype-specific T cells may also be clonally deleted, causing a tumor escape of the T-cell immunosurveillance.[58]

Antigens other than the idiotype are also being tested. Isolated myeloma plasma cells tranduced with the appropriate cytokines, e.g. GM-CSF, might be an attractive alternative. Myeloma plasma cells expressing the whole repertoire of tumor antigens might induce a strong polyclonal rejection immunity. The sperm-17 protein (see earlier) is also in its early development.

Vaccination in myeloma has shown promising results. It remains to be seen which is the best immunizing structure: the idiotype, other tumor-related antigens, or whole tumor cells with the complete antigen repertoire (cell-based vaccines). Are ex vivo loaded DCs better than protein antigens themselves? Is DNA vaccination better than protein vaccination with the optimal additions? Which cytokines or other chemoattractive factors should be added? When the best vaccine has been identified, the optimal vaccination schedule and then the best patient population must be defined, which is probably those where maximum cytoreduction has been induced or very early during the course of the disease, i.e. in MGUS patients with a high risk of switching to myeloma. Ten years from now we might have a clinical vaccination protocol in routine use.

MONOCLONAL ANTIBODY-BASED THERAPY

There are a number of ongoing studies using monoclonal antibody therapy in patients with multiple myeloma but, at present, published data are limited.

IL-6 is an essential growth factor for myeloma cells. A mouse monoclonal antibody against human IL-6 has been used to treat 10 patients with myeloma. In several patients, an antiproliferative effect was characterized by reduction in the plasma-cell labeling index within the bone-marrow. One patient achieved a 30% reduction in tumor mass but no other patients had a significant clinical response.[59]

Many myeloma cell-specific antigens have been identified as targets for antibody therapy, including CD19, CD20, CD38, CD138, MUC-1, and HM1.24. In a phase II trial, a mouse monoclonal antibody against CD19 was used, coupled with blocked ricin to inhibit non-specific binding. CD19 is expressed not on the malignant myeloma plasma cells but on the putative clonogenic myeloma tumor cells appearing early in the B-cell ontogeny. Considerable side effects were noted, including elevation of hepatic transaminases, myalgia, trombocytopenia, nausea, vomiting, capillary syndromes, and neurotoxicity. No clinical effects were seen.[60]

CD20 is expressed in about 20% of patients with MM, often in a heterogeneous fashion, although its expression can be induced in vitro with interferon-γ. None the less, following the demonstration of a transient partial response to rituximab in a patient with relapsed CD20+ light-chain myeloma, rituximab has been evaluated in several clinical studies in myeloma. Rituximab was combined with melphalan and prednisolone (MP) in a study of patients with newly diagnosed myeloma, the rationale being chemosensitization and B-cell depletion in vivo.[61] Five of 22 patients demonstrated response to initial rituximab prior to the initiation of MP, four of whom had CD20+ plasma cells. The influence of rituximab on the achievment of CR following MP and progression-free survival can, however, not be evaluated. In another report, 19 patients with previously treated myeloma received single-agent rituximab.[62] Only one of 18 evaluable patients achieved PR and five patients had stable disease with a median time to treatment failure of 5 months. Five of these six patients had CD20+ bone marrow plasma cells.

On the basis that circulating CD20+ B cells represent the proliferative compartment associated with myeloma plasma cell overproduction in myeloma, rituximab has also been used as an in vivo B-cell 'purge' prior to the collection of autologous stem cells. This approach is feasible and is associated with prolonged B-cell depletion clinical trial.[63,64] It appears that rituximab had limited activity in myeloma. Interferon-γ may increase the expression of CD20, although its feasibility has not yet been demonstrated in vivo.

A humanized monoclonal antibody to the plasma cell antigen HM1.24 is in a phase I trial. No clinical information is yet available.

Angiogenesis is of fundamental importance for the growth of tumor cells including myeloma plasma cells in the bone marrow. Treatment approaches directed against neoangiogenesis is attracting great interest. A key function in angiogenesis is vascular endothelial growth factor (VEGF) and its receptors. A monoclonal antibody has been produced against VEGF, bevacizumab, which is

Table 20.1 *Summary of immunotherapeutic approaches in multiple myeloma*

Type of immunotherapy	Immunotherapeutics		Phase of disease
Active specific immunotherapy (vaccination)	Current studies	Idiotypic Ig protein coupled with KLH or alum; also idiotype loaded *ex vivo* on to dendritic cells. GM-CSF seems mandatory; other cytokines to be added are IL-2 and IL-12	Early phase of the disease, advanced disease, or in complete remission after chemotherapy
	Future prospects	scFv DNA vaccines fused with helper structures, such as tetanus toxin, chemokines, cytokines, defensins, etc.	
Passive specific immunotherapy (monoclonal antibodies)	Anti-IL-6 Anti-CD20 Anti-HM1.24 Anti-VEGF		Advanced disease

GM-CSF, granulocyte–macrophage colony-stimulating factor; Ig, immunoglobulin; KLH, keyhole limpet hemocyanin; IL, interleukin; scFv, single-chain antibody of VH and VL fragments; VEGF, vascular endothelial growth factor.

currently in testing for treatment of relapsed myeloma patients with or without thalidomide.

Although a number of monoclonal antibodies have been tested in human plasma cell myeloma and others are under evaluation, so far there is no effective antibody for therapy of multiple myeloma in man, such as exists for other B-cell malignancies like non-Hodgkin's lymphomas and chronic lymphocytic leukemia.

DONOR LYMPHOCYTE INFUSION

Donor lymphocyte infusion (DLI) has been reviewed extensively in Chapter 17. However, it is appropriate also to mention it in this chapter, as DLI is an immunotherapeutic approach with well-documented clinical effect. In patients treated with allogeneic stem cell transplantation, reinfusion of donor lymphocytes at signs of relapse induces a donor T-lymphocyte recognition of the myeloma cells via minor histocompatibility complex structures inducing myeloma cell death through the Fas/Fas L or granzym B/perforin systems.

CONCLUDING REMARKS

Immunotherapy of malignant diseases is an expanding therapeutic field. Multiple myeloma could be an ideal tumor for immunotherapy as the tumor cells express the unique idiotypic antigen in addition to other shared self-tumor antigens. A summary of ongoing immunotherapeutic approaches is shown in Table 20.1. Idiotypic vaccination can induce a relevant cellular immunity but clinical responses are so far limited. However, immunization in B-cell non-Hodgkin's lymphoma using the

autologous idiotype has shown encouraging clinical results, which might provide hope for myeloma patients. Therapeutic vaccination will probably be most effective in the minimal residual disease setting or early during the course of the disease. At present, there are no promising monoclonal antibodies. Given time, immunotherapy may become part of the therapeutic arsenal in multiple myeloma but, at present, immunotherapy in myeloma remains experimental and should not be undertaken outside clinical trials.

KEY POINTS

- Myeloma tumor cells express many tumor-associated antigens, including the clone-specific idiotypic immuoglobulin, which can be used for immunotherapeutic approaches.
- Myeloma cells express MHC class I as well as class II molecules, which makes them susceptible to attack by CD4 as well as by CD8 T cells.
- Donor lymphocyte infusion is a clinically well-documented cellular immunotherapeutic approach.
- Idiotypic myeloma protein is, so far, the most commonly exploited antigen for vaccination, but others, such as cancer testis antigens (e.g. MAGE, sperm protein-17), MUC-1, etc., are also being explored.
- The idiotypic protein, together with granulocyte–macrophage colony-stimulating factor or loaded on to autologous dendritic cells, can induce a specific T-cell response in the majority of patients. The reported clinical effects are so far limited but

15% of the patients seemed to have some kind of a clinical response.

- Improvement in the idiotype vaccination might be obtained by using a DNA vaccine consisting of idiotype scFv fragments and fusion proteins, which might elicit a better immune response.
- Idiotype immunization should preferentially be performed early during the course of the disease or in remission after high-dose chemotherapy.
- Measures should be taken to restore T-cell dysfunction.
- Large prospective clinical trials are required urgently.
- There is at present no clinically effective monoclonal antibody in the treatment of multiple myeloma, but a number of different target structures are being exploited, including CD20, CD38, MUC-1, HMI-24, IL-6, and IL-6R.

REFERENCES

● = Key primary paper
♦ = Major review article

1. Stevenson GT, Stevenson FK. Antibody to a molecularly-defined antigen confined to a tumour cell surface. *Nature* 1975; **254**:714–16.
2. Paglia P, Chiodoni C, Rodolfo M, Colombo MP. Murine dendritic cells loaded in vitro with soluble protein prime cytotoxic T lymphocytes against tumor antigen in vivo. *J Exp Med* 1996; **183**:317–22.
♦3. Pardoll DM, Topalian SL. The role of CD4+ T cell responses in antitumor immunity, *Curr Opin Immunol* 1998; **10**:588–94.
●4. Samanci A, Yi Q, Fagerberg J, Strigard K, Smith G, Ruden U, *et al*. Pharmacological administration of granulocyte/macrophage-colony- stimulating factor is of significant importance for the induction of a strong humoral and cellular response in patients immunized with recombinant carcinoembryonic antigen. *Cancer Immunol Immunother* 1998; **47**:131–42.
5. Engering AJ, Cella M, Fluitsma D, Brockhaus M, Hoefsmit EC, Lanzavecchia A, *et al*. The mannose receptor functions as a high capacity and broad specificity antigen receptor in human dendritic cells. *Eur J Immunol* 1997; **27**:2417–25.
6. Guyre PM, Graziano RF, Goldstein J, Wallace PK, Morganelli PM, Wardwell K, *et al*. Increased potency of Fc-receptor-targeted antigens. *Cancer Immunol Immunother* 1997; **45**:146–8.
●7. Biragyn A, Tani K, Grimm MC, Weeks S, Kwak LW. Genetic fusion of chemokines to a self tumor antigen induces protective, T-cell dependent antitumor immunity. *Nat Biotechnol* 1999; **17**:253–8.
8. Sirisinha S, Eisen HN. Autoimmune-like antibodies to the ligand-binding sites of myeloma proteins. *Proc Natl Acad Sci USA* 1971; **68**:3130–5.

●9. Lynch RG, Graff RJ, Sirisinha S, Simms ES, Eisen HN. Myeloma proteins as tumor-specific transplantation antigens. *Proc Natl Acad Sci USA* 1972; **69**:1540–4.
10. Hannestad K, Kao MS, Eisen HN. Cell-bound myeloma proteins on the surface of myeloma cells: potential targets for the immune system. *Proc Natl Acad Sci USA* 1972; **69**:2295–9.
11. Jorgensen T, Gaudernack G, Hannestad K. Immunization with the light chain and the VL domain of the isologous myeloma protein 315 inhibits growth of mouse plasmacytoma MOPC315. *Scand J Immunol* 1980; **11**:29–35.
12. Sugai S, Palmer DW, Talal N, Witz IP. Protective and cellular immune responses to idiotypic determinants on cells from a spontaneous lymphoma of NZB-NZW F1 mice. *J Exp Med* 1974; **140**:1547–58.
13. George AJ, Tutt AL, Stevenson FK. Anti-idiotypic mechanisms involved in suppression of a mouse B cell lymphoma, BCL1. *J Immunol* 1987; **138**:628–34.
14. Kaminski MS, Kitamura K, Maloney DG, Levy R. Idiotype vaccination against murine B cell lymphoma. Inhibition of tumor immunity by free idiotype protein. *J Immunol* 1987; **138**:1289–96.
●15. Campbell MJ, Esserman L, Byars NE, Allison AC, Levy R. Idiotype vaccination against murine B cell lymphoma. Humoral and cellular requirements for the full expression of antitumor immunity. *J Immunol* 1990; **145**:1029–36.
16. Lauritzsen GF, Weiss S, Bogen B. Anti-tumour activity of idiotype-specific, MHC-restricted Th1 and Th2 clones in vitro and in vivo. *Scand J Immunol* 1993; **37**:77–85.
●17. Lauritzsen GF, Weiss S, Dembic Z, Bogen B. Naive idiotype-specific CD4+ T cells and immunosurveillance of B-cell tumors. *Proc Natl Acad Sci USA* 1994; **91**:5700–4.
18. Lauritzsen GF, Bogen B. The role of idiotype-specific, CD4+ T cells in tumor resistance against major histocompatibility complex class II molecule negative plasmacytoma cells. *Cell Immunol* 1993; **148**:177–88.
19. Cao W, Myers-Powell BA, Braciale TJ. Recognition of an immunoglobulin VH epitope by influenza virus-specific class I major histocompatibility complex-restricted cytolytic T lymphocytes. *J Exp Med* 1994; **179**:195–202.
●20. Kwak LW, Young HA, Pennington RW, Weeks SD. Vaccination with syngeneic, lymphoma-derived immunoglobulin idiotype combined with granulocyte/macrophage colony-stimulating factor primes mice for a protective T-cell response. *Proc Natl Acad Sci USA* 1996; **93**:10972–7.
21. Wolff JA, Malone RW, Williams P, Chong W, Acsadi G, Jani A, *et al*. Direct gene transfer into mouse muscle in vivo. *Science* 1990; **247**:1465–8.
22. Hawkins RE, Winter G, Hamblin TJ, Stevenson FK, Russel SJ. A genetic approach to idiotypic vaccination. *J Immunother* 1993; **14**:273–8.
23. Chen TT, Tao MH, Levy R. Idiotype-cytokine fusion proteins as cancer vaccines. Relative efficacy of IL-2, IL-4, and granulocyte-macrophage colony-stimulating factor. *J Immunol* 1994; **153**:4775–87.
24. Medzhitov R, Janeway CJ. Innate immunity. *N Engl J Med* 2000; **343**:338–44.
♦25. Matzinger P. An innate sense of danger. *Semin Immunol* 1998; **10**:399–415.

●26. King CA, Spellerberg MB, Zhu D, Rice J, Sahota SS, Thompsett AR, et al. DNA vaccines with single-chain Fv fused to fragment C of tetanus toxin induce protective immunity against lymphoma myeloma. Nat Med 1998; 4:1281–6.

27. Biragyn A, Surenhu M, Yang D, Ruffini PA, Haines BA, Klyushnenkova E, et al. Mediators of innate immunity that target immature, but not mature, dendritic cells induce antitumor immunity when genetically fused with nonimmunogenic tumor antigens. J Immunol 2001; 167:6644–53.

28. Bergmann L, Mitrou PS, Kelker W, Weber KC. T-cell subsets in malignant lymphomas and monoclonal gammopathies. Scand J Haematol 1985; 34: 170–6.

29. Mellstedt H, Holm G, Pettersson D, Bjorkholm M, Johansson B, Lindemalm C, Peest D, Ahre A. T cells in monoclonal gammopathies. Scand J Haematol 1982; 29: 57–64.

30. Shapira R, Froom P, Kinarty A, Aghai E, Lahat N. Increase in the suppressor-inducer T cell subset in multiple myeloma and monoclonal gammopathy of undetermined significance. Br J Haematol 1989; 71:223–5.

31. Serra HM, Mant MJ, Ruether BA, Ledbetter JA, Pilarski LM. Selective loss of CD4+ CD45R+ T cells in peripheral blood of multiple myeloma patients. J Clin Immunol 1988; 8:259–65.

32. Massaia M, Attisano C, Peola S, Montacchini L, Omede P, Corradini P, et al. Rapid generation of antiplasma cell activity in the bone marrow of myeloma patients by CD3-activated T cells. Blood 1993; 82:1787–97.

33. Janson CH, Grunewald J, Osterborg A, DerSimonian H, Brenner MB, Mellstedt H, et al. Predominant T cell receptor V gene usage in patients with abnormal clones of B cells. Blood 1991; 77:1776–80.

34. Moss P, Gillespie G, Frodsham P, Bell J, Reyburn H. Clonal populations of CD4+ and CD8+ T cells in patients with multiple myeloma and paraproteinemia. Blood 1996; 87:3297–306.

35. Halapi E, Werner A, Wahlstrom J, Osterborg A, Jeddi-Tehrani M, Yi, Q, et al. T cell repertoire in patients with multiple myeloma and monoclonal gammopathy of undetermined significance: clonal CD8+ T cell expansions are found preferentially in patients with a low tumor burden. Eur J Immunol 1997; 27:2245–52.

36. Paglieroni T, MacKenzie MR. In vitro cytotoxic response to human myeloma plasma cells by peripheral blood leukocytes from patients with multiple myeloma and benign monoclonal gammopathy. Blood 1979; 54:226–37.

37. Massaia M, Borrione P, Attisano C, Barral P, Beggiato E, Montacchini L, et al. Dysregulated Fas and Bcl-2 expression leading to enhanced apoptosis in T cells of multiple myeloma patients. Blood 1995; 85:3679–87.

38. Frassanito MA, Silvestris F, Cafforio P, Dammacco F. CD8+/CD57 cells and apoptosis suppress T-cell functions in multiple myeloma. Br J Haematol 1998; 100:469–77.

●39. Osterborg A, Yi Q, Bergenbrant S, Holm G, Lefvert AK, Mellstedt H. Idiotype-specific T cells in multiple myeloma stage I: an evaluation by four different functional tests. Br J Haematol 1995; 89:110–6.

40. Yi Q, Osterborg A, Bergenbrant S, Mellstedt H, Holm G, Lefvert AK. Idiotype-reactive T-cell subsets and tumour

load in monoclonal gammopathies. Blood 1995; 86:3043–9.

41. Yi Q, Eriksson I, He W, Holm G, Mellstedt H, Osterborg A. Idiotype-specific T lymphocytes in monoclonal gammopathies: evidence for the presence of CD4+ and CD8+ subsets. Br J Haematol 1997; 96:338–45.

42. Fagerberg J, Yi Q, Gigliotti D, Harmenberg U, Ruden U, Persson B, et al. T-cell-epitope mapping of the idiotypic monoclonal IgG heavy and light chains in multiple myeloma. Int J Cancer 1999; 80:671–80.

43. Wen YJ, Ling M, Lim SH. Immunogenicity and cross-reactivity with idiotypic IgA of VH CDR3 peptide in multiple myeloma. Br J Haematol 1998; 100:464–8.

44. Dabadghao S, Bergenbrant S, Anton D, He W, Holm G, Yi Q. Anti-idiotypic T-cell activation in multiple myeloma induced by M-component fragments presented by dendritic cells. Br J Haematol 1998; 100:647–54.

45. Bergenbrant S, Osterborg A, Holm G, Mellstedt H, Lefvert AK. Anti-idiotypic antibodies in patients with monoclonal gammopathies: relation to the tumour load. Br J Haematol 1991; 78:66–70.

●46. Chiriva-Internati M, Wang Z, Salati E, Bumm K, Barlogie B, Lim SH. Sperm protein 17 (Sp17) is a suitable target for immunotherapy of multiple myeloma. Blood 2002; 100:961–5.

●47. Kwak LW, Taub DD, Duffey PL, Bensinger WI, Bryant EM, Reynolds CW, et al. Transfer of myeloma idiotype-specific immunity from an actively immunised marrow donor. Lancet 1995; 345:1016–20.

●48. Bergenbrant S, Yi Q, Osterborg A, Bjorkholm M, Osby E, Mellstedt H, et al. Modulation of anti-idiotypic immune response by immunization with the autologous M-component protein in multiple myeloma patients. Br J Haematol 1996; 92:840–6.

●49. Osterborg A, Yi Q, Henriksson L, Fagerberg J, Bergenbrant S, Jeddi-Tehrani M, et al. Idiotype immunization combined with granulocyte–macrophage colony-stimulating factor in myeloma patients induced type I, major histocompatibility complex-restricted, CD8- and CD4-specific T-cell responses. Blood 1998; 91:2459–66.

●50. Bendandi M, Gocke CD, Kobrin CB, Benko FA, Sternas LA, Pennington R, et al. Complete molecular remissions induced by patient-specific vaccination plus granulocyte-monocyte colony-stimulating factor against lymphoma. Nat Med 1999; 5:1171–7.

51. Wen YJ, Ling M, Bailey-Wood, R, Lim SH. Idiotypic protein-pulsed adherent peripheral blood mononuclear cell-derived dendritic cells prime immune system in multiple myeloma. Clin Cancer Res 1998; 4:957–62.

52. Liso A, Stockerl-Goldstein KE, Reichardt VL, Okada CY, Benike CJ, Engelman EG, et al. Idiotype vaccination using dendritic cells after autologous peripheral blood progenitor cell trans-plantation for multipla myeloma. Blood 1998; 92(Suppl 1): Abstract 428, p105a.

●53. Reichard VL, Okada CY, Liso A, Benike CJ, Stockerl-Goldste in KE, Engleman E, et al. Idiotype vaccination using dendritic cells after autologous peripheral blood stem cell transplantation for multiple myelom – a feasibility study. Blood 1999; 93:2411–9.

54. Liso A, Stockerl-Goldstein KE, Auffermann-Gretzinger S, Benike C, Reichardt V, van Beckhoven A, et al. Idiotype

vaccination using dendritic cells after autologous peripheral blood progenitor cell transplantation for multiple myeloma. *Biol Blood Marrow Transplant* 2000; **6**:621-7.

55. Lim SH, Bailey-Wood R. Idiotypic protein-pulsed dendritic cell vaccination in multiple myeloma. *Int J Cancer* 1999; **83**:215-22.

◆56. Adelchi Ruffini P, Neelapu SS, Kwak LW, Biragyn A. Idiotypic vaccination for B-cell malignancies as a model for therapeutic cancer vaccines: from prototype protein to second generation vaccines. *Trends Hematol Oncol* 2002; **87**:989-1001.

●57. Bogen B. Peripheral T cell tolerance as a tumor escape mechanism: deletion of CD4+ T cells specific for a monoclonal immunoglobulin idiotype secreted by a plasmacytoma. *Eur J Immunol* 1996; **26**:2671-9.

58. Lauritzsen GF, Hofgaard PO, Schenck K, Bogen B. Clonal deletion of thymocytes as a tumor escape mechanism. *Int J Cancer* 1998; **78**:216-22.

●59. Bataille R, Barlogie B, Lu ZY, Rossi JF, Lavabre-Bertrand T, Beck T, *et al.* Biologic effects of anti-interleukin-6 murine monoclonal antibody in advanced multiple myeloma. *Blood* 1995; **86**:685-91.

60. Grossbard ML, Fidias P, Kinsella J, O'Toole J, Lambert JM, Blattler WA, *et al.* Anti-B4-blocked ricin: a phase II trial of 7 day continuous infusion in patients with multiple myeloma. *Br J Haematol* 1998; **102**:509-15.

61. Hussein MA, Carma MA, Maclain DA, Elson P, His E. Biological and clinical evaluation of rituxan in the management of newly diagnosed multiple myeloma patients. *Blood* 1999; **94**(Suppl 1):331A.

62. Treon SP, Radji N, Andersen KC. Immunotherapy strategies for a treatment of plasma cell malignancies. *Semin Oncol* 2000; **27**:598-613.

63. Waples IM, Guaeltieri RJ, Hoon JK, Schreeder MT, Prasthofer ES, Heffelfinger R, *et al.* High dose chemotherapy in stem cell transplantation in patients with multiple myeloma treated with monoclonal antibody against CD20 prior to stem cell collection. *Blood* 2000; **96**(Suppl 1): 326B.

64. Cremer FV, Gemmel C, Witzens M, Moldenhauser G, Ho AD, Moos M, *et al.* Treatment with the anti-CD20 antibody rituximab as consideration therapy for patients with multiple myeloma after proliferate stem cell transplantation. *Blood* 2000; **96**(Suppl 1):298B.

PART 5

Complications

21

Management of bone disease

EUGENE V. McCLOSKEY

INTRODUCTION

Bone destruction and its clinical sequelae are a significant cause of morbidity in patients with multiple myeloma. Furthermore, despite progress in antitumor therapy and the use of more aggressive regimens, the incidence of skeletal disease remains high. Bone pain, pathological fracture, and hypercalcemia are all direct consequences of osteolysis, with compelling evidence that this bone destruction is mediated by normal osteoclasts (bone-resorbing cells) stimulated by factors produced by the tumor or by stromal cells in response to the presence of tumor (see also Chapter 6).[1,2]

The bisphosphonates are potent inhibitors of osteoclast-mediated bone resorption (for reviews see Fleisch[3,4]). At least ten bisphosphonates are currently available or in development. The newer bisphosphonates have markedly higher potency than earlier agents but current clinical data suggest that they may not differ in their ultimate therapeutic effect. The greatest experience in malignancy-associated bone disease has been gained with the bisphosphonates etidronate, clodronate, ibandronate, and pamidronate. These agents are now the treatment of choice for the management of hypercalcemia due to malignancy.[5–9] Their efficacy in this setting has prompted placebo-controlled studies to examine their ability to decrease the incidence of skeletal complications in malignancies, particularly breast cancer and myeloma.[10–21] This chapter focuses on studies addressing the long-term efficacy of bisphosphonates in multiple myeloma, but it also addresses the potential of new drugs for treating bone disease and the treatment of fractures, including novel orthopedic/radiological interventions.

THE BURDEN OF SKELETAL COMPLICATIONS IN MULTIPLE MYELOMA

Unlike solid tumors where bone metastatic disease is a relatively late feature, complications secondary to skeletal destruction are a prominent feature at the time of diagnosis of multiple myeloma.[17] The most common skeletal complications of neoplasia are hypercalcemia, bone pain, and fractures at both axial and appendicular sites. Some estimate of the incidence can be derived from the control arms of placebo-controlled studies of bisphosphonates in myeloma, which demonstrate vertebral fractures occurring in 15–30% of patients annually and peripheral fractures in approximately 10%.[22] There are obvious difficulties in extrapolating such data to the routine clinical setting, since selection criteria for studies can exclude patients with severe or mild disease, leading respectively to underestimation or overestimation of the incidence. Furthermore, the methods of reporting incidence are not uniform across the studies. Bearing these limitations in mind, the incidence of skeletal complications is high despite apparent responses to systemic therapy. Furthermore, multiple complications within an individual are common, so that estimates based on events per 100 patient years are usually two- to three-fold higher than estimates of incidence computed as the proportion of patients with events.

Irrespective of whether focal or generalized osteolysis occurs, the pathogenesis for increased bone resorption involves disturbances in the normal remodeling mechanisms. It is of relevance that the destruction of bone tissue is mediated largely, if not exclusively, by authentic osteoclasts rather than tumor cells directly, and this provides the rationale for the use of anti-osteoclastic agents, such as the bisphosphonates.

BISPHOSPHONATES

Although a number of studies have examined the effects of bisphosphonates in myeloma bone disease, many have only involved small numbers of patients or examined short-term efficacy and others have been open and uncontrolled studies. In the past 5–10 years, several randomized, placebo-controlled studies of bisphosphonates have been reported for the bisphosphonates clodronate and pamidronate. Two other double-blind, placebo-controlled studies have also examined the utility of oral etidronate in myeloma,[23,24] but this agent has never been licensed for this disease, largely due to the knowledge that therapy can lead to osteomalacia[25,26] and may even increase the risk of pathological fracture.[27] More recently, the first randomized, placebo-controlled study of ibandronate and an active treatment comparison study of pamidronate with zoledronic acid have been published.[28,29] The use of bisphosphonates, particularly of clodronate and pamidronate, is well established and has been the subject of a recent Cochrane Review.[30]

Clodronate

In the Finnish Leukaemia Group study,[10] oral clodronate 2400 mg daily was compared with placebo over a 2-year period in 336 patients with stage I–III multiple myeloma. Treatment was associated with a significant 50% reduction in radiographic progression of osteolytic disease (12% vs. 24% of patients; $P = 0.026$) and a 25% reduction in the incidence of vertebral fracture (30% vs. 40%; ns). The incidence of non-vertebral fractures and mortality was similar in both groups. It is now recognized that the administration of clodronate (800 mg three times daily) in this study was suboptimal owing to the effect of food on the absorption of bisphosphonates. Intestinal absorption is maximized if clodronate is taken with water as a single daily dose, and the rate of absorption and bioavailability is reduced to one-third when clodronate is taken after a fat-loaded meal.[31]

In the Medical Research Council (MRC)` VIth Myelomatosis Trial, over 530 patients with newly diagnosed multiple myeloma were randomized to receive placebo or oral clodronate 1600 mg daily in addition to systemic chemotherapy (largely ABCM (Adriamycin and BCNU given intravenously at a dose of 30 mg/m² on day 1, and cyclophosphamide 100 mg/m² and melphalan 6 mg/m² given orally on days 21 and 22 of a repeating 6-week cycle) regimen with or without prednisolone).[17] Treatment with clodronate was associated with a 50% decrease in the proportion of patients with severe hypercalcemia (5.1% vs. 10.1%; $P = 0.064$) and a similar reduction in reported non-vertebral fractures (6.8% vs. 13.2%; $P = 0.036$). Fewer patients receiving clodronate sustained incident vertebral fractures (38% vs. 55%; $P = 0.012$) and patients also lost less height over 3 years compared with those receiving placebo (2.0 ± 0.7 vs. 3.4 ± 0.7 cm; $P = 0.011$). The incidences of pathological fracture and hypercalcemia were consistently lower in the clodronate groups throughout 4 years of follow-up. No overall effect of clodronate on survival was observed but in a *post-hoc* analysis, patients without vertebral fracture at entry survived significantly longer on clodronate. In a recent report of extended follow-up, the possible effect of clodronate on mortality in this subgroup was confirmed with a median survival that was 23 months longer than in similar patients receiving placebo[32] (Fig. 21.1). It is important to note that, while this effect may represent a chance observation, it persisted following adjustment for other prognostic factors.

Pamidronate

The publication of the first report of a double-blind, placebo-controlled study by Berenson and colleagues had a major influence on the consideration of bisphosphonate usage by hematologists treating multiple myeloma.[13] In this study, 392 patients with stage III myeloma were randomized to receive either placebo or pamidronate

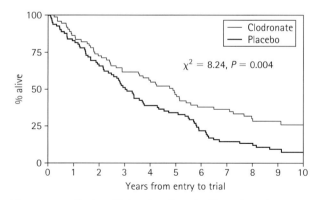

Figure 21.1 *Kaplan–Meier plot of survival in patients in the MRC VIth Myelomatosis Trial without vertebral fractures at entry/diagnosis. Median survival was increased by 23 months in patients treated with clodronate compared with placebo. The two groups were well matched for other prognostic factors, e.g. serum creatinine, bone marrow plasma cells, Durie–Salmon stage, and serum β_2-microglobulin.*

90 mg intravenously administered at 4-week intervals over nine cycles initially[13] but ultimately over 21 cycles of treatment.[14] Treatment over the first nine cycles of treatment was associated with a marked reduction (44%) in the incidence of pathological fracture (at vertebral but not non-vertebral sites), a 36% reduction in radiotherapy requirements to bone, but no significant effect on the incidence of severe hypercalcemia.[13] During the next 12 cycles, the incidences of pathological fracture and skeletal radiotherapy were similar or greater in the pamidronate group.[14] While the proportion of patients with any skeletal complication remained lower in the pamidronate group, most of this reduction occurred during the first nine cycles of treatment. Interestingly, survival in the patients with more advanced disease was significantly increased in the pamidronate group (median 21 vs. 14 months; $P = 0.041$ adjusted for baseline serum β_2-microglobulin and Eastern Cooperative Oncology Group (ECOG) performance status)[14] (Fig. 21.2).

In 1998, Brincker and colleagues studied the effect of oral pamidronate 300 mg daily (two divided doses of 150 mg) vs. placebo in 300 patients with newly diagnosed, previously untreated multiple myeloma.[18] Treatment was associated with a significant reduction in bone pain (0.58 vs. 0.80 mean events/year; $P = 0.04$) and a significant prolongation of the time to first severe bone pain (1003 vs. 565 days; $P = 0.005$) as judged by the investigators. However, there was no statistically significant difference in the number of pathological fractures (vertebral and non-vertebral) and requirement for surgery. These somewhat disappointing results may have reflected a relatively low incidence of skeletal events in this study combined with probable impairment of absorption of pamidronate due to the splitting of the daily dose.

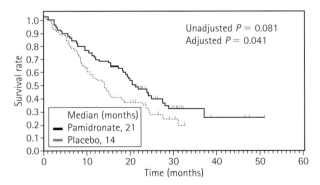

Figure 21.2 *Kaplan–Meier plot of survival in patients in the study of pamidronate in myeloma. In patients with stable disease on second-line or salvage chemotherapy, pamidronate was associated with a significant increase in median survival of 7 months compared with placebo. The difference persisted following adjustment for other prognostic factors (adjusted* P *value). (Reproduced from Berenson et al., J Clin Oncol 1998;* **16***:593–602.)*

Ibandronate

Ibandronate is one of a number of new, highly potent bisphosphonates that have entered clinical development. A short infusion or bolus injection[33] has been shown to be effective in the acute management of tumor-associated hypercalcemia.[8,34] Long term, it can be administered orally or intravenously, and the latter route has recently been tested in myeloma. In a relatively small study, patients with stage II ($n = 33$) or III ($n = 164$) multiple myeloma were randomized to receive placebo ($n = 99$) or 2 mg ibandronate ($n = 99$) as a monthly bolus injection in addition to chemotherapy.[28] Treatment was given for at least 12 months and up to a maximum of 24 months.

Ibandronate therapy was associated with significantly greater suppression of bone turnover as judged by biochemical markers, but the time to first skeletal event was similar in the two study groups (438 and 462 days for ibandronate and placebo, respectively). The proportions of patients experiencing complications were also similar (54% vs. 52%) and there was no difference in changes of bone pain scores or quality of life. Thus, a monthly injection of ibandronate 2 mg was ineffective in reducing skeletal morbidity in myeloma and it is likely that this simply represents a suboptimal dose. Certainly, 2 mg has been shown to be less effective in the acute management of hypercalcemia.[8]

Risedronate

Risedronate is currently licensed for the treatment of Paget's disease of bone (30 mg daily for 2 months)[35] and osteoporosis (5 mg daily).[36,37] In a small open study in multiple myeloma, 11 patients with bone lesions were treated orally with 30 mg/day of risedronate for 6 months, and monitored for an additional 6 months.[38] The treatment was associated with a marked suppression of bone resorption within the first week as judged by fasting urinary excretion of pyridinoline and deoxypyridinoline, markers of type 1 collagen degradation. The markers were reduced by 50% of their basal value at the end of treatment. In the absence of a control group, it is not clear how long the effect persisted for, but marker values were still 22% below baseline at the end of the follow-up period. A similar but, as expected, delayed effect was observed on markers of bone formation. Histomorphometric analysis showed a significant reduction of osteoclast number and erosion depth without mineralization defects. Spinal bone mineral density measured by dual-energy X-ray absorptiometry increased (5.3%) at the end of treatment.[38] To date, no published double-blind, placebo, or active controlled studies with risedronate have been published, but it may add to the choice of bisphosphonates for clinical use if appropriate evidence becomes available.

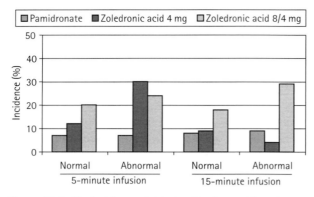

Figure 21.3 *The incidence of deterioration in renal function following intravenous infusions of zoledronic acid in patients with normal or moderately impaired renal function. Both 4 mg and 8 mg doses, diluted in 50 mL of solution, were associated with deterioration of renal function following infusions over 5 minutes. When infused in 100 mL solution over 15 minutes, the lower dose was comparable to pamidronate while the higher dose continued to cause problems. The dose was reduced to 4 mg in the 8 mg group, hence 8 mg/4 mg.*[29]

Zoledronic acid

Zoledronic acid is a new, highly potent bisphosphonate. A direct comparative study of long-term pamidronate with zoledronic acid has been published.[29] This study enrolled both women with breast cancer and patients with multiple myeloma. Patients were randomized to receive pamidronate 90 mg, zoledronic acid 4 mg, or zoledronic acid 8 mg. The treatments were given intravenously at 3–4-week intervals depending on chemotherapy schedules, and were initially infused over 2 hours in 250 mL of solution (pamidronate 90 mg) or over 5 minutes in 50 mL (zoledronic acid 4 mg or 8 mg). Two subsequent protocol amendments were required because of a higher incidence of deterioration in renal function in the patients receiving zoledronic acid (Fig. 21.3). The first amendment increased the infusion volume and time for zoledronic acid to 100 mL and 15 minutes, while the second required discontinuation of the higher dose (8 mg) and the use of the 4 mg dose in this arm of the study.

The trial was designed to show non-inferiority of zoledronic acid compared with pamidronate. Despite marked differences in potency, the incidence of skeletal events (excluding hypercalcemia) over the 12 months of treatment was similar in all three treatment groups (47%, 49% and 49% of patients experiencing events for 4 mg zoledronic acid, 8/4 mg zoledronic acid, and 90 mg pamidronate, respectively). The median times to first event were also similar (373 days vs. 363 days for zoledronic acid 4 mg and pamidronate, respectively) and there were no detectable differences in pain scores, analgesic use, or performance status. Zoledronic acid 4 mg is now the

indicated dose for prevention of skeletal complications in myeloma. Except for differing effects on renal function (see later), the side-effect profiles of zoledronic acid 4 mg and pamidronate 90 mg were also similar. The main advantage of zoledronic acid over pamidronate is the shorter infusion time (15 minutes) for zoledronic acid 4 mg. The fact that the same dose can cause renal impairment when administered over a shorter time period, particularly in the presence of pre-existing poor renal function, suggests that caution needs to be exercised during its administration in patients with multiple myeloma. It has been recommended that serum creatinine is measured routinely prior to each infusion.

Cochrane Review

In addition to the studies described above, the recently published Cochrane Review[30] also included data from the two studies of etidronate,[23,24] a small placebo-controlled study of clodronate,[39] and three small, non-placebo-controlled studies.[40–42] The meta-analysis demonstrated a highly significant reduction in the incidence of pathological vertebral fractures (25% vs. 35%; odds ratio (OR) 0.59, 95% confidence interval (CI) 0.45–0.78, $P = 0.0001$) during treatment with a bisphosphonate (Fig. 21.4). The reduction in absolute risk of 10% equates to a number needed to treat (NNT) of ten for vertebral fracture (i.e. for every ten patients treated with bisphosphonates, one patient will avoid a vertebral fracture).[30] In contrast, the meta-analysis did not show any overall significant effect of bisphosphonates on non-vertebral fracture risk (OR 1.05; 95%CI 0.77–1.44; $P = 0.7$). However, some heterogeneity was noted among the trials, with clodronate showing a non-significant benefit and pamidronate and ibandronate showing non-significant adverse effects. For the prevention of hypercalcemia, the meta-analysis revealed an incidence of 8% during bisphosphonate therapy compared with 10.1% in patients receiving standard therapy alone (control group), equating to an odds ratio of 0.76 (95%CI 0.56–1.03; $P = 0.07$) (Fig. 21.4). Difficulties in interpreting the effects on bone pain resulted from the different mechanisms of collecting and reporting pain data across the studies, but the meta-analysis suggested a reduction in incidence from 51% to 42% by bisphosphonate usage. Thus, on average, for every 11 patients treated with bisphosphonate, one patient will not experience pain.

Comparison across the different potencies of tested bisphosphonates showed no convincing evidence for improved efficacy for more potent bisphosphonates. The effects of clodronate and pamidronate were similar and either could be used, depending on the needs of the patient. The analysis is consistent with the conclusion that, if one uses an adequate dosage of any particular

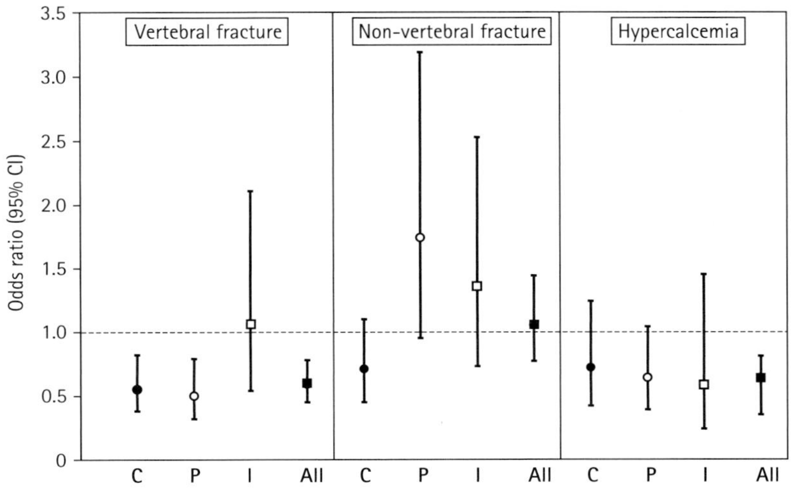

Figure 21.4 *Data derived from the meta-analysis of bisphosphonates in myeloma.[30] The effect of treatment with clodronate (C), pamidronate (P), and ibandronate (I), and for combined data from studies of all three bisphosphonates (All), are shown. Odds ratios below 1 represent a beneficial effect of treatment.*

bisphosphonate, then the efficacy will be similar and mirrors the results of the comparative study of pamidronate and zoledronic acid.[29]

It is clear that the results of the meta-analysis would have been even more favorable for bisphosphonates if etidronate had been excluded from the analysis. The recent guidelines published by the UK Myeloma Forum recommend long-term treatment with clodronate or pamidronate for all patients with myeloma requiring treatment for their disease, regardless of the presence or absence of bone lesions.[43] These recommendations have subsequently been updated (www.ukmf.org.uk) to include zoledronic acid as an alternative to pamidronate. This is in line with recommendations from the USA (American Society for Clinical Oncology; ASCO).[44]

Bisphosphonate side effects and safety

The inhibition of bone resorption by bisphosphonates consistently lowers serum calcium values, but symptomatic hypocalcemia is rare, usually only occurring in the presence of subnormal parathyroid activity,[45,46] abnormal magnesium levels,[47] or other concomitant therapies, such as aminoglycoside antibiotics.[48] In the presence of tumor-associated hypercalcemia, serum levels of parathyroid hormone (PTH) are suppressed but increase in response to the decrease in serum calcium caused by bisphosphonates.[49] In long-term therapy, serum PTH values usually increase slightly during therapy but long-term significant elevation of PTH does not occur.[29] The concomitant use of other specific inhibitors of bone resorption (e.g. other bisphosphonates, calcitonin, and mithramycin) has shown more rapid rather than more profound responses in patients with hypercalcemia.[50] Clodronate, pamidronate, and alendronate have been associated with transient rises in hepatic transaminases,

but the increases in adenine aminotransferase (ALT) and aspartate aminotransferase (AST) are not marked and rarely exceed twice the laboratory reference range.[51]

Unwanted effects of nitrogen-containing bisphosphonates include transient fever, bone pain, episcleritis, iritis, myalgia, malaise, and thrombophlebitis at the infusion site,[52-55] some of which appear to occur more frequently during zoledronic acid compared with pamidronate treatment.[29] They do not readily impair the mineralization of bone and pamidronate has not shown adverse effects on bone formation during oral use in myeloma.[56] Osteomalacia has, however, been reported after multiple high-dose intravenous therapy in Paget's disease of bone.[57] The use of pamidronate and other aminobisphosphonates is associated with a transient leukopenia during the early phase of treatment. Lymphopenia occurs more consistently than fever and is evident by 24 hours, followed later by a fall in neutrophil counts. The effect is usually transient and the clinical significance of decreases in subpopulations of circulating lymphocytes (natural killer cells, T cells, and CD4+ and CD8+ T-cell subsets) is not clear.[55] It is thought to represent an acute-phase reaction and is associated with the expected changes in serum zinc and in acute-phase proteins.[54] Finally, data from the Aredia study suggested that there may be a greater degree of bone marrow suppression in myeloma patients receiving long-term intravenous pamidronate with more frequent development or worsening of anemia (38% vs. 25%; $P = 0.017$).[14] While the oral administration of nitrogen-containing bisphosphonates is associated with an increased risk of upper gastrointestinal (GI) side effects such as esophagitis,[18,58,59] clodronate has only been reported to increase the incidence of lower-bowel side effects, with diarrhea being reported significantly more frequently during treatment.[17,21,60] The absence of significant upper GI tract side effects has led to the clinical use of doses of clodronate taken during the night when patients awaken for other reasons, a suggestion that may improve compliance but has not been formally tested.

Renal impairment

Renal impairment is a frequent finding at first diagnosis of multiple myeloma. This raises two questions about the use of bisphosphonates – does renal impairment require an alteration in the dose of a bisphosphonate and can bisphosphonate therapy have a detrimental effect on renal function?

Pharmacokinetic studies of bisphosphonates demonstrate that the clearance of bisphosphonate from the serum is dependent on skeletal uptake and renal function. There is some evidence that renal excretion of bisphosphonates includes tubular secretion of bisphosphonate, since the renal clearance of clodronate may exceed the glomerular filtration rate by up to 50% in experimental animals[61,62] and possibly also in man.[63,64] The elimination of bisphosphonates is reduced in the presence of renal impairment,[65,66] but this is largely offset by increases in skeletal retention of bisphosphonates in high bone turnover states, such as that seen in tumor bone disease,[64] so that the contribution of renal clearance to the total clearance of clodronate is decreased. For example, in malignant diseases affecting the skeleton, the amount of clodronate retained by the skeleton is found to be similar to that excreted through the kidneys.[64] Since the range of skeletal retention is large and dependent on the rate of skeletal turnover, adjustments in dose for moderate decreases in renal function are thought to be unnecessary.[64–66] In severe and endstage renal disease, there is only relatively limited experience with bisphosphonates and this has largely been restricted to short-term treatment of hypercalcemia[67] or severe parathyroid bone disease.[68,69] In patients requiring hemodialysis, intravenous clodronate has been administered either at the end of dialysis or 2 hours before dialysis, with the latter resulting in approximately one-third of the dose being removed during dialysis.[70] Long-term safety in such patients will need to be monitored closely and may even require histological assessments of bone biopsies, if skeletal disease appears unresponsive or worsens on treatment.[71]

Early in the development of the bisphosphonates, concerns were raised that intravenous bisphosphonates may impair renal function when given by bolus injection.[72] No systematic change in renal function has been reported during intravenous pamidronate or oral clodronate in multiple myeloma as judged by sequential measurements of serum creatinine. For example, in the MRC VIth Myeloma Trial, the number of patients showing improvements (serum creatinine decreased by 50 μmol/L or more) or deteriorations (serum creatinine increased by 50 μmol/L or more) between diagnosis and plateau were similar in clodronate- and placebo-treated patients. There was no difference if the changes were examined in those with baseline serum creatinine values less than or greater than 265 mmol/L.

Significant impairment of renal function was observed in the recent comparative study of zoledronic acid and pamidronate,[29] but it is not clear to what extent this was observed in patients with myeloma (Fig. 21.3). During the first phase of the study, both zoledronic acid 4 mg and 8 mg treatments were associated with a higher incidence of renal deterioration than pamidronate 90 mg. The effect was most marked in patients with mild renal impairment (serum creatinine $\geq$ 124 mmol/L) but it was also observed in those with normal renal function.[29] Increasing the infusion time to 15 minutes and the volume of infusion to 100 mL appeared to prevent renal deterioration secondary to zoledronic acid 4 mg, but problems persisted with the 8 mg dose, leading to its discontinuation. Care needs to be taken in routine clinical practice to ensure that the infusion time for the 4 mg dose is not faster than recommended. Regular monitoring of renal function is required, preferably before each infusion. The effects of zoledronic acid in patients with moderate to severe renal impairment are unknown and it should be avoided in these patients until further information is made available.

Costs of long–term bisphosphonate therapy

Long-term bisphosphonate therapy in multiple myeloma is commonly regarded as relatively expensive. Only two economic studies have been published, both of which have addressed the use of oral clodronate.[73,74] Neither study had access to information on quality of life to allow derivation of costs per quality-adjusted life year.

The use of clodronate in the Finnish Myeloma Study[10] was not found to increase treatment costs significantly in an analysis published by Laakso and colleagues.[73] They noted that the benefits of clodronate on the skeleton (a 50% reduction in patients with progressive osteolysis) were associated with a non-significant 12% reduction in hospital costs due to a lower requirement for hospitalization. The concomitant use of clodronate was associated with a 22% increase in overall costs of treatment (278 Finnish marks vs. 227 Finnish marks daily).

A more robust analysis of the costs of treatment with clodronate in myeloma was undertaken more recently,[74] using data derived from the MRC VIth Myeloma Trial.[17] Using a state-transition model for the first 4 years of the study and resource utilization data from trial investigators, the authors estimated the mean costs of each transition state and each skeletal complication. Clodronate was

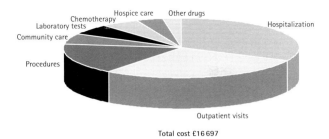

Total cost £16 697

Figure 21.5 *Breakdown of the costs of management of multiple myeloma. Data were derived from an analysis of subjects recruited to the MRC VIth Myeloma Trial.[74] Hospitalization and outpatient visits accounted for almost two-thirds of the total costs.*

found to reduce the mean costs of skeletal complications by 50% from £2860 to £1376 over the 4 years of treatment. The costs of clodronate itself increased the overall management costs by £3377 (from £19 557 to £22 934), an increase of 17%. This estimate was shown to be robust (£2605–£4150) by sensitivity analysis.[74] It should be borne in mind that the additional cost does not take into account any additional benefits over and above a reduction in the costs of skeletal complications, most notably any gains in quality of life.

Hospitalization is the major component of treatment costs in the management of multiple myeloma, accounting for 32% of the total cost of managing patients over the first 4 years following diagnosis[74] (Fig. 21.5). Additionally, outpatient and day-ward attendances accounted for a further 28% of the overall cost of managing patients, whereas chemotherapy accounted for only 5%. Therefore, treatment regimens that reduce the use of secondary care resources will minimize the increase in overall costs of managing multiple myeloma, even if they do not lead to cost savings. It is clear that the numbers needed to treat to prevent skeletal complications in multiple myeloma compare very favorably with the use of treatments as secondary prevention in other diseases, such as stroke reductions in patients with a previous stroke or transient ischemic attack.[75,76]

Reductions in the cost of treatment could be achieved if it was possible to target treatment at selected groups of patients with myeloma or if it was possible to define the optimum time in the course of disease to commence treatment. It is clear that long-term bisphosphonate therapy shows benefits when given early in the course of the disease[10,17,77] or at later stages in myeloma.[13,14] The progression of skeletal disease is probably at its most active at or around the time of diagnosis as judged by biochemical markers of bone turnover and the high prevalence of baseline fractures, despite a relatively short period of symptoms preceding the diagnosis.[17] These observations combined with the possible survival benefit

in patients with a lower burden of skeletal disease at diagnosis support the notion that treatment should be commenced as early as possible.[17,43]

The decision of if and when to stop treatment is also difficult.[44] It is important to remember that myeloma is presently an incurable disease and osteolysis will continue throughout its course. The speed of offset of the action of the bisphosphonates is unknown but is likely to be greater in malignancy than in other diseases associated with lower rates of bone turnover. At present, it would seem reasonable to continue treatment with bisphosphonates indefinitely. It is important to remember that the occurrence of complications is reduced but not totally prevented by bisphosphonates. The onset of a complication in a treated patient should, therefore, be regarded as an indication to consider more aggressive bisphosphonate therapy rather than to deem it a treatment failure and to discontinue therapy. The use of biochemical markers of bone resorption to monitor osteolysis and adequacy of response to bisphosphonates is undergoing evaluation and may improve clinical decision making.[78–80]

Bisphosphonate therapy and survival

It is important to state that none of the studies of bisphosphonates in myeloma have shown an overall improvement in survival.[30] Several studies have suggested that inhibition of skeletal disease may be associated with improved survival in certain subgroups of patients. For example, there was no difference in overall survival between the clodronate- and placebo-treated patients in the VIth MRC Trial, but in patients without vertebral fracture at entry clodronate was associated with increased survival (median survival 1362 vs. 1094 days; $P < 0.05$).[17] This effect has persisted with increased follow-up and following adjustment for other prognostic variables.[32] Intermittent pamidronate has been associated with improved survival in patients receiving second-line chemotherapy.[14] Similar survival benefits have been observed in subgroups of patients with early or late metastatic bone disease in breast cancer.[81,82] Finally, a 23% reduction in overall mortality has recently been reported in a large double-blind, placebo-controlled study of clodronate in women with primary breast cancer,[21] suggesting that maximum benefit can be obtained when these agents are used as early as possible in the course of the disease.

These potential survival advantages of bisphosphonates in subgroups of myeloma patients ideally require confirmation in appropriately designed clinical trials. Such confirmation may, however, not be possible given the unethical nature of further placebo-controlled studies in the presence of compelling evidence that bisphosphonates reduce skeletal complications in myeloma.[43]

CLINICAL UTILITY OF BIOCHEMICAL MARKERS OF BONE METABOLISM

The interaction between myeloma cells and bone cells, combined with the concurrent use of antimyeloma and antiosteolytic therapy, requires a means to monitor bone disease independently of tumor response or progression. Potential clinical roles of such measures would include the ability to measure bone turnover to determine the severity of disease and to monitor response to therapy. A variety of biochemical markers have been developed (see Chapter 6). In recent years, they have been used in large epidemiologic or clinical trials in patients with a wide variety of metabolic bone diseases, including osteoporosis and cancer.[83,84] However, analytical and biological variability remains a significant problem within individuals and it is difficult to translate the trial results into everyday clinical management.[84–86]

Several cross-sectional studies have correlated biochemical markers of bone resorption with disease severity. Urine excretion of deoxypyridinoline (DPD/DPyr) is significantly higher in myeloma than in monoclonal gammopathy of undetermined significance (MGUS) or control subjects, respectively.[87,88] In addition, urine levels of free DPD, total pyridinolines, and the N-terminal telopeptide of type I collagen (NTx) increase with greater degrees of bone involvement.[88,89] For example, mean values of resorption markers are significantly higher in stages II and III compared with stage I, and correlate positively with other markers of disease severity, including β_2-microglobulin, C-reactive protein (CRP), and osteolytic lesions.[87–89] In contrast, markers of bone formation in myeloma tend to be lower than values in healthy subjects, and correlate inversely with disease severity and bone resorption.[89] Thus, serum osteocalcin (OC; or bone gla protein, BGP) or bone-specific alkaline phosphatase (bALP) are significantly lower in multiple myeloma patients than in MGUS patients or healthy controls.[87,90] Within myeloma patients, both serum OC and bALP are reported to be lower in stage III disease compared with I and II, but these results are not always consistent.[87,89,90]

It is not yet clear whether changes in markers of bone turnover may be used clinically as early indicators of osteolytic progression or response to bisphosphonates or other therapies. Even in post-menopausal osteoporosis, where the markers have been investigated extensively, controversy remains over the possible benefit of monitoring individual patients.[91,92] There are very limited published data to assess similar use in myeloma. One recent study has shown that biochemical markers are able to demonstrate a reduction of high bone turnover rates present before transplantation to within the normal range following high-dose chemotherapy and autografting.[93] Several studies have reported changes in biochemical markers during bisphosphonate therapy. For example, in the Finnish Myeloma Study, serum markers of bone formation (alkaline phosphatase (ALP) and N-terminal pro-peptide of type I collagen (PINP)) and resorption (carboxyterminal telopeptide of type I collagen – ICTP) were both significantly reduced by clodronate therapy compared with placebo.[94] High baseline markers indicated a poor prognosis and suppression of the markers by clodronate was more marked in survivors than in non-survivors. Similar prognostic information with serum ICTP and other markers was subsequently reported from other small observational studies.[88,95,96] Studies of the relationship between bisphosphonate-induced changes in biochemical markers and clinical outcome are much needed. In a relatively small study of patients with osteolytic bone disease from a variety of cancers, treatment with intravenous pamidronate induced significant reductions in a wide range of markers, including urinary free pyridinoline and deoxypyridinoline, NTx, CTx (an assay for a different epitope on the carboxy-terminal telopeptide than ICTP), calcium excretion, and ICTP. Despite the reductions, not all of the markers showed significant correlations with outcomes including pain reduction.[97] In the ibandronate study, while there was no significant difference in the effects of treatment on changes in biochemical markers due to a wide variability within individuals, the bisphosphonate was associated with a highly significant increase in the numbers of patients showing a biochemical response.[28] Furthermore, patients showing a response in either serum osteocalcin or CTx had a significantly lower rate of skeletal complications (Fig. 21.6), suggesting that markers may provide useful information about the adequacy of suppression of bone turnover during bisphosphonate treatment.[28]

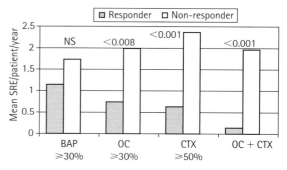

Figure 21.6 *Relationship between decreases in biochemical markers of bone turnover and the incidence of skeletal complications derived from the placebo-controlled study of ibandronate.[28] The patients (responders) in whom the bisphosphonate induced the greatest decreases in biochemical markers, such as osteocalcin (OC), carboxy-terminal telopeptide of type I collagen (CTX), and bone-specific alkaline phosphatase (BAP), experienced a significantly lower incidence of skeletal complications. SRE, skeletal-related events.*

Despite relatively promising results in groups of patients, uncertainties remain over the impact that biochemical monitoring will have on clinical practice. The recently updated ASCO guidelines have recommended that until these issues are resolved, the use of markers should remain within research protocols and they do not have a current role in routine care.[44]

NEW DEVELOPMENTS FOR TREATING BONE DISEASE

Recent advances in our knowledge of the factors involved in osteoclast proliferation and activity, particularly the interaction of receptor activator of NF-κB ligand (RANKL) and osteoprotegerin (OPG), have led to the study of new therapies, which are as yet in an early but promising stage of clinical development. These developments are described in more detail in Chapter 6 and will only be discussed briefly here.

Receptor activator of nuclear factor-κB ligand is an essential factor for osteoclast formation and activation and enhances bone resorption.[98–100] RANKL is also involved in mediating immune cell communication, dendritic cell survival, and lymph node organogenesis.[101] OPG functions as a soluble decoy receptor for RANKL and shares homologies with other members of the tumor necrosis factor receptor superfamily.[102,103] Myeloma cells appear to be able to induce an imbalance in the OPG/RANKL system in favor of bone resorption.[104–106] Furthermore, it is of interest that bisphosphonates administered to osteoblast cultures *in vitro* have induced increased expression of OPG, suggesting an alternative mechanism for bisphosphonate-induced anti-osteoclastic activity.[107] OPG itself has been demonstrated to be an effective inhibitor of bone resorption by preventing osteoporosis when administered to ovariectomized rats and results in osteopetrosis (increased bone mass) when overexpressed in transgenic mice. In contrast, reductions in OPG might be expected to lead to bone loss, and serum OPG levels in myeloma patients are apparently reduced compared with healthy controls.[108] A recent study in a mouse model of multiple myeloma showed that recombinant OPG could prevent the development of osteolytic lesions, preserve cancellous bone volume, and increase bone mineral density at several skeletal sites in animals with established disease.[109] A note of caution is required, however, as OPG has also been demonstrated to bind to and inhibit the apoptotic effects of tumor necrosis factor-related apoptosis-inducing ligand (TRAIL) on tumor cells,[110] an effect that may have a detrimental outcome on tumor cell survival and proliferation in myeloma and other tumors, including prostate cancer.[111,112]

Alternative strategies have included the development of an immune response to RANKL by incorporating a 'promiscuous' T-helper epitope into RANKL. This epitope forces the immune system to respond with antibody production to RANKL despite it being a self-protein. Such an approach has been shown to reduce bone loss in ovariectomized mice and in a mouse model of rheumatoid arthritis.[113] A different approach has been the use of a genetically engineered soluble form of RANK (RANK.Fc; Immunex), which acts as a decoy receptor and binds to RANKL.[114]

Both OPG and RANK.Fc have been shown to reduce overall tumor burden as assessed by skeletal tumor volume or serum IgG levels, respectively,[105,109,115] but it remains unclear whether RANKL is a facilitator of myeloma cell growth or whether the effect is mediated indirectly by other factors, perhaps altered by the changes in bone turnover. The latter may be supported by the evidence of survival benefits in some subgroups of patients in human studies of bisphosphonates in multiple myeloma.[13,14,17,32] Long-term studies will be required to determine the efficacy and safety of therapies that reduce levels of RANKL, or interfere with its binding to RANK. For example, RANKL plays an important role in both cellular and humoral immune responses by stimulation of dendritic cells, interference with which may lead to increased susceptibility to opportunistic infections.[116,117]

MANAGEMENT OF BONE PAIN

Bone pain is the predominant symptom in approximately three-quarters of patients at first diagnosis of multiple myeloma.[17,118] Alleviation of bone pain has a marked effect to improve the quality of life, even in advanced disease. Vertebral fractures are a major contributor to back pain, with increasing pain severity in those with multiple fractures. The management of bone pain depends on an accurate assessment to characterize the pain, its relation to the disease, and its impact on the patient's quality of life. Pain is inherently subjective so that the patient's perception should be the major driver to the need for interventions. Chronic pain is also frequently associated with other physical and psychological symptoms, particularly fatigue and psychological distress. Provision of adequate information to patients of their underlying disease processes and susceptibility to fragility fractures can help to modify behavior to decrease the risk of increased pain or fractures, and to improve adherence with therapy. In addition, adequate analgesia is obligatory with progression through the World Health Organization (WHO) three-step analgesic ladder for cancer pain (see Chapter 18). Finally, as myeloma remains an essentially incurable disease, palliative care should aim to improve the quality of life of the patient and their family throughout the course of the disease, and especially at the end of life. Effective treatment for pain is an essential part of this care and referral to specialists in palliative care is appropriate whenever bone pain is unresponsive to standard strategies.

Radiotherapy

When the bone pain is localized to specific areas, for example the spine or ribs, local radiotherapy is frequently used and may be very effective (see Chapter 15). Patients may get immediate pain relief following the first fraction of radiotherapy, but it is more usual for there to be an improvement in pain 2 weeks after radiotherapy, and improvement may take up to 6 weeks. The optimal radiotherapy schedules are those that give maximum short- and long-term benefit with minimum morbidity and disruption of the patient's remaining life. While pain relief is the most common treatment endpoint, any comparison of regimens is difficult owing to a lack of consensus in the methods for capturing this endpoint.[119] For localized bone pain, a single fraction of radiotherapy, repeated if necessary, appears to fulfill these criteria, but there are very few published data on which to base decisions about dose, frequency, and duration of radiotherapy in multiple myeloma. In a recent Cochrane Review of radiotherapy for the palliation of bone metastases,[120] only one study in myeloma was identified and it was not included in the final analysis. In the absence of controlled trials, several centers have reported their experiences with the use of radiotherapy. In a review of 59 patients with multiple myeloma and referred for treatment of painful bony lesions, pain relief was reportedly obtained in practically all of the irradiated regions with most lesions treated to doses of 3000 cGy in 10–15 fractions.[121] In the same series, patients with generalized pain due to multiple site involvement were treated with single-dose hemi-body irradiation, to doses of 600 cGy to the upper and 800 cGy to the lower hemi-body, respectively. The treatment was deemed to be well tolerated with minimal side effects. Experience with double hemi-body irradiation (DHBI) over a 6-year period was also evaluated by McSweeney and colleagues in 55 patients with multiple myeloma.[122] Of these, 42 had relapsed post-plateau and 13 were chemoresistant to initial therapy. Symptomatic improvement of bone pain was reported in 95% of patients, with one in five patients being able to discontinue opiate analgesics altogether.[122] Cytopenia was, however, a significant problem. Long bones are less frequently involved in myeloma but radiotherapy appears equally effective. Local recurrence appears to be uncommon (approximately ≤10%) if the symptomatic lesion plus a margin of 1–2 cm is irradiated.[123]

These reports suggest a possibly higher response rate in myeloma than in solid tumors with bone metastases.[120,124] Questions remain, however, regarding fraction size and the adequacy of one fraction for long-term control. If the conclusions from the Cochrane Review can be applied to the use of radiotherapy for bone pain in myeloma, then there is no evidence of any difference in efficacy between different fractionation schedules. Conventionally, treatment has been administered over one to five fractions but, in many patients, a single fraction of 8 Gy is adequate for pain relief.[125] In breast and prostate cancer, several radioisotopes have been investigated for use as radiopharmaceuticals in painful bone metastases.[126] In general, they are β-emitters with a short-range effect and are taken up at sites of new bone formation (either alone or attached to a bisphosphonate).[127] In contrast, there are very limited data on the use of radioisotopes such as strontium-89, rhenium-186, and samarium-153 for bone pain in myeloma.[128,129] There is a need for good-quality randomized trials to address some of the uncertainties related to radiotherapy use in myeloma and other malignant bone diseases.

Bisphosphonates

While radiotherapy remains the treatment of choice for localized pain, it is limited in the management of widespread pain or recurrent pain in patients who have already received maximal doses at affected sites. There is a substantial body of evidence that intravenous bisphosphonates are of value in the acute treatment of bone pain in malignancy, but many of the randomized controlled trials have not included patients with myeloma[130] or have only included small numbers of such patients.[131] Open studies suggest that intravenous bisphosphonates can reduce bone pain in myeloma[132–134] (Fig. 21.7). It has not been convincingly demonstrated that oral administration of bisphosphonates can significantly reduce acute bone pain,[135] but in long-term studies the incidence and severity of bone pain can be reduced.[10,17,30]

The rate of onset of the analgesic effect is similar to that of the inhibition of bone resorption, suggesting that the two effects might be related. In solid tumors with skeletal metastases, there appears to be a relationship between pretreatment bone resorption measured by urinary excretion of N-telopeptide of type I collagen and subsequent symptomatic response to intravenous pamidronate.[130] It is possible that bisphosphonates may reduce pain by other mechanisms. For example, in two recent studies using a mouse model, several bisphosphonates, including clodronate and pamidronate, have been demonstrated to have apparent central anti-nociceptive effects.[136,137] Further well-controlled studies are required to document the utility of intravenous bisphosphonates in the acute management of bone pain in multiple myeloma.

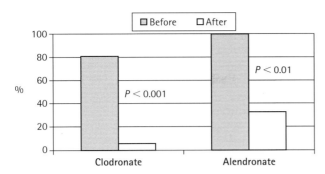

Figure 21.7 *Prevalence of bone pain before and after intravenous infusions of clodronate or alendronate in patients with myelomatosis.[133] Inhibition of bone resorption was associated with a significant reduction in bone pain.*

Table 21.1 *The Mirels scoring system to predict the likelihood of pathological fracture in cortical bone. The scores for site, pain, lesion, and size are summed, and scores greater than nine indicate the need for fixation to prevent an imminent pathological fracture. Scores less than seven are associated with a low risk of fracture (<5%).[142]*

Variable	Score 1	2	3
Site	Upper limb	Lower limb	Peritrochanter
Pain	Mild	Moderate	Functional
Lesion	Blastic	Mixed	Lytic
Size	<1/3[a]	1/3–2/3[a]	>2/3[a]

[a] Refers to the proportion (on a radiograph) of a single cortical layer destroyed.

MANAGEMENT OF PATHOLOGICAL FRACTURES

The axial skeleton, particularly the spine, is the most frequent site of pathological fractures in multiple myeloma and other diseases associated with bone metastases. In the absence of specific complications, such as spinal instability or spinal cord compression, the management of vertebral fractures has usually been limited to the treatment of bone pain, as discussed above. More recently, a number of surgical techniques have been developed that offer other options for the acute and long-term treatment of patients with symptomatic vertebral fractures. Non-weight-bearing bones, such as the ribs, fibula, and much of the pelvis, can safely be treated with radiotherapy alone in almost all cases. In contrast, surgical interventions have played an important role in the management of appendicular fractures, both after the event and in prophylactic procedures in those patients with impending fractures. Optimum treatment must, wherever possible, be aimed at identifying patients who are, or may be, at risk of fracture and should be performed as part of a multidisciplinary team approach.

The orthopedic management of pathological fracture is markedly different from that of routine traumatic or osteoporotic fracture and is best undertaken by orthopedic specialists in the field. Orthopedic treatment with non-specialized equipment may achieve the initial goal of treatment (immediate stabilization of the fracture) but may fail because the fracture is unlikely to unite. Thus, fixation should aim to last the lifetime of the patient.[138,139]

Appendicular fractures

While the incidence of long bone fractures is relatively low compared with vertebral fracture in multiple myeloma, appendicular pathological fractures have a significant impact on the patient and health care resources, as they usually require hospitalization and surgical fixation.[74] The efficacy of bisphosphonates to reduce the incidence of appendicular or non-vertebral (appendicular plus ribs and pelvis) has not been convincingly demonstrated across myeloma studies.[30] Oral clodronate was associated with an 82% reduction in upper and lower limb fractures in the MRC trial.[17] Reductions in appendicular fractures have been reported with bisphosphonates in other diseases, particularly post-menopausal osteoporosis.[37,140,141]

For patients with known osteolytic disease in the long bones, prophylactic surgery should be strongly considered.[138] As a general rule, pathological fracture should be regarded as inevitable when 50% or more of a single cortex has been destroyed. In addition, avulsion of the lesser trochanter should be regarded as an indication of imminent hip fracture. Where there is less than 50% cortical erosion, radiotherapy may be considered without prophylactic fixation, the exception being the femoral neck, where any degree of cortical erosion should be considered as an indication for prophylactic fixation. Several scoring systems have been developed to estimate fracture risk and that derived by Mirels, based on lesion site, associated pain, degree of lysis, and size of cortical destruction, is widely utilized (Table 21.1).[142] In the original study, a score of seven or less was found to be associated with low fracture risk (<5%) and was deemed to be compatible with a more conservative management policy, including radiotherapy without prior fixation. Prophylactic fixation is recommended for those lesions that score nine or above, while those scoring eight have an intermediate risk of fracture (15%) with the decision about surgical intervention depending on other clinical grounds.[142] Prophylactic internal fixation should usually be followed by radiotherapy, once the wound has healed, to inhibit further tumor growth and bone destruction.

For pathological fractures in the lower limbs, treatment with load-bearing devices (e.g. intramedullary nailing) is preferred to load-sharing devices (e.g. plates and screws), as failure owing to fracture of the plate or screws, or pulling out of screws, occurs frequently within a short period of time.[143,144] The use of dynamic hip screws should be avoided in the management of hip fractures, while more extensive destruction of the proximal femur (or the proximal humerus) is best managed by the use of endoprosthetic reconstructions. The latter may require referral to a recognized center for orthopedic oncology, but the immediate costs of more expensive interventions will be offset at least partially by the avoidance of costly revision surgery and prolonged hospital stays.

Spinal fractures

In contrast to appendicular sites, the definition of impending spinal fracture is not as well characterized, but greater than 50% destruction of a vertebral body, with associated pain, is thought to be a clinically useful indicator. Established vertebral fractures in myeloma are associated with significant height loss and back pain.[145] The debilitating pain can last for weeks or months and is often unresponsive to conventional conservative therapy. This has resulted in the development of specialist orthopedic and interventional radiological procedures that may play a significant role in the future management of complicated patients. Certainly, the possibility of palliation should be assessed and discussed with a surgeon or radiologist experienced in modern spinal practice.

VERTEBROPLASTY AND KYPHOPLASTY

Percutaneous vertebroplasty is an interventional radiological procedure for the treatment of pain in patients with vertebral compressions caused by osteoporosis, metastases, or hemangioma.[146,147] First introduced in the mid-1980s for the treatment of vertebral hemangiomata,[148] it consists of percutaneous injection of bone cement (polymethylmethacrylate; PMMA) into the vertebral body under fluoroscopy guidance (Fig. 21.8). Newer developments include the use of balloon vertebroplasty (kyphoplasty; see later) with calcium phosphate cement.

The principal indication for vertebroplasty is pain and the greatest benefits are seen in patients with pain localized to a vertebral compression fracture. There is no doubt that vertebroplasty can reduce pain in patients with vertebral fractures complicating myeloma. In one small series of metastatic disease and myeloma patients, the response rate for pain reduction was 97% (36 of 37 patients).[149,150] Radiological evaluation should include lateral plain X-rays and a computed tomography (CT) or magnetic resonance imaging (MRI) scan. The latter provides the most useful information, with sagittal T2-weighted images with fat suppression helping to discriminate bone edema from relatively recent fractures. Isotope bone scans can also be useful to identify recent fractures, but vertebroplasty may be effective in giving pain relief regardless of the age of fracture, at least in osteoporosis.[151] Contraindications to vertebroplasty include coagulopathies, infection, and spinal cord or nerve root compression by bone or epidural neoplastic disease. Relative contraindications include vertebral bodies showing collapse of greater than 75% of height or destruction of the posterior vertebral wall. Above the eighth thoracic vertebra, the risks of damage due to decreasing size of the pedicles makes the procedure of less value, but recent experience suggests that good benefit can be obtained at these high levels.[152] Although minimally invasive, this procedure can be dangerous if the proper technique is not utilized and can cause complications largely related to migration of the cement.[153,154] For example, migration into the spinal canal can compress the spinal cord and/or nerve roots with severe consequences, while pulmonary embolus of PMMA is not uncommon. Other complications include death, bleeding, major vascular injury, infection, pneumothorax, hemothorax, and failure of pain relief. A number of techniques, particularly improved use of imaging techniques, appear to reduce the risk of complications.[153]

Kyphoplasty represents a modification of vertebroplasty that, in addition to stabilizing the vertebra and relieving pain, aims to restore the vertebral body back toward its original height.[155] This is achieved by the insertion of inflatable bone tamps (balloons) into the vertebral body, which can create a cavity into which bone cement can be introduced. However, in order to correct the spine deformity maximally, the procedure should ideally be performed within a few days of the fracture before impaction occurs, whereas vertebroplasty has been used to treat vertebral fractures that continue to cause pain despite appropriate prolonged conservative therapy.[156] The impact of a delay on the vertebral height regained during kyphoplasty was documented in a recent report of 2194 fractures treated in almost 1500 osteoporosis patients (mean age 74 years) in the USA.[157] Where the duration of symptoms at the initial visit was under 3 months, the average fractured vertebral body height was 71% before treatment and 92% after treatment ($P = 0.002$). In fractures over 3 months, the average fractured vertebral body height was 74% before treatment and 84% after treatment ($P = 0.05$). The average lost height restored for all fractures was 57%.

In a recent study, 55 consecutive kyphoplasty procedures were performed in 18 patients (mean age 64 years) with osteolytic vertebral compression fractures resulting from multiple myeloma.[158] The mean duration of back pain and other symptoms was 11 months prior to the procedure, and follow-up was reported during a mean of

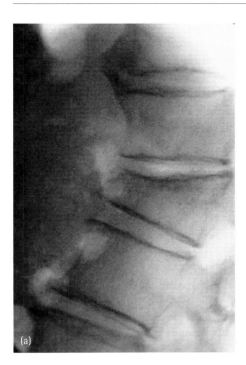
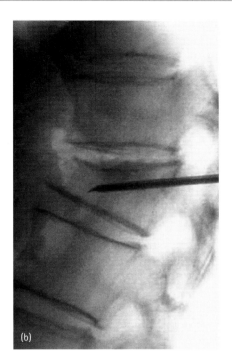
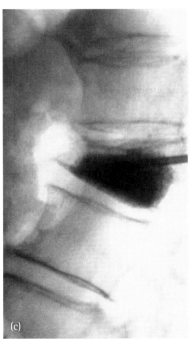

Figure 21.8 *Sequence of radiographs demonstrating a vertebroplasty for a painful wedge fracture in a single vertebra at the thoracolumbar junction (a). Under fluoroscopic guidance, a trochar has been introduced across one of the pedicles into the anterior third of the vertebral body (b). Polymethylmethacrylate was then injected under pressure into the vertebra to stabilize the vertebral body and give pain relief (c). (Reproduced from www.massgeneralimaging.com.)*

7 months. There were no major complications related directly to use of this technique. On average, 34% of vertebral height loss, estimated from lateral spine radiographs, was restored by the procedure. There were highly significant improvements in the quality of life, as judged by comparing pre-operative SF36 scores with those from the last follow-up visit, in the domains for bodily pain (23.2 to 55.4; $P = 0.0008$), physical function (21.3 to 50.6; $P = 0.0010$), vitality (31.3 to 47.5; $P = 0.010$), and social functioning (40.6 to 64.8; $P = 0.014$). The procedure was reported to be relatively safe with asymptomatic cement leakage reported at only two of the 55 levels involved in the procedures (4%).[158] The authors concluded that kyphoplasty is efficacious in the

treatment of osteolytic vertebral compression fractures resulting from multiple myeloma, and is associated with early clinical improvement of pain and function as well as some restoration of vertebral body height.

The complication profile of kyphoplasty is obviously similar to that of vertebroplasty, but the frequency of cement leakage into extravertebral structures and the vasculature seems lower during kyphoplasty.[159] This may result from the prior construction of a cavity within the bone that allows the injection of PMMA under a much lower pressure than that used in vertebroplasty. The possibility that either procedure might predispose to problems in adjacent vertebrae (i.e. increase the risk of further fracture) has not been adequately addressed. As with vertebroplasty, most of the published data for kyphoplasty are retrospective series with no prospective controlled studies yet available. Biomechanical comparisons of kyphoplasty and vertebroplasty in cadavers have found no significant mechanical differences.[160,161] As it is likely that most patients may not get treatment within a reasonable timeframe, vertebroplasty may offer similar benefits in terms of improved quality of life, particularly in those with a reduced life expectancy. This argument may be countered by a potentially lower complication rate in kyphoplasty.[159] Further controlled studies of both vertebroplasty and kyphoplasty are required to realize their full potential in the management of vertebral compression fractures in myeloma.

SPINAL CORD COMPRESSION

Spinal cord compression is one of the most serious complications of multiple myeloma and may affect up to 20% of patients at some time during the course of their disease.[162,163] Early consideration of the diagnosis of spinal cord compression in patients with back pain, leg weakness or paralysis, numbness, and dysesthesia is essential to successful rehabilitation. It is important to remember that patients may also present with symptoms related to the upper limbs. More than 60% of patients with skeletal metastases presenting with severe back pain and an abnormal plain spinal radiograph are shown to have MRI evidence of epidural disease, emphasizing the importance of early consideration of potential spinal problems. Rarely, compression vertebral fractures can also cause acute cord compression. Spinal radiographs are rarely diagnostic and MRI is the investigation of choice. If MRI is unavailable, either CT imaging or myelography may be useful in confirming cord compression and defining the level and extent of the lesion.

Where spinal cord compression is suspected, high-dose corticosteroids (dexamethasone 16 mg/day[164]) should be initiated, followed by a rapid assessment and urgent referral for radiotherapy or surgery. Surgery is only indicated as first-line management if there is evidence of spinal instability[43,164]), in which case pre-operative radiotherapy may increase the complication rate.[165] In the absence of spinal instability, the outcome is probably not improved by surgery,[166] and radiotherapy alone remains the preferred treatment option.[43,164] The long-term outcome is relatively poor. In a retrospective review of 24 historical patients treated with radiotherapy (alone or post-surgical decompression) between 1979 and 1989, the median durations of local control and survival were only 4.5 and 10 months, respectively.[166]

SUMMARY

The rationale for the use of the bisphosphonates in myeloma-induced osteolysis is well established. The evidence to date supports the view that whilst systemic chemotherapy is effective in reducing bone resorption, bone destruction continues in myeloma so that supplementary bone protection should be considered. Long-term treatment with clodronate, pamidronate, or zoledronic acid has been shown to modify the progression of skeletal disease. The efficacies of oral and intravenous bisphosphonates seem similar, and the numbers needed to treat compare very favorably with the use of treatments as secondary prevention in other diseases. Further research is required to determine whether we can better identify subgroups of patients who will derive particular benefit, or perhaps not benefit at all, from bisphosphonate therapy. The use of biochemical markers of bone resorption and formation to evaluate the risk of skeletal disease, and its response to treatment, also requires further study.

KEY POINTS

- Long-term treatment with clodronate, pamidronate, or zoledronic acid has been shown to modify the progression of skeletal disease.
- The efficacies of oral and intravenous bisphosphonates appear similar.
- All patients with myeloma requiring treatment for their disease should receive long-term treatment with a bisphosphonate.
- The use of biochemical markers of bone resorption and formation in a clinical setting requires further study.
- Effective treatment for bone pain includes adequate analgesia, radiotherapy, and bisphosphonates.
- The management of pathological fractures differs from that of routine traumatic fractures and is best undertaken by specialists in the field.

- Vertebroplasty can stabilize compressed vertebrae and reduce pain. Kyphoplasty is a new procedure that also aims to restore vertebral height.

REFERENCES

● = Key primary paper
◆ = Major review article
* = Paper that represents the first formal publication of a management guideline

1. Taube T, Beneton MN, McCloskey EV, Rogers S, Greaves M, Kanis JA. Abnormal bone remodelling in patients with myelomatosis and normal biochemical indices of bone resorption. *Eur J Haematol* 1992; **49**:192–8.
◆2. Croucher PI, Apperley JF. Bone disease in multiple myeloma. *Br J Haematol* 1998; **103**:902–10.
3. Fleisch H. Bisphosphonates: mechanisms of action. *Endocrinol Rev* 1998; **19**:80–100.
◆4. Fleisch H. From polyphosphates to bisphosphonates and their role in bone and calcium metabolism. *Prog Mol Subcell Biol* 1999; **23**:197–216.
5. O'Rourke NP, McCloskey EV, Vasikaran S, Eyres K, Fern D, Kanis JA. Effective treatment of malignant hypercalcaemia with a single intravenous infusion of clodronate. *Br J Cancer* 1993; **67**:560–3.
6. Body JJ, Dumon JC. Treatment of tumour-induced hypercalcaemia with the bisphosphonate pamidronate: dose-response relationship and influence of tumour type. *Ann Oncol* 1994; **5**:359–63.
7. Purohit OP, Radstone CR, Anthony C, Kanis JA, Coleman RE. A randomised double-blind comparison of intravenous pamidronate and clodronate in the hypercalcaemia of malignancy. *Br J Cancer* 1995; **72**:1289–93.
8. Ralston SH, Thiebaud D, Herrmann Z, Steinhauer EU, Thurlimann B, Walls J, *et al.* Dose-response study of ibandronate in the treatment of cancer- associated hypercalcaemia. *Br J Cancer* 1997; **75**:295–300.
9. Zojer N, Keck AV, Pecherstorfer M. Comparative tolerability of drug therapies for hypercalcaemia of malignancy. *Drug Saf* 1999; **21**:389–406.
●10. Lahtinen R, Laakso M, Palva I, Virkkunen P, Elomaa I. Randomised, placebo-controlled multicentre trial of clodronate in multiple myeloma. Finnish Leukaemia Group [published erratum: *Lancet* 1992; **340**:1420]. *Lancet* 1992; **340**:1049–52.
11. Paterson AH, Powles TJ, Kanis JA, McCloskey E, Hanson J, Ashley S. Double-blind controlled trial of oral clodronate in patients with bone metastases from breast cancer. *J Clin Oncol* 1993; **11**:59–65.
12. Kanis JA, Powles T, Paterson AH, McCloskey EV, Ashley S. Clodronate decreases the frequency of skeletal metastases in women with breast cancer. *Bone* 1996; **19**:663–7.

●13. Berenson JR, Lichtenstein A, Porter L, Dimopoulos MA, Bordoni R, George S, *et al.* Efficacy of pamidronate in reducing skeletal events in patients with advanced multiple myeloma. Myeloma Aredia Study Group. *N Engl J Med* 1996; **334**:488–93.
●14. Berenson JR, Lichtenstein A, Porter L, Dimopoulos MA, Bordoni R, George S, *et al.* Long-term pamidronate treatment of advanced multiple myeloma patients reduces skeletal events. Myeloma Aredia Study Group. *J Clin Oncol* 1998; **16**:593–602.
15. Hortobagyi GN, Theriault RL, Porter L, Blayney D, Lipton A, Sinoff C, *et al.* Efficacy of pamidronate in reducing skeletal complications in patients with breast cancer and lytic bone metastases. Protocol 19 Aredia Breast Cancer Study Group. *N Engl J Med* 1996; **335**:1785–91.
16. Hortobagyi GN, Theriault RL, Lipton A, Porter L, Blayney D, Sinoff C, *et al.* Long-term prevention of skeletal complications of metastatic breast cancer with pamidronate. Protocol 19 Aredia Breast Cancer Study Group. *J Clin Oncol* 1998; **16**:2038–44.
●17. McCloskey EV, MacLennan IC, Drayson MT, Chapman C, Dunn J, Kanis JA. A randomized trial of the effect of clodronate on skeletal morbidity in multiple myeloma. MRC Working Party on Leukaemia in Adults. *Br J Haematol* 1998; **100**:317–25.
●18. Brincker H, Westin J, Abildgaard N, Gimsing P, Turesson I, Hedenus M, *et al.* Failure of oral pamidronate to reduce skeletal morbidity in multiple myeloma: a double-blind placebo-controlled trial. Danish-Swedish co-operative study group. *Br J Haematol* 1998; **101**:280–6.
19. Theriault RL, Lipton A, Hortobagyi GN, Leff R, Gluck S, Stewart JF, *et al.* Pamidronate reduces skeletal morbidity in women with advanced breast cancer and lytic bone lesions: a randomized, placebo-controlled trial. Protocol 18 Aredia Breast Cancer Study Group. *J Clin Oncol* 1999; **17**:846–54.
20. Hultborn R, Gundersen S, Ryden S, Holmberg E, Carstensen J, Wallgren UB, *et al.* Efficacy of pamidronate in breast cancer with bone metastases: a randomized, double-blind placebo-controlled multicenter study. *Anticancer Res* 1999; **19**:3383–92.
●21. Powles T, Paterson S, Kanis JA, McCloskey E, Ashley S, Tidy A, *et al.* Randomized, placebo-controlled trial of clodronate in patients with primary operable breast cancer. *J Clin Oncol* 2002; **20**:3219–24.
22. McCloskey EV, Guest JF, Kanis JA. The clinical and cost considerations of bisphosphonates in preventing bone complications in patients with metastatic breast cancer or multiple myeloma. *Drugs* 2001; **61**:1253–74.
23. Belch AR, Bergsagel DE, Wilson K, O'Reilly S, Wilson J, Sutton D, *et al.* Effect of daily etidronate on the osteolysis of multiple myeloma. *J Clin Oncol* 1991; **9**:1397–402.
24. Daragon A, Humez C, Michot C, Le LX, Grosbois B, Pouyol F, *et al.* Treatment of multiple myeloma with etidronate: results of a multicentre double-blind study. Groupe d'Etudes et de Recherches sur le Myelome (GERM). *Eur J Med* 1993; **2**:449–52.
25. Preston CJ, Yates AJ, Beneton MN, Russell RG, Gray RE, Smith R, *et al.* Effective short term treatment of Paget's disease with oral etidronate. *Br Med J (Clin Res Ed)* 1986; **292**:79–80.

26. McCloskey EV, Yates AJ, Beneton MN, Galloway J, Harris S, Kanis JA. Comparative effects of intravenous diphosphonates on calcium and skeletal metabolism in man. *Bone* 1987; **8**(Suppl 1):S35–S41.

27. Eyres KS, Marshall P, McCloskey E, Douglas DL, Kanis JA. Spontaneous fractures in a patient treated with low doses of etidronic acid (disodium etidronate). *Drug Saf* 1992; 7:162–5.

●28. Menssen HD, Sakalova A, Fontana A, Herrmann Z, Boewer C, Facon T, et al. Effects of long-term intravenous ibandronate therapy on skeletal-related events, survival, and bone resorption markers in patients with advanced multiple myeloma. *J Clin Oncol* 2002; **20**:2353–9.

●29. Rosen LS, Gordon D, Antonio BS, Kaminski M, Howell A, Belch A, et al. Zoledronic acid versus pamidronate in the treatment of skeletal metastases in patients with breast cancer or osteolytic lesions of multiple myeloma: a phase III, double-blind, comparative trial. *Cancer J* 2001; 7:377–87.

◆30. Djulbegovic B, Wheatley K, Ross J, Clark O, Bos G, Goldschmidt H, et al. Bisphosphonates in multiple myeloma (Cochrane Review). Oxford: The Cochrane Library Issue 3. Update Software. 2002.

31. Laitinen K, Patronen A, Harju P, Loyttyniemi E, Pylkkanen L, Kleimola T, et al. Timing of food intake has a marked effect on the bioavailability of clodronate. *Bone* 2000; **27**:293–6.

●32. McCloskey EV, Dunn JA, Kanis JA, MacLennan IC, Drayson MT. Long-term follow-up of a prospective, double-blind, placebo-controlled randomized trial of clodronate in multiple myeloma. *Br J Haematol* 2001; **113**:1035–43.

33. Pecherstorfer M, Ludwig H, Schlosser K, Buck S, Huss HJ, Body JJ. Administration of the bisphosphonate ibandronate (BM 21.0955) by intravenous bolus injection. *J Bone Miner Res* 1996; **11**:587–93.

34. Pecherstorfer M, Herrmann Z, Body JJ, Manegold C, Degardin M, Clemens MR, et al. Randomized phase II trial comparing different doses of the bisphosphonate ibandronate in the treatment of hypercalcemia of malignancy. *J Clin Oncol* 1996; **14**:268–76.

35. Miller PD, Brown JP, Siris ES, Hoseyni MS, Axelrod DW, Bekker PJ. A randomized, double-blind comparison of risedronate and etidronate in the treatment of Paget's disease of bone. Paget's Risedronate/Etidronate Study Group. *Am J Med* 1999; **106**:513–20.

36. Reginster J, Minne HW, Sorensen OH, Hooper M, Roux C, Brandi ML, et al. Randomized trial of the effects of risedronate on vertebral fractures in women with established postmenopausal osteoporosis. Vertebral Efficacy with Risedronate Therapy (VERT) Study Group. *Osteoporos Int* 2000; **11**:83–91.

37. McClung MR, Geusens P, Miller PD, Zippel H, Bensen WG, Roux C, et al. Effect of risedronate on the risk of hip fracture in elderly women. Hip Intervention Program Study Group. *N Engl J Med* 2001; **344**:333–40.

38. Roux C, Ravaud P, Cohen-Solal M, de Vernejoul MC, Guillemant S, Cherruau B, et al. Biologic, histologic and densitometric effects of oral risedronate on bone in patients with multiple myeloma. *Bone* 1994; **15**:41–9.

39. Delmas PD, Charhon S, Chapuy MC, Vignon E, Briancon D, Edouard C, et al. Long-term effects of dichloromethylene diphosphonate (Cl2MDP) on skeletal lesions in multiple myeloma. *Metab Bone Dis Relat Res* 1982; **4**:163–8.

40. Heim ME, Clemens MR, Queisser W, Pecherstorfer M, Boewer C, Herold M, et al. Prospective randomized trial of dichloromethilene bisphosphonate (clodronate) in patients with multiple myeloma. *Onkologie* 1995; **18**:439–48.

41. Terpos E, Palermos J, Tsionos K, Anargyrou K, Viniou N, Papassavas P, et al. Effect of pamidronate administration on markers of bone turnover and disease activity in multiple myeloma. *Eur J Haematol* 2000; **65**:331–6.

42. Kraj M, Poglod R, Pawlikowski J, Maj S, Nasilowska B. Effect of pamidronate on skeletal morbidity in myelomatosis. Part 1. The results of the first 12 months of pamidronate therapy. *Acta Pol Pharm* 2000; **57**(Suppl.):113–16.

*43. Guidelines Working Group of the UK Myeloma Forum. Diagnosis and management of multiple myeloma. *Br J Haematol* 2001; **115**:522–40.

*44. Berenson JR, Hillner BE, Kyle RA, Anderson K, Lipton A, Yee G, et al. American Society of Clinical Oncology Clinical Practice Guidelines: the role of bisphosphonates in multiple myeloma. *J Clin Oncol* 2002; **20**:3719–36.

45. Sims EC, Rogers PB, Besser GM, Plowman PN. Severe prolonged hypocalcaemia following pamidronate for malignant hypercalcaemia. *Clin Oncol (R Coll Radiol)* 1998; **10**:407–9.

46. Comlekci A, Biberoglu S, Hekimsoy Z, Okan I, Piskin O, Sekeroglu B, et al. Symptomatic hypocalcemia in a patient with latent hypoparathyroidism and breast carcinoma with bone metastasis following administration of pamidronate. *Intern Med* 1998; **37**:396–7.

47. Johnson MJ, Fallon MT. Symptomatic hypocalcemia with oral clodronate. *J Pain Symptom Manage* 1998; **15**:140–2.

48. Mayordomo JI, Rivera F. Severe hypocalcaemia after treatment with oral clodronate and aminoglycoside [letter]. *Ann Oncol* 1993; **4**:432–3.

49. Fraser WD, Logue FC, Gallacher SJ, O'Reilly DS, Beastall GH, Ralston SH, et al. Direct and indirect assessment of the parathyroid hormone response to pamidronate therapy in Paget's disease of bone and hypercalcaemia of malignancy. *Bone Miner* 1991; **12**:113–21.

50. Ralston SH, Gardner MD, Dryburgh FJ, Jenkins AS, Cowan RA, Boyle IT. Comparison of aminohydroxypropylidene diphosphonate, mithramycin, and corticosteroids/calcitonin in treatment of cancer-associated hypercalcaemia. *Lancet* 1985; **2**:907–10.

51. Laitinen K, Taube T. Clodronate as a cause of aminotransferase elevation. *Osteoporos Int* 1999; **10**:120–2.

52. Adami S, Zamberlan N. Adverse effects of bisphosphonates. A comparative review. *Drug Safety* 1996; **14**:158–70.

53. Thiebaud D, Jaeger P, Gobelet C, Jacquet AF, Burckhardt P. A single infusion of the bisphosphonate AHPrBP (APD) as treatment of Paget's disease of bone. *Am J Med* 1988; **85**:207–12.

54. Adami S, Bhalla AK, Dorizzi R, Montesanti F, Rosini S, Salvagno G, et al. The acute-phase response after bisphosphonate administration. *Calcif Tissue Int* 1987; **41**:326–31.

55. Pecherstorfer M, Jilch R, Sauty A, Horn E, Keck AV, Zimmer-Roth I, et al. Effect of first treatment with

aminobisphosphonates pamidronate and ibandronate on circulating lymphocyte subpopulations. *J Bone Miner Res* 2000; **15**:147–54.

56. Abildgaard N, Rungby J, Glerup H, Brixen K, Kassem M, Brincker H, *et al.* Long-term oral pamidronate treatment inhibits osteoclastic bone resorption and bone turnover without affecting osteoblastic function in multiple myeloma. *Eur J Haematol* 1998; **61**:128–34.

57. Adamson BB, Gallacher SJ, Byars J, Ralston SH, Boyle IT, Boyce BF. Mineralisation defects with pamidronate therapy for Paget's disease. *Lancet* 1993; **342**:1459–60.

58. van Holten-Verzantvoort AT, Bijvoet OL, Hermans J, *et al.* Reduced morbidity from skeletal metastases in breast cancer patients during long-term bisphosphonate (APD) treatment. *Lancet* 1987; **2**:983–5.

59. De Groen P, Lubbe DF, Hirsch LJ, *et al.* Esophagitis associated with the use of alendronate. *N Engl J Med* 1996; **335**:1016–21.

60. Jalava T, Sarna S, Pylkkänen L, Mawer EB, Kanis J, Selby P, *et al.* Association between vertebral fracture and increased mortality in osteoporotic patients. *J Bone Miner Res* 2003; **18**:1254–60.

61. Troehler U, Bonjour JP, Fleisch H. Renal secretion of diphosphonates in rats. *Kidney Int* 1975; **8**:6–13.

62. Yakatan GJ, Poynor WJ, Talbert RL, Floyd BF, Slough CL, Ampulski RS, *et al.* Clodronate kinetics and bioavailability. *Clin Pharmacol Ther* 1982; **31**:402–10.

63. Pentikainen PJ, Elomaa I, Nurmi AK, Karkkainen S. Pharmacokinetics of clodronate in patients with metastatic breast cancer. *Int J Clin Pharmacol Ther Toxicol* 1989; **27**:222–8.

●64. O'Rourke N, McCloskey EV, Neugebauer G, Kanis JA. Renal and non-renal clearance of clodronate in malignancy and renal impairment. *Drug Invest* 1994; **7**:26–33.

65. Saha H, Castren-Kortekangas P, Ojanen S, Juhakoski A, Tuominen J, Tokola O, *et al.* Pharmacokinetics of clodronate in renal failure. *J Bone Miner Res* 1994; **9**:1953–8.

●66. Berenson JR, Rosen L, Vescio R, Lau HS, Woo M, Sioufi A, *et al.* Pharmacokinetics of pamidronate disodium in patients with cancer with normal or impaired renal function. *J Clin Pharmacol* 1997; **37**:285–90.

67. Machado CE, Flombaum CD. Safety of pamidronate in patients with renal failure and hypercalcemia. *Clin Nephrol* 1996; **45**:175–9.

68. Hamdy NA, Gray RE, McCloskey E, Galloway J, Rattenbury JM, Brown CB, *et al.* Clodronate in the medical management of hyperparathyroidism. *Bone* 1987; **8**(Suppl 1):S69–77.

69. Hamdy NA, McCloskey EV, Brown CB, Kanis JA. Effects of clodronate in severe hyperparathyroid bone disease in chronic renal failure. *Nephron* 1990; **56**:6–12.

70. Beigel AE, Rienhoff E, Olbricht CJ. Removal of clodronate by haemodialysis in end-stage renal disease patients. *Nephrol Dial Transplant* 1995; **10**:2266–8.

71. Ring T, Sodemann B, Nielsen C, Melsen F, Kornerup HJ. Mineralization defect but no effect on hypercalcemia during clodronate treatment in secondary hyperparathyroidism. *Clin Nephrol* 1995; **44**:209–10.

72. Bounameaux HM, Schifferli J, Montani JP, Jung A, Chatelanat F. Renal failure associated with intravenous diphosphonates. *Lancet* 1983; **1**:471.

●73. Laakso M, Lahtinen R, Virkkunen P, Elomaa I. Subgroup and cost–benefit analysis of the Finnish multicentre trial of clodronate in multiple myeloma. Finnish Leukaemia Group. *Br J Haematol* 1994; **87**:725–9.

●74. Bruce NJ, McCloskey EV, Kanis JA, Guest JF. Economic impact of using clodronate in the management of patients with multiple myeloma. *Br J Haematol* 1999; **104**:358–64.

75. Gent M, Blakely JA, Easton JD, Ellis DJ, Hachinski VC, Harbison JW, *et al.* The Canadian American Ticlopidine Study (CATS) in thromboembolic stroke. *Lancet* 1989; **1**:1215–20.

76. Diener HC, Cunha L, Forbes C, Sivenius J, Smets P, Lowenthal A. European Stroke Prevention Study. 2. Dipyridamole and acetylsalicylic acid in the secondary prevention of stroke. *J Neurol Sci* 1996; **143**:1–13.

77. Riccardi A, Ucci G, Brugnatelli S, Mora O, Merlini G, Piva N, *et al.* Prospective, controlled, non randomised study on prophylactic parenteral dichloremethylene bisphosphonate (clodronate) in multiple myeloma. *Int J Oncol* 1994; **5**:833–9.

78. Elomaa I, Risteli L, Laakso M, Lahtinen R, Virkkunen P, Risteli J. Monitoring the action of clodronate with type I collagen metabolites in multiple myeloma. *Eur J Cancer* 1996; **32A**:1166–70.

79. Vinholes J, Guo CY, Purohit OP, Eastell R, Coleman RE. Evaluation of new bone resorption markers in a randomized comparison of pamidronate or clodronate for hypercalcemia of malignancy. *J Clin Oncol* 1997; **15**:131–8.

●80. Vinholes J, Coleman R, Lacombe D, Rose C, Tubiana-Hulin M, Bastit P, *et al.* Assessment of bone response to systemic therapy in an EORTC trial: preliminary experience with the use of collagen cross-link excretion. European Organization for Research and Treatment of Cancer. *Br J Cancer* 1999; **80**:221–8.

81. Lipton A, Theriault RL, Hortobagyi GN, Simeone J, Knight RD, Mellars K, *et al.* Pamidronate prevents skeletal complications and is effective palliative treatment in women with breast carcinoma and osteolytic bone metastases: long term follow-up of two randomized, placebo-controlled trials. *Cancer* 2000; **88**:1082–90.

82. Diel IJ, Solomayer EF, Costa SD, Gollan C, Goerner R, Wallwiener D, *et al.* Reduction in new metastases in breast cancer with adjuvant clodronate treatment. *N Engl J Med* 1998; **339**:357–63.

83. Garnero P, Delmas PD. Biochemical markers of bone turnover. Applications for osteoporosis. *Endocrinol Metab Clin North Am* 1998; **27**:303–23.

◆84. Seibel MJ. Molecular markers of bone turnover: biochemical, technical and analytical aspects. *Osteoporos Int* 2000; **11**(Suppl 6):S18–29.

85. Kanis JA, McCloskey EV. Bone turnover and biochemical markers in malignancy. *Cancer* 1997; **80**:1538–45.

◆86. Woitge HW, Seibel MJ. Biochemical markers to survey bone turnover. *Rheum Dis Clin North Am* 2001; **27**:49–80.

87. Corso A, Arcaini L, Mangiacavelli S, Astori C, Orlandi E, Lorenzi A, *et al.* Biochemical markers of bone disease in asymptomatic early stage multiple myeloma. A study on their role in identifying high risk patients. *Haematologica* 2001; **86**:394–8.

●88. Jakob C, Zavrski I, Heider U, Brux B, Eucker J, Langelotz C. *et al.* Bone resorption parameters [carboxy-terminal telopeptide of type-I collagen (ICTP), amino-terminal collagen type-I telopeptide (NTx), and deoxypyridinoline (Dpd)] in MGUS and multiple myeloma. *Eur J Haematol* 2002; **69**:37–42.

89. Alexandrakis MG, Passam FH, Malliaraki N, Katachanakis C, Kyriakou DS, Margioris AN. Evaluation of bone disease in multiple myeloma: a correlation between biochemical markers of bone metabolism and other clinical parameters in untreated multiple myeloma patients. *Clin Chim Acta* 2002; **325**:51–7.

90. Woitge HW, Horn E, Keck AV, Auler B, Seibel MJ, Pecherstorfer M. Biochemical markers of bone formation in patients with plasma cell dyscrasias and benign osteoporosis. *Clin Chem* 2001; **47**:686–93.

91. Delmas PD, Hardy P, Garnero P, Dain M. Monitoring individual response to hormone replacement therapy with bone markers. *Bone* 2000; **26**:553–60.

92. Bauer DC, Sklarin PM, Stone KL, Black DM, Nevitt MC, Ensrud KE, et al. Biochemical markers of bone turnover and prediction of hip bone loss in older women: the study of osteoporotic fractures. *J Bone Miner Res* 1999; **14**:1404–10.

93. Clark RE, Flory AJ, Ion EM, Woodcock BE, Durham BH, Fraser WD. Biochemical markers of bone turnover following high-dose chemotherapy and autografting in multiple myeloma. *Blood* 2000; **96**:2697–702.

●94. Elomaa I, Risteli L, Laakso M, Lahtinen R, Virkkunen P, Risteli J. Monitoring the action of clodronate with type I collagen metabolites in multiple myeloma. *Eur J Cancer* **32A**:1166–70.

95. Abildgaard N, Bentzen SM, Nielsen JL. Serum markers of bone metabolism in multiple myeloma: prognostic value of the carboxy-terminal telopeptide of type I collagen (ICTP). Nordic Myeloma Study Group. *Br J Haematol* 1997; **96**:103–10.

●96. Abildgaard N, Brixen K, Kristensen JE, Eriksen EF, Nielsen JL, et al. Comparison of five biochemical markers of bone resorption in multiple myeloma: elevated pre-treatment levels of S-ICTP and U-Ntx are predictive for early progression of the bone disease during standard chemotherapy. *Br J Haematol* 2003; **120**:235–42.

97. Engler H, Koeberle D, Thuerlimann B, Senn HJ, Riesen WF. Diagnostic and prognostic value of biochemical markers in malignant bone disease: a prospective study on the effect of bisphosphonate on pain intensity and progression of malignant bone disease. *Clin Chem Lab Med* 1998; **36**:879–85.

98. Arai F, Miyamoto T, Ohneda O, Inada T, Sudo T, Brasel K, et al. Commitment and differentiation of osteoclast precursor cells by the sequential expression of c-Fms and receptor activator of nuclear factor kappaB (RANK) receptors. *J Exp Med* 1999; **190**:1741–54.

◆99. Suda T, Takahashi N, Udagawa N, Jimi E, Gillespie MT, Martin TJ. Modulation of osteoclast differentiation and function by the new members of the tumor necrosis factor receptor and ligand families. *Endocrine Rev* 1999; **20**:345–57.

100. Takahashi N, Udagawa N, Suda T. A new member of tumor necrosis factor ligand family, ODF/OPGL/TRANCE/RANKL, regulates osteoclast differentiation and function. *Biochem Biophys Res Commun* 1999; **256**:449–55.

101. Kong YY, Boyle WJ, Penninger JM. Osteoprotegerin ligand: a common link between osteoclastogenesis, lymph node formation and lymphocyte development. *Immunol Cell Biol* 1999; **77**:188–93.

102. Yasuda H, Shima N, Nakagawa N, Mochizuki SI, Yano K, Fujise N, et al. Identity of osteoclastogenesis inhibitory factor (OCIF) and osteoprotegerin (OPG): a mechanism by which OPG/OCIF inhibits osteoclastogenesis in vitro. *Endocrinology* 1998; **139**:1329–37.

◆103. Hofbauer LC, Khosla S, Dunstan CR, Lacey DL, Boyle WJ, Riggs BL. The roles of osteoprotegerin and osteoprotegerin ligand in the paracrine regulation of bone resorption. *J Bone Miner Res* 2000; **15**:2–12.

104. Giuliani N, Bataille R, Mancini C, Lazzaretti M, Barille S. Myeloma cells induce imbalance in the osteoprotegerin/ osteoprotegerin ligand system in the human bone marrow environment. *Blood* 2001; **98**:3527–33.

105. Pearse RN, Sordillo EM, Yaccoby S, Wong BR, Liau DF, Colman N, et al. Multiple myeloma disrupts the TRANCE/ osteoprotegerin cytokine axis to trigger bone destruction and promote tumor progression. *Proc Natl Acad Sci USA* 2001; **98**:11581–86.

106. Giuliani N, Colla S, Sala R, Moroni M, Lazzaretti M, La Monica S, et al. Human myeloma cells stimulate the receptor activator of nuclear factor-kappaB ligand (RANKL) in T lymphocytes: a potential role in multiple myeloma bone disease. *Blood* 2002; **100**:4615–21.

107. Viereck V, Emons G, Lauck V, Frosch KH, Blaschke S, Grundker C, et al. Bisphosphonates pamidronate and zoledronic acid stimulate osteoprotegerin production by primary human osteoblasts. *Biochem Biophys Res Commun* 2002; **291**:680–6.

108. Seidel C, Hjertner O, Abildgaard N, Heickendorff L, Hjorth M, Westin J, et al. Serum osteoprotegerin levels are reduced in patients with multiple myeloma with lytic bone disease. *Blood* 2001; **98**:2269–71.

●109. Croucher PI, Shipman CM, Lippitt J, Perry M, Asosingh K, Hijzen A, et al. Osteoprotegerin inhibits the development of osteolytic bone disease in multiple myeloma. *Blood* 2001; **98**:3534–40.

110. Emery JG, McDonnell P, Burke MB, Deen KC, Lyn S, Silverman C, et al. Osteoprotegerin is a receptor for the cytotoxic ligand TRAIL. *J Biol Chem* 1998; **273**:14363–7.

111. Mariani SM, Matib M, Armandola EA, Krammer PH. Interleukin-1β-converting enzyme related protease/caspases are involved in TRAIL-induced apoptosis of myeloma and leukemia cells. *J Exp Med* 1995; **137**:221–9.

112. Holen I, Croucher PI, Hamdy FC, Eaton CL. Osteoprotegerin (OPG) is a survival factor for human prostate cancer cells. *Cancer Res* 2002; **62**:1619–23.

113. Juji T, Hertz M, Aoki K, Horie D, Ohya K, Gautam A, et al. A novel therapeutic vaccine approach, targeting RANKL, prevents bone destruction in bone-related disorders. *J Bone Miner Metab* 2002; **20**:266–8.

●114. Oyajobi BO, Anderson DM, Traianedes K, Williams PJ, Yoneda T, Mundy GR. Therapeutic efficacy of a soluble receptor activator of nuclear factor kappaB-IgG Fc fusion protein in suppressing bone resorption and hypercalcemia in a model of humoral hypercalcemia of malignancy. *Cancer Res* 2001; **61**:2572–8.

● 115. Yaccoby S, Pearse RN, Johnson CL, Barlogie B, Choi Y, Epstein J. Myeloma interacts with the bone marrow microenvironment to induce osteoclastogenesis and is dependent on osteoclast activity. *Br J Haematol* 2002; **116**:278–90.

◆ 116. Hofbauer LC, Khosla S, Dunstan CR, Lacey DL, Boyle WJ, Riggs BL. The roles of osteoprotegerin and osteoprotegerin ligand in the paracrine regulation of bone resorption. *J Bone Miner Res* 2000; **15**:2–12.

◆ 117. Hofbauer LC, Neubauer A, Heufelder AE. Receptor activator of nuclear factor-kappaB ligand and osteoprotegerin: Potential implications for the pathogenesis and treatment of malignant bone diseases. *Cancer* 2001; **92**:460–70.

118. Kyle RA. Multiple myeloma: review of 869 cases. *Mayo Clin Proc* 1975; **50**:29–40.

119. Wu JS, Bezjak A, Chow E, Kirkbride P. Primary treatment endpoint following palliative radiotherapy for painful bone metastases: need for a consensus definition? *Clin Oncol (R Coll Radiol)* 2002; **14**:70–7.

◆ 120. McQuay HJ, Collins SL, Carroll D, Moore RA. Radiotherapy for the palliation of painful bone metastases. *Cochrane Database Syst Rev* 2000; CD001793.

121. Bosch A, Frias Z. Radiotherapy in the treatment of multiple myeloma. *Int J Radiat Oncol Biol Phys* 1988; **15**:1363–9.

122. McSweeney EN, Tobias JS, Blackman G, Goldstone AH, Richards JD. Double hemibody irradiation (DHBI) in the management of relapsed and primary chemoresistant multiple myeloma. *Clin Oncol (R Coll Radiol)* 1993; **5**:378–83.

123. Catell D, Kogen Z, Donahue B, Steinfeld A. Multiple myeloma of an extremity: must the entire bone be treated? *Int J Radiat Oncol Biol Phys* 1998; **40**:117–19.

124. Chow E, Wong R, Hruby G, Connolly R, Franssen E, Fung KW, *et al.* Prospective patient-based assessment of effectiveness of palliative radiotherapy for bone metastases. *Radiother Oncol* 2001; **61**:77–82.

125. Steenland E, Leer JW, van Houwelingen H, Post WJ, van den Hout WB, Kievit J, *et al.* The effect of a single fraction compared to multiple fractions on painful bone metastases: a global analysis of the Dutch Bone Metastasis Study. *Radiother Oncol* 1999; **52**:101–9.

126. Ben Josef E, Porter AT. Radioisotopes in the treatment of bone metastases. *Ann Med* 1997; **29**:31–5.

127. Janjan NA. Radiation for bone metastases: conventional techniques and the role of systemic radiopharmaceuticals. *Cancer* 1997; **80**:1628–45.

128. Charkes ND, Durant J, Barry WE. Bone pain in multiple myeloma. Studies with radioactive 87m Sr. *Arch Intern Med* 1972; **130**:53–8.

129. Edwards GK, Santoro J, Taylor A Jr. Use of bone scintigraphy to select patients with multiple myeloma for treatment with strontium-89. *J Nucl Med* 1994; **35**:1992–93.

130. Vinholes JJ, Purohit OP, Abbey ME, Eastell R, Coleman RE. Relationships between biochemical and symptomatic response in a double-blind randomised trial of pamidronate for metastatic bone disease. *Ann Oncol* 1997; **8**:1243–50.

131. Ernst DS, Brasher P, Hagen N, Paterson AH, MacDonald RN, Bruera E. A randomized, controlled trial of intravenous

clodronate in patients with metastatic bone disease and pain. *J Pain Symptom Manage* 1997; **13**:319–26.

132. Ascari E, Attardo-Parrinello G, Merlini G. Treatment of painful bone lesions and hypercalcemia. *Eur J Haematol Suppl* 1989; **51**:135–9.

133. Attardo-Parrinello G, Merlini G, Pavesi F, Crema F, Fiorentini ML, Ascari E. Effects of a new aminodiphosphonate (aminohydroxybutylidene diphosphonate) in patients with osteolytic lesions from metastases and myelomatosis. Comparison with dichloromethylene diphosphonate. *Arch Intern Med* 1987; **147**:1629–33.

134. Fulfaro F, Casuccio A, Ticozzi C, Ripamonti C. The role of bisphosphonates in the treatment of painful metastatic bone disease: a review of phase III trials. *Pain* 1998; **78**:157–69.

135. Robertson AG, Reed NS, Ralston SH. Effect of oral clodronate on metastatic bone pain: a double-blind, placebo-controlled study. *J Clin Oncol* 1995; **13**:2427–30.

136. Goicoechea C, Porras E, Alfaro MJ, Martin MI. Alendronate induces antinociception in mice, not related with its effects in bone. *Jpn J Pharmacol* 1999; **79**:433–7.

137. Bonabello A, Galmozzi MR, Bruzzese T, Zara GP. Analgesic effect of bisphosphonates in mice. *Pain* 2001; **91**:269–75.

138. Tillman RM. The role of the orthopaedic surgeon in metastatic disease of the appendicular skeleton. Working Party on Metastatic Bone Disease in Breast Cancer in the UK. *J Bone Joint Surg Br* 1999; **81**:1–2.

＊ 139. The Breast Specialty Group of the British Association of Surgical Oncology. British Association of Surgical Oncology Guidelines. The management of metastatic bone disease in the United Kingdom. *Eur J Surg Oncol* 1999; **25**:3–23.

140. Black DM, Cummings SR, Karpf DB, Cauley JA, Thompson DE, Nevitt MC. *et al.* Randomised trial of effect of alendronate on risk of fracture in women with existing vertebral fractures. Fracture Intervention Trial Research Group. *Lancet* 1996; **348**:1535–41.

141. Harris ST, Watts NB, Genant HK, McKeever CD, Hangartner T, Keller M, *et al.* Effects of risedronate treatment on vertebral and nonvertebral fractures in women with postmenopausal osteoporosis: a randomized controlled trial. Vertebral Efficacy With Risedronate Therapy (VERT) Study Group. *J Am Med Assoc* 1999; **282**:1344–52.

142. Mirels H. Metastatic disease in long bones. A proposed scoring system for diagnosing impending pathologic fractures. *Clin Orthop* 1989; **249**:256–64.

143. Harrington KD. Orthopaedic management of extremity and pelvic lesions. *Clin Orthop* 1995; **312**:136–47.

144. Damron TA, Sim FH. Surgical treatment for metastatic disease of the pelvis and the proximal end of the femur. *Instr Course Lect* 2000; **49**:461–70.

145. McCloskey EV, Kanis JA. The assessment of vertebral deformity. In: Genant HK, Jergas M, van Kuijk C (eds) *Vertebral fractures in osteoporosis.* San Francisco: UCSF, 1996:215–33.

● 146. Deramond H, Depriester C, Toussaint P, Galibert P. Percutaneous vertebroplasty. *Semin Musculoskelet Radiol* 1997; **1**:285–96.

147. Jensen ME, Kallmes DE. Percutaneous vertebroplasty in the treatment of malignant spine disease. *Cancer J* 2002; **8**:194–206.

148. Galibert P, Deramond H, Rosat P, Le Gars D. [Preliminary note on the treatment of vertebral angioma by percutaneous acrylic vertebroplasty.] *Neurochirurgie* 1987; **33**:166–8.

149. Cortet B, Cotten A, Boutry N, Dewatre F, Flipo RM, Duquesnoy B, *et al.* Percutaneous vertebroplasty in patients with osteolytic metastases or multiple myeloma. *Rev Rhum Engl Ed* 1997; **64**:177–83.

150. Cotten A, Dewatre F, Cortet B, Assaker R, Leblond D, Duquesnoy B, *et al.* Percutaneous vertebroplasty for osteolytic metastases and myeloma: effects of the percentage of lesion filling and the leakage of methyl methacrylate at clinical follow-up. *Radiology* 1996; **200**:525–30.

151. Kaufmann TJ, Jensen ME, Schweickert PA, Marx WF, Kallmes DF. Age of fracture and clinical outcomes of percutaneous vertebroplasty. *AJNR Am J Neuroradiol* 2001; **22**:1860–3.

152. Kallmes DF, Schweickert PA, Marx WF, Jensen ME. Vertebroplasty in the mid- and upper thoracic spine. *AJNR Am J Neuroradiol* 2002; **23**:1117–20.

153. Moreland DB, Landi MK, Grand W. Vertebroplasty: techniques to avoid complications. *Spine J* 2001; **1**:66–71.

154. Levine SA, Perin LA, Hayes D, Hayes WS. An evidence-based evaluation of percutaneous vertebroplasty. *Manag Care* 2000; **9**:56–60, 63.

155. Hardouin P, Fayada P, Leclet H, Chopin D. Kyphoplasty. *Joint Bone Spine* 2002; **69**:256–61.

156. Cortet B, Cotten A, Boutry N, Flipo RM, Duquesnoy B, Chastanet P, *et al.* Percutaneous vertebroplasty in the treatment of osteoporotic vertebral compression fractures: an open prospective study. *J Rheumatol* 1999; **26**:2222–28.

157. Garfin SR. A retrospective review of early outcomes of balloon kyphoplasty. Proceedings of the NASS 16th Annual Meeting. *Spine J* 2002; **2**:18S.

●158. Dudeney S, Lieberman IH, Reinhardt MK, Hussein M. Kyphoplasty in the treatment of osteolytic vertebral compression fractures as a result of multiple myeloma. *J Clin Oncol* 2002; **20**:2382–7.

159. Phillips FM, McNally TA, Liberman IH, Truumees E. Does kyphoplasty reduce potential for extra-vertebral and intravascular polymethylmethacrylate leakage when compared with vertebroplasty? Proceedings of the NASS 16th Annual Meeting. *Spine J* 2002; **2**:19S.

160. Belkoff SM, Maroney M, Fenton DC, Mathis JM. An in vitro biomechanical evaluation of bone cements used in percutaneous vertebroplasty. *Bone* 1999; **25**:23S–6S.

161. Belkoff SM, Mathis JM, Jasper LE, Deramond H. An ex vivo biomechanical evaluation of a hydroxyapatite cement for use with vertebroplasty. *Spine* 2001; **26**:1542–6.

162. Spiess JL, Adelstein DJ, Hines JD. Multiple myeloma presenting with spinal cord compression. *Oncology* 1988; **45**:88–92.

163. Woo E, Yu YL, Ng M, Huang CY, Todd D. Spinal cord compression in multiple myeloma: who gets it? *Aust N Z J Med* 1986; **16**:671–5.

164. Loblaw DA, Laperriere NJ. Emergency treatment of malignant extradural spinal cord compression: an evidence-based guideline. *J Clin Oncol* 1998; **16**:1613–24.

165. Ghogawala Z, Mansfield FL, Borges LF. Spinal radiation before surgical decompression adversely affects outcomes of surgery for symptomatic metastatic spinal cord compression. *Spine* 2001; **26**:818–24.

166. Wallington M, Mendis S, Premawardhana U, Sanders P, Shahsavar-Haghighi K. Local control and survival in spinal cord compression from lymphoma and myeloma. *Radiother Oncol* 1997; **42**:43–7.

22

Management of myeloma patients with renal failure

JOAN BLADÉ AND LAURA ROSIÑOL

INCIDENCE

The incidence of renal failure in patients with multiple myeloma (MM) varies from series to series. This variation is probably due to the differences between the patient populations included, which obviously depend on both the characteristics of the institutions where the patients are seen and the criteria for definition of renal failure. Thus, between 20 and 25% of the patients seen in a tertiary hospital have a serum creatinine equal to or higher than 2 mg/dL (177 μmol/L).[1–6] In two recently published large multicenter studies, in which renal failure was defined by a serum creatinine higher than 1.5 mg/dL (133 μmol/L), the frequency of renal failure was 31% and 29%, respectively.[7,8] The degree of renal failure is usually moderate, with a serum creatinine lower than 4 mg/dL (354 μmol/L).[1–8] However, in a series from a tertiary hospital, the proportion of patients with newly diagnosed MM and renal failure severe enough to require dialysis was as high as 13% (30 of 236).[9] In contrast, only 19 of 586 patients (3%) seen at the Mayo Clinic during a 6-year period had a serum creatinine higher than 8 mg/dL (707 μmol/L),[10] while in the series by Alexanian et al.,[3] the proportion of patients with a serum creatinine level greater than 7 mg/dL (619 μmol/L) was about 2% (10 of 561). As already mentioned, it is likely that these differences are explained by a referral bias to different institutions. It is usually stated that in addition to the patients presenting with impairment of renal function at

diagnosis, an additional 25% develop renal failure later in the course of the disease. Although its real incidence is difficult to assess, in our experience the number of patients developing renal insufficiency during the course of the disease is less than 25%, and is usually due to episodes of hypercalcemia or to the use of nephrotoxic antibiotics employed in the treatment of bacterial infections in advanced phases of the disease.

CAUSES OF RENAL FAILURE

The causes of renal function impairment in patients with MM are summarized in Table 22.1. The commonest cause

Table 22.1 *Causes of renal function impairment in multiple myeloma*

- Urinary light-chain excretion
  - Myeloma kidney (cast nephropathy)
- Immunoglobulin tissue deposition
  - Amyloid – AL (light chains)
  - Immunoglobulin deposition disease – MIDD (light and/or heavy chains)
- Tubular dysfunction
  - Fanconi syndrome
- Immunoglobulin-unrelated renal damage, including:
  - Hypercalcemia
  - Nephrotoxic drugs
  - Infection

of renal damage is cast nephropathy (myeloma kidney), which results from the production and excretion of free light chains (Bence Jones protein) and leads to tubular damage and progressive renal failure that may suddenly be worsened by precipitating factors. In contrast, the clinical pattern of deposition of light chains in the glomeruli is a nephrotic syndrome with or without renal failure. The structural differences in the light chains are responsible for the different potential toxicity for the glomerular basement membranes or the distal tubules; for this reason, the kidney usually shows only one pattern of involvement.[11,12]

Light–chain excretion

The main cause of renal insufficiency in patients with MM is the so-called 'myeloma kidney' owing to light-chain tubular damage. More than 50% of patients with multiple myeloma have light-chain urine protein excretion.[2] Light chains have a low molecular weight, with a half-life of less than 1 day, and are filtered through the glomerulus and catabolized by proximal tubular renal cells. If the filtered load is too great to be catabolized by the proximal tubule, it passes to the distal collecting tubule, where it combines with Tamm–Horsfall protein and precipitates as the urine becomes more concentrated. The characteristic features of myeloma kidney are the presence of myeloma casts, consisting of eosinophilic, frequently lamellated material composed of light chains within renal tubule lumens, surrounded by multinucleated giant cells of foreign-body type in the distal tubules and collecting ducts (Fig. 22.1, Plate 6).[11–13] Tubular atrophy is usually prominent. Interstitial fibrosis and interstitial inflammatory reaction may also be observed. Typically, there are no prominent glomerular abnormalities. In addition, by immunofluorescence or ultrastructural

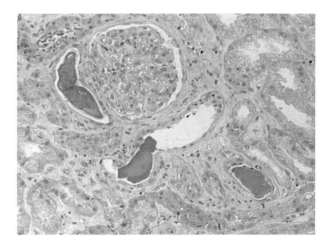

Figure 22.1 *Myeloma kidney (cast nephropathy). Typical intratubular lesions consisting of large, dense proteinaceous casts composed of immunoglobulin light chains (Masson's Trichrome, ×100).*

studies, the Tamm–Horsfall protein, a mucoprotein synthesized by the distal tubular cells, can also be identified in the tubular casts.[11] The presence of the Tamm–Horsfall protein within the tubules may lead to the precipitation of the light chains and subsequent cast formation. However, the role of Tamm–Horsfall in myeloma cast formation is not well established. Precipitation is facilitated by increased concentration of light chain and low pH of the tubular fluid.[14] There is a close correlation between the degree of cast formation and the severity of renal failure.[10–12,15]

The reason why some light chains are nephrotoxic while others are not is basically unknown and the mechanism by which the nephrotoxic light chains damage the kidney structures is also unclear. It has been suggested that the isoelectric point could play an important role in the light-chain toxicity.[16,17] However, in four studies no relationship between the light-chain isoelectric point and nephrotoxicity was found.[18–21] It has been suggested that certain light-chain immunochemical properties could be involved in the pathogenesis of cast formation and renal damage.[11–14,22] It is also worth noting that several authors have failed to find a correlation between the amount of urinary light-chain excretion and the development of renal failure. In fact, there are patients who never develop renal failure even if their urine light-chain protein excretion is very high. Kyle and Greipp[23] reported a patient with 'idiopathic' light-chain proteinuria who was excreting 9–13 g of Bence Jones proteinuria per day for more than 9 years (more than 45 kg in total) without developing nephropathy. In our experience, patients with multiple myeloma and renal failure are usually diagnosed simultaneously with both conditions, with only a few patients developing renal failure later in the course of the disease. This supports the notion that the light chains cause severe renal failure from the beginning, even before other clinical manifestations of myeloma are apparent.[6,9] Most of the patients who develop severe renal failure during the course of the disease have precipitating factors, such as serious infection.[9] At our institution, we observed three patients with relapsed or refractory myeloma and normal renal function treated with salvage therapy with thalidomide who developed acute severe renal failure, two of them requiring dialysis, while receiving amikacin because of a concurrent bacterial infection.[24] According to this observation, the possibility that thalidomide potentiates the nephrotoxicity of amikacin can not be excluded. It is our practice to try to avoid aminoglycoside antibiotics in patients with MM receiving thalidomide. In addition, unexplained and, in some cases, fatal hyperkalemia in patients with renal impairment on thalidomide treatment has been observed.[25] Thus, it is recommended that renal function and potassium levels are checked regularly in patients receiving thalidomide.

Light–chain tissue deposition

Light-chain tissue deposition consists of glomerular deposits of immunoglobulins, usually light chains, leading to amyloid or non-amyloid glomerulopathy. In both instances, the clinical consequence is the development of a picture of nephrotic syndrome.

In AL amyloid the deposits consist of fibrillar structures composed of light chains, more frequently of λ type, characterized by positive staining with Congo red.[11,12] Amyloid deposition is found in mesangial and/or glomerular basement membranes (Figs 22.2 and 22.3, Plates 7 and 8). It is usually stated that the frequency of associated AL in patients with MM is about 10%. In a report of 1705 patients with MM from the Mayo Clinic,[26] the frequency of associated AL varied according to the M-protein type: 5% in IgG, 2% in IgA, 13% in light chain only (Bence Jones), and 19% in IgD myeloma. When a patient with MM has associated systemic amyloidosis, the amyloid involvement is usually extrarenal (macroglossia, carpal tunnel syndrome, cardiac involvement) and, in the author's experience, the development of nephrotic syndrome owing to renal amyloid deposition in a patient with MM is uncommon. The finding of an M-protein in serum or urine in an adult with nephrotic syndrome is highly suspicious of AL amyloid, which may or may not be associated with multiple myeloma.[27] Renal involvement in AL amyloidosis is discussed in more detail in Chapter 27.

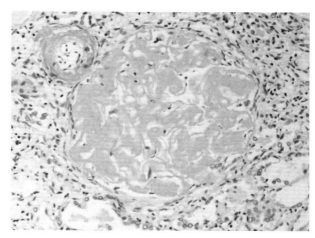

Figure 22.2 *Extensive glomerular involvement by amyloid deposition (Congo red, × 200).*

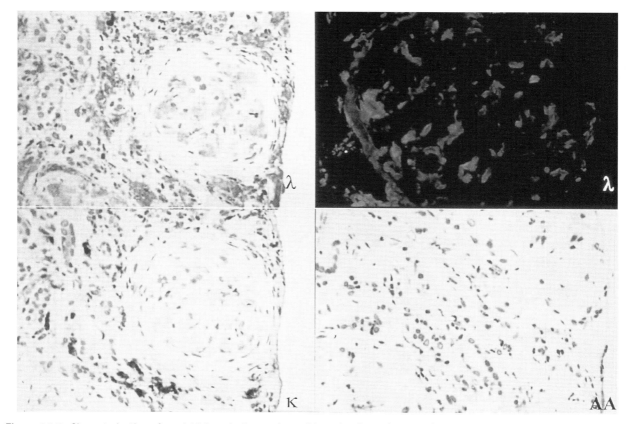

Figure 22.3 *Characterization of amyloid deposits in a patient with nephrotic syndrome and primary amyloidosis. λ light-chain positivity by immunohistochemical and immunofluorescence studies, and negativity for κ light chain and amyloid A (original, × 200).*

More recently, another form of renal light-chain deposition has been recognized. It is characterized by the deposition of non-fibrillar (Congo red negative) material and was initially termed light-chain deposition disease (LCDD).[28] However, in some cases, the tissue deposits may also contain immunoglobulin heavy-chain fragments. For this reason, the term 'monoclonal immunoglobulin deposition disease' (MIDD) is more appropriate.[29,30] In contrast with amyloidosis, the light chain in MIDD is usually of κ type. MIDD, like AL amyloid, is usually associated with subtle B-cell dyscrasias rather than overt MM and the incidence of clinically evident MIDD in patients with MM is low. Renal involvement, resulting in nephrotic syndrome, is usually prominent in MIDD. Renal function may rapidly deteriorate, resembling a picture of glomerulonephritis. These patients may also have involvement of the heart, liver, or other organs, mimicking AL amyloidosis.[30] Nodular glomerulosclerosis, resembling diabetic lesions or membranoproliferative glomerulonephritis, is the most typical histological feature of MIDD. Interestingly, glomerular lesions may be minimal in early phases of the disease. In these cases, the diagnostic clue comes from conspicuous tubular changes (i.e. deposition of eosinophilic, periodic acid Schiff (PAS)-positive material along the outer part of the tubular basement membrane consisting of monoclonal immunoglobulin chains, as demonstrated by immunofluorescence studies).[29] In addition to the characteristic glomerular and tubular changes, interstitial fibrosis is a constant finding.

Tubular dysfunction

Acquired Fanconi's syndrome is a rare condition characterized by a failure in the reabsorptive capacity of the proximal renal tubules, resulting in glycosuria, aminoaciduria, hypophosphatemia, and hypouricemia.[31] Acquired Fanconi's syndrome can be due to inherited-enzyme disorders, toxic drug reactions, or monoclonal gammopathies. It seems that in monoclonal gammopathies, the renal damage is caused by partially catabolized light chains, which form crystalline inclusions within the proximal tubular cells, which ultimately interfere with membrane transporters. In over 90% of cases the light chain is of κ type. Slowly progressive renal insufficiency and bone pain from Fanconi-induced osteoporosis are the most common clinical features in patients with MM and acquired Fanconi's syndrome. However, most patients are asymptomatic and the diagnosis is usually made when finding glycosuria, proteinuria, hypokalemia, renal tubular acidosis, mild renal failure, or unexplained hypouricemia during the investigation of a patient with monoclonal gammopathy of undetermined significance (MGUS). It has recently been shown in a murine model that limited sequence peculiarities of the light-chain variable regions can lead to the development of tubular lesions, such as those typically seen in acquired Fanconi's syndrome or those of myeloma cast nephropathy.[22]

Other causes of renal failure

There are a number of other causes of renal damage in MM.[11,12] Infiltration by myeloma cells can be observed occasionally. Hypercalcemia is a common precipitating cause of renal failure in patients with MM. Hyperuricemia, nephrotoxic antibiotics, non-steroidal anti-inflamatory drugs, and infectious interstitial nephritis can also precipitate renal failure.

Impairment of renal function is unusual in patients with Waldenström's macroglobulinemia (WM).[32] Cast formation is uncommon since the light-chain urine protein excretion, although present in 70% of patients, is usually at a very low level. Nephrotic syndrome is seen in patients with WM, and may be due to either glomerular amyloid deposition or glomerular proliferative changes consisting of subendothelial deposits or thrombi.[33,34] With immunofluorescence, these deposits are shown to be constituted exclusively of IgM. This picture is particularly observed in patients with high IgM serum levels and hyperviscosity. Interestingly, this complication may be reversible with plasma exchange.

Renal involvement in POEMS (polyneuropathy, organomegaly, endocrinopathy, M-protein, and skin lesions) syndrome is rare. However, microangiopathic glomerulonephritis, with evidence of endothelial damage, which is probably mediated by vascular endothelial growth factor (VEGF), may cause endstage renal failure.[35,36]

RENAL BIOPSY IN PATIENTS WITH MULTIPLE MYELOMA

In patients with symptomatic MM and renal failure in whom proteinuria mainly consists of light chains, the histopathologic picture of myeloma kidney is so likely that renal biopsy is not necessary and should be avoided. In cases where the clinical finding is of a nephrotic syndrome with or without renal failure, the first diagnostic possibility is associated AL amyloid, with MIDD being possible but less likely. In this situation, a subcutaneous fat aspirate should be done; if negative for amyloid, a rectal biopsy may be helpful. If there is no demonstration of amyloid in the above locations, a renal biopsy would be the next step searching for AL, MIDD, or an unrelated glomerular nephropathy, such as glomerulonephritis.

REVERSIBILITY OF RENAL IMPAIRMENT

When defining recovery of renal function as a decrease in serum creatinine level to less than 1.5 mg/dL

(133 μmol/L), the reversibility rate of renal failure in patients with MM varies from 20 to 58%.[3,5–8,15,37–39] The reversibility mainly depends on the degree of renal insufficiency. Thus, more than 50% of patients with serum creatinine levels lower than 4 mg/dL (354 μmol/L) completely recover their renal function.[3,6,8] In contrast, in the authors' experience, the reversibility rate in patients with a serum creatinine greater than 4 mg/dL (354 μmol/L), the recovery rate is less than 10%.[6] In a series including 94 patients with MM and initial renal failure, logistic regression analysis showed that the factors associated with renal function recovery were a serum creatinine level lower than 4 mg/dL (354 μmol/L), a total urine protein excretion of less than 1 g/24 hours, and a serum calcium level higher than 11.5 mg/dL (2.86 mmol/L).[6] There are, however, other studies reporting no significant correlation between the serum creatinine levels and reversibility of renal failure.[5,37] The average time taken for recovery of renal function is usually less than 2 months with only a minority of patients requiring more than 4 months to recover their renal function. Recovery of renal function is unlikely to occur if it has not already recovered by 4 months.

The likelihood of improvement of renal function in patients with severe renal failure is very low.[9] In fact, in our experience, it is very unusual that patients with myeloma kidney needing dialysis recover their renal function and, when this occurs, it is usually within the first weeks (see p. 345). Plasma exchange may increase the likelihood of renal recovery, particularly in patients not yet requiring dialysis (see later).

STANDARD-DOSE CHEMOTHERAPY IN PATIENTS WITH RENAL FAILURE

In five series in which the response to therapy in patients with MM and renal failure was analyzed, the response rate ranged from 39 to 50%.[6,8,38,40,41] In one of these studies, the response in patients receiving combination chemotherapy was significantly higher than that observed in those given melphalan and prednisone.[6] In our experience, the response rate in patients with impaired renal function is lower than in those with normal renal function (39% vs. 56%). However, the lower response rate is because of the early mortality rate in patients with renal failure as compared with those with normal renal function (30% vs. 7%).[6] If patients who die within the first 2 months of initiation of treatment are excluded, the response to therapy is similar regardless of whether there is renal function impairment.[6] In consequence, renal failure per se does not indicate resistance to chemotherapy. In fact, even for patients on a chronic hemodialysis program and who survive the first 2 months on dialysis, the

response rate is similar to that of those with normal renal function.[9] However, renal failure is a bad prognostic factor in MM. In a single-institution study, the median survival of 94 patients with initial renal failure was 9 months.[6] However, it is of interest that the median survival of patients with reversible renal failure was 28 months in contrast with 5 months for those with non-reversible renal function impairment.[6]

It has been widely considered that in patients with renal failure, conventional chemotherapy with melphalan and prednisone is not the most appropriate treatment approach because the need for dose adjustment of melphalan in order to avoid severe myelosuppression may imply the risk of suboptimal treatment. However, the use of melphalan and the need for dose adjustment in patients with renal failure is a matter of controversy. It is well known that the absorption of melphalan varies from patient to patient, the serum levels of melphalan being extremely variable following oral administration.[42] In addition, the pharmacokinetics of melphalan are difficult to assess, since the drug is extensively bound to serum proteins, particularly to serum albumin, and it is spontaneously hydrolyzed in aqueous media.[43] It has been shown by several investigators that spontaneous degradation and not renal excretion is the main via for melphalan elimination. In fact, two studies have shown that the urinary excretion of melphalan during the 24 hours following administration was only 13% and 14%, respectively.[43,44] This suggests that renal function in not crucial in the elimination of melphalan. Taking into account all the above, it has been suggested that there is no need for dose reduction of melphalan in patients with renal failure.

However, occasional patients with renal failure treated with melphalan develop severe long-lasting myelosuppression. In addition, one study from the Cancer and Acute Leukemia Group B showed that patients with renal function impairment treated with intravenous melphalan had higher myelosuppression than patients with normal renal function.[45] Furthermore, patients with renal failure undergoing autotransplantation and given high-dose melphalan had significant toxicity, particularly those on dialysis and low serum albumin, thus leading to the recommendation of decreasing the dose of melphalan for high-dose therapy intensification from 200 mg/m^2 to 140 or 100 mg/m^2 (see p. 344).[46] In the light of these observations, it seems that the use of melphalan should be avoided in the conventional treatment of patients with MM and renal failure.

On the other hand, combination chemotherapy could produce a more rapid response with a quicker reduction in the light-chain protein production, thereby avoiding further renal damage. In this regard, it has been suggested that chemotherapy with a 4-day continuous infusion of Adriamycin and vincristine plus high-dose dexamethasone (VAD)[47] or high-dose methylprednisolone (VAMP)[48] could be more effective than more conventional approaches (i.e. single alkylating agents plus standard-dose steroids) in patients with MM and renal failure. In addition, no dosage modification is required and toxicity is not increased in patients with renal failure. Although it has not been investigated in prospective trials, VAD is the best approach for patients with severe renal failure. For patients in whom treatment with VAD is not feasible (associated cardiac disorders, very advanced age, poor clinical condition), in the authors' experience, treatment with pulsed intravenous cyclophosphamide (800–1000 mg every 3 weeks), which produces only a transient granulocytopenia, plus high-dose dexamethasone on days 1–4, also at 3-week intervals, would be the most appropriate therapy. In patients who show significant myelotoxicity to cyclophosphamide, with severe granulocytopenia or thrombocytopenia, dexamethasone alone is a very useful treatment in renal failure.

HIGH–DOSE THERAPY AND STEM CELL TRANSPLANTATION

One question that frequently arises is whether patients with persistent renal failure should be excluded from high-dose therapy/stem cell transplantation (HDT/SCT) programs. Several case reports and studies including small numbers of patients have shown the feasibility of HDT/SCT in patients with MM and renal failure.[49–52] The Spanish Registry reported a series of 14 patients with non-reversible renal failure undergoing HDT/SCT and compared the results with those achieved in patients with normal renal function at transplantation.[53] The median serum creatinine level of the 14 patients with abnormal renal function at transplantation was 2.5 mg/dL, range 2.1–9.3 (221 μmol/L, range 186–822), and four of them were on long-term dialysis. The stem cell collection and engraftment were similar to those of patients with normal renal function. However, the transplant-related mortality (TRM) was significantly higher in patients with impaired renal function (29% vs. 4%). The factors significantly associated with TRM were a serum creatinine level >5 mg/dL (442 μmol/L), a hemoglobin level <9.5 mg/dL, and poor performance status (Eastern Cooperative Oncology Group score; ECOG >2). The overall event-free survival (EFS) and overall survival (OS) were not significantly different in patients with or without renal failure. From this small series, it was concluded that patients with MM and renal failure with a serum creatinine level >5 mg/dL (442 μmol/L) and poor performance status should be excluded from HDT/SCT programs.

Badros et al.[46] reported the results of HDT/SCT with melphalan 200 mg/m^2 (MEL-200) or melphalan 140 mg/m^2 (MEL-140) in 81 patients with non-reversible renal failure, 38 of them on dialysis at the time of transplant. The engraftment and the complete remission rate (CR) were similar to those observed in patients with normal renal function. However, TRM was 6% and 13% after a single and double transplant, respectively. The main cause of death was multiorgan failure. In addition, non-hematological toxicity, particularly in dialysis-dependent patients receiving MEL-200, was very high. Thus, severe bacterial infections were documented in 48% of the patients. Other frequent complications were pneumonitis (eight patients required mechanic ventilation) and atrial dysrhythmias. Of note, encephalopathy, including coma, was observed in a number of patients, particularly in those on dialysis, as compared with those not requiring renal replacement (47% vs. 6%). The cause of the encephalopathy is not clear. It has been postulated that altered drug metabolism might be the cause. Low serum albumin and high serum concentration of melphalan increased toxicity and mortality, and significantly influenced overall survival. The incidence of complications was significantly higher in patients receiving MEL-200 than in those given MEL-140. Of interest, patients given MEL-140 had a similar outcome (CR, EFS, and OS) to those receiving MEL-200. Chemoresistant disease, low serum albumin, and older age were associated with a significantly higher TRM and shorter overall survival. Considering the above results, in patients with renal failure HDT/SCT should be individually considered and only performed in younger patients (<55 years) with chemosensitive disease and good general condition, and the intensification regimen should consist of MEL-140 or MEL-100 rather than MEL-200.[46]

When MIDD or AL is associated with overt MM, the treatment approach should be the same as for patients with myeloma. In AL patients younger than 65 years and with fewer than three organs involved and no symptomatic cardiopathy, HDT/SCT should be considered (see Chapter 27). This approach may be particularly helpful when nephrotic syndrome is the predominant feature of AL. In patients with MIDD and with no symptomatic cardiac involvement, HDT/SCT should also be considered. It is of interest that patients without overt myeloma and in whom the plasma cell burden is low and the organ dysfunction is the result of tissue deposition, as occurs in AL, MIDD, POEMS, and scleromyxoedema (generalized lichen myxoedematosus – papules and plaques infiltrating the skin, usually associated with a cathodal IgGλ monoclonal protein), the likelihood of response to high-dose therapy is high.[30,54–56] In addition, in these circumstances there is no need for tumor reduction before stem cell mobilization. Furthermore, in these patients, mobilization with granulocyte colony stimulating factor (G-CSF) alone usually provides enough CD34+ cells for bone marrow rescue.

In patients with non-reversible renal failure requiring chronic dialysis and who achieve complete remission (disappearance of malignant bone marrow plasma cells with no evidence of serum/urine M-protein on immunofixation) after conventional or high-dose therapy, a kidney transplant may be offered. However, most patients will show recurrence of their nephropathy at relapse.[57]

PLASMA EXCHANGE

It has been suggested that a rapid removal of light chains with plasma exchange, along with chemotherapy, could prevent irreversible renal failure by avoiding further renal damage.[15,17,37,58] Misiani et al.[38] reported that 22% (two of 23) patients treated with chemotherapy and plasma exchange completely recovered from their acute renal failure. In a non-randomized study including 50 patients, Pozzi et al.[15] showed that in patients treated with chemotherapy and plasma exchange, the recovery of renal function was significantly higher than in those treated with chemotherapy alone (61% vs. 27%). Zucchelli et al.[59] reported the results of a controlled trial comparing chemotherapy plus plasma exchange versus chemotherapy alone in 29 patients with MM and severe renal failure (24 of them on dialysis plus the remaining five with a serum creatinine higher than 442 μmol/L (5 mg/dL) and light-chain urine protein excretion higher than 1 g/24 hours. In the plasma exchange group, the light-chain urine protein excretion was significantly reduced when compared with the no plasma exchange arm. More importantly, in 13 of the 15 patients in the plasma exchange arm, the serum creatinine level decreased to less than 221 μmol/L (2.5 mg/dL), while only two of the 14 patients treated with chemotherapy alone could stop dialysis. Finally, the 1-year survival was significantly longer in the plasma exchange arm (66% vs. 28%). However, there are problems with interpreting the results of this trial. The patients randomized to plasma exchange received hemodialysis while those in the control arm received peritoneal dialysis, and there were baseline differences between the two groups, particularly in the proportion of patients needing dialysis at entry. The Mayo Clinic group compared, in a small randomized trial, forced diuresis and chemotherapy (ten patients) versus forced diuresis, chemotherapy, and plasma exchange (11 patients).[10] They only found a statistical trend in favor of the plasma exchange group. The survival was not significantly different between both treatment arms. These two small trials have, therefore, not provided conclusive evidence for the benefit or otherwise of plasma exchange. A larger randomized controlled trial is under way in Canada and another is about to open in the UK.

In our experience, patients with renal failure severe enough to require dialysis do not benefit from plasma exchange. This is in agreement with the findings by Johnson et al.[10] and Pozzi et al.,[15] who recognized the severity of myeloma cast formation as the major factor associated with non-reversible renal failure, even in patients undergoing plasma exchange.[9,10,15] On the other hand, the Oxford Renal Unit group treated 16 patients with myeloma and acute renal failure with plasma exchange, achieving significant renal function improvement in six, with dialysis discontinuation in three. In contrast, only one of 26 patients not treated with plasma exchange improved;[60] however, these data are not from a randomized or controlled study.

It is our practice to perform plasma exchange with 5% albumin in saline solution with a total volume of about 5 L in each session in patients with MM and non-oliguric severe renal failure. Serum and M-protein are measured before and after each plasma exchange procedure, and the sessions are repeated every 2 or 3 days to a maximum of four to five sessions. With this approach, replacement with coagulation factors is usually not necessary. Owing to the background immunoglobulin removal with plasma exchange, intravenous immunoglobulins are given after the end of plasma exchange in order to prevent bacterial infections in these high-risk patients (multiple myeloma with severe renal failure receiving their initial chemotherapy and undergoing plasma exchange with depletion of immunoglobulins).

DIALYSIS-DEPENDENT RENAL FAILURE

The proportion of patients with MM and renal failure severe enough to require renal replacement with dialysis has been reported in a number of studies. As already mentioned, the frequency varies from 2% to 13% depending on the characteristics of the institutions where the patients are seen (myeloma reference centers vs. general hospitals).[3,9,10,61] It is of interest that in about three-quarters of the patients, the diagnosis of both conditions is simultaneous and only one-quarter of myeloma patients who will require dialysis develop renal failure late in the course of the disease.[5,9,15,16,62] Severe renal failure is more commonly seen in light-chain and IgD myeloma than in IgG and IgA myeloma types.[26] Thus, in patients with renal failure, the frequency of light-chain myeloma ranges from 20 to 62%, while in the general myeloma series, it represents about 15% of cases.[5,10,15–17,38,40,41,61–64] It is sometimes suggested that in patients with renal failure, the proportion of patients with λ light chain is higher than expected, but this is not clearly established.[9]

In four series, the response rate to chemotherapy in patients with MM on a long-term dialysis program ranged from 40 to 60%.[9,38,40,41] At our institution, we found a response rate of 40% in patients on dialysis versus 43% in a group of 105 patients with stage III myeloma who did not require dialysis and who had survived the first 2 months from the initiation of chemotherapy.[9] Thus, the response to chemotherapy is not influenced by renal function *per se*.

In patients requiring dialysis, the reversibility of renal failure is usually less than 10%.[9,10,40,41,62–65] Although recovery rarely occurs after 4 months on dialysis, at least three cases of delayed partial recovery after more than 1 year on dialysis have been recognized.[9,66,67] Contrasting with most reported series, two studies reported that 75% (12 of 16) and 43% (13 of 30) of patients were able to discontinue dialysis replacement, respectively.[17,38]

Despite improvements in survival during recent years, the mortality rate among patients with MM and dialysis-dependent renal failure during the first 2 months from diagnosis is still around 30%.[5,6,9,17,63] If patients do not die during the initiation of dialysis, survival appears to be not significantly different from that of other myeloma patients. The Mayo Clinic group[59] reported that five of 11 patients on long-term dialysis had a survival from 7 to 48 months from the initiation of dialysis. Iggo *et al.*[40] found that the survival at 1 year was 45%. In two other series, the median survival was about 2 years, with one-third of patients surviving for more than 3 years.[9,41] Thus, the need for dialysis does not adversely affect survival. The issue of quality of life, measured by the need of hospitalization, in patients with MM and on a long-term dialysis program has been assessed in several studies. In the series by Korzets *et al.*,[41] the number of hospital admissions was 6.1 per year and the total number of days in hospital was 75 per patient per year, mainly due to peritonitis related to chronic peritoneal dialysis. In contrast, in two series, the average of hospitalization was 12 and 19 days per patient-year, respectively.[9,63] In addition, in the authors' experience, patients who survive for more than 1 year spend less than 10 days per year in hospital, a figure similar to that observed in patients on chronic dialysis because of diabetic nephropathy.[9] It seems that there are no significant differences between chronic peritoneal dialysis (CAPD) and hemodialysis. In this regard, Shetty *et al.*[68] reported a relatively low incidence of CAPD-related peritonitis (one case per 14.4 months) and the need for hospitalization was comparable to that observed in patients on long-term hemodialysis.[9,59] Taking into account all the above, long-term dialysis is a worthwhile treatment for patients with myeloma and severe endstage renal failure.

OVERALL TREATMENT APPROACH IN PATIENTS WITH MULTIPLE MYELOMA AND RENAL FAILURE

Patients with a moderate increase in serum creatinine levels or reversible renal failure should receive standard chemotherapy with or without HDT/SCT according to the patient's age and clinical condition. Patients with a serum creatinine higher than 4 mg/dL (354 μmol/L) should be treated with VAD, or cyclophosphamide plus dexamethasone, or dexamethasone alone. High-dose therapy is not generally recommended in these patients but, if performed, the intensification regimen should consist of MEL-140 or MEL-100. In non-oliguric patients who are not requiring dialysis, an early plasma exchange program, along with forced diuresis and chemotherapy, may be of benefit. However, in patients with advanced myeloma kidney already requiring dialysis, plasma exchange does not seem to be beneficial. Renal replacement with dialysis is a worthwhile palliative measure for myeloma patients with endstage renal failure.

KEY POINTS

- Twenty-five percent of patients with multiple myeloma have renal function impairment at the time of diagnosis and, in approximately 10% of newly diagnosed patients, the degree of renal failure is severe enough to require renal replacement with dialysis.
- The main cause of renal failure is 'myeloma kidney' or 'cast nephropathy,' resulting from tubular damage by urinary free light chains.
- Glomerular involvement leading to nephrotic syndrome is uncommon. If present, it is suggestive of AL amyloid or monoclonal immunoglobulin deposition disease.
- Renal biopsy is only indicated when the cause of renal function impairment is unclear.
- Renal failure is reversible in about 50% of patients. Reversibility mainly depends on the degree of renal failure (serum creatinine < or > 4 mg/dL (<or>354 μmol/L) and the amount of light-chain urine protein excretion (<1 g/24 hours) and the presence of hypercalcemia (>2.86 mmol/L (11.5 mg/dL)).
- The response to initial chemotherapy ranges from 40 to 50%, because of early mortality.
- In patients with serum creatinine higher than >4 mg/dL (354 μmol/L), VAD, or cyclophosphamide plus dexamethasone, or dexamethasone, alone appear to be better approaches than melphalan-containing regimens.
- In patients with renal failure, high-dose therapy/ stem cell transplantation should be considered only in younger patients (<55 years) with chemosensitive disease and good performance status.
- In non-oliguric patients with a serum creatinine level >4 mg/dL (<354 μmol/L), early plasma exchange is probably of benefit.

- In patients with advanced myeloma kidney requiring dialysis, the benefit of plasma exchange is doubtful.
- Renal replacement with dialysis is a worthwhile palliative approach for myeloma patients with advanced non-reversible renal failure.

REFERENCES

● = Key primary paper
◆ = Major review article
✳ = Paper that represents the first formal publication of a management guideline

✳1. DeFronzo RA, Humphrey RL, Wright JR, Cooke CR. Acute renal failure in multiple myeloma. *Medicine (Baltimore)* 1975; **54**:209–23.

●2. Kyle RA. Multiple myeloma: review of 869 cases. *Mayo Clin Proc* 1975; **50**:29–40.

✳3. Alexanian R, Barlogie, Dixon D. Renal failure in multiple myeloma: pathogenesis and prognostic implications. *Arch Intern Med* 1990; **150**:1693–5.

●4. Bernstein SP, Humes HD. Reversible renal insufficiency in multiple myeloma. *Arch Intern Med* 1982; **142**:2083–6.

●5. Cohen DJ, Sherman W, Osserman EF, Appel GB. Acute renal failure in patients with multiple myeloma. *Am J Med* 1984; **76**:247–56.

●6. Bladé J, Frenéndez-Llama P, Bosch F, Montoliu J, Lens XM, Montoto S, *et al.* Renal failure in multiple myeloma. Presenting features and predictors of outcome in 94 patients from a single institution. *Arch Intern Med* 1998; **158**:1889–93.

●7. Knudsen LM, Hippe E, Hjorth M, Holmberg E, Westin J. Renal function in newly diagnosed multiple myeloma. A demographic study of 1353 patients. *Eur J Haematol* 1994; **53**:207–12.

●8. Knudsen LM, Hjorth M, Hippe E. Renal failure in multiple myeloma: reversibility and impact on prognosis. *Eur J Haematol* 2000; **65**:175–81.

●9. Torra R, Bladé J, Cases A, López-Pedret J, Montserrat E, Rozman C, *et al.* Patients with multiple myeloma and renal failure requiring long-term dialysis: presenting features, response to therapy, and outcome in a series of 20 cases. *Br J Haematol* 1995; **91**:854–9.

●10. Johnson WJ, Kyle RA, Pineda AA, O'Brien PC, Holley KE. Treatment of renal failure associated to multiple myeloma. *Arch Intern Med* 1990; **150**:863–9.

◆11. Hill GS, Morel-Maroger L, Méry JP, Brouet JC, Mignon F. Renal lesions in multiple myeloma: their relationship to associated protein abnormalities. *Am J Kidney Dis* 1983; **4**:423–38.

◆12. Verroust P, Morel-Maroger L, Preud'Homme JL. Renal lesions in dysproteinemia. *Semin Immunopathol* 1982; **5**:333–56.

◆13. Sanders PW. Pathogenesis and treatment of myeloma kidney. *J Lab Clin Med* 1994; **124**:484–8.

●14. Boege F, Merkle M, Werle E, Röckle H. Structural features related to the nephropathogenicity of Bence-Jones protein. *Kidney Int* 1994; **46**:S93–6.

●15. Pozzi C, Pasquali S, Donini U, Casanova S, Banfi G, Tiraboschi G, *et al.* Prognostic factors and effectiveness of treatment in acute renal failure due to multiple myeloma: review of 50 cases. *Clin Nephrol* 1987; **28**:1–9.

●16. Rota S, Mougenot B, Baudouin B, De Meyer-Brasseur M, Lemaitre V, Michel C, *et al.* Multiple myeloma and severe renal failure: a clinicopathologic study of outcome and prognosis in 34 patients. *Medicine* 1987; **66**:126–37.

●17. Pasqualli, Casanova S, Zuchelli A, Zuchelli P. Long-term survival in patients with acute and severe renal failure due to multiple myeloma. *Clin Nephrol* 1990; **34**:247–54.

18. Coward RA, Delamore IW, Mallick NP, Robinson EL. The importance of urinary immunoglobulin light chain isoelectric point (pI) in nephrotoxicity in multiple myeloma. *Clin Sci* 1984; **66**:229–32.

19. Melcion C, Mougenot B, Baudouin B, Ronco P, Moulonguet-Doleris L, Vanhille P, *et al.* Renal failure in myeloma: relationship with isoelectric point of immunoglobulin light chains. *Clin Nephrol* 1984; **22**:138–43.

20. Johns EA, Turner R, Cooper EH, MacLennan ICM. Isoelectric points of urinary light chains in myelomatosis: analysis in relation to nephrotoxicity. *J Clin Pathol* 1986; **39**:833–7.

21. Palant CE, Bonitati J, Bartholomew WR, Brentjens JR, Walshe JJ, Bentzel CJ. Nodular glomerulosclerosis associated with multiple myeloma. Role of light chain isoelectric point. *Am J Med* 1986; **80**:98–102.

22. Decourt C, Rocca A, Bridoux F, Vrtovsnik F, Preud'homme JL, Cogne M, *et al.* Mutational analysis in murine models for myeloma-associated Fanconi's syndrome or cast myeloma nephropathy. *Blood* 1999; **94**:3559–66.

●23. Kyle RA, Greipp PR. 'Idiopathic' Bence Jones proteinuria: long-term follow-up in seven patients. *N Engl J Med* 1982; **306**:564–7.

24. Bladé J, Esteve J, Rosiñol L, Perales M, Montoto S, Tuset M, *et al.* Thalidomide in refractory and relapsing multiple myeloma. *Semin Oncol* 2001; **28**:588–92.

25. Harris E, Behrens J, Samson D, Rahemtulla A, Russell NH, Byrne JL. Use of thalidomide in patients with myeloma and renal failure may be associated with unexplained hyperkalaemia. *Br J Haematol* 2003; **122**:160–1.

26. Bladé J, Lust JA, Kyle RA. Immunoglobulin D multiple myeloma: presenting features, response to therapy, and survival in a series of 53 cases. *J Clin Oncol* 1994; **12**:2398–404.

◆27. Gertz MA, Lacy MQ, Dispenzieri A. Amyloidosis. *Hematol Oncol Clin North Am* 1999; **13**:1211–34.

✳28. Randall RE, Williamson WC, Mullinax F, Tung MY, Still WJS. Manifestations of systemic light chain deposition. *Am J Med* 1976; **60**:293–9.

◆29. Preud'Homme JL, Aucouturier P, Touchard G, Striker L, Khamlichi AA, Rocca A, *et al.* Monoclonal immunoglobulin deposition disease (Randall type). Relationship with structural abnormalities of immunoglobulin chains. *Kidney Int* 1994; **46**:965–72.

◆30. Dhodapkar MV, Merlini G, Solomon A. Biology and therapy of immunoglobulin deposition diseases. *Hematol Oncol Clin North Am* 1997; **11**:89–110.

◆31. Lacy MQ, Gertz MA. Acquired Fanconi's syndrome associated with monoclonal gammopathies. *Hematol Oncol Clin North Am* 1999; **13**:1273–80.

◆32. Dimopoulos MA, Galani E, Matsouka C, Verroust P, Richet G. Waldenström's macroglobulinemia. *Hematol Oncol Clin North Am* 1999; **13**:1351–66.

33. Morel-Maroger L, Bash A, Danon F, Verroust P, Richet G. Pathology of the kidney in Waldenström's macroglobulinemia. *N Engl J Med* 1970; **283**:123–127.

34. Fudenberg HH, Virella G. Multiple myeloma and Waldenström's macroglobulinemia: unusual presentations. *Semin Hematol* 1980; **17**:63–90.

35. Modesto-Segonds A, Rey JP, Orfila C, Huchard G, Suc JM. Renal involvement in POEMS syndrome. *Clin Nephrol* 1995; **43**:342–5.

36. Nakamoto Y, Imai H, Yasuda T, Wakui H, Miura AB. A spectrum of clinicopathological features of nephropathy associated with POEMS syndrome. *Nephrol Dial Transplant* 1999; **14**:2370–8.

●37. Cavo M, Baccarani M, Galieni P, Gobbi M, Tura S. Renal failure in multiple myeloma: a study of the presenting findings, response to treatment and prognosis in 26 patients. *Nouv Rev Fr Hematol* 1986; **28**:147–52.

●38. Misiani R, Tiraboschi G. Mingardi G, Mecca G. Management of myeloma kidney: an anti-light-chain approach. *Am J Kidney Dis* 1987; **10**:28–33.

●39. Medical Research Council Working Party on Leukemia in Adults. Analysis and management of renal failure in the fourth myelomatosis trial. *Br Med J* 1984; **288**:1411–16.

●40. Iggo N, Palmer ABD, Severn A, Trafford JAP, Mufti GJ, Taube D, et al. Chronic dialysis in patients with multiple myeloma and renal failure: a worthwhile treatment. *Q J Med* 1989; **270**:903–10.

●41. Korzets A, Tam F, Russell G, Feehally J, Walls J, Moon TE, et al. The role of continuous ambulatory peritoneal dialysis in en-stage renal failure due to multiple myeloma. *Am J Kidney Dis* 1990; **6**:216–23.

*42. Alberts DS, Chang SY, Chen H-SG, Moon TE, Enas TL, Furner RL, et al. Oral melphalan kinetics. *Clin Pharmacol Ther* 1979; **26**:737–45.

◆43. Sarosy G, Leyland-Jones B, Soochan P, Cheson BD. The systemic administration of intravenous melphalan. *J Clin Oncol* 1988; **11**:1768–82.

44. Bosanquet AG, Gilby E. Pharmacokinetics of oral and intravenous melphalan during routine treatment of multiple myeloma. *Eur J Cancer Clin Oncol* 1982; **18**:355–62.

●45. Cornwell GG III, Pajak TF, McIntyre OR, Kochwa S, Dosik H. Influence of renal failure on myelosuppressive effects of melphalan: Cancer and Acute Leukemia Group B experience. *Cancer Treat Rep* 1982; **66**:475–81.

●46. Badros A, Barlogie B, Siegel E, Roberts J, Langmaid C, Zangari M, et al. Results of autologous stem cell transplant in multiple myeloma patients with renal failure. *Br J Haematol* 2001; **114**:822–9.

*47. Barlogie B, Smith L, Alexanian R. Effective treatment of advanced myeloma refractory to alkylating agents. *N Engl J Med* 1984; **310**:1353–6.

*48. Aitchison RG, Reilly IAG, Morgan AG, Russell NH. Vincristine, adriamycin and high dose steroids in myeloma complicated by renal failure. *Br J Cancer* 1990; **61**:765–6.

49. Ballester OF, Tummala R, Janssen WE, Fields KK, Hiemenz JW, Goldstein SC, et al. High-dose chemotherapy and autologous peripheral blood stem cell transplantation in patients with multiple myeloma and renal failure. *Bone Marrow Transplant* 1997; **20**:653–6.

50. Rebibou JM, Caillot D, Casasnovas RO, Tanter Y, Maillard N, Solary E, et al. Peripheral blood stem cell transplantation in a myeloma patient with endstage renal failure. *Bone Marrow Transplant* 1997; **20**:63–5.

51. Reiter E, Kalhs P, Keil F, Rabitsch W, Gisslinger H, Mayer G, et al. Effects of high-dose melphalan and peripheral blood stem cell transplantation on renal function in patients with multiple myeloma and renal insufficiency: a case report and review of the literature. *Ann Hematol* 1999; **78**:189–91.

52. Tosi F, Zamagni E, Ronconi S, et al. Safety of autologous hematopoietic stem cell transplantation in patients with multiple myeloma and chronic renal failure. *Leukemia* 2000; **14**:1310–13.

●53. San Miguel JF, LaHuerta JJ, Garía-Sanz R, Alegre A, Bladé J, Martínez R, et al. Are myeloma patients with renal failure candidates for autologous stem cell transplantation? *Hematol J* 2000; **1**:28–36.

◆54. Comenzo RL, Gertz MA. Autologous stem cell transplantation for primary systemic amyloidosis. *Blood* 2002; **99**:4276–82.

*55. Rovira M, Carreras E, Bladé J, Graus F, Valls J, Fernández-Avilés F, et al. Dramatic improvement of POEMS syndrome following haematopoietic cell transplantation. *Br J Haematol* 2001; **115**:373–5.

●56. Jaccard A, Royer B, Dordessoule D, Brouet JC, Fermand JP. High-dose therapy and autologous stem cell transplantation in POEMS syndrome. *Blood* 2002; **99**:3057–9.

◆57. Gerlag PGG, Koene RAP, Berden JHM. Renal transplantation in light chain nephropathy: case report and review of the literature. *Clin Nephrol* 1986; **25**:101–4.

58. Vhalin A, Löfvenberg E, Holm J. Improved survival in multiple myeloma with renal failure. *Acta Med Scand* 1987; **221**:205–9.

●59. Zucchelli P, Pasquali S, Cagnoli L, Ferrari G. Controlled plasma exchange trial in acute renal failure due to multiple myeloma. *Kidney Int* 1988; **33**:1175–80.

60. Winearls CG. Acute myeloma kidney. *Kidney Int* 1995; **48**:1347–61.

●61. Sharland A, Snowdon L, Joshua DE, Gibson J, Tiller DJ. Hemodialysis: an appropriate therapy in myeloma-induced renal failure. *Am J Kidney Dis* 1997; **30**:786–92.

●62. Cosio FG, Pence TV, Shapiro FL, Kjellstrand CM. Severe renal failure in multiple myeloma. *Clin Nephrol* 1981; **15**:206–10.

*63. Johnson WJ, Kyle RA, Dahlberg PJ. Dialysis in the treatment of multiple myeloma. *Mayo Clin Proc* 1980; **55**:65–72.

●64. Lazarus HM, Adelstein DJ, Herzig RH, Smith MC. Long-term survival of patients with multiple myeloma and acute renal failure at presentation. *Am J Kidney Dis* 1983; **2**:521–5.

●65. Coward RA, Mallick NP, Delamore IW. Should patients with renal failure associated to multiple myeloma be dialysed? *Br Med J* 1983; **287**:1575–8.

66. Brown WW, Hebert LA, Piering WF, Piciotta AV, Lemann J Jr, Garancis JC. Reversal of chronic endstage renal failure due to myeloma kidney. *Ann Intern Med* 1979; **90**:793–4.

67. Dahlberg PJ, Newcomer KL, Yutuc WR, Smith MJ. Myeloma kidney: improved renal function following long-term chemotherapy and hemodialysis. *Am J Nephrol* 1983; **3**:242–3.

68. Shetty A, Oreopoulos DG. Myeloma patients do well on CAPD tool. *Br J Haematol* 1997; **96**:654–7.

23

Neurologic aspects of monoclonal gammopathy of undetermined significance, multiple myeloma, and related disorders

ROBERT A. KYLE AND ANGELA DISPENZIERI

INTRODUCTION

Radiculopathy is the single most frequent neurologic complication of multiple myeloma. It usually involves the thoracic or lumbosacral area, and results from compression of the nerve root by a paravertebral plasmacytoma or by the collapsed bone itself. Compression of the spinal cord from an extramedullary plasmacytoma occurs in 5% of patients with myeloma during the course of their disease. Rarely, myeloma cells diffusely infiltrate the meninges. Intracranial plasmacytomas most commonly arise in the base of the skull and represent myelomatous lesions from bone. Soft-tissue plasmacytomas of the central nervous system are rare. Peripheral sensorimotor peripheral neuropathy is uncommon in multiple myeloma; when present, it is usually caused by amyloidosis or osteosclerotic myeloma.

The neurologic complications of monoclonal gammopathy of undetermined significance (MGUS) consist mainly of a sensorimotor peripheral neuropathy. The differential diagnosis includes primary systemic amyloidosis (AL), POEMS syndrome (polyneuropathy, organomegaly, endocrinopathy, monoclonal protein, and skin changes; osteosclerotic myeloma), and neuropathy associated with multiple myeloma, Waldenström's macroglobulinemia, or lymphoma.

MONOCLONAL GAMMOPATHY OF UNDETERMINED SIGNIFICANCE

Monoclonal gammopathy of undetermined significance is characterized by the presence of a monoclonal (M) protein without evidence of multiple myeloma, macroglobulinemia, primary amyloidosis, or related disorders (see Chapter 24). MGUS is defined by the presence of a serum M-protein value less than 30 g/L, less than 10% plasma cells in the bone marrow, absence of lytic lesions, and no or only small amounts of M-protein (monoclonal light chain, Bence Jones protein) in the urine. In addition, anemia, hypercalcemia, and renal insufficiency are absent, unless caused by an unrelated disease. MGUS is common; more than 650 patients with newly diagnosed MGUS were seen at Mayo Clinic in 2001. MGUS is found in more than 1% of patients older than 50 years. It has been reported in 3% of persons older than 70 years in Sweden,[1] in the USA,[2] and in France.[3]

In a series of 241 patients with MGUS seen at Mayo Clinic from 1956 to 1970, multiple myeloma, primary amyloidosis, macroglobulinemia, or a related lymphoproliferative disorder developed in 26% during a follow-up of 24–38 years (see Chapter 24). A population-based long-term follow-up of 1384 patients with MGUS in southeastern Minnesota was recently reported.[4] During follow-up, multiple myeloma, primary amyloidosis, lymphoma with an IgM serum M-protein, macroglobulinemia, plasmacytoma, or chronic lymphocytic leukemia developed in 115 patients. The cumulative probability of progression to one of these disorders was 10% at 10 years, 21% at 20 years, and 26% at 25 years. The risk of progression was about 1% per year. The number of patients with progression to a serious plasma cell disorder (115 patients) was 7.3 times the number expected on the basis of incidence rates for those conditions in the general population. Only the concentration and type of M-protein were independent predictors of progression. The presence of a monoclonal urine protein (κ or λ) and a reduction of one or more uninvolved immunoglobulins were not risk factors for progression. Patients with IgM or IgA M-protein had an increased risk of progression to disease compared with patients who had IgG M-protein ($P = 0.001$). The risk of progression to multiple myeloma or a related disorder 20 years after diagnosis of MGUS was 15% for an initial M-protein level of 5 g/L or less, 16% for 10 g/L, 25% for 15 g/L, 41% for 20 g/L, 49% for 25 g/L, and 64% for 30 g/L (Fig. 23.1). The risk of progression with an M-protein value of 25 g/L was 4.6 times more than with a 5 g/L spike. The number of plasma cells in the bone marrow also may be of some help in the prediction of progression. Cesana et al.[5] reported that more than 5% bone marrow plasma cells was an independent risk factor for progression.

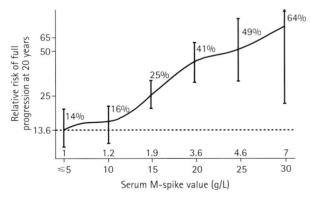

Figure 23.1 *Actuarial risk of full progression, according to serum monoclonal (M) protein value at diagnosis of monoclonal gammopathy of undetermined significance in patients from southeastern Minnesota. Numbers above the horizontal axis are the risk of progression at each monoclonal protein value. Reproduced from Kyle RA, Rajkumar SV. Monoclonal gammopathies of undetermined significance: a review.* Immunol Rev *2003;**194**:112–39, with permission.*

Baldini et al.[6] reported that the malignant transformation rate at 4–6 years was 6.8% when the bone marrow plasma cell level was less than 10% compared with 37% in the group who met the criteria of MGUS but who had a bone marrow plasma cell value of 10–30%.

Peripheral neuropathy and MGUS

During a 1-year period, 692 patients with a clinically apparent neuropathy were identified in the electromyography laboratory at Mayo Clinic. Of these, 358 patients had an associated systemic disease known to cause neuropathy, such as diabetes mellitus, or alcoholism. Of the remaining 334 patients, 279 had had serum protein electrophoresis. Twenty-eight patients (10%) had an M-protein. MGUS was found in 16 patients, primary amyloidosis in seven, multiple myeloma in three, Waldenström's macroglobulinemia in one, and γ heavy-chain disease in one. There was a statistically significant increase in the prevalence of M-proteins in patients with peripheral neuropathy compared with the normal population in Minnesota, France, and Sweden. It must be emphasized that the diagnosis of peripheral neuropathy was based on the clinical diagnosis. The incidence would have been greater if the diagnosis was based on only electrophysiologic evidence.[7]

In another series, 16 of 58 patients with MGUS had a peripheral neuropathy. These patients were identified from a group of 1400 patients admitted to a large neurologic referral hospital.[8] Seven of the nine patients with a slow nerve conduction velocity had an IgM κ M-protein. In other reports, peripheral neuropathy was found in four of 132 consecutive patients with a monoclonal gammopathy,[9] and eight of 19 patients with MGUS had a clinical polyneuropathy.[10] In an unselected series of patients with MGUS, neuropathy was noted in two of 34 patients with IgG (6%), two of 14 with IgA (15%), and eight of 26 (31%) with IgM; the neuropathy was subclinical in six patients.[11] In another study, 14 of 31 patients with an IgM MGUS had peripheral neuropathy.[12] Isobe and Osserman[13] reported MGUS in 5.4% of 239 patients with peripheral neuropathy or myelopathy. In a group of 104 patients with polyneuropathy and monoclonal gammopathy, 23 had a hematologic malignancy: six had stage I multiple myeloma, two had stage III myeloma, ten had low-grade lymphoma, three had a plasmacytoma, one had Castleman's disease, and one had POEMS syndrome.[14]

There is no question that an association exists between MGUS and peripheral neuropathy. The incidence is variable and depends on patient selection bias, the vigor with which the presence of an M-protein is sought, and whether peripheral neuropathy is diagnosed on clinical or electrophysiologic grounds. A monograph on neurologic disorders associated with plasma cell dyscrasias has been published.[15] Neuropathy and monoclonal gammopathy were recently reviewed.[16]

ETIOLOGY AND PATHOGENESIS

The cause of peripheral neuropathy in MGUS is unknown. In some instances, a genetic role may be evident. In one report, a mother and son had an IgM M-protein and peripheral neuropathy.[17] In another report, a brother and sister had an IgM monoclonal gammopathy and a demyelinating peripheral neuropathy.[18]

The injection of monoclonal IgG from patients with polyneuropathy associated with monoclonal gammopathy or myeloma produced a demyelinating peripheral neuropathy with slowed nerve conduction velocities in mice. The injection of Fab fragments from monoclonal IgG produced a similar demyelination.[19] Demyelination of the sciatic nerve of cats occurred after intraneural injection of an IgM protein reacting with myelin-associated glycoprotein (MAG) from three patients with peripheral neuropathy. The M-protein and complement were detected on the surface of the myelin sheath, suggesting that the M-protein reacted with an epitope of myelin.[20] Alternatively, injection of serum from three patients with monoclonal gammopathy and chronic sensorimotor polyneuropathy revealed no evidence of demyelination or nerve conduction abnormalities when injected into rat sciatic nerves.[21] Intraneural injection of serum from a patient with MGUS and sensorimotor polyneuropathy produced myelino-axonal degeneration.[22]

In 1980, Latov et al.[23] described a patient with sensorimotor peripheral neuropathy and an IgM M-protein. The M-protein activity was directed against peripheral nerve myelin. This was documented by complement fixation and immunoabsorption. Dellagi et al.[24] also reported that the IgM M-protein with anti-MAG activity is bound to the myelin sheaths of patients with peripheral neuropathy. Direct electron microscopic immunohistochemical studies with colloidal gold revealed deposition of IgM within the myelin, and extending throughout the compact myelin in both large and small myelinated fibers. This is additional evidence that deposition of the IgM protein plays a role in pathogenesis. It is unknown whether IgM initiates the myelin damage or simply precipitates in an already damaged nerve. Single-fiber preparations show myelin swelling of internodes. Localization of myelin thickening and widening of myelin lamellae suggest a link between the two abnormalities.[25]

In approximately half of the patients with an IgM monoclonal gammopathy and peripheral neuropathy, the M-protein binds to MAG.[26,27] Dellagi et al.[24] described ten patients who had an IgM protein value less than 10 g/L and peripheral neuropathy with antibody against the myelin sheath. Bollensen et al.[28] suggested that IgM proteins with anti-MAG activity may react with Po, which is the major protein of myelin in human peripheral nerves. IgM κ deposition has been noted in areas of splitting of the myelin lamellae and bound to the internalized myelin debris,[29] as

well as throughout the compact myelin. Binding of the IgM protein to MAG is specific because it can be completely blocked by MAG isolated from human myelin.[30] In 16 patients with peripheral neuropathy and an IgM M-protein reacting with MAG, the anti-MAG IgM titers ranged from 1:12 800 to 1:100 000. Low antibody titers to MAG (1:400 or less) were found in eight of 24 patients with an IgM M-protein but no peripheral neuropathy. Very low titers (1:200 or less) were found in 17% of control patients without monoclonal gammopathy.[31] Ilyas et al.[32] reported that an IgM M-protein in three patients with peripheral neuropathy bound to the carbohydrate portion of MAG and also to a single ganglioside of sciatic nerve. The IgM proteins do not bind to deglycosylated MAG, a finding that suggests that the reactive determinants contain carbohydrate moieties.[33,34]

In addition to MAG, other target antigen determinants have been recognized. Freddo et al.[35] reported that monoclonal IgM from 16 patients with anti-MAG activity bound to two glycolipids in the peripheral nerve. Antiglycolipid antibodies have been associated with IgM neuropathies and multifocal neuropathies.[36] Gangliosides represent other target antigens.[37] Ilyas et al.[38] reported a reaction with antibody to GD_{1b} or disialosyl gangliosides. Carpo et al.[39] reported high titers of anti-GD_{1a} ganglioside antibodies in 5% of patients with chronic inflammatory demyelinating polyneuropathy, 18% with multifocal motor neuropathy, 3.8% with lower motor neuron disease, and 1.8% with amyotrophic lateral sclerosis. Clinical improvement was associated with some reduction of antibody titer.[39] In another report, antiganglioside antibodies were found in 15% of 87 patients with polyneuropathy associated with a monoclonal gammopathy. Antiganglioside antibodies were significantly associated with demyelinating neuropathy and with IgM monoclonal gammopathy.[40] The IgM protein may be reactive with chondroitin sulfate and produce axonal rather than myelin damage. In one patient, clusters of thinly myelinated fibers consistent with regeneration after axonal degeneration were seen. Sherman et al.[41] and Yee et al.[42] also reported binding of the IgM protein to chondroitin sulfate C. Monoclonal IgM antibodies may be directed against sulfatide. An extensive review of antibodies associated with peripheral neuropathy has been published.[43]

Although the relationship of the M-protein and demyelinating neuropathy is unclear, it is apparent that the immunoglobulin plays some role in demyelination.

CLINICAL FEATURES

Typically, MGUS-associated neuropathy has the following features:

- it is associated with the occurrence of an M-protein in the serum;
- POEMS syndrome is not present;

- an asymmetric sensorimotor polyradiculopathy or neuropathy begins insidiously, and is usually slowly progressive;
- it occurs more often in the sixth to seventh decades of life;
- it affects males more frequently than females;
- paresthesias, ataxia, and pain may be permanent features;
- cranial nerves are not involved.

IgM is the most frequent monoclonal gammopathy, followed by IgG and IgA. The association of neuropathies and monoclonal gammopathies has been the subject of several reviews.[44–46]

Nerve conduction is characteristically abnormal in both motor and sensory fibers. The conduction velocity of motor fibers is decreased by approximately 20%.[47] The amplitude of the compound muscle action potential is markedly decreased in the lower extremities. Frequently, responses from the sensory fibers of the upper and lower limb nerves cannot be elicited. Needle electromyography reveals findings of denervation in 80% of patients. Both demyelination and denervation may be present.[48] The sural nerve is usually more severely involved than the median nerve.

We reviewed our experience with 65 patients with MGUS and sensorimotor peripheral neuropathy at Mayo Clinic. Thirty-one patients had IgM, 24 had IgG, and ten had IgA. IgM was over-represented in the group and was associated with sensory symptoms, ataxia, slower nerve conduction, and more frequent dispersion of the compound muscle action potential than IgG or IgA neuropathies. There was no correlation between the size of the M-protein and the severity of the neuropathy. Furthermore, the type and severity of neuropathy with anti-MAG activity were not significantly different from those without anti-MAG activity. The course of the neuropathy was progressive in more than two-thirds of patients.[49] In another report of 39 patients with MGUS, it was suggested that those with neuropathy associated with IgM were different and should be distinguished from those with IgG or IgA.[50]

In a review of 40 patients with polyneuropathy associated with an IgM gammopathy, all but one had symmetric polyneuropathy. It was purely sensory in 17 and predominantly sensory in 13. Electrophysiologic studies revealed demyelination in 83%. Anti-MAG antibodies were found in 65% and were associated with only demyelinating neuropathies.[51] In a series of 52 symptomatic patients with IgM monoclonal gammopathy, symptomatic neuropathy occurred in three of four patients with a high anti-MAG titer and in three of 21 patients with a low anti-MAG titer.[52] In a cohort of 65 patients with polyneuropathy and a monoclonal IgM gammopathy, multivariate analysis revealed that only the initial findings on the electrophysiologic studies were independent prognostic factors. The presence of anti-MAG or anti-SGPG (sulfoglucuronyl paragloboside) specificity did not yield any additional prediction of outcome.[53]

IgG AND IgA MGUS

The relationship of IgG and IgA M-proteins to peripheral neuropathy is less well documented than that of IgM.[15] Read et al.[54] described three patients with an IgG M-protein and peripheral neuropathy. Bleasel et al.[55] described five patients with peripheral neuropathy and IgG MGUS. In a comparison of 19 patients with IgM MGUS and 15 with IgG MGUS, Simovic et al.[56] reported prolongation of distal latencies of the median and ulnar motor nerves, greater slowing of peroneal nerve conduction velocity, and more severe demyelination in IgM MGUS. IgA monoclonal gammopathy has been reported in several patients with peripheral neuropathy.[57–59]

DIFFERENTIAL DIAGNOSIS

MGUS neuropathy must be distinguished from amyloidosis, POEMS syndrome (osteosclerotic myeloma), chronic inflammatory demyelinating polyneuropathy, multiple myeloma, T-cell and B-cell lymphomas, paraneoplastic neuropathies, and metabolic and toxic neuropathies.

MGUS neuropathies differ from those associated with primary amyloidosis in the following respects: (1) the lower extremities are peripherally affected in MGUS, but the upper and lower extremities tend to be affected to a greater degree in amyloidosis, with the exception of carpal tunnel syndrome, which is a common finding in amyloidosis; (2) the course in amyloidosis is always slowly progressive; and (3) although amyloidosis may present as a sensorimotor peripheral neuropathy, autonomic features, such as postural hypotension, sphincter dysfunction, anhidrosis, and heart or kidney failure, often occur. Autonomic features and organ failure are not a part of MGUS neuropathy.

The relationship between chronic inflammatory demyelinating polyradiculopathy (CIDP) and CIDP with MGUS is unclear. In a comparison of 77 patients with CIDP and 26 with CIDP and MGUS, the latter group had a more indolent course, less severe weakness, and more frequent sensory loss. The outcome in the two groups was similar.[60] In a comparison of 45 patients with CIDP and 15 with MGUS-associated neuropathy, Gorson et al.[61] reported that the latter group had less severe weakness, more ataxia, vibration loss in the hands, and absent median and ulnar sensory potentials. In another report, the clinical course was progressive in most patients with MGUS, whereas those with CIDP were more likely to have a relapsing course. Impairment appeared to develop more slowly in the patients with MGUS, and they also had less severe functional impairment and a lesser degree of weakness and sensory changes.[62] In contrast, one study noted no significant clinical or electrophysiologic

Table 23.1 *Clinical and laboratory features of plasma cell dyscrasia associated with peripheral neuropathy*

Characteristic	MGUS	POEMS	Multiple myeloma	AL amyloidosis
Peripheral neuropathy	~5%	100%	1–8%	15–20%
Sensory versus motor predominance	Sensory, ataxia	Motor	Sensory	Sensory
Type of neuropathy	Demyelinating	Demyelinating > axonal	Demyelinating	Axonal and small fiber neuropathy
Autonomic involvement	No	+	No	+ to ++
Organomegaly	−	++	+	++
Skin involvement	−	++	+	+
Other symptoms	Asymptomatic	Edema, fatigue, endocrine abnormalities	Bone pain, fatigue, infections	Fatigue, edema, cardiomyopathy, nephrotic syndrome
Monoclonal heavy chain	IgM > IgG > IgA	IgG > IgA > IgM	IgG > IgA	IgG > IgA > IgM
Monoclonal light chain	κ 67% of cases	λ > 95% of cases	κ 66% of cases	λ 66% of cases
Serum M-protein spike (g/L)	<30	Usually <20	Usually >30	Usually <20
BM plasma cells (%)	<10	Usually <5	>10	Usually <10
Skeletal lesions	−	+++ (sclerotic, mixed sclerotic and lytic)	+++ (lytic, osteoporotic, or fracture)	−
Thrombocytosis	−	++	−	+ to ++
Anemia	−	+	++	+

BM, bone marrow; M, monoclonal; MGUS, monoclonal gammopathy of undetermined significance; POEMS, polyneuropathy, organomegaly, endocrinopathy, monoclonal protein, skin changes; −, absent; +, rare; ++, occurs frequently; +++, almost always present.

difference between patients with CIDP and those with CIDP and MGUS.[63] They reported that patients with anti-MAG antibody had more pronounced slowing of the peroneal motor nerve conduction velocity, a lower frequency of conduction block, and the distal accentuation of conduction slowing. Cocito *et al.*[64] reported that the terminal latency index was lower in MAG-associated neuropathy than in CIDP. In summary, CIDP may occur at any age, motor symptoms tend to predominate over sensory symptoms, and there is a greater tendency for the course to be relapsing. M-proteins are not found. The characteristics of peripheral neuropathy associated with MGUS, POEMS syndrome, multiple myeloma, and AL amyloidosis are shown in Table 23.1.

THERAPY

Treatment of patients with peripheral neuropathy and monoclonal gammopathy has been disappointing. In ten patients with polyneuropathy and monoclonal gammopathy, Sherman *et al.*[65] reported that plasma exchange produced improvement in neuropathy in six and stabilization in three. The neuropathy progressed with cessation of plasma exchange. In a randomized trial, 39 patients with MGUS and peripheral neuropathy received either plasma exchange twice weekly or sham plasma exchange in a double-blind trial. Those who had sham plasma exchange subsequently underwent plasma exchange in an open trial. The average neuropathy disability score improved by two points

in the sham exchange group and by 12 points in the plasma exchange group. The neuropathy disability score, weakness score, and summed compound muscle action potentials improved more with plasma exchange than with sham exchange. In both the double-blind and the open trials, IgG or IgA gammopathy had a better response to plasma exchange than IgM gammopathy.[66] Mazzi *et al.*[67] reported that eight of 13 patients with peripheral neuropathy and a monoclonal gammopathy obtained benefit with plasma exchange. However, in a prospective study of 44 patients with an IgM monoclonal gammopathy and peripheral neuropathy, patients were randomized to receive either chlorambucil (0.1 mg/kg daily) orally or chlorambucil plus 15 courses of plasma exchange during the first 4 months of therapy. There was no difference in the two treatment groups, a finding suggesting that plasma exchange added no additional benefit to chlorambucil therapy.[68] In another report, cyclophosphamide plus prednisone produced improvement in eight of 16 patients with monoclonal gammopathy and a sensorimotor peripheral neuropathy. In six other patients, the neuropathy stabilized.[69]

We have also used chlorambucil for patients with IgM monoclonal gammopathy and melphalan for those with IgG and IgA monoclonal gammopathies and peripheral neuropathy. Some of these patients have obtained benefit. In one report, nine of ten patients with peripheral neuropathy and an IgM M-protein responded to prednisone, cyclophosphamide, chlorambucil, azathioprine, or plasmapheresis.[70]

Table 23.2 *Treatment of peripheral neuropathy*

| Treatment | Effect of therapy | | | |
	MGUS	POEMS	MM	Amyloidosis
Plasmapheresis	Impr in >30%[65-67]	Not effective[2]	Unknown	Not effective
Intravenous gamma globulin	Impr in ~20%[75]	Not effective[2]	Unknown	Not effective
Corticosteroids	Impr in 2/6, but significant side effects[1]	Effective in ~15–20%[2]	Possibly effective if used at high doses to treat the underlying PCD	Possibly effective if used at high doses to treat the underlying PCD
Oral or intravenous alkylators	Impr in 50%, but risk of alkylator exposure	Effective in <50%[2]	Stabilization and impr possible	Stabilization and impr possible
Fludarabine	Impr in 70% of IgM patients[71,72]	Unknown	Not applicable	Not applicable
Rituximab	Impr in 5/5 patients[73]	Unknown	Not applicable	Unknown
Interferon-α	Impr in 8/10 IgM patients[3]	Unknown	Unknown	Unknown
High-dose chemotherapy with PBSCT	Unknown	Effective in >50–100%[2]	Stabilization and impr possible	Stabilization and impr possible
Radiation to dominant bone lesion	Not applicable	Effective in >50%[2]	Stabilization and impr possible	Not applicable

Impr, improvement; MGUS, monoclonal gammopathy of undetermined significance; MM, multiple myeloma; PBSCT, peripheral blood stem cell transplantation; PCD, plasma cell dyscrasia; POEMS, polyneuropathy, organomegaly, endocrinopathy, monoclonal protein, skin changes.

Fludarabine, a purine analog, produced benefit in seven out of ten patients with an IgM monoclonal gammopathy and neuropathy.[71] In another report, three of four patients with an IgM monoclonal gammopathy and peripheral neuropathy obtained clinical and neurophysiologic benefit from fludarabine.[72] Rituximab (Rituxan) is a monoclonal antibody directed against CD20, which is frequently expressed on the surface membrane of lymphocytes in lymphoma. In one study, it produced benefit in all five patients with an IgM monoclonal gammopathy and neuropathy.[73] In all five patients, previous treatment with plasma exchange and cyclophosphamide had been successful, but relapse had occurred. Thus, responses have been achieved with chemotherapy but data are insufficient to draw definite conclusions.

Intravenous gamma globulin produces benefit in some patients with CIDP, and may be used for patients with sensorimotor peripheral neuropathy and monoclonal gammopathy.[74] In a randomized crossover study comparing intravenous gamma globulin with placebo, strength improved in two patients and sensory symptoms improved in one other. Antibody titers to MAG or gangliosides did not change. Less than 20% of the treated patients had any benefit.[75] Gabapentin was helpful for a patient with severe tremor due to chronic demyelinating neuropathy associated with an IgM M protein.[76]

The patient with MGUS and peripheral neuropathy should be treated with simple analgesics or amytriptyline. If symptoms are severe enough to warrant additional treatment, we begin with plasmapheresis. Total exchange is done three times weekly for 2–3 weeks (40–50 mL/kg; replacement: 4% normal serum albumin to replace 70% and normal saline for the remainder). If the patient responds, plasmapheresis is repeated as needed to maintain the benefit. If the patient does not respond, corticosteroids or intravenous gammaglobulin can be used, but these have been disappointing. One may then proceed with melphalan if the patient has an IgG or IgA monoclonal gammopathy. If the patient has an IgM monoclonal gammopathy, rituximab or chlorambucil is a reasonable choice (Table 23.2).

Motor neuron disease

Although several instances of monoclonal gammopathy and motor neuron disease have been reported, there is little evidence that a causal effect exists. Eleven of 120 patients (9% with motor neuron disease) had an associated M-protein. Of the 11 patients, ten had amyotrophic lateral sclerosis and one had progressive spinal muscle atrophy.[77] Other reports of amyotrophic lateral sclerosis and MGUS have been published (Merlini *et al.*, read at International Conference on Multiple Myeloma, Bologna, Italy, June 19–22, 1989).[78]

MULTIPLE MYELOMA

Multiple myeloma is characterized by the proliferation of a clone of plasma cells, which produces pain, weakness, and fatigue. Hypercalcemia and renal insufficiency are often present. Anemia eventually occurs in almost every patient. An M-protein is found in the serum or urine in 97% of patients at diagnosis. Radiographic abnormalities, including lytic lesions, osteoporosis, or pathologic fractures, are present in 80% of patients at diagnosis. The diagnosis of multiple myeloma depends on the demonstration of increased numbers of plasma cells in the bone marrow.

Neurologic involvement is most often manifested by nerve root pain. Compression of the spinal cord or cauda equina, usually caused by myeloma arising in the marrow cavity of a vertebral body and extending into the extradural space, occurs in at least 5% of patients at some time during the course of their disease. This may result in severe back pain with radicular features, weakness, or paralysis of the lower extremities. Incontinence of stool and urine is common. Peripheral neuropathy is infrequent in multiple myeloma; when present, it is usually associated with amyloidosis.

A patient with peripheral neuropathy of the upper extremities and multiple myeloma was reported in 1937.[79] There was no evidence of myelomatous invasion of the nerves. Peripheral neuropathy was noted in ten (3.6%) of 277 hospitalized patients with multiple myeloma. Three of the ten patients had systemic amyloidosis.[80] In a series of 23 patients with multiple myeloma, three had clinical neuropathy and six had electrophysiologic evidence of peripheral neuropathy.[81] We described ten patients with multiple myeloma and peripheral neuropathy.[7] Four had systemic amyloidosis. Four of the remaining six patients presented with peripheral neuropathy and myeloma was discovered during evaluation of the neuropathy. The neuropathy involved the lower extremities and was slowly progressive. Chemotherapy for the myeloma produced no benefit. The fifth patient had a predominantly sensory neuropathy, and the sixth patient had severe muscle weakness, bilateral facial palsies, and respiratory insufficiency. In another report, three patients with multiple myeloma and progressive sensorimotor neuropathy had no response to melphalan and prednisone.[82] The presence of a λ light chain within the neurons was reported in the patient with multiple myeloma.[83]

Spinal cord compression

Compression of the spinal cord or cauda equina is usually produced by a plasmacytoma arising in the marrow cavity of the vertebra with extension to the extradural area. It occurs in 5–10% of patients with myeloma.[84] The incidence of spinal cord compression decreased from 10% before 1960 to 3.8% between 1960 and 1970,[85] and to less than 2% in the late 1980s.[86] The reduction in spinal cord compression is most likely due to better management of multiple myeloma. The thoracic cord is most commonly

involved and paraplegia frequently occurs. Back pain is usually a prominent feature and may be radicular. Weakness of the lower extremities may develop gradually but often there is an abrupt onset with paralysis developing over a few hours. This is accompanied by loss of potency, bladder control, and fecal continence. Ataxia and spasticity may be prominent. Sensation is lost below the level of the lesion. Compression of the cauda equina is associated with pain in the buttocks and weakness of the legs. Loss of sensation in the saddle area is found. Clinical suspicion is vital and magnetic resonance imaging (MRI) with gadolinium is the most effective method of determining the site of involvement. Computed tomography (CT) is also a useful procedure. A CT- or MRI-guided needle biopsy of the tumor may be helpful for diagnosis. Patients with spinal cord compression must be recognized quickly.

Patients should be treated immediately with high-dose corticosteroids followed by radiation. High-dose corticosteroids may provide both immediate pain palliation and improvement in neurologic function.[87,88] The optimal corticosteroid dose has not been established, but common dose schedules for metastatic disease include dexamethasone in an initial bolus of 100 mg intravenously followed by 4 mg orally 4 times daily,[89] or a 100-mg intravenous bolus followed by 96 mg in four divided doses for 3 days and then tapered.[87,88]

If the deficit is due to compression by the plasma cell tumor (rather than a bone fragment retropulsed by a pathologic compression fracture), the outcome with radiation therapy appears to be superior to that of surgical intervention.[90,91] One small trial randomized 29 patients either to laminectomy plus radiation or to radiation alone. Half of the surgically treated patients who were ambulatory before treatment remained so after treatment, whereas all retained ambulation after radiotherapy.[91] Most myelomatous lesions involve the anterior spinal cord because the tumor typically arises from the vertebral body rather than the lamina or spinous process; these anatomical proclivities and the inherent radiosensitivity of plasma cell tumors usually make radiation the treatment of choice. The optimal dose and fractionation schedule have not been established by randomized controlled trials, but a standard dose would be the equivalent of 4000 cGy in 20 fractions over 4 weeks.[87,91]

Leptomeningeal myeloma

Penetration of the dura and involvement of the leptomeninges are uncommon features of multiple myeloma.[92] Fassas et al.[93] reported that 18 of 1586 patients with multiple myeloma had central nervous system involvement – 15 of whom had cerebrospinal fluid plasma cells or leptomeningeal enhancement or both on MRI. This was associated with unfavorable cytogenetic abnormalities, high tumor mass, plasmablastic morphology, extramedullary myeloma, and circulating plasma cells. Patients may present with focal weakness, cranial nerve palsies, lethargy or stupor, and papilledema. Lesions may be visualized with gadolinium-enhanced MRI.[94] Examination of the cerebrospinal fluid shows increased numbers of abnormal plasma cells and is an essential part of the evaluation.[95] Involvement of the dura and leptomeninges is found. Treatment consists of intrathecal injection of methotrexate or cytosine arabinoside. Radiation of the skull and spinal cord also may be of temporary benefit. Responses are usually of short duration and survival is short – typically less than 6–9 months.[93,96] There are no prospective studies comparing intrathecal injection of methotrexate or cytosine arabinoside or radiation therapy.

Radiculopathy

Radiculopathy is the single most frequent neurologic complication and usually occurs in the lumbosacral area. Root pain results from compression of the nerve by direct extension of the vertebral plasmacytoma lesion, foraminal stenosis due to the collapsed bone itself, or, least commonly, leptomeningeal disease. Although painful, radiculopathy poses a much less serious threat than spinal cord compression. MRI of the affected area commonly clarifies the cause and guides therapy. Unless there is concomitant spinal cord compression or threat thereof, radiation may not be indicated. Corticosteroids followed by systemic chemotherapy may provide immediate palliation. If there is no soft-tissue component causing the foraminal stenosis, radiation will be of no benefit.

Cranial nerve abnormalities and intracranial plasmacytomas

Intracranial plasmacytomas or myelomas can be classified into four groups: (1) those extending from the skull and pressing inward; (2) those growing from the dura mater or the leptomeninges; (3) those arising from the mucous membranes of a nasopharyngeal plasmacytoma; and (4) intraparenchymal lesions without evidence of extension from any of the three other sites.[97–99] This last group is distinctly unusual.[97,100,101] Base-of-the-skull plasmacytomas and leptomeningeal studding are most apt to cause symptoms, including cranial nerve palsies. Solitary extramedullary dural-based plasmacytomas appear to have a different immunophenotype than intramedullary cranial plasmacytomas and are at lower risk for progression to myeloma.[99]

Involvement of cranial nerves and their divisions is a rare complication of myeloma, and occurs most commonly at the time of progressive disease. The cranial nerves are typically not infiltrated by plasma cells, but rather are locally distorted or compressed. Sixth nerve

and eighth nerve palsies may be caused by plasmacytoma, involving the petrous bones and the sella.[97] The 'numb chin syndrome' manifests as objective or subjective sensory disorders, or both in the distribution of the mental nerve or inferior alveolar nerve.[102] Lytic lesions of the mandible occur in about 10% of patients,[103] and can compress the mandibular nerve or its tributaries. CT scanning of the skull is most helpful for delineating bony destruction. MRI is more useful for defining soft tissue.

Orbital involvement may occur in multiple myeloma. The majority of patients present with proptosis but visual loss can also occur.[104]

SOLITARY PLASMACYTOMA

The diagnosis of solitary plasmacytoma of bone is based on histologic evidence of a tumor consisting of monoclonal plasma cells identical to those in multiple myeloma (see Chapter 25). In addition, complete skeletal radiographs must show no other lesions of myeloma, and the bone marrow aspirate must contain no evidence of multiple myeloma. Typically, immunofixation of the serum and concentrated urine shows no M-protein, but up to half of patients do have an M-protein in the serum or urine. There should be no evidence of anemia, hypercalcemia, or renal insufficiency related to the plasmacytoma. Treatment consists of radiation in the range of 40–50 cGy (see Chapter 25).

Solitary plasmacytoma of bone may be associated with peripheral neuropathy. If the plasmacytoma has a sclerotic rim and there are other features besides neuropathy, the POEMS syndrome must be considered within the differential diagnosis (see later). A sacral plasmacytoma produced a severe peripheral neuropathy in one patient. Surgical removal and irradiation produced improvement of the peripheral neuropathy.[105] Read and Warlow[106] described three patients with solitary plasmacytoma and peripheral neuropathy. They also reviewed 13 previously reported cases from the literature.

POEMS SYNDROME (OSTEOSCLEROTIC MYELOMA)

POEMS syndrome is characterized by polyneuropathy, organomegaly, endocrinopathy, M-protein, and skin changes.[107] Radiographs reveal osteosclerotic lesions in more than 95% of patients.[108]

Clinical features

Symptoms of peripheral neuropathy usually dominate the clinical picture. Symptoms begin in the feet and consist of tingling, paresthesias, and coldness. Motor involvement follows the sensory symptoms. Both are distal, symmetric, and progressive with a gradual proximal spread. Severe weakness occurs in more than half of patients and results in inability to climb stairs, arise from a chair, or grip objects firmly with their hands. The course is usually progressive and patients may be confined to a wheelchair. Impotence occurs but autonomic symptoms are not a feature. Bone pain and fractures rarely occur.

Physical examination reveals a symmetric sensorimotor neuropathy involving the extremities. Muscle weakness is more marked than sensory loss. Touch, pressure, vibratory, and joint position senses are usually involved. Loss of temperature discrimination and nociception is less frequent. The cranial nerves are not involved except for papilledema.

The liver is palpable in almost half of patients, but splenomegaly and lymphadenopathy are found in only a minority. The skin changes include hyperpigmentation, Raynaud's phenomenon, white nails, and clubbing. The skin may be thickened. Angiomas of the skin are common. Coarse black hair often appears on the extremities. Pitting edema of the lower extremities is common. Occasionally, ascites and pleural effusion occur. Testicular atrophy and gynecomastia may be present. Pulmonary hypertension may occur.[109]

Laboratory and radiological features

Anemia is not a feature and, in fact, polycythemia may occur. Thrombocytosis is common.[110] Hypercalcemia and renal insufficiency are rarely present. Bone marrow usually contains fewer than 10% plasma cells. The concentration of the M-protein on electrophoresis is small (median 11 g/L) and is rarely more than 30 g/L. The M-protein is usually IgG or IgA, and almost always of the λ type.[111] Bence Jones proteinuria is uncommon.

Diabetes mellitus and gonadal dysfunction are the most common endocrinopathies. Serum luteinizing hormone and follicle-stimulating hormone levels may be increased. Hyperprolactinemia may account for hypogonadism or galactorrhea. Hypothyroidism may occur but is usually mild. Adrenal insufficiency also may occur.

Osteosclerotic lesions occur in approximately 95% of patients; half have a solitary sclerotic lesion and at least a third have multiple sclerotic lesions. The lesions may be modest in size and misinterpreted as benign bony sclerosis. Both osteosclerotic and osteolytic lesions may be found. One can easily overlook a small sclerotic rim surrounding a large lytic lesion. The pelvis, spine, ribs, and proximal extremities are most often involved.

Protein levels in the cerebrospinal fluid are increased in virtually all patients. More than half of our patients had a cerebrospinal fluid protein value more than 1 g/L.[110] Plasma cells are not present in the cerebrospinal fluid.

Electromyography shows moderate slowing of nerve conduction, and prolonged distal latencies and progressive dispersion of the compound muscle action potentials. The slowing of motor conduction is proportionately greater than the reduction in the compound muscle action potential amplitude. Distal fibrillation potentials are found on needle electromyography. Biopsy of the sural nerve usually shows both axonal degeneration and demyelination. A loss of myelinated fibers and an increased frequency of axonal degeneration in teased fibers was reported by Ono et al.[112]

Pathogenesis

The cause of osteosclerotic myeloma is unknown. Patients frequently have higher levels of interleukin-1β, tumor necrosis factor α, and interleukin-6 than patients with multiple myeloma.[113] Levels of vascular endothelial growth factor are frequently increased and often decrease with successful therapy.[114] Antibodies to human herpesvirus 8 were reported in 78% of patients with POEMS syndrome and Castleman's disease and in 22% of those with POEMS syndrome without Castleman's disease.[115] The plasma cells may secrete an immunoglobulin or another substance that is toxic to peripheral nerves. It is tempting to incriminate the presence of λ light chains in the pathogenesis because of their unexpected frequency. Castleman's disease (giant lymph node hyperplasia, angiofollicular lymph node hyperplasia) and osteosclerotic myeloma have been reported.[116] Gherardi et al.[117] found angiofollicular lymph node hyperplasia in two of three patients with POEMS syndrome. In our experience, about 15% of patients with POEMS syndrome also have Castleman's disease. Lambotte et al.[118] described a patient with nephrotic syndrome, from light-chain deposition disease, in whom a POEMS syndrome subsequently developed.

Diagnosis and course

The diagnosis of POEMS syndrome depends on the demonstration of increased numbers of monoclonal plasma cells in a biopsy specimen from the osteosclerotic lesion. Patients with POEMS syndrome usually present with sensory motor peripheral neuropathy. A metastatic radiologic bone survey must be done to detect osteosclerotic lesions. Lesions can be subtle and easily confused with benign fibrous dysplasia or a vertebral hemangioma. The M-protein in the serum and urine is small and may easily be overlooked.

The course of POEMS syndrome is chronic, and patients survive for years in contrast to patients with multiple myeloma. The cause of death in POEMS syndrome is not the excessive proliferation of plasma cells and a large tumor mass. The natural history is one of progressive peripheral neuropathy until the patient is bedridden. Death usually occurs from inanition or a terminal bronchopneumonia.

Therapy

Single or multiple osteosclerotic lesions in a limited area should be treated with radiation in a dose of 40–50 cGy. More than half of patients show substantial improvement of the neuropathy. The improvement may be very slow and not apparent for 6 months. We have seen patients who have continued to improve for 2–3 years after radiation therapy.

If the patient has widespread osteosclerotic lesions, systemic therapy is necessary. In contrast to CIDP, plasmapheresis and intravenous immunoglobulin do not produce clinical benefit. Melphalan and prednisone therapy has produced benefit in some patients. Autologous stem cell transplantation after high-dose melphalan therapy is a consideration for younger patients with widespread osteosclerotic lesions. The stem cells should be collected before the patient is exposed to alkylating agents because they will damage the hematopoietic stem cells. The mortality rate associated with the procedure is currently only 1–2%.[119,120]

WALDENSTRÖM'S MACROGLOBULINEMIA

Waldenström's macroglobulinemia is characterized by the proliferation of lymphocytes and plasma cells producing an IgM M-protein (see Chapter 29). Examination of the fundus frequently shows retinal dilation and hemorrhages. Serum protein electrophoresis reveals a tall narrow peak or dense band that represents the IgM M-protein. Seventy-five percent of the IgM M-proteins have a κ light chain. A small monoclonal light chain is found in the urine in 80% of patients. Increased numbers of lymphocytes and plasma cells are found in the bone marrow. A normocytic normochromic anemia is usually present. Lytic bone lesions occur in less than 5% of patients (see Chapter 29). Sensorimotor peripheral neuropathy in association with macroglobulinemia does not differ from that occurring in patients with MGUS of the IgM type (see earlier).

HYPERVISCOSITY

Hyperviscosity is characterized by blurring or loss of vision and neurological symptoms, including headache, dizziness, vertigo, nystagmus, loss of hearing, ataxia, paresthesias, or diplopia. Chronic nasal bleeding or oozing of the gums is characteristic and post-surgical or gastrointestinal bleeding may also occur. Sleepiness, stupor, coma, or cerebral hemorrhage may develop. Congestive heart failure may also occur. Physical examination shows retinal vein engorgement and flame-shaped hemorrhages. Papilledema may also be present.

The serum viscosity level should be measured if a patient has any symptoms suggestive of hyperviscosity syndrome or if the IgM value is more than 40 g/L. This can be determined with a Wells–Brookfield viscometer (Brookfield Engineering Laboratory, Stoughton, MA, USA) or an Ostwald-100 viscometer. The Wells–Brookfield viscometer is preferred because it requires less serum and is more accurate, and testing can be performed at different shear rates and temperatures. In addition, the determination can be made much more quickly, particularly when the serum viscosity level is increased.

The relationship between serum viscosity and clinical manifestations is not precise. Symptoms rarely occur from hyperviscosity when the relative viscosity is less than 4 cp (normal ⩽1.8 cp). Most patients have symptoms when the viscosity reaches 6–7 cp but exceptions do occur. The decision to perform plasmapheresis must be based on the patient's symptoms and fundoscopic findings.

A relationship between the amount of the serum M-protein spike and symptoms of hyperviscosity is not linear. At low serum IgM levels an increase of 10–20 g/L produces only a minimal change in the serum viscosity, but when the IgM concentration is 40–50 g/L an increase of only 10–20 g/L greatly increases the relative viscosity.[121] The specific viscosity level at which clinical symptoms occur varies from one patient to the next. The molecular characteristics of the protein, aggregation of protein molecules, the presence of disease involving the small blood vessels, hematocrit level, and cardiac output may all be factors in producing symptoms of hyperviscosity.[122] Plasmapheresis should be performed for symptomatic hyperviscosity. One or two exchanges is usually sufficient to lower the serum viscosity.

AL AMYLOIDOSIS

Amyloid appears homogeneous and amorphous under the light microscope and stains pink with hematoxylin–eosin. When stained with Congo red, it produces an apple-green birefringence when viewed under polarized light. The amyloid actually consists of linear, non-branching aggregated fibrils that are 7.5–10.0 nm wide and of indefinite length. The fibrils consist of the variable portions of monoclonal (κ or λ) immunoglobulin light chains in primary amyloidosis (AL) or, very rarely, heavy chains. In secondary amyloidosis (AA), the fibrils consist of protein A, a non-immunoglobulin. In familial amyloidosis (AF), the fibrils are composed of mutant transthyretin (pre-albumin) or, occasionally, fibrinogen, lysozyme, or apolipoprotein. In senile systemic amyloidosis, the fibrils consist of normal transthyretin. The amyloid fibrils associated with long-term dialysis arthropathy consist of β_2-microglobulin. Peripheral neuropathy is rare in AA amyloidosis or dialysis-associated amyloidoses, whereas it may be a major feature of AL and AF. The incidence of AL is 0.89 per 100 000 (8.9 per million person-years).[123] The median age at diagnosis is 65 years, and only 1% of patients are younger than 40 years (see Chapter 27).

Weakness, fatigue, and weight loss are the most frequent symptoms and occur in more than half of patients. The major physical findings include ankle edema, hepatomegaly, purpura, and macroglossia. The liver is palpable in about a fifth of patients, and splenomegaly is found in less than 5%. Macroglossia may be prominent but it is found in only 10% of patients. Purpura is common and usually involves the neck and face, particularly the upper eyelids. The skin may be fragile and easily traumatized. Multiple organs are involved and may produce nephrotic syndrome, congestive heart failure, carpal tunnel syndrome, orthostatic hypotension, or peripheral neuropathy (see Chapter 27).[124]

Peripheral neuropathy and AL amyloidosis

Sensorimotor peripheral neuropathy is found at the time of diagnosis in approximately 15% of patients with AL. Symptoms are usually present for more than a year before the diagnosis is made. The initial symptoms of neuropathy are usually due to sensory rather than motor nerve dysfunction and usually affect the lower extremities before the upper limbs. Symptoms consist of loss of feeling, altered sensation, prickling numbness, and pain. The pain may be burning or lancinating. Muscle weakness usually occurs after a variable period. Occasionally, amyloid neuropathy presents with autonomic symptoms, such as postural hypotension, syncope, or impotence. On examination, one may find sensory, motor, or autonomic (decreased sweating or altered regulation of cardiovascular responses) features. Neuropathy is progressive, but death is usually due to cardiac or renal involvement.

In a series of 26 patients with sural nerve biopsy-proven amyloid neuropathy at Mayo Clinic and an M-protein in the serum or urine, 81% had paresthesias, 65% had muscle weakness, and 58% had numbness. Autonomic neuropathy was present in 17 of 26 patients at the time of diagnosis. The median duration of symptoms before diagnosis was 29 months and the median survival was 25 months.[125]

Involvement of small-diameter sensory fibers (particularly loss of pain, warm, and cold sensation) is characteristic of amyloid neuropathy. We reviewed the clinical characteristics of 18 immunohistochemically confirmed cases of AL.[126] Loss of sensation, paresthesias, and pain were present initially in 14 patients. In the four remaining patients, the first symptoms were weakness in two, weight loss in one, and postural hypotension in one. The sensory loss began in the feet more frequently than in the hands,

but it was soon present in both. The first sensory symptom was paresthesias in more than half of the patients, and lancinating pains, usually in the distal limbs, occurred in approximately a quarter. Typically, sensory, motor, and autonomic deficits developed in all the patients over time.

Motor nerve conduction velocities are usually just below normal values, and compound muscle action potential amplitudes are decreased or absent. Distal motor latencies tend to be normal. In most cases, sensory nerve action potentials cannot be recorded. Fibrillation is found in most patients with needle electromyography.

Sural nerve biopsy is the only certain way to recognize amyloidosis in the peripheral nerve. Axonal degeneration, sometimes with predominant involvement of the small myelinated and unmyelinated fibers, is seen. Rajani et al.[127] reported that 13 (1.2%) of 1098 sural nerve biopsy specimens were positive for amyloid deposition. The neuropathy was predominantly sensory in six patients, motor in two, and mixed in five. Amyloid was identified in the endoneurium in 12 of the 13 biopsy specimens. Axonal loss was moderate or severe in 12 of the 13 patients. Histologically, there is loss of small myelinated and unmyelinated fibers.[128] Amyloid deposits infiltrate epineural and endoneural connective tissue. Blood vessel walls of the epineurium and endoneurium are frequently thickened by amyloid deposits, and there is a gross loss of myelin fibers, which often show signs of active axonal degeneration. Teased fiber studies show a predominance of axonal degeneration. Amyloid may also infiltrate the proximal dorsal root and sympathetic ganglia.

Carpal tunnel syndrome is an initial presenting finding in about a quarter of patients with AL. The symptoms consist of paresthesias in the distribution of the median nerve, which supplies the skin of the first three fingers and the lateral half of the fourth finger on the palmar aspect. The symptoms are frequently worse at night and also may be aggravated by use of the wrist. The median nerve is entrapped by swelling from synovitis or deposition of amyloid in the tenosynovium or the transverse carpal ligament. Subsequently, atrophy of the thenar muscles may occur. The diagnosis may be confirmed by electromyography.

Other clinical features and laboratory investigations are discussed in Chapter 27. The median duration of survival in 474 patients with AL seen at Mayo Clinic within 1 month of diagnosis was 13.2 months. Only 7% survived for 5 or more years. Patients with peripheral neuropathy but no evidence of congestive heart failure, orthostatic hypotension, or nephrotic syndrome at diagnosis have a median duration of survival of 26 months.

Therapy of AL is unsatisfactory (see Chapter 27). In a prospective study of 220 patients, melphalan and prednisone were superior to colchicine alone.[129] The use of a combination of alkylating agents is not superior to treatment with melphalan and prednisone.[130] Autologous

KEY POINTS

- There is a definite association between peripheral neuropathy and monoclonal gammopathy of undetermined significance (MGUS), particularly with IgM paraproteins. The paraprotein may show antimyelin activity.
- POEMS syndrome (polyneuropathy, organomegaly, endocrinopathy, monoclonal protein, and skin changes; osteosclerotic myeloma) and primary amyloidosis must be excluded before making a diagnosis of MGUS with peripheral neuropathy.
- Treatment of MGUS with peripheral neuropathy consists of plasmapheresis, intravenous gamma-globulin, chemotherapy, or corticosteroids, but frequently these are ineffective.
- Radiculopathy is the commonest neurological problem in myeloma.
- Spinal cord compression must be urgently considered in the patient with back pain, weakness and paresthesias of the lower extremities, and difficulty with bowel or urinary function.
- Sensorimotor peripheral neuropathy is found at the time of diagnosis in approximately 15% of patients with primary systemic amyloidosis.
- The diagnosis of primary amyloidosis depends on the demonstration of amyloid in tissue. Abdominal fat aspiration or bone marrow biopsy is positive for amyloid in 90% of patients. A sural nerve biopsy may be needed for a definitive diagnosis.
- POEMS syndrome (osteosclerotic myeloma) must be considered in any patient with severe sensorimotor peripheral neuropathy. A radiographic survey shows an osteosclerotic lesion in more than 95% of patients.

peripheral blood stem cell transplantation is currently available for AL. Comenzo et al.[131] reported that 17 of 25 patients given an autologous stem cell transplant were alive at 24 months. Eleven of the 17 had improved or had amyloid-related involvement. Four of five patients with peripheral neuropathy obtained neurologic improvement after peripheral stem cell transplantation.

Familial amyloidosis (AF)

Familial or inherited amyloidosis has been reviewed by Buxbaum and Tagre.[132]

ACKNOWLEDGMENT

This is supported in part by grant CA62242 from the National Cancer Institute.

REFERENCES

- ● = Key primary paper
- ◆ = Major review article
- ＊ = Paper that represents the first formal publication of a management guideline

●1. Axelsson U, Bachmann R, Hallen J. Frequency of pathological proteins (M-components) in 6,995 sera from an adult population. *Acta Med Scand* 1966; **179**:235–47.
2. Kyle RA, Finkelstein S, Elveback LR, Kurland LT. Incidence of monoclonal proteins in a Minnesota community with a cluster of multiple myeloma. *Blood* 1972; **40**:719–24.
3. Saleun JP, Vicariot M, Deroff P, Morin JF. Monoclonal gammopathies in the adult population of Finistère, France. *J Clin Pathol* 1982; **35**:63–8.
●4. Kyle RA, Terneau TM, Rajkumar SV, Offord JR, Larson DR, Plevak MF, *et al.* A long-term study of prognosis in monoclonal gammopathy of undetermined significance. *N Engl J Med* 2002; **346**:564–9.
5. Cesana C, Klersy C, Barbarano L, Nosari AM, Crugnola M, Pungolino E, *et al.* Prognostic factors for malignant transformation in monoclonal gammopathy of undetermined significance and smoldering multiple myeloma. *J Clin Oncol* 2002; **20**:1625–34.
6. Baldini L, Guffanti A, Cesana BM, Colombi M, Chiorboli O, Damilano I, *et al.* Role of different hematologic variables in defining the risk of malignant transformation in monoclonal gammopathy. *Blood* 1996; **87**:912–8.
7. Kelly JJ Jr, Kyle RA, O'Brien PC, Dyck PJ. Prevalence of monoclonal protein in peripheral neuropathy. *Neurology* 1981; **31**:1480–3.
8. Kahn SN, Riches PG, Kohn J. Paraproteinaemia in neurological disease: incidence, associations, and classification of monoclonal immunoglobulins. *J Clin Pathol* 1980; **33**:617–21.
9. Johansen P, Leegaard OF. Peripheral neuropathy and paraproteinemia: an immunohistochemical and serologic study. *Clin Neuropathol* 1985; **4**:99–104.
10. Vrethem M, Cruz M, Wen-Xin H, Malm C, Holmgren H, Ernerudh J. Clinical, neurophysiological and immunological evidence of polyneuropathy in patients with monoclonal gammopathies. *J Neurol Sci* 1993; **114**:193–9.
11. Nobile-Orazio E, Barbieri S, Baldini L, Marmiroli P, Carpo M, Premoselli S, *et al.* Peripheral neuropathy in monoclonal gammopathy of undetermined significance: prevalence and immunopathogenetic studies. *Acta Med Scand* 1992; **85**:383–90.
12. Baldini L, Nobile-Orazio E, Guffanti A, Barbieri S, Carpo M, Cro L, *et al.* Peripheral neuropathy in IgM monoclonal gammopathy and Waldenström's macroglobulinemia: a frequent complication in elderly males with low MAG-reactive serum monoclonal component. *Am J Hematol* 1994; **45**:25–31.
●13. Isobe T, Osserman EF. Pathologic conditions associated with plasma cell dyscrasias: a study of 806 cases. *Ann N Y Acad Sci* 1971; **190**:507–18.
14. Eurelings M, Notermans NC, Van de Donk NW, Lokhorst HM. Risk factors for hematological malignancy in polyneuropathy associated with monoclonal gammopathy. *Muscle Nerve* 2001; **24**:1295–302.

◆15. Kelly JJ Jr, Kyle RA, Latov N (eds). *Polyneuropathies associated with plasma cell dyscrasias*. Boston: Nijhoff, 1987.

16. Nobile-Orazio E, Carpo M. Neuropathy and monoclonal gammopathy. *Curr Opin Neurol* 2001; **14**:615–20.

17. Busis NA, Halperin JJ, Stefansson K, Kwiatkowski DJ, Sagar SM, Schiff SR, *et al.* Peripheral neuropathy, high serum IgM, and paraproteinemia in mother and son. *Neurology* 1985; **35**:679–83.

18. Jonsson V, Schroder HD, Staehelin Jensen T, Nolsoe C, Stigsby B, Trojaborg W, *et al.* Autoimmunity related to IgM monoclonal gammopathy of undetermined significance: peripheral neuropathy and connective tissue sensibilization caused by IgM M-proteins. *Acta Med Scand* 1988; **223**:255–61.

19. Besinger UA, Toyka KV, Anzil AP, Fateh-Mognadam A, Rouscher R, Heininger K. Myeloma neuropathy: passive transfer from man to mouse. *Science* 1981; **213**:1027–30.

20. Dalakas MC, Flaum MA, Rick M, Engel WK, Gralnick HR. Treatment of polyneuropathy in Waldenström's macroglobulinemia: role of paraproteinemia and immunologic studies. *Neurology* 1983; **33**:1406–10.

21. Bosch EP, Ansbacher LE, Goeken JA, Cancilla PA. Peripheral neuropathy associated with monoclonal gammopathy: studies of intraneural injections of monoclonal immunoglobulin sera. *J Neuropathol Exp Neurol* 1982; **41**:446–59.

22. Lawlor MW, Richards MP, Fisher MA, Stubbs EB Jr. Sensory nerve conduction deficit in experimental monoclonal gammopathy of undetermined significance (MGUS) neuropathy. *Muscle Nerve* 2001; **24**:809–16.

●23. Latov N, Sherman WH, Nemni R, Galassi G, Shyong JS, Penn AS, *et al.* Plasma-cell dyscrasia and peripheral neuropathy with a monoclonal antibody to peripheral-nerve myelin. *N Engl J Med* 1980; **303**:618–21.

24. Dellagi K, Dupouey P, Brouet JC, Billecocq A, Gomez D, Clauvel JP, *et al.* Waldenström's macroglobulinemia and peripheral neuropathy: a clinical and immunologic study of 25 patients. *Blood* 1983; **62**:280–5.

25. Rebai T, Mhiri C, Heine P, Charfi H, Meyrignac C, Gherardi R. Focal myelin thickenings in a peripheral neuropathy associated with IgM monoclonal gammopathy. *Acta Neuropathol* 1989; **79**:226–32.

26. Latov N, Hays AP, Sherman WH. Peripheral neuropathy and anti-MAG antibodies. *Crit Rev Neurobiol* 1988; **3**:301–32.

27. Hafler DA, Johnson D, Kelly JJ, Panitch H, Kyle R, Weiner HL. Monoclonal gammopathy and neuropathy: myelin-associated glycoprotein reactivity and clinical characteristics. *Neurology* 1986; **36**:75–8.

28. Bollensen E, Steck AJ, Schachner M. Reactivity with the peripheral myelin glycoprotein PO in serum from patients with monoclonal IgM gammopathy and polyneuropathy. *Neurology* 1988; **38**:1266–70.

29. Lach B, Rippstein P, Atack D, Afar DE, Gregor A. Immunoelectron microscopic localization of monoclonal IgM antibodies in gammopathy associated with peripheral demyelinative neuropathy. *Acta Neuropathol* 1993; **85**:298–307.

30. Steck AJ, Murray N, Meier C, Page N, Perruisseau G. Demyelinating neuropathy and monoclonal IgM antibody to myelin-associated glycoprotein. *Neurology* 1983; **33**:19–23.

31. Nobile-Orazio E, Francomano E, Daverio R, Barbieri S, Marmiroli P, Manfredini E, *et al.* Anti-myelin-associated glycoprotein IgM antibody titers in neuropathy associated with macroglobulinemia. *Ann Neurol* 1989; **26**:543–50.

32. Ilyas AA, Quarles RH, MacIntosh TD, Dobersen MJ, Trapp BD, Dalakas MC, *et al.* IgM in a human neuropathy related to paraproteinemia binds to a carbohydrate determinant in the myelin-associated glycoprotein and to a ganglioside. *Proc Natl Acad Sci USA* 1984; **81**:1225–9.

33. Shy ME, Vietorisz T, Nobile-Orazio E, Latov N. Specificity of human IgM M-proteins that bind to myelin-associated glycoprotein: peptide mapping, deglycosylation, and competitive binding studies. *J Immunol* 1984; **133**:2509–12.

34. Frail DE, Edwards AM, Braun PE. Molecular characteristics of the epitope in myelin-associated glycoprotein that is recognized by a monoclonal IgM in human neuropathy patients. *Molec Immunol* 1984; **21**:721–5.

35. Freddo L, Ariga T, Saito M, Macala LC, Yu RK, Latov N. The neuropathy of plasma cell dyscrasia: binding of IgM M-proteins to peripheral nerve glycolipids. *Neurology* 1985; **35**:1420–4.

36. Fredman P. The role of antiglycolipid antibodies in neurological disorders. *Ann N Y Acad Sci* 1998; **845**:341–52.

37. Steck AJ, Murray N, Dellagi K, Brouet JC, Seligmann M. Peripheral neuropathy associated with monoclonal IgM autoantibody. *Ann Neurol* 1987; **22**:764–7.

38. Ilyas AA, Quarles RH, Dalakas MC, Fishman PH, Brady RO. Monoclonal IgM in a patient with paraproteinemic polyneuropathy binds to gangliosides containing disialosyl groups. *Ann Neurol* 1985; **18**:655–9.

39. Carpo M, Nobile-Orazio E, Meucci N, Gamba M, Barbieri S, Allaria S, *et al.* Anti-GD1a ganglioside antibodies in peripheral motor syndromes. *Ann Neurol* 1996; **39**:539–43.

40. Eurelings M, Ang CW, Notermans NC, Van Doorn PA, Jacobs BC, Van den Berg LH. Antiganglioside antibodies in polyneuropathy associated with monoclonal gammopathy. *Neurology* 2001; **57**:1909–12.

41. Sherman WH, Latov N, Hays AP, Takatsu M, Nemni R, Galassi G, *et al.* Monoclonal IgM kappa antibody precipitating with chondroitin sulfate C from patients with axonal polyneuropathy and epidermolysis. *Neurology* 1983; **33**:192–201.

42. Yee WC, Hahn AF, Hearn SA, Rupar AR. Neuropathy in IgM lambda paraproteinemia: immunoreactivity to neural proteins and chondroitin sulfate. *Acta Neuropathol* 1989; **78**:57–64.

◆43. Quarles RH, Weiss MD. Autoantibodies associated with peripheral neuropathy. *Muscle Nerve* 1999; **22**:800–22.

44. Latov N. Pathogenesis and therapy of neuropathies associated with monoclonal gammopathies. *Ann Neurol* 1995; **37**(Suppl 1):S32–42.

45. Kissel JT, Mendell JR. Neuropathies associated with monoclonal gammopathies. *Neuromuscul Disord* 1995; **6**:3–18.

46. Ropper AH, Gorson KC. Neuropathies associated with paraproteinemia. *N Engl J Med* 1998; **338**:1601–7.

47. Smith IS, Kahn SN, Lacey BW, King RH, Eames RA, Whybrew DJ, *et al.* Chronic demyelinating neuropathy associated with benign IgM paraproteinaemia. *Brain* 1983; **106**:169–95.

48. Kelly JJ Jr. The electrodiagnostic findings in peripheral neuropathy associated with monoclonal gammopathy. *Muscle Nerve* 1983; **6**:504–9.

●49. Gosselin S, Kyle RA, Dyck PJ. Neuropathy associated with monoclonal gammopathies of undetermined significance. *Ann Neurol* 1991; **30**:54–61.

50. Suarez GA, Kelly JJ Jr. Polyneuropathy associated with monoclonal gammopathy of undetermined significance: further evidence that IgM-MGUS neuropathies are different than IgG-MGUS. *Neurology* 1993; **43**:1304–8.

51. Chassande B, Leger JM, Younes-Chennoufi AB, Bengoufa D, Maisonobe T, Bouche P, *et al.* Peripheral neuropathy associated with IgM monoclonal gammopathy: correlations between M-protein antibody activity and clinical/electrophysiological features in 40 cases. *Muscle Nerve* 1998; **21**:55–62.

52. Meucci N, Baldini L, Cappellari A, Di Troia A, Allaria S, Scarlato G, *et al.* Anti-myelin-associated glycoprotein antibodies predict the development of neuropathy in asymptomatic patients with IgM monoclonal gammopathy. *Ann Neurol* 1999; **46**:119–22.

53. Eurelings M, Moons KG, Notermans NC, Sasker LD, De Jager AE, Wintzen AR, *et al.* Neuropathy and IgM M-proteins: prognostic value of antibodies to MAG, SGPG, and sulfatide. *Neurology* 2001; **56**:228–33.

54. Read DJ, Vanhegan RI, Matthews WB. Peripheral neuropathy and benign IgG paraproteinaemia. *J Neurol Neurosurg Psychiatry* 1978; **41**:215–19.

55. Bleasel AF, Hawke SH, Pollard JD, McLeod JG. IgG monoclonal paraproteinaemia and peripheral neuropathy. *J Neurol Neurosurg Psychiatry* 1993; **56**:52–7.

56. Simovic D, Gorson KC, Ropper AH. Comparison of IgM-MGUS and IgG-MGUS polyneuropathy. *Acta Neurol Scand* 1998; **97**:194–200.

57. Dhib-Jalbut S, Liwnicz BH. Binding of serum IgA of multiple myeloma to normal peripheral nerve. *Acta Neurol Scand* 1986; **73**:381–7.

58. Bailey RO, Ritaccio AL, Bishop MB, Wu AY. Benign monoclonal IgAκ gammopathy associated with polyneuropathy and dysautonomia. *Acta Neurol Scand* 1986; **73**:574–80.

59. Simmons Z, Bromberg MB, Feldman EL, Blaivas M. Polyneuropathy associated with IgA monoclonal gammopathy of undetermined significance. *Muscle Nerve* 1993; **16**:77–83.

60. Simmons Z, Albers JW, Bromberg MB, Feldman EL. Presentation and initial clinical course in patients with chronic inflammatory demyelinating polyradiculo-neuropathy: comparison of patients without and with monoclonal gammopathy. *Neurology* 1993; **43**:2202–9.

61. Gorson KC, Allam G, Ropper AH. Chronic inflammatory demyelinating polyneuropathy: clinical features and response to treatment in 67 consecutive patients with and without a monoclonal gammopathy. *Neurology* 1997; **48**:321–8.

62. Simmons Z, Albers JW, Bromberg MB, Feldman EL. Long-term follow-up of patients with chronic inflammatory demyelinating polyradiculoneuropathy, without and with monoclonal gammopathy. *Brain* 1995; **118**:359–68.

63. Maisonobe T, Chassande B, Verin M, Jouni M, Leger JM, Bouche P. Chronic dysimmune demyelinating polyneuropathy: a clinical and electrophysiological study of 93 patients. *J Neurol Neurosurg Psychiatry* 1996; **61**:36–42.

64. Cocito D, Isoardo G, Ciaramitaro P, Migliaretti G, Pipieri A, Barbero P, *et al.* Terminal latency index in polyneuropathy with IgM paraproteinemia and anti-MAG antibody. *Muscle Nerve* 2001; **24**:1278–82.

65. Sherman WH, Olarte MR, McKiernan G, Sweeney K, Latov N, Hays AP. Plasma exchange treatment of peripheral neuropathy associated with plasma cell dyscrasia. *J Neurol Neurosurg Psychiatry* 1984; **47**:813–19.

*●66. Dyck PJ, Low PA, Windebank AJ, Jeradeh SS, Gosselin S, Bourque P. Plasma exchange in polyneuropathy associated with monoclonal gammopathy of undetermined significance. *N Engl J Med* 1991; **325**:1482–6.

67. Mazzi G, Raineri A, Zucco M, Passadore P, Pomes A, Orazi BM. Plasma-exchange in chronic peripheral neurological disorders. *Int J Artif Organs* 1999; **22**:40–6.

68. Oksenhendler E, Chevret S, Leger JM, Louboutin JP, Bussel A, Brouet JC. Plasma exchange and chlorambucil in polyneuropathy associated with monoclonal IgM gammopathy: IgM-associated Polyneuropathy Study Group. *J Neurol Neurosurg Psychiatry* 1995; **59**:243–7.

69. Notermans NC, Lokhorst HM, Franssen H, Van der Graaf Y, Teunissen LL, Jennekens FG, *et al.* Intermittent cyclophosphamide and prednisone treatment of polyneuropathy associated with monoclonal gammopathy of undetermined significance. *Neurology* 1996; **47**:1227–33.

70. Kelly JJ, Adelman LS, Berkman E, Bhan I. Polyneuropathies associated with IgM monoclonal gammopathies. *Arch Neurol* 1988; **45**:1355–9.

71. Sherman WH, Latov N, Lange D, Hays R, Younger D. Fludarabine for IgM antibody-mediated neuropathies. *Ann Neurol* 1994; **36**:326–7.

72. Wilson HC, Lunn MP, Schey S, Hughes RA. Successful treatment of IgM paraproteinaemic neuropathy with fludarabine. *J Neurol Neurosurg Psychiatry* 1999; **66**:575–80.

73. Levine TD, Pestronk A. IgM antibody-related polyneuropathies: B-cell depletion chemotherapy using Rituximab. *Neurology* 1999; **52**:1701–4.

74. Faed JM, Day B, Pollock M, Taylor PK, Nukada H, Hammond-Tooke GD. High-dose intravenous human immunoglobulin in chronic inflammatory demyelinating polyneuropathy. *Neurology* 1989; **39**:422–5.

*75. Dalakas MC, Quarles RH, Farrer RG, Dambrosia J, Soueidan S, Stein DP, *et al.* A controlled study of intravenous immunoglobulin in demyelinating neuropathy with IgM gammopathy. *Ann Neurol* 1996; **40**:792–5.

76. Saverino A, Solaro C, Capello E, Trompetto C, Abbruzzese G, Schenone A. Tremor associated with benign IgM paraproteinaemic neuropathy successfully treated with gabapentin. *Mov Disord* 2001; **16**:967–8.

77. Younger DS, Rowland LP, Latov N, Sherman W, Pesce M, Lange DJ, *et al.* Motor neuron disease and amyotrophic lateral sclerosis: relation of high CSF protein content to paraproteinemia and clinical syndromes. *Neurology* 1990; **40**:595–9.

78. Patten BM. Neuropathy and motor neuron syndromes associated with plasma cell disease. *Acta Neurol Scand* 1984; **70**:47–61.

79. Davison C, Balser BH. Myeloma and its neural complications. *Arch Surg* 1937; **35**:913–36.

80. Silverstein A, Doniger DE. Neurologic complications of myelomatosis. *Arch Neurol* 1963; **9**:534–44.

81. Walsh JC. The neuropathy of multiple myeloma: an electrophysiological and histological study. *Arch Neurol* 1971; **25**:404–14.

82. Delauche MC, Clauvel JP, Seligmann M. Peripheral neuropathy and plasma cell neoplasias: a report of 10 cases. *Br J Haematol* 1981; **48**:383–92.

83. Borges LF, Busis NA. Intraneuronal accumulation of myeloma proteins. *Arch Neurol* 1985; **42**:690–4.

84. Svien HF, Price RD, Bayrd ED. Neurosurgical treatment of compression of the spinal cord caused by myeloma. *J Am Med Assoc* 1953; **153**:784–6.

85. Callis MN, Sheets RF. Multiple myeloma in Iowa. *J Iowa Med Soc* 1974; **64**:429–33.

86. Riccardi A, Gobbi PG, Ucci G, Bertoloni D, Luoni R, Rutigliano L, et al. Changing clinical presentation of multiple myeloma. *Eur J Cancer* 1991; **27**:1401–5.

87. Greenberg HS, Kim JH, Posner JB. Epidural spinal cord compression from metastatic tumor: results with a new treatment protocol. *Ann Neurol* 1980; **8**:361–6.

88. Sorensen S, Helweg-Larsen S, Mouridsen H, Hansen HH. Effect of high-dose dexamethasone in carcinomatous metastatic spinal cord compression treated with radiotherapy: a randomised trial. *Eur J Cancer* 1994; **1**:22–7.

89. Vecht CJ, Haaxma-Reiche H, van Putten WL, de Visser M, Vries EP, Twijnstra A. Initial bolus of conventional versus high-dose dexamethasone in metastatic spinal cord compression. *Neurology* 1989; **39**:1255–7.

90. Gilbert RW, Kim JH, Posner JB. Epidural spinal cord compression from metastatic tumor: diagnosis and treatment. *Ann Neurol* 1978; **3**:40–51.

91. Young RF, Post EM, King GA. Treatment of spinal epidural metastases: randomized prospective comparison of laminectomy and radiotherapy. *J Neurosurg* 1980; **53**:741–8.

●92. Maldonado JE, Kyle RA, Ludwig J, Okazaki H. Meningeal myeloma. *Arch Int Med* 1970; **126**:660–3.

93. Fassas AB, Muwalla F, Berryman T, Benramdane R, Joseph L, Anaissie E, et al. Myeloma of the central nervous system: association with high-risk chromosomal abnormalities, plasmablastic morphology and extramedullary manifestations. *Br J Haematol* 2002; **117**:103–8.

94. Leifer D, Grabowski T, Simonian N, Demirjian ZN. Leptomeningeal myelomatosis presenting with mental status changes and other neurologic findings. *Cancer* 1992; **70**:1899–904.

95. Patriarca F, Zaja F, Silvestri F, Sperotto A, Scalise A, Gigli G, et al. Meningeal and cerebral involvement in multiple myeloma patients. *Ann Hematol* 2001; **80**:758–62.

96. Petersen SL, Wagner A, Gimsing P. Cerebral and meningeal multiple myeloma after autologous stem cell transplantation: a case report and review of the literature. *Am J Hematol* 1999; **62**:228–33.

97. Clarke E. Cranial and intracranial myelomas. *Brain* 1954; **77**:61–81.

98. Toland J, Phelps PD. Plasmacytoma of the skull base. *Clin Radiol* 1971; **22**:93–6.

99. Schwartz TH, Rhiew R, Isaacson SR, Orazi A, Bruce JN. Association between intracranial plasmacytoma and multiple myeloma: clinicopathological outcome study. *Neurosurgery* 2001; **49**:1039–44.

100. Husain MM, Metzer WS, Binet EF. Multiple intraparenchymal brain plasmacytomas with spontaneous intratumoral hemorrhage. *Neurosurgery* 1987; **20**:619–23.

101. Krumholz A, Weiss HD, Jiji VH, Bakal D, Kirsh MB. Solitary intracranial plasmacytoma: two patients with extended follow-up. *Ann Neurol* 1982; **11**:529–32.

102. Massey EW, Moore J, Schold SC Jr. Mental neuropathy from systemic cancer. *Neurology* 1981; **31**:1277–81.

103. Scutellari PN, Orzincolo C, Bagni B, Feggi L, Franceschini F, Spanedda R. Bone disease in multiple myeloma: a study of 237 cases [in Italian]. *Radiol Med* 1992; **83**:542–60.

104. Hogan MC, Lee A, Solberg LA, Thome SD. Unusual presentation of multiple myeloma with unilateral visual loss and numb chin syndrome in a young adult. *Am J Hematol* 2002; **70**:55–9.

105. Davidson S. Solitary myeloma with peripheral polyneuropathy: recovery after treatment. *Calif Med* 1972; **116**:68–71.

106. Read D, Warlow C. Peripheral neuropathy and solitary plasmacytoma. *J Neurol Neurosurg Psychiatry* 1978; **41**:177–84.

●107. Bardwick PA, Zvaifler NJ, Gill GN, Newman D, Greenway GD, Resnick DL. Plasma cell dyscrasia with polyneuropathy, organomegaly, endocrinopathy, M protein, and skin changes: the POEMS syndrome. Report on two cases and a review of the literature. *Medicine (Baltimore)* 1980; **59**:311–22.

108. Dispenzieri A, Kyle RA, Lacy MQ, Rajkumar SV, Therneau TM, Larson DR, et al. POEMS syndrome: definitions and long-term outcome. *Blood* 2003; **101**:2496–506.

109. Lesprit P, Godeau B, Authier FJ, Soubrier M, Zuber M, Larroche C, et al. Pulmonary hypertension in POEMS syndrome: a new feature mediated by cytokines. *Am J Respir Crit Care Med* 1998; **157**:907–11.

◆110. Kelly JJ Jr, Kyle RA, Miles JM, Dyck PJ. Osteosclerotic myeloma and peripheral neuropathy. *Neurology* 1983; **33**:202–10.

111. Takatsuki K, Sanada I. Plasma cell dyscrasia with polyneuropathy and endocrine disorder: clinical and laboratory features of 109 reported cases. *Jap J Clin Oncol* 1983; **13**:543–55.

112. Ono K, Ito M, Hotchi M, Katsuyama T, Komiya I, Yamada T. Polyclonal plasma cell proliferation with systemic capillary hemangiomatosis, endocrine disturbance, and peripheral neuropathy. *Acta Pathol Jpn* 1985; **35**:251–67.

113. Gherardi RK, Bélec L, Soubrier M, Malapert D, Zuber M, Viard JP, et al. Overproduction of proinflammatory cytokines imbalanced by their antagonists in POEMS syndrome. *Blood* 1996; **87**:1458–65.

114. Watanabe O, Maruyama I, Arimura K, Kitajima I, Arimura H, Hanatani M, et al. Overproduction of vascular endothelial growth factor/vascular permeability factor is causative in Crow-Fukase (POEMS) syndrome. *Muscle Nerve* 1998; **21**:1390–7.

115. Bélec L, Mohamed AS, Authier FJ, Hallouin MC, Soe AM, Cotigny S, et al. Human herpesvirus 8 infection in patients with POEMS syndrome-associated multicentric Castleman's disease. *Blood* 1999; **93**:3643–53.

116. Bitter MA, Komaiko W, Franklin WA. Giant lymph node hyperplasia with osteoblastic bone lesions and the POEMS (Takatsuki's) syndrome. *Cancer* 1985; **56**:188–94.

117. Gherardi R, Baudrimont M, Kujas M, Malapert D, Lange F, Gray F, *et al.* Pathological findings in three non-Japanese patients with the POEMS syndrome. *Virchows Arch* 1988; **413**:357–65.

118. Lambotte O, Durrbach A, Ammor M, Paradis V, Djeffal R, Machover D, *et al.* Association of a POEMS syndrome and light chain deposit disease: first case report. *Clin Nephrol* 2001; **55**:482–6.

119. Jaccard A, Royer B, Bordessoule D, Brouet JC, Fermand JP. High-dose therapy and autologous blood stem cell transplantation in POEMS syndrome. *Blood* 2002; **99**:3057–9.

120. Dispenzieri A, Lacy MQ, Litzow MR, Tefferi A, Inwards DJ, Micallef IN, *et al.* Peripheral blood stem cell transplant (PBSCT) in patients with POEMS syndrome (abstract). *Blood* 2001; **98**:391b.

●121. Fahey JL, Barth WF, Solomon A. Serum hyperviscosity syndrome. *J Am Med Assoc* 1965; **192**:464–7.

122. Bloch KJ, Maki DG. Hyperviscosity syndromes associated with immunoglobulin abnormalities. *Semin Hematol* 1973; **10**:113–24.

●123. Kyle RA, Linos A, Beard CM, Linke RP, Gertz MA, O'Fallon WM, *et al.* Incidence and natural history of primary systemic amyloidosis in Olmsted County, Minnesota, 1950 through 1989. *Blood* 1992; **79**:1817–22.

◆124. Kyle RA, Gertz MA. Primary systemic amyloidosis: clinical and laboratory features in 474 cases. *Semin Hematol* 1995; **32**:45–59.

125. Rajkumar SV, Gertz MA, Kyle RA. Prognosis of patients with primary systemic amyloidosis who present with dominant neuropathy. *Am J Med* 1998; **104**:232–7.

126. Li K, Kyle RA, Dyck PJ. Immunohistochemical characterization of amyloid proteins in sural nerves and clinical associations in amyloid neuropathy. *Am J Pathol* 1992; **141**:217–26.

127. Rajani B, Rajani V, Prayson RA. Peripheral nerve amyloidosis in seral nerve biopsies: a clinicopathologic analysis of 13 cases. *Arch Pathol Lab Med* 2000; **124**:114–18.

128. Quattrini A, Nemni R, Sferrazza B, *et al.* Amyloid neuropathy simulating lower motor neuron disease. *Neurology* 1998; **51**:600–2.

✳129. Kyle RA, Gertz MA, Greipp PR, Ricevuti G, Dell'Antonio G, Lazzerini A, *et al.* A trial of three regimens for primary amyloidosis: colchicine alone, melphalan and prednisone, and melphalan, prednisone, and colchicine. *N Engl J Med* 1997; **336**:1202–7.

130. Gertz MA, Lacy MQ, Lust JA, Greipp PR, Witzig TE, Kyle RA. Prospective randomized trial of melphalan and prednisone versus vincristine, carmustine, melphalan, cyclophosphamide, and prednisone in the treatment of primary systemic amyloidosis. *J Clin Oncol* 1999; **17**:262–7.

✳131. Comenzo RL, Vosburgh E, Falk RH, Sanchorawala V, Reisinger J, Dubrey S, *et al.* Dose-intensive melphalan with blood stem-cell support for the treatment of AL (amyloid light-chain) amyloidosis: survival and responses in 25 patients. *Blood* 1998; **91**:3662–70.

◆132. Buxbaum JN, Tagoe CE. The genetics of the amyloidoses. *Ann Rev Med* 2000; **51**:543–69.

PART 6

Related disorders

Monoclonal gammopathies of undetermined significance: the transition from MGUS to myeloma

JOHN A. LUST, KATHLEEN A. DONOVAN AND PHILIP R. GREIPP

INTRODUCTION

Monoclonal gammopathies are disorders characterized by a monoclonal protein (M-protein) detected in the serum or urine by electrophoresis. The M-protein is produced by monoclonal plasma cells in the bone marrow. Multiple myeloma (MM) is the malignant expression of an IgG, IgA, IgD, IgE, or free light-chain monoclonal gammopathy. Marrow plasma cells accumulate and patients die of progressive disease related to bone destruction, renal failure, anemia, infection, or bleeding. Multiple myeloma has a clinically benign precursor condition termed monoclonal gammopathy of undetermined significance (MGUS). Patients are typically asymptomatic and have stable M-protein measurements. The term MGUS has been adopted because approximately 1% of patients per year develop a serious disease, such as multiple myeloma or a related disorder.

There is now a wealth of information in the literature that postulates a role for cytokines, oncogenes, chromosomal abnormalities, and other genetic/phenotypic changes in the monoclonal plasma cells as well as alterations in the marrow microenvironment in the pathogenesis of monoclonal gammopathies. In this chapter, much of these data will be reviewed in the context of the clinical progression of MGUS to active myeloma. A greater understanding of the biology of monoclonal gammopathies may provide a rational basis for the development of novel biologic therapies to treat or prevent myeloma in the future.

CLINICAL DIFFERENCES BETWEEN MGUS AND MYELOMA

Multiple myeloma is recognized clinically by the proliferation of malignant plasma cells in the bone marrow. Specific criteria exist that serve as useful guidelines to allow clinicians to differentiate between MM, MGUS, and other related plasmaproliferative disorders. As shown in Table 24.1, patients with MGUS usually have <10% marrow plasma cells, a serum monoclonal protein <30 g/L, no urinary Bence Jones protein, and no anemia, renal failure, lytic bone lesions, or hypercalcemia. In contrast, patients with active myeloma typically present with a marrow plasmacytosis of ≥10%, a serum monoclonal protein of ≥30 g/L (although no specific value is required for the diagnosis if end-organ damage is present; see Chapter 12), or a 24-hour urine monoclonal protein of ≥1 g, and end-organ damage including one or more of the following: anemia, hypercalcemia, renal insufficiency, and lytic bone lesions. Myeloma patients often present with back pain, severe fatigue, pneumonia, or other bone pain.[1] MGUS is more common than

Table 24.1 *Clinical characteristics of patients with monoclonal gammopathy of undetermined significance (MGUS), smoldering multiple myeloma (SMM), indolent multiple myeloma (IMM), and active multiple myeloma (MM)*

Characteristic	MGUS[a]	SMM[a] (asymptomatic myeloma)	IMM[b]	MM[a]
Marrow plasma cells	<10%	≥10%	≥10%	≥10%
Serum M-spike	<30 g/L	≥30 g/L	≥30 g/L	Usually but not necessarily ≥30 g/L
Bence Jones protein	<1 g/24 hours	<1 g/24 hours	<1 g/24 hours	≥1 g/24 hours
Anemia	Absent	Absent	May be present	Usually present
Hypercalcemia, renal insufficiency	Absent	Absent	Absent	May be present
Lytic bone lesions	Absent	Absent	A few may be present	Usually present
Requires chemotherapy	No	No	No	Yes

[a] International Working Group Diagnostic Criteria.[84]
[b] Not included in the International Working Group Diagnostic Criteria.

myeloma, occurring in 1% of the population over age 50 and 3% over age 70.[2] Most patients with myeloma probably have undetected prior MGUS. In a retrospective study of patients with MM in Olmsted County, Minnesota, USA, 58% had prior MGUS or plasmacytoma.[3] It is of great clinical importance to distinguish between patients with MGUS or MM because MGUS patients may be safely observed off chemotherapy. Unnecessary treatment can lead to acute leukemia or morbidity/mortality from chemotherapy. However, during long-term follow-up of 241 patients with MGUS, approximately 17% of patients went on to develop multiple myeloma.[4]

Between these two extremes of the disease, two clinically intermediate stages have been described called smoldering multiple myeloma (SMM) and indolent multiple myeloma (IMM). Patients with SMM are usually asymptomatic. They have a marrow plasmacytosis of ≥10% and/or a serum monoclonal protein of ≥30 g/L. Lytic bone lesions are absent and they have stable disease.[5] Patients with IMM are similar to those with SMM, except a small number of bone lesions may be present on bone survey studies. In contrast to MM patients who receive chemotherapy, patients with MGUS, SMM, and IMM have stable disease and are followed off chemotherapy.

Ancillary tests, such as β_2-microglobulin, peripheral blood labeling index, urinary light chain <500 mg/24 hours, and detection of plasmablasts on bone marrow examination, are typically negative in MGUS and SMM. However, one or more of these tests may be positive in myeloma and must not be attributable to another cause (i.e. increased β_2-microglobulin in renal insufficiency). Computed tomography (CT) or magnetic resonance imaging (MRI) may be needed to rule out skeletal lesions in patients with suspected disease and who have a negative radiographic bone survey. Newer assays, such as the detection of monoclonal free light chains, may be useful in the differentiation of MGUS from disorders such as light-chain myeloma or primary amyloidosis.[6]

In a large study of 1384 patients with MGUS reported by Kyle *et al.*[7] the median age at diagnosis of MGUS was 72 years; 2% were younger than 40 years at diagnosis. Of the monoclonal proteins found in these patients 24% were ≤5.0 g/L, 19% 5.1–10.0 g/L, 33% 10.1–15.0 g/L, 18% 15.1–20.0 g/L, 5% 20.1–25.0 g/L, and 1% 25.1–30.0 g/L. Seventy percent were IgG, 12% IgA, and 15% IgM; a biclonal was found in 3%. The light-chain was κ in 61% and λ in 39%. The concentrations of uninvolved immunoglobulins were reduced in 38% of patients whose immunoglobulin concentrations were determined quantitatively. Only 17% had a urinary monoclonal protein value greater than 150 mg per 24 hours. The bone marrow of 160 patients (12%) was examined and the median percentage of plasma cells was 3% (range 0–10%).[7]

FOLLOW-UP OF MONOCLONAL GAMMOPATHIES

If the patient has no other features of plasma cell dyscrasia and a serum spike value less than 15 g/L, serum protein electrophoresis should be repeated at annual intervals.[8] A bone marrow examination, skeletal roentgenograms, and a 24-hour urine specimen for immunofixation are not necessary in this setting. If the asymptomatic patient has an M-protein level of 15–25 g/L, additional studies should include quantification of immunoglobulins and collection of a 24-hour urine specimen for electrophoresis and immunofixation. The serum protein electrophoretic pattern should be repeated in 3–6 months and, if stable, should be repeated in 6 months and then annually, or sooner if any symptoms occur. If the IgG or IgA serum M-spike value is more than 25 g/L, a metastatic bone survey, including single views of the humeri and femurs, should be done. Bone marrow aspiration and biopsy also should be performed. If the patient has an IgM

Table 24.2 *Miscellaneous monoclonal gammopathies*[a]

Solitary plasmacytoma of bone (SPB) and extramedullary plasmacytoma (EMP):
- Biopsy-proven plasmacytoma (medullary or extramedullary)
- Exclusion of MM[a]

Idiopathic Bence Jones proteinuria:
- Free light-chain in the urine >1 g/24 hours
- Exclusion of MM or amyloidosis[a]

AL amyloidosis:[b,c]
- Tissue biopsy confirming amyloidosis
- M-protein in the serum or urine
- Clinical features of amyloidosis

Monoclonal immunoglobulin deposition disease:[c]
- Renal glomerular deposition and excretion of monoclonal light chain (often κ) or heavy chains

Adult-acquired Fanconi's syndrome:[c]
- Renal tubular deposition and excretion of monoclonal light chain (usually κ)

Scleromyxedema (lichen myxedematosus):
- Mucinous deposition in the skin and M-protein in the serum (usually IgGλ)

Monoclonal gammopathy with peripheral neuropathy:[c]
- IgM M-protein; may also occur with IgG and IgA

Osteosclerotic myeloma:
- Single or multiple osteosclerotic bone lesions
- Usually a λ-isotype M-protein
- May have associated POEMS or Castleman's disease

Heavy-chain disease (γ, α, μ):
- Free heavy-chain in the urine in γ, heavy- and light-chain in μ diverse clinical and pathologic presentations

Monoclonal IgM-associated lymphoproliferative disease or lymphoma:
- Includes Waldenström's macroglobulinemia

Cold agglutinin disease:
- IgM-κ M-protein on erythrocytes

Type I and II monoclonal cryoglobulinemia:
- Type I IgG, IgA, or IgM M-protein
- Type II IgM or IgG M-protein immune complex with polyclonal immunoglobulin

Systemic capillary leak syndrome:
- Usually an IgGκ M-protein with intermittent edema and effusions

Acquired C_1 esterase-inhibitor deficiency:
- Usually IgM M-protein with angioedema

---

[a] MM must be excluded initially but may develop during follow-up, especially in patients with SPB or idiopathic Bence Jones proteinuria.
[b] Serum amyloid A and familial (transthyretin) amyloidosis and senile or localized amyloidosis must be excluded.
[c] Typical MM infrequently may be associated with these conditions.
MM, multiple myeloma; POEMS, polyneuropathy, organomegaly, endocrinopathy, monoclonal gammopathy, and skin changes.

M-protein, an aspirate and biopsy of the bone marrow and a CT scan of the abdomen may be useful in recognizing Waldenström's macroglobulinemia (WM) or lymphoproliferative disorders. Levels of β_2-microglobulin and C-reactive protein should be determined. If all the results of these studies are satisfactory, serum electrophoresis should be repeated in 2 or 3 months and, if the finding is stable, the test should be repeated at 6–12-month intervals.

Electrophoresis and immunofixation of a 24-hour urine specimen should be performed if the serum M-protein value is >15 g/L. They also should be done if the serum M-protein value increases, or if other evidence of evolving MM or WM occurs. Determination of the plasma cell labeling index and a search for circulating plasma cells in the peripheral blood may be helpful in this situation.[8]

In addition to myeloma, several syndromes are associated with monoclonal gammopathy (Table 24.2). The clinician involved in the care of patients with monoclonal gammopathy will need to include these syndromes in the differential of MGUS. Review of each of these syndromes in detail is beyond the scope of this chapter.

PROGRESSION OF HIGH–RISK MGUS, SMM, AND IMM TO ACTIVE MM

In the analysis of 1384 patients with MGUS detailed above, Kyle *et al.*[7] found that during follow-up multiple myeloma, lymphoma with an IgM monoclonal protein, primary amyloidosis, macroglobulinemia, chronic lymphocytic leukemia, or plasmacytoma developed in 115 patients (8%). The cumulative probability of progression to one of these disorders was 10% at 10 years, 21% at 20 years, and 26% at 25 years. Only the concentration and type of monoclonal protein were independent predictors of progression. The presence of a monoclonal urinary light-chain or a reduction in one or more uninvolved immunoglobulins was not a risk factor for progression. Patients with IgM or IgA monoclonal protein had an increased risk of progression to disease, as compared with patients who had an IgG monoclonal protein. The risk of progression to multiple myeloma or a related disorder at 20 years was 14% for an initial monoclonal protein value of 5 g/L or less, 25% for an initial monoclonal protein value of 15 g/L, 41% for an initial monoclonal protein value of 20 g/L, 49% for an initial monoclonal protein value of 25 g/L, and 64% for an initial monoclonal protein value of 30 g/L (see Fig. 23.1, p. 351).[7]

For SMM and IMM the risk of progression is even higher. In several studies, patients with indolent MM and who had the presence of one or more lytic bone lesions were found to have a short median time to progression of 8–10 months.[9–11] Weber *et al.*[12] reported on 101 patients with stage I asymptomatic multiple myeloma (or SMM) out of a total of 695 consecutive, previously untreated patients with MM evaluated between October 1974 and October 1995. Patients with MGUS were excluded. Factors associated with disease progression included a serum M-protein >30 g/L, IgA heavy-chain type, and Bence Jones protein excretion >50 mg/24-hour urine collection. Patients with at least two of these risk factors (high risk) had a median time to disease progression of 17 months. In contrast, patients with none of the risk factors (low risk) had a median time to progression of 95 months. Patients with one risk factor (intermediate risk) had a median time to progression of 39 months and could be further subclassified based on MRI imaging of the thoracic and lumbar spine. Patients with abnormal MRI imaging had significantly earlier disease progression (median 21 months) than those with a normal pattern (median 57 months).[12] Although the above clinical features are helpful in the classification of patients, additional biomarkers are still needed to identify those patients with high-risk MGUS and SMM who are at high risk for disease progression. These are likely to arise from an improved understanding of the biology of myeloma pathogenesis.

GENETIC AND PHENOTYPIC DIFFERENCES BETWEEN PLASMA CELLS IN MGUS AND MYELOMA

With the advent of fluorescence *in situ* hybridization (FISH), it has been shown that virtually all myeloma cells from patients are cytogenetically abnormal and aneuploidy is the most common abnormality.[13–17] Plasma cells in myeloma frequently have trisomy of chromosomes 7, 9, 11, 15, and 18.[13,15,16] Recent data suggest that most MGUS plasma cells are aneuploid as well.[18–20] The incidence of trisomy for at least one chromosome was 61% in one study of MGUS cells using four chromosomal probes by FISH analysis[19] and 100% in a second study that used six probes to analyze MGUS cells.[17,20] By FISH analysis, myeloma cells appear to differ from those found in patients with MGUS in that the results for myeloma may be somewhat more heterogeneous for a given patient. In any event, it does appear that karyotypic instability begins in MGUS and continues throughout the course of the disease. Chromosome 13 deletions (13q−) by FISH or by karyotype has been associated with an adverse prognosis in myeloma.[21,22] This abnormality can be present in up to 50% of patients and the pathogenetic mechanism remains to be determined.[21–24] For MGUS, chromosome 13 abnormalities appear to be restricted primarily to a small subpopulation of clonal cells, suggesting that it is a secondary genetic event.[17,25,26]

Chromosomal translocations into the immunoglobulin heavy-chain locus on chromosome 14q32 are seen in approximately 60–70% of cases of myeloma.[14,17,27,28] Errors in VDJ recombination, somatic hypermutation, or switch recombination can mediate the immunoglobulin translocation.[14,17] Translocations may occur involving the light-chain loci as well. These immunoglobulin translocations are usually into IgH switch regions.[14] They involve several loci including 11q13 (*bcl-1*), 4p16 (FGFR3), 16q23 (c-*maf*), 6p21 (cyclin D3), and several other chromosome partners.[17,29,30] By interface FISH analysis, it has been reported that IgH translocations are present in approximately 47% of MGUS tumors, in 60–70% of patients with intramedullary multiple myeloma, and in greater than 80% of patients with plasma cell leukemia.[17] It has been hypothesized that a translocation involving an immunoglobulin heavy- or light-chain gene may be the initial cause of MGUS, and that other genotypic and phenotypic changes in the monoclonal plasma cell are important in the clinical manifestation of the plasma cell process.[17]

A higher percentage of myeloma patients appear to have activating mutations of N-*ras* or K-*ras* when compared with individuals with MGUS. In one study the incidence of N- and K-*ras* mutations was found to be 39% in 160 newly diagnosed patients.[31] No significant association was observed between any *ras* mutation and stage of disease, β_2-microglobulin, labeling index, or survival. However, the median survival of patients with a K-*ras* mutation was significantly shorter compared with patients with no *ras* mutation. In another study, N-*ras* and K-*ras* mutations were found in 55% of myeloma patients at diagnosis but in only 12.5% of patients with MGUS and indolent MM.[32] K-*ras* mutations were more frequent than N-*ras* mutations.

Plasma cells from patients with MGUS and MM have also been analyzed by gene expression profiling.[33] Using clustering analysis, normal and MM plasma cells were differentiated and four subgroups of MM (MM1, MM2, MM3, and MM4) were identified. The expression pattern of MM1 was similar to normal plasma cells, whereas MM4 was similar to MM cell lines. MM2 and MM3 represented patients with less aggressive disease when compared with MM4. Interestingly, clinical parameters linked to poor prognosis, such as abnormal karyotype and high serum β_2-microglobulin, were most prevalent in MM4.[33] More recently, analysis using CD138+ selected MGUS or MM plasma cells found that only 28 genes were differentially expressed, suggesting that MGUS plasma cells are more like myeloma plasma cells than normal plasma cells.[34]

The plasma cell labeling index (PCLI), which measures synthesis of DNA, is useful for differentiating MGUS or smoldering myeloma from active myeloma.[35] Bone marrow plasma cells are exposed to bromodeoxyuridine for 1 hour. Plasma cells are identified by intracytoplasmic immunofluorescence using anti-κ or anti-λ light-chain antibodies bound to fluorescein. The percentage of myeloma cells in S-phase are determined using an anti-bromodeoxyuridine monoclonal antibody (BU-1) and a rhodamine-labeled goat antimouse antibody in a double fluorescence technique. Slides are read with a fluorescence microscope containing both fluorescein and rhodamine filters. Among newly diagnosed untreated patients, a high immunofluorescence labeling index distinguished those with multiple myeloma from those with stable monoclonal gammopathies ($P < 0.002$).[35] An increased PCLI is good evidence that myeloma either is present or will soon develop.

The presence of circulating plasma cells of the same isotype in the peripheral blood is also a good marker of active myeloma. In a series of 57 patients with newly diagnosed smoldering myeloma, 16 had progression within 12 months. Sixty-three percent of patients who have progressed had an increased number of peripheral blood plasma cells. In contrast, only four of 41 patients who remained stable for 1 year had an increase in peripheral blood plasma cells at diagnosis.[36–38]

Angiogenesis appears to be important in hematologic malignancies as well as solid tumors.[39,40] A recent report demonstrated that myeloma cells produce vascular endothelial growth factor and that this can stimulate interleukin-6 (IL-6) in a paracrine fashion leading to myeloma cell growth.[41] There is evidence that increased bone marrow angiogenesis occurs in myeloma and is related to disease activity.[40,42–45] Rajkumar et al.[46] studied 400 patients with MGUS, MM, and AL amyloidosis. The median microvessel density (MVD) per high-power field was 1.3 in controls, 3 in MGUS, 4 in SMM, 11 in newly diagnosed MM, and 20 in relapsed MM. The authors concluded that bone marrow angiogenesis progressively increases from MGUS to advanced myeloma, indicating that angiogenesis may be related to disease progression.[46] Angiogenesis in myeloma also appears to be correlated with the plasma cell labeling index,[47] a measure of the proliferative activity of the neoplastic plasma cells, as described above, and is an independent predictor of poor survival in myeloma.[48]

IL-1β-induced IL-6 production differentiates MGUS, SMM, and active MM: relevance to the transition from MGUS to SMM to active MM

Interleukin-6 has been shown to be a central growth factor for myeloma cells.[49–53] Both autocrine and paracrine mechanisms of IL-6 production have been hypothesized.[49,54,55] Carter et al.[56] found that human myeloma cells produce IL-1β that can induce IL-6 production by marrow stromal cells. Based on this work, we investigated whether differences in IL-6 and IL-1β expression could

be detected in monoclonal plasma cells from patients with MGUS or MM.[57] Expression of IL-6 and IL-1β in bone marrow cells was determined using cell sorting to enrich for plasma cells followed by reverse transcriptase/polymerase chain reaction (RT-PCR). IL-6 mRNA expression was detectable in the sorted CD38+/CD45− plasma cell populations from none of six MGUS and five of 11 MM patients. All five MM patients with autocrine IL-6 expression demonstrated an elevated plasma cell labeling index. IL-1β mRNA was detectable in the sorted CD38+/CD45− plasma cell populations from one of six MGUS and ten of 11 MM patients. In situ hybridization (ISH) confirmed that the IL-1β-producing cells were plasma cells.[57] These results suggested that IL-1β production appeared to distinguish MGUS from MM better than IL-6 and, therefore, we focused our investigation on IL-1β.

Subsequently, ISH for IL-1β was performed using bone marrow aspirates from 51 MM, seven smoldering MM, 21 MGUS, and five normal control samples.[58] Using the ISH technique, IL-1β mRNA was detectable in the plasma cells from 49 of 51 patients with active myeloma and seven of seven patients with smoldering myeloma. In contrast, five of 21 patients with MGUS and none of five normal controls had detectable IL-1β message. Bone lesions were present in 40 of the 51 MM patients analyzed and all 40 patients had IL-1β mRNA by ISH. These results demonstrate that >95% of MM patients but <25% of MGUS patients are positive for IL-1β production.[58]

Although the ISH was very useful at detecting IL-1β, it did not allow us to differentiate SMM from active MM. Therefore, we measured the ability of IL-6 production by bone marrow stromal cells to serve as a highly sensitive surrogate marker for IL-1β functional activity. We hypothesized that patients with MM or SMM at risk for progression to active MM may have higher IL-1β bioactivity than patients with stable SMM or MGUS. IL-1β bioactivity was determined by quantifying IL-1β-specific IL-6 production by cultured bone marrow stromal cells, in the presence or absence of an IL-1β-neutralizing antibody, using an IL-6 enzyme-linked immunosorbant assay (ELISA). IL-6 results by ELISA from six representative patients with either MGUS, SMM or myeloma are detailed in Fig. 24.1. Supernatants from two MGUS patients generated low levels of IL-6 not significantly different from the media control. In contrast, the IL-6 levels measured in the supernatants of the bone marrow cells from the two myeloma patients were approximately 50–80 ng/mL and clearly distinguishable from those with MGUS. Both myeloma patients had bone lesions evident on X-ray. The SMM patients appear to fall into two groups, those with high values similar to patients with myeloma and those with low values like patients with MGUS. We have now observed that several patients with SMM and high IL-6 values have subsequently progressed to active

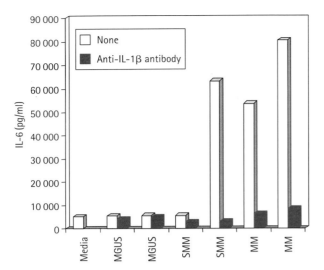

Figure 24.1 *Interleukin-1β (IL-1β) bioassay/interleukin-6 (IL-6) stromal cell co-culture assay. The interleukin-1β bioassay utilizes production by bone marrow stromal cells as a surrogate marker for IL-1β functional activity. Ficoll purified bone marrow cells from six representative patients with monoclonal gammopathy of undetermined significance (MGUS), smoldering multiple myeloma (SMM), or multiple myeloma (MM) are cultured at 2×10^6 cells/mL for 48 hours. Supernatants are pooled, aliquoted, and frozen at $-80°C$. Normal stromal cells are plated at 1×10^5 cells/mL and incubated at $37°C$ for 48 hours. After 48 hours, the stromal cells are washed and either IL-1β standards or a patient's supernatant (0.5 mL) are added with or without anti-IL-1β antibody. Cultures are incubated at $37°C$ for another 48 hours. Supernatants are harvested and frozen at $-80°C$ for analysis. Supernatants are analyzed for IL-6 using the Biosource ELISA kits according to the manufacturer's specifications.*

myeloma with a median time of 2–3 years. Finally, in the three patients with elevated IL-6 levels, anti-IL-1β antibody is able to inhibit paracrine IL-6 production by the marrow stromal cells by >90%. Our results demonstrate that stromal cell IL-6 production is induced predominantly by IL-1β in this model, is useful in differentiating patients with active myeloma from those with clinically benign disease, and may be helpful at identifying those patients at high risk who may benefit from novel chemoprevention trials.

In summary, the biologic effects of IL-1β closely parallel several of the clinical features of human myeloma. IL-1β has potent osteoclast activating factor activity, can increase the expression of adhesion molecules, and can induce paracrine IL-6 production.[56,59–63] The increased production of adhesion molecules could explain why myeloma cells are found predominantly in the bone marrow. Subsequently, these 'fixed' monoclonal plasma cells could now stimulate osteoclasts through the production of IL-1β and paracrine generation of IL-6, resulting

in osteolytic disease. The paracrine generation of IL-6 by marrow stromal cells may further support the growth and survival of the myeloma cells. The importance of IL-1β in myeloma pathogenesis is a result of its ability to induce IL-6. Because IL-6 production by IL-1β follows a sigmoid curve, small amounts of IL-1β may act as a trigger to induce IL-6 and other cytokine cascades, resulting in progression to active myeloma.

Chronic inflammation and cancer: a potential mechanism for human myelomagenesis

There is a substantial body of literature that supports the hypothesis that chronic inflammation can predispose an individual to cancer.[64–68] For example, chronic ulcerative colitis may predispose to colon cancer, hepatitis may lead to liver cancer, esophageal adenocarcinoma is associated with Barrett's esophagus, and chronic *Helicobacter* infection can lead to cancer of the stomach.[65–68] Inflammation can contribute to the development of neoplasia through the generation of reactive oxygen and nitrogen species, resulting in DNA mutations and the production of inflammatory cytokines that can support and perpetuate these genetically altered cells (Fig. 24.2).[64,69]

Pristane can induce plasmacytomas in genetically susceptible BALB/c mice. The tumors develop in peritoneal granulomas and are chacterized by c-*myc* activating t(12;15) chromosomal translocations and by secretion of IgA.[70,71] Pristane induces a chronic inflammatory state leading to the production of IL-6, which has been shown to be critical for plasmacytomagenesis.[70,72] Of interest, pristane can also induce rheumatoid arthritis (RA) in BALB/c mice and, in certain cases, both diseases may coexist in the same mouse.[71] In humans, patients with rheumatoid arthritis have increased serum levels of IL-1β and IL-6 manifested clinically by an elevated CRP and often show polyclonal plasmacytosis on bone marrow examination. RA patients have an increased risk of the development of both MGUS and MM.[73–77] Agents such as prednisone, thalidomide, and anti-IL-6 monoclonal antibody therapies, which all have anti-inflammatory/anticytokine effects, have all been shown to have activity in both RA and MM.[53,78–82] In the pristane mouse model, indomethacin can inhibit the development of plasmacytomas.[83] The above observations suggest that chronic inflammation that activates the IL-1b/NF-kB/IL-6 pathway may play a dominant role in the pathogenesis of myeloma as well. Inflammation can contribute to the development of neoplasia through the generation of reactive oxygen and nitrogen species resulting in DNA mutations and the production of inflammatory cytokines that can support and perpetuate these genetically altered cells. Ongoing molecular and cellular changes in the monoclonal

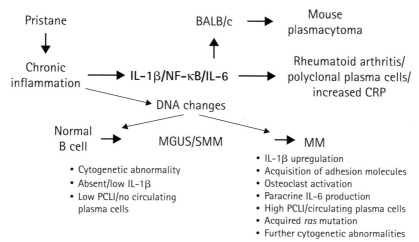

Figure 24.2 *Chronic inflammation and myeloma. Pristane can induce plasmacytomas in genetically susceptible BALB/c mice. Pristane induces a chronic inflammatory state leading to the production of interleukin-6 (IL-6), which has been shown to be critical for plasmacytomagenesis. Of interest, pristane can also induce rheumatoid arthritis (RA) in BALB/c mice and, in certain cases, both diseases may co-exist in the same mouse. In humans, patients with RA have increased serum levels of IL-1β and IL-6, manifested clinically by an elevated C-reactive protein (CRP), and often show polyclonal plasmacytosis on bone marrow examination. RA patients have an increased risk of the development of both monoclonal gammopathy of undetermined significance (MGUS) and multiple myeloma (MM). The above observations suggest that chronic inflammation that activates the IL-1β/NF-κB/IL-6 pathway may play a dominant role in the pathogenesis of myeloma as well. Inflammation can contribute to the development of neoplasia through the generation of reactive oxygen and nitrogen species, resulting in DNA mutations and the production of inflammatory cytokines that can support and perpetuate these genetically altered cells. Ongoing molecular and cellular changes in the monoclonal plasma cells lead to the transition from MGUS to SMM to active MM. NF-κB, nuclear factor κ B; PCLI, plasma cell labeling index.*

plasma cells lead to the transition from MGUS to SMM to active MM.

CONCLUSION

Comparison of the spectrum of clinical disease between MM and its clinically benign precursor condition, MGUS, has provided direction into the investigation of those changes that may be important in the pathogenesis of myeloma. MGUS and MM have major biologic differences, including increased cell proliferation, cytokine changes, cytogenetic abnormalities, oncogene mutations, and alterations in the marrow microenvironment. One of these changes that appears relevant is upregulation of IL-1β expression in the progression from MGUS to SMM to active MM. IL-1β has potent osteoclast activating factor activity, can increase the expression of adhesion molecules, and can induce paracrine IL-6 production. The paracrine generation of IL-6 by marrow stromal cells supports the growth and survival of the myeloma cells. It is important to understand the biology of the transition from MGUS to SMM to MM because it may be possible to intervene therapeutically and prevent progression to active disease. Chemoprevention trials are currently under way for patients with high-risk MGUS

and SMM/IMM. These prospective studies, in which high-risk patients are followed over time, are likely to provide a great deal of information about the biology of the progression from MGUS to MM and its therapeutic management.

KEY POINTS

- Monoclonal gammopathies are disorders, characterized by a monoclonal protein (M-protein) detected in the serum or urine by electrophoresis, that include multiple myeloma and its clinically benign precursor condition, monoclonal gammopathy of undetermined significance (MGUS).
- Approximately 1% of MGUS patients per year develop a serious disease, such as multiple myeloma or a related disorder.
- In an analysis of 1384 patients with MGUS, only the concentration and type of monoclonal protein were independent predictors of progression.
- Additional biologic parameters such as *ras* mutations, plasma cell labeling index, and

interleukin-1β (IL-1β) production may also be useful at distinguishing MGUS from myeloma.

- Chronic inflammation, typical of diseases such as rheumatoid arthritis, may play a dominant role in the pathogenesis of myeloma.
- Chemoprevention trials are now in progress for patients with high-risk MGUS and smoldering multiple myeloma/indolent multiple myeloma because it may be possible to minimize or prevent progression to active myeloma.

ACKNOWLEDGMENTS

Supported by grants PO1 CA62242, U10 CA 21115 (Eastern Cooperative Oncology Group), N01 CN65125 from the National Institutes of Health, and the Multiple Myeloma Research Foundation (Senior Research Grant to JAL).

REFERENCES

● = Key primary paper

1. Kyle RA, Lust JA. Monoclonal gammopathies of undetermined significance, *Semin Hematol* 1989; **26**:176–200.
2. Greipp PR, Lust JA. Pathogenetic relation between monoclonal gammopathies of undetermined significance and multiple myeloma, *Stem Cells* 1995; **13**:10–21.
3. Kyle RA, Beard CM, O'Fallon WM, Kurland LT. Incidence of multiple myeloma in Olmsted County, Minnesota: 1978 through 1990, with a review of the trend since 1945, *J Clin Oncol* 1994; **12**:1577–83.
4. Kyle RA. 'Benign' monoclonal gammopathy – after 20 to 35 years of follow-up, *Mayo Clinic Proc* 1993; **68**:26–36.
5. Kyle RA, Greipp PR. Smoldering multiple myeloma. *N Engl J Med* 1980; **302**:1347–9.
6. Katzmann JA, Clark RJ, Abraham RS, Bryant S, Lymp JF, Bradwell AR, *et al.* Serum reference intervals and diagnostic ranges for free kappa and free lambda immunoglobulin light chains: relative sensitivity for detection of monoclonal light chains. *Clin Chem* 2002; **48**:1437–44.
●7. Kyle RA, Therneau TM, Rajkumar SV, Offord JR, Larson DR, Plevak MF, *et al.* A long-term study of prognosis in monoclonal gammopathy of undetermined significance, *N Engl J Med* 2002; **346**:564–9.
8. Kyle RA, Rajkumar SV. Monoclonal gammopathies of undetermined significance. *Hematol Oncol Clinics North Am* 1999; **13**:1181–202.
9. Dimopoulos MA, Moulopoulos A, Smith T, Delasalle KB, Alexanian R. Risk of disease progression in asymptomatic multiple myeloma. *Am J Med* 1993; **94**:57–61.
10. Facon T, Menard JF, Michaux JL, Euller-Ziegler L, Bernard JF, Grosbois B, *et al.* Prognostic factors in low tumour mass asymptomatic multiple myeloma: a report on 91 patients. The Groupe d'Etudes et de Recherche sur le Myelome (GERM). *Am J Hematol* 1995; **48**:71–5.
11. Wisloff F, Andersen P, Andersson TR, Brandt E, Eika C, Fjaestad K, *et al.* Incidence and follow-up of asymptomatic multiple myeloma. The myeloma project of health region I in Norway. II. *Eur J Haematol* 1991; **47**:338–41.
12. Weber DM, Dimopoulos MA, Moulopoulos LA, Delasalle KB, Smith T, Alexanian R. Prognostic features of asymptomatic multiple myeloma. *Br J Haematol* 1997; **97**:810–4.
13. Fonseca R, Coignet LJ, Dewald GW. Cytogenetic abnormalities in multiple myeloma. *Hematol Oncol Clin North Am* 1999; **13**:1169–80, viii.
14. Hallek M, Bergsagel PL, Anderson KC. Multiple myeloma: increasing evidence for a multistep transformation process. *Blood* 1998; **91**:3–21.
15. Drach J, Schuster J, Nowotny H, Angerler J, Rosenthal F, Fiegl M, *et al.* Multiple myeloma: high incidence of chromosomal aneuploidy as detected by interphase fluorescence in situ hybridization. *Cancer Res* 1995; **55**:3854–9.
16. Flactif M, Zandecki M, Lai JL, Bernardi F, Obein V, Bauters F, *et al.* Interphase fluorescence in situ hybridization (FISH) as a powerful tool for the detection of aneuploidy in multiple myeloma. *Leukemia* 1995; **9**:2109–14.
17. Dalton WS, Bergsagel PL, Kuehl WM, Anderson KC, Harousseau JL. Multiple myeloma. *Hematology (Am Soc Hematol Educ Program.* 2001: 157–177.
18. Drach J, Angerler J, Schuster J, Rothermundt C, Thalhammer R, Haas OA, *et al.* Interphase fluorescence in situ hybridization identifies chromosomal abnormalities in plasma cells from patients with monoclonal gammopathy of undetermined significance. *Blood* 1995; **86**:3915–21.
19. Avet-Loiseau H, Facon T, Daviet A, Godon C, Rapp MJ, Harousseau JL, Grosbois B, *et al.* 14q32 translocations and monosomy 13 observed in monoclonal gammopathy of undetermined significance delineate a multistep process for the oncogenesis of multiple myeloma. Intergroupe Francophone du Myelome. *Cancer Res* 1999; **59**:4546–50.
20. Fonseca R, Ahmann GJ, Jalal SM, Dewald GW, Larson DR, Therneau TM, *et al.* Chromosomal abnormalities in systemic amyloidosis. *Br J Haematol* 1998; **103**:704–10.
21. Zojer N, Konigsberg R, Ackermann J, Fritz E, Dallinger S, Kromer E, *et al.* Deletion of 13q14 remains an independent adverse prognostic variable in multiple myeloma despite its frequent detection by interphase fluorescence in situ hybridization. *Blood* 2000; **95**:1925–30.
22. Facon T, Avet-Loiseau H, Guillerm G, Moreau P, Genevieve F, Zandecki M, *et al.* and Intergroupe Francophone du Myelome. Chromosome 13 abnormalities identified by FISH analysis and serum beta2-microglobulin produce a powerful myeloma staging system for patients receiving high-dose therapy. *Blood* 2001; **97**:1566–71.
23. Fonseca R, Oken MM, Harrington D, Bailey RJ, Van Wier SA, Henderson KJ, *et al.* Deletions of chromosome 13 in multiple myeloma identified by interphase FISH usually denote large deletions of the q arm or monosomy. *Leukemia* 2001; **15**:981–6.

24. Shaughnessy J, Barlogie B. Chromosome 13 deletion in myeloma. *Curr Top Microbiol Immunol* 1999; **246**:199–203.

25. Avet-Loiseau H, Li JY, Morineau N, Facon T, Brigaudeau C, Harousseau JL, *et al.* Monosomy 13 is associated with the transition of monoclonal gammopathy of undetermined significance to multiple myeloma. Intergroupe Francophone du Myelome. *Blood* 1999; **94**:2583–9.

26. Konigsberg R, Ackermann J, Kaufmann H, Zojer N, Urbauer E, Kromer E, *et al.* Deletions of chromosome 13q in monoclonal gammopathy of undetermined significance, *Leukemia* 2000; **14**:1975–9.

27. Bergsagel PL, Nardini E, Brents, L, Chesi, M, Kuehl WM. IgH translocations in multiple myeloma: a nearly universal event that rarely involves c-myc. *Curr Top Microbiol Immunol* 1997; **224**:283–7.

28. Chesi M, Kuehl WM, Bergsagel PL. Recurrent immunoglobulin gene translocations identify distinct molecular subtypes of myeloma. *Ann Oncol* 2000; **11**:131–5.

29. Bergsagel PL, Chesi M, Nardini E, Brents LA, Kirby SL, Kuehl WM. Promiscuous translocations into immunoglobulin heavy chain switch regions in multiple myeloma. *Proc Natl Acad Sci USA* 1996; **93**:13931–6.

30. Chesi M, Nardini E, Brents LA, Schrock E, Ried T, Kuehl WM, *et al.* Frequent translocation t(4;14)(p16.3;q32.3) in multiple myeloma is associated with increased expression and activating mutations of fibroblast growth factor receptor 3. *Nat Genet* 1997; **16**:260–4.

31. Liu P, Leong T, Quam L, Billadeau D, Kay NE, Greipp P, Kyle RA, *et al.* Activating mutations of N- and K-ras in multiple myeloma show different clinical associations:analysis of the Eastern Cooperative Oncology Group Phase III Trial. *Blood* 1996; **88**:2699–706.

32. Bezieau S, Devilder MC, Avet-Loiseau H, Mellerin MP, Puthier D, Pennanin E, *et al.* High incidence of N and K-Ras activating mutations in multiple myeloma and primary plasma cell leukemia at diagnosis. *Hum Mutat* 2001; **18**:212–24.

●33. Zhan F, Hardin J, Kordsmeier B, Bumm K, Zheng M, Tian E, *et al.* Global gene expression profiling of multiple myeloma, monoclonal gammopathy of undetermined significance, and normal bone marrow plasma cells. *Blood* 2002; **99**:1745–57.

●34. Davies FE, Dring AM, Li C, Rawstron AC, Shammas M, Hideshima T, *et al.* The molecular basis of the transition of MGUS to multiple myeloma. *Blood* 2002; **100**:102a.

●35. Greipp PR, Witzig TE, Gonchoroff NJ, Habermann TM, Katzmann JA, O'Fallon WM, *et al.* Immunofluorescence labeling indices in myeloma and related monoclonal gammopathies. *Mayo Clin Proc* 1987; **62**:969–77.

36. Witzig TE, Gonchoroff NJ, Katzmann JA, Therneau TM, Kyle RA, Greipp PR. Peripheral blood B cell labeling indices are a measure of disease activity in patients with monoclonal gammopathies. *J Clin Oncol* 1988; **6**:1041–6.

37. Witzig TE, Kyle RA, Greipp PR. Circulating peripheral blood plasma cells in multiple myeloma. *Curr Top Microbiol Immunol* 1992; **182**:195–9.

38. Witzig TE, Kyle RA, O'Fallon WM, Greipp PR. Detection of peripheral blood plasma cells as a predictor of disease course in patients with smouldering multiple myeloma. *Br J Haematol* 1994; **87**:266–72.

39. Folkman J. Angiogenesis-dependent diseases. *Semin Oncol* 2001; **28**:536–42.

40. Rajkumar SV, Kyle RA. Angiogenesis in multiple myeloma. *Semin Oncol* 2001; **28**:560–4.

41. Dankbar B, Padro T, Leo R, Feldmann B, Kropff M, Mesters RM, *et al.* Vascular endothelial growth factor and interleukin-6 in paracrine tumor-stromal cell interactions in multiple myeloma. *Blood* 2000; **95**:2630–6.

42. Rajkumar SV, Witzig TE. A review of angiogenesis and antiangiogenic therapy with thalidomide in multiple myeloma. *Cancer Treat Rev* 2000; **26**:351–62.

43. Rajkumar SV, Fonseca R, Witzig TE, Gertz MA, Greipp PR. Bone marrow angiogenesis in patients achieving complete response after stem cell transplantation for multiple myeloma. *Leukemia* 1999; **13**:469–72.

44. Rajkumar SV, Leong T, Roche PC, Fonseca R, Dispenzieri A, Lacy MQ, *et al.* Prognostic value of bone marrow angiogenesis in multiple myeloma. *Clin Cancer Res* 2000; **6**:3111–16.

45. Rajkumar SV, Greipp PR. Angiogenesis in multiple myeloma. *Br J Haematol* 2001; **113**:565.

46. Rajkumar SV, Mesa RA, Fonseca R, Schroeder, G, Plevak MF, Dispenzieri A, *et al.* Bone marrow angiogenesis in 400 patients with monoclonal gammopathy of undetermined significance, multiple myeloma, and primary amyloidosis. *Clin Cancer Res* 2002; **8**:2210–6.

47. Vacca A, Ribatti D, Roncali L, Ranieri G, Serio G, Silvestris F, *et al.* Bone marrow angiogenesis and progression in multiple myeloma. *Br J Haematol* 1994; **87**:503–8.

48. Greipp PR, Lust JA, O'Fallon WM, Katzmann JA, Witzig TE, Kyle RA. Plasma cell labeling index and beta 2-microglobulin predict survival independent of thymidine kinase and C-reactive protein in multiple myeloma. *Blood* 1993; **81**:3382–7.

49. Kawano M, Hirano T, Matsuda T, Taga T, Horii Y, Iwato K, *et al.* Autocrine generation and requirement of BSF-2/IL-6 for human multiple myelomas. *Nature* 1988; **332**:83–5.

50. Schwab G, Siegall CB, Aarden LA, Neckers LM, Nordan RP. Characterization of an interleukin-6-mediated autocrine growth loop in the human multiple myeloma cell line, U266. *Blood* 1991; **77**:587–93.

51. Bataille R, Jourdan M, Zhang XG, Klein B. Serum levels of interleukin 6, a potent myeloma cell growth factor, as a reflect of disease severity in plasma cell dyscrasias. *J Clin Invest* 1989; **84**:2008–11.

52. Zhang XG, Klein B, Bataille R. Interleukin-6 is a potent myeloma-cell growth factor in patients with aggressive multiple myeloma. *Blood* 1989; **74**:11–13.

53. Bataille R, Barlogie B, Lu ZY, Rossi JF, Lavabre-Bertrand T, Beck T, *et al.* Biologic effects of anti-interleukin-6 murine monoclonal antibody in advanced multiple myeloma. *Blood* 1995; **86**:685–91.

54. Klein B, Zhang XG, Jourdan M, Content J, Houssiau F, Aarden L, *et al.* Paracrine rather than autocrine regulation of myeloma-cell growth and differentiation by interleukin-6. *Blood* 1989; **73**:517–26.

55. Portier M, Rajzbaum G, Zhang XG, Attal M, Rusalen C, Wijdenes J, *et al.* In vivo interleukin 6 gene expression in the tumoral environment in multiple myeloma. *Eur J Immunol* 1991; **21**:1759–62.

●56. Carter A, Merchav S, Silvian-Draxler I, Tatarsky I. The role of interleukin-1 and tumour necrosis factor-alpha in human multiple myeloma. *Br J Haematol* 1990; **74**:424–31.

57. Donovan KA, Lacy MQ, Kline MP, Ahmann GJ, Heimbach JK, Kyle RA, et al. Contrast in cytokine expression between patients with monoclonal gammopathy of undetermined significance or multiple myeloma. *Leukemia* 1998; **12**:593–600.

58. Lacy MQ, Donovan KA, Heimbach JK, Ahmann GJ, Lust JA. Comparison of interleukin-1 beta expression by in situ hybridization in monoclonal gammopathy of undetermined significance and multiple myeloma. *Blood* 1999; **93**:300–5.

59. Collins T, Read MA, Neish AS, Whitley MZ, Thanos D, Maniatis T. Transcriptional regulation of endothelial cell adhesion molecules:NF-kappa B and cytokine-inducible enhancers. *FASEB J* 1995; **9**:899–909.

60. Dustin ML, Rothlein R, Bhan AK, Dinarello CA, Springer TA. Induction by IL 1 and interferon-gamma: tissue distribution, biochemistry, and function of a natural adherence molecule (ICAM-1). *J Immunol* 1986; **137**:245–54.

61. Terry RW, Kwee L, Levine JF, Labow MA. Cytokine induction of an alternatively spliced murine vascular cell adhesion molecule (VCAM) mRNA encoding a glycosylphosphatidylinositol-anchored VCAM protein. *Proc Natl Acad Sci USA* 1993; **90**:5919–23.

62. Torcia M, Lucibello M, Vannier E, Fabiani S, Miliani A, Guidi G, et al. Modulation of osteoclast-activating factor activity of multiple myeloma bone marrow cells by different interleukin-1 inhibitors. *Exp Hematol* 1996; **24**:868–74.

63. Yamamoto I, Kawano M, Sone T, Iwato K, Tanaka H, Ishikawa H, et al. Production of interleukin 1 beta, a potent bone resorbing cytokine, by cultured human myeloma cells. *Cancer Res* 1989; **49**:4242–6.

64. Shacter E, Weitzman SA. Chronic inflammation and cancer. *Oncology (Huntingt)* 2002; **16**:217–26, 229; discussion 230–2.

65. Correa P. Helicobacter pylori as a pathogen and carcinogen. *J Physiol Pharmacol* 1997; **48**:19–24.

66. Choi PM, Zelig MP. Similarity of colorectal cancer in Crohn's disease and ulcerative colitis: implications for carcinogenesis and prevention. *Gut* 1994; **35**:950–4.

67. Hayashi PH, Zeldis JB. Molecular biology of viral hepatitis and hepatocellular carcinoma. *Comprehens Ther* 1993; **19**:188–96.

68. Pera M, Trastek VF, Pairolero PC, Cardesa A, Allen MS, Deschamps C. Barrett's disease: pathophysiology of metaplasia and adenocarcinoma. *Ann Thorac Surg* 1993; **56**:1191–7.

69. Miwa H, Kanno H, Munakata S, Akano Y, Taniwaki M, Aozasa, K. Induction of chromosomal aberrations and growth-transformation of lymphoblastoid cell lines by inhibition of reactive oxygen species-induced apoptosis with interleukin-6. *Lab Invest* 2000; **80**:725–34.

70. Potter M. Perspectives on the origins of multiple myeloma and plasmacytomas in mice, *Hematol Oncol Clin North Am* 1992; **6**:211–23.

●71. Potter M, Wax JS. Genetics of susceptibility to pristane-induced plasmacytomas in BALB/cAn:reduced susceptibility in BALB/cJ with a brief description of pristane-induced arthritis. *J Immunol* 1981; **127**:1591–5.

72. Hilbert DM, Kopf M, Mock BA, Kohler G, Rudikoff S. Interleukin 6 is essential for in vivo development of B lineage neoplasms. *J Exp Med* 1995; **182**:243–8.

73. Bataille R, Robinet-Levy M, Barchechath-Flaisler F, Peres S, Aznar R, Sany J. Immunofixation improves the detection of monoclonal gammopathy of undetermined significance (M.G.U.S.) in patients with rheumatoid arthritis. *Clin Exp Rheumatol* 1987; **5**:259–61.

74. Eriksson M. Rheumatoid arthritis as a risk factor for multiple myeloma:a case-control study. *Eur J Cancer* 1993; **29A**:259–63.

75. Matteson EL, Hickey AR, Maguire L, Tilson HH, Urowitz MB. Occurrence of neoplasia in patients with rheumatoid arthritis enrolled in a DMARD Registry. Rheumatoid Arthritis Azathioprine Registry Steering Committee. *J Rheumatol* 1991; **18**:809–14.

76. Kelly C, Baird G, Foster H, Hosker H, Griffiths I. Prognostic significance of paraproteinaemia in rheumatoid arthritis. *Ann Rheumat Dis* 1991; **50**:290–4.

77. Linet MS, McLaughlin JK, Harlow SD, Fraumeni JF. Family history of autoimmune disorders and cancer in multiple myeloma. *Int J Epidemiol* 1988; **17**:512–3.

78. Lehman TJ, Striegel KH, Onel KB. Thalidomide therapy for recalcitrant systemic onset juvenile rheumatoid arthritis. *J Pediatr* 2002; **140**:125–7.

79. Scoville CD. Pilot study using the combination of methotrexate and thalidomide in the treatment of rheumatoid arthritis. *Clin Exp Rheumatol* 2001; **19**:360–1.

80. Wendling D, Racadot E, Wijdenes J. Treatment of severe rheumatoid arthritis by anti-interleukin 6 monoclonal antibody. *J Rheumatol* 1993; **20**:259–62.

81. Singhal S, Mehta J, Desikan R, Ayers D, Roberson P, Eddlemon P, et al. Antitumor activity of thalidomide in refractory multiple myeloma. *N Engl J Med* 1999; **341**:1565–71.

82. Kyle RA. Diagnosis and management of multiple myeloma and related disorders. *Prog Hematol* 1986; **14**:257–82.

83. Potter M, Wax JS, Anderson AO, Nordan RP. Inhibition of plasmacytoma development in BALB/c mice by indomethacin. *J Exp Med* 1985; **161**:996–1012.

84. International Myeloma Working Group. Criteria for the classification of monoclonal gammopathies, multiple myeloma and related disorders: a report of the International Myeloma Working Group. *Br J Haematol* 2003; **121**:749–57.

25

Solitary bone and extramedullary plasmacytoma

MELETIOS A. DIMOPOULOS AND LIA A. MOULOPOULOS

INTRODUCTION

Most patients with multiple myeloma present with symptoms, show evidence of generalized disease, and require systemic treatment promptly in order to reduce the malignant clone. Some patients with plasma cell tumors present with a single bone lesion or with an extramedullary mass owing to a monoclonocal plasma cell infiltrate, and further studies show no evidence of myeloma elsewhere. Such patients with solitary bone plasmacytoma (SBP) or solitary extramedullary plasmacytoma (SEP) usually become symptom-free with local radiotherapy. Although the exact incidence of solitary plasmacytoma is not clear, this entity affects less than 5% of patients with plasma cell tumors treated at one large referral center.[1]

SOLITARY BONE PLASMACYTOMA

Diagnosis

The diagnosis of SBP requires histologic evidence of a monoclonal plasma cell infiltrate in a single bone lesion, absence of other bone lesions on skeletal survey, and lack of marrow plasmacytosis elsewhere. Furthermore, there should be no evidence of anemia, hypercalcemia, or renal dysfunction that could be attributed to the plasma cell proliferative disorder (Table 25.1). Some older series have included patients with two bone lesions or patients with up to 10% bone marrow plasma cells, while others have excluded patients who developed multiple myeloma within 2 years of diagnosis or in whom monoclonal protein persisted after local treatment.[2-4] Such broad and ill-defined inclusion criteria have created confusion regarding the

Table 25.1 *Diagnostic criteria for solitary bone plasmacytoma*

- Single area of bone destruction due to monoclonal plasma cells
- Normal bone marrow aspiration and biopsy
- Normal results on a complete skeletal survey, and magnetic resonance imaging of the spine and pelvis
- No anemia, hypercalcemia, or renal impairment attributable to a plasma cell proliferative disorder

outcome of patients with SBP. Advances in imaging modalities have improved the precision of diagnosis of SBP. Computed tomography (CT) and particularly magnetic resonance imaging (MRI) depict the extent of the plasmacytoma more clearly than plain radiographs. Furthermore, MRI can sample a large volume of bone marrow and is a very sensitive procedure for detecting unsuspected involvement of bone marrow in patients with apparent SBP.[5] A recent update of the MD Anderson series indicated that 26% of patients initially referred for SBP were excluded when MRI of the spine revealed abnormal lesions that had not been detected on skeletal survey.[6] Thus, a normal MRI of the spine and pelvis is also required for the accurate diagnosis of SBP (Table 25.1). With more sensitive staging procedures and with more strict diagnostic criteria, the diagnosis of SBP should become less common. Further studies are needed in order to assess whether evaluations such as flow cytometry of normal-appearing marrow, fluorescent *in situ* hybridization, or positron emission tomography (PET) scanning may improve further our ability to detect truly localized plasmacytoma.

Clinical and laboratory features

Clinical features of SBP from three representative series are shown in Table 25.2. SBP is a rare disease and almost

Table 25.2 *Characteristics of patients with solitary bone plasmacytoma*

Series	Number of patients	Median age (years)	Spine disease (% of patients)	Monoclonal protein (% of patients)
Galieni et al.[7]	32	52	40	47
Frassica et al.[8]	46	56	54	54
Wilder et al.[6]	60	54	40	75

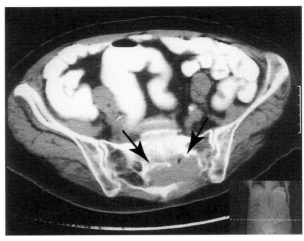

Figure 25.1 *A 63-year-old woman with solitary bone plasmacytoma of the sacrum. Axial computed tomography scan at the level of the sacrum shows a lytic lesion in the left site of the sacrum (arrows), which has invaded the sacral canal and the left sacral foramen.*

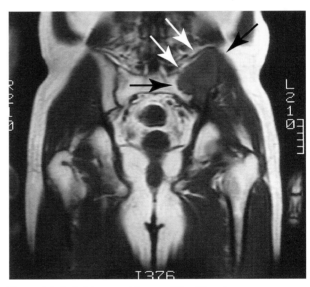

Figure 25.2 *A 44-year-old man with solitary bone plasmacytoma of the sacrum. Coronal T1-weighted magnetic resonance image of the pelvis shows a low-signal-intensity mass (arrows) involving the left sacral wing and iliac bone.*

all series are retrospective, including patients seen over a long period; thus MRI was not used for the staging of all patients in any of the reported series. In the MD Anderson series,[6] MRI was used to stage patients presenting after 1990, but the patients presenting prior to this date are also included. All the published series will, therefore, include some patients who with MRI would be classified as myeloma rather than SBP.

The majority of patients are men and their median age is about a decade younger than that of patients with multiple myeloma.[6–14] Although SBP may arise from any bone, the axial skeleton is affected most often, particularly the spine. The most common presenting symptom is pain at the site of the skeletal lesion. Patients with vertebral involvement may present with symptoms and signs of spinal cord or nerve root compression, and patients with solitary plasmacytoma of long bones may present with a fracture. In occasional patients with SBP, symptoms and signs of peripheral neuropathy may be the primary presenting feature. This polyneuropathy is a demyelinating process, which, in some cases, is due to the deposition of monoclonal protein in the endoneurium of the affected nerves.[15]

With conventional radiographs most patients show a purely lytic bone destruction with a clear margin. Occasional patients show sclerotic bone involvement. With CT scannning of the affected bone the extent of SBP is depicted more clearly (Fig. 25.1). The MRI of the bone marrow in patients with solitary bone plasmacytoma may include T1-weighted, T2-weighted, and contrast-enhanced T1-weighted sequences, depending on the circumstances. The primary tumor is imaged initially with sagittal and axial images of the involved bone. A search for additional lesions can be achieved with coronal short inversion-time inversion-recovery (STIR) images of the spine and pelvis, and sagittal T1-weighted and STIR or T2-weighted fast spin echo with fat saturation images of the spine. A T1-weighted spin echo sequence remains the most important sequence for depiction of bone marrow plasmacytoma. The tumor is shown as an area of bone marrow replacement with signal intensity lower than that of yellow bone marrow, slightly lower than or similar to that of red bone marrow, and similar to muscle (Fig. 25.2). For T2 imaging either a fast spin echo T2-weighted image with fat saturation or a STIR can be used. For imaging of a large area of the skeleton (such as the entire spine), STIR images are preferred because they are less prone to artifacts due to field heterogeneity. T1-weighted contrast-enhanced images can be used to better demonstrate any associated epidural or paraspinal soft-tissue component and in cases of questionable bone marrow involvement on T1- and T2-weighted images (Figs 25.3 and 25.4). Lesions will enhance to a variable degree depending on tumor vascularity. In adults, normal red

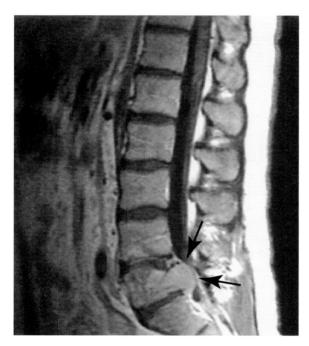

Figure 25.3 *A 31-year-old man with solitary bone plasmacytoma of the lumbar spine. Contrast-enhanced T1-weighted sagittal magnetic resonance image shows involvement of L5 with extraosseous component in the anterior epidural space (arrows).*

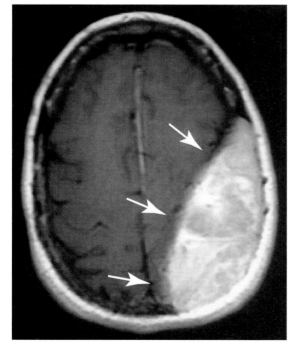

Figure 25.4 *A 62-year-old woman with solitary bone plasmacytoma of the skull. Axial contrast-enhanced T1-weighted magnetic resonance image shows osseous involvement of the left frontoparietal area associated with a large enhancing extra-axial mass (arrows).*

marrow enhances minimally. Contrast-enhanced T1-weighted images with fat saturation provide excellent contrast between the enhancing areas of bone marrow infiltration and the dark signal of the saturated bone marrow.[5,16] The utility of MRI in the staging of SBP is further supported by the higher rate of relapse of patients who showed unsuspected and asymptomatic lesions. In a group of 23 patients with solitary plasmacytoma of the thoracolumbar spine, multiple myeloma developed in seven of eight patients with a solitary lesion on plain radiography alone but in only one of seven patients who also had negative results on MRI.[17]

Electrophoresis and immunofixation of serum and urine samples should be performed in all patients with SBP before any treatment is administered. A monoclonal protein is detected in the serum and/or the urine of most patients with SBP (Table 25.2), but the levels of the monoclonal protein are much lower than those of patients with multiple myeloma. In a recent MD Anderson series, a serum monoclonal protein was present in 37 of 60 patients (62%); in 26 of 37 patients (70%), the monoclonal protein levels were ≤10 g/L and in 30% of patients the levels were 11–22 g/L. In an additional eight of 60 patients (13%), only Bence Jones protein was present in the urine (range 0.2–7.0 g/L).[6] The uninvolved immunoglobulins are preserved in the overwhelming majority of patients with SBP. The low levels of monoclonal protein, the significant fraction of patients with non-secretory disease, and the preservation of uninvolved immunoglobulins are all features consistent with the very low tumor load of patients with SBP. Serum monoclonal protein above 20 g/L and depressed uninvolved immunoglobulins are consistent with occult but disseminated myeloma and should trigger a more extensive work-up to confirm this suspicion.

Treatment and response

RADIATION THERAPY

Radiation therapy is the appropriate treatment for SBP (see also Chapter 15). Treatment fields should be designed to include all disease shown by MRI or CT scanning, and should include a margin of normal tissue. For vertebral plasmacytoma, the margin should include at least one uninvolved vertebra. Thoracic plasmacytomas may be treated with a single posterior field, and cervical or lumbar plasmacytomas may be treated with two parallel opposed fields. The clinical target volume for a long bone should normally include the gross disease with a 2–5 cm margin. Although the optimal dose of radiation therapy has not been prospectively defined, most series indicate that a dose of at least 4000 cGy in 200 cGy fractions provides the best local control. For spinal lesions, the dose should be limited to 4000 cGy. For other lesions of the axial skeleton (femora, humeri, pelvis), the radiotherapy dose can be increased to 5000 cGy.[6] After radiotherapy, virtually all patients have relief of symptoms. With serial, post-radiotherapy plain radiography assessments, radiologic response includes sclerosis and bone remineralization, and is observed in approximately 50% of patients.[11,17] When CT scanning or MRI is used, in most cases of SBP the soft tissue mass does not disappear.[6]

In most patients with adequately staged SBP (i.e. where MRI shows no disease elsewhere), the monoclonal protein is reduced significantly after completion of radiation therapy.[18] Serial follow-up studies are necessary because the rate of reduction may be slow and a continuous decrease of the protein may be observed for several years.[19] With the use of post-treatment immunofixation studies, disappearance of monoclonal protein is observed in 20–50% of patients with evaluable monoclonal protein at baseline. This suggests that all disease was included within the radiotherapy field. However, in other patients the paraprotein persists, indicating that tumor is present outside the field of radiotherapy. Wilder et al.[6] reported persistence of monoclonal protein in 71% of patients and this was found to be a risk factor for subsequent progression. The probability of disappearance of monoclonal protein is higher when the pretreatment levels are low. In one series, the disappearance rates for serum monoclonal proteins of 1–10 g/L and $\geqslant$11 g/L were 41% and 0%, respectively.[17] There is, however, no obvious relation between radiation dose and disappearance of monoclonal protein.[17]

SURGERY

Although fine needle aspiration is usually sufficient to establish the diagnosis of SBP, a limited surgical procedure (incisional biopsy) may be required in occasional patients for diagnostic purposes. In some patients with vertebral lesions when the diagnosis has not yet been made and when there is rapid neurologic deterioration, a laminectomy may be indicated for both diagnostic and therapeutic purposes.[4] In such instances, radiotherapy should be administered after the surgery to consolidate eradication of tumor. Surgical fixation of a pathologic fracture of a long bone may also be required in some instances. Surgical intervention may also be necessary when there is instability of the bone and in the unusual situation of tumor resistance to radiotherapy.

ADJUVANT SYSTEMIC THERAPY

The value of adjuvant systemic therapy after radiotherapy has not been evaluated systematically. There are several retrospective series in which some patients received adjuvant chemotherapy and their outcome was compared with that of other patients who did not. Mayr et al.[20] found that adjuvant chemotherapy may prevent progression to multiple myeloma. Holland et al.[13] found that adjuvant chemotherapy prolonged the time to progression to myeloma but did not affect the overall rate of progression. In the series reported by Shih et al., the percentages of patients who remained with no evidence of disease at last follow-up were 55% for those who received adjuvant chemotherapy and 64% for those who did not.[21] Tsang et al.[14] reported that among their five patients who were selected to receive adjuvant chemotherapy, four patients failed. On the basis of available data, there is no evidence that adjuvant systemic therapy is of benefit in patients with SBP, while the use of systemic chemotherapy or corticosteroids may induce the evolution of resistant malignant cells and may expose the patients to the risks of myelodysplastic syndrome and secondary leukemia.[22] Because chemotherapy or corticosteroids when administered during or after radiotherapy may affect the rate of monoclonal protein reduction, they may obscure the recognition of patients in whom myeloma protein disappears after radiotherapy.

Prognostic factors and outcome

PATTERNS OF PROGRESSION

After treatment with radiotherapy, patients with SBP may experience local failure within the radiotherapy fields, may develop systemic disease, or may remain free of disease for many years and thus may be considered cured.

Local control, defined as long-term clinical and radiographic stability, has been achieved in at least 90% of patients with SBP. In some series, local control was more likely to be achieved in patients with plasmacytomas <5 cm,[14] but this observation was not confirmed in other series.[6] Some series have suggested a radiotherapy dose–response relationship for local control. Medenhall et al.[23] reported a 31% incidence of local failure for doses less than 4000 cGy and 6% incidence for higher doses. Mill and Griffith[24] observed a trend toward higher local recurrence in SBP patients treated with radiotherapy doses <5000 cGy. Frassica et al.[8] observed that all their local failures occurred in patients receiving less than 4500 cGy. In some series, local failure appeared to be higher in patients with vertebral plasmacytomas.[3] However, several series have not confirmed a dose–response relationship for local control.[6,11,14] This may be due in part to the small number of local recurrences and to the practice of delivering higher doses of radiation to larger lesions.[6] With modern radiotherapy planning and techniques, and with doses of 4000 cGy or greater, the probability of local failure should become negligible.

The outcome of patients with SBP who received local radiotherapy without adjuvant chemotherapy is shown in Table 25.3. The majority of patients with SBP develop distant recurrence. The most common pattern

Table 25.3 *Progression and survival of patients with solitary bone plasmacytoma*

Series	Number of patients	10 year disease–free survival (%)	Median survival (years)
Knowling et al.[9]	25	16	7.5
Bolek et al.[11]	27	46	10.0
Frassica et al.[8]	46	25	9.3
Wilder et al.[6]	60	38	11.0

of progression consists of new bone lesions, diffuse marrow plasmacytosis, and rising of monoclonal protein levels. In several patients, however, new bone lesions develop without involvement of the intervening marrow, consistent with a pattern of multiple plasmacytomas or macrofocal myeloma. The median time to systemic progression is 2–4 years, but myeloma may develop in occasional patients 10 or more years after the original diagnosis of SBP. However, the available data relate to series of patients who were not generally staged by MRI. As already noted, in a small series of patients the risk of progression was much higher in those with positive MRI examinations.[17] It is, therefore, probable that as MRI examination becomes an established part of the staging criteria for the diagnosis of SBP, the risk of progression will be lower and the event-free survival longer than in current series.

Finally, in a few patients with SBP, recurrent isolated plasmacytomas develop several months or years after treatment of the original lesion. Careful evaluations with plain radiographs, MRI, and bone marrow biopsies still do not reveal systemic disease. The best management of these patients is not established. We believe that when isolated lesions develop at long intervals (>2 years), systemic treatment may be withheld and such patients may be treated with localized radiotherapy.[6,18] The remaining patients may be appropriate candidates for systemic treatment.

PROGNOSTIC FACTORS AND SURVIVAL

In many series, several clinical and laboratory parameters were assessed for their possible correlation with the likelihood of distant failure. In some series, no factors predictive of systemic recurrence could be identified.[8,9,21,25,26] Most authors agree that the dose of local radiotherapy does not affect the chance of distant progression.[1] Bataille and Sany reported that multiple myeloma developed more commonly in patients with impaired performance status, in older patients, and in patients with vertebral involvement.[3] These observations were not confirmed from several other series.[1] Tsang et al.[14] performed a Cox-regression analysis, which indicated that the only factor associated with disease-free survival was older age.[14] Age was not predictive in several series.[6,11,13,20,21] The two main parameters that have been associated with a higher risk of progression are the depression of uninvolved immunoglobulins and the persistence of monoclonal protein after radiotherapy.[1] The MD Anderson group was the first to show that disappearance of monoclonal protein after radiotherapy was associated with prolonged stability and even cure.[18] An update of the MD Anderson series, which included 61 patients with carefully staged SBP, indicated that, among 11 patients with disappearance of monoclonal protein, myeloma developed in only two patients after 4 and 12 years, respectively. Myeloma developed in 57% of patients with persistent monoclonal protein and in 63% of those with non-secretory plasmacytoma ($P = 0.02$).[17] In a more recent report from the same institution, the following parameters were assessed for their impact on myeloma-free survival and cause-specific survival: disappearance versus persistence of monoclonal protein after radiotherapy, secretory versus non-secretory disease at diagnosis, tumor size, spinal versus non-spinal location, presence versus absence of an associated soft tissue mass on CT or MRI, magnitude of serum monoclonal protein elevation at diagnosis, performance status, and total radiotherapy dose. Although not statistically significant, the prognosis of patients with secretory SBP appeared to be better than that of non-secretory tumors. The 10-year myeloma-free survival rates were 46% and 16% for patients with secretory and non-secretory disease, respectively. On multivariate analysis, persistence of monoclonal protein more than 1 year after radiotherapy was the only independent adverse prognostic factor for myeloma-free and cause-specific survival.[6]

The median overall survival of patients with SBP averages 10 years and up to 20% of patients die of unrelated causes. This long survival is due partly to the prolonged stability of several patients who may be cured with local radiotherapy and partly to the relatively long survival of patients who develop multiple myeloma. Liebross et al.[17] reported that their patients with SBP who progressed to myeloma had features of low-tumor mass disease, a 77% response rate to chemotherapy, and a subsequent median survival of 5.3 years. As previously discussed, the overall survival of patients with SBP may improve further as MRI examination becomes an established part of the staging criteria for the diagnosis.

EXTRAMEDULLARY PLASMACYTOMA

Diagnosis

Solitary extramedullary plasmacytoma is a plasma cell tumor that arises outside the bone marrow. SEP is even less common than SBP. The diagnosis of SEP is based on histologic confirmation of a single extramedullary mass infiltrated by monoclonal plasma cells with no evidence of multiple myeloma elsewhere, i.e. there is no evidence of bone lesions on skeletal survey, there is lack of marrow plasmacytosis, and there is no evidence of anemia, hypercalcemia, or renal dysfunction that could be attributed to the plasma cell proliferative disorder (Table 25.4). The role of MRI in the staging of SEP has not been studied.

On light microscopy, SEP must be differentiated from reactive plasmacytosis, plasma cell granuloma, poorly differentiated neoplasms, immunoblastic lymphoma, lymphoplasmacytic lymphoma, and mucosa-associated lymphoid tissue (MALT) lymphoma.[26–31] Immunohistochemistry and flow cytometry may help to distinguish SEP from these other entities, since it is comprised of plasma cells that co-express CD38 and cytoplasmic light chains of either κ or λ type. Negative staining for CD20 and positive staining for CD79 may strengthen further the diagnosis of SEP. Hotz et al.[29] reported that among 24 patients with morphologically diagnosed SEP of the head and neck area, only 14 patients had monoclonal lesions after immunohistochemistry for light chain was applied. In the remaining ten patients, reactive polyclonal plasmacytosis was confirmed. Hussong et al.[32] have recently suggested that SEP may represent a form of extranodal marginal zone lymphoma that has undergone extensive plasmacytic differentiation. They examined a small number of cases with presumed SEP and reported that in addition to the predominant plasma cell component, many features of marginal zone lymphoma, such as reactive follicles, lymphoepithelial lesions, centrocyte-like cells, and monocytoid cells, were observed within the tumors.[32] These authors suggested that SEP, in fact, represent marginal zone lymphomas that have undergone extensive plasmacytic differentiation. Whether this statement applies to all patients with SEP requires detailed studies. Nevertheless, this concept is consistent with the original report of Wiltshaw,[33] who, 25 years ago, described the natural history of SEP and its relationship to SBP and to multiple myeloma. She emphasized several features that distinguished SEP from the other two entities, such as

Table 25.4 *Diagnostic criteria for solitary extramedullary plasmacytoma*

- Single extramedullary mass infiltrated by monoclonal plasma cells
- Absence of morphologic and immunophenotypic findings suggestive of reactive plasmacytosis, poorly differentiated epithelial tumors, immunoblastic lymphoma, and lymphoplasmatic lymphoma
- Normal bone marrow aspiration and biopsy
- Normal results on a full skeletal survey and magnetic resonance imaging of the spine and pelvis
- No anemia, hypercalcemia, or renal impairment attributable to a plasma cell proliferative disorder

a marked predilection for mucosal surfaces, a high incidence of spread to other soft tissue sites, and infrequent involvement of the bone marrow.

Clinical and laboratory features

The median age at presentation is 55 years and 75% of patients are male. A monoclonal protein is detected in the serum and/or urine in a minority of patients (25% or less). These tumors can occur at any site, but more than 80% develop in the head and neck area, especially in the upper respiratory tract (nasal cavity, paranasal sinuses, and nasopharynx) (Table 25.5, Fig. 25.5). The plasmacytomas are usually submucosal lesions and the patients may present with symptoms such as epistaxis, nasal dicharge or obstruction, sore throat, hoarseness, and hemoptysis.[34–42]

Table 25.5 *Characteristics of patients with solitary extramedullary plasmacytoma*

Series	Number of patients	Median age	Head and neck disease (% of patients)	Monoclonal protein (%)
Knowling et al.[9]	25	59	–	32
Brinch et al.[10]	18	56	94	18
Liebross et al.[37]	22	55	86	23
Galieni et al.[42]	46	55	80	21

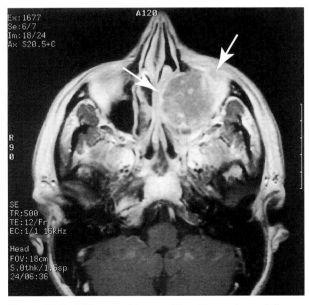

Figure 25.5 *A 32-year-old man with solitary extramedullary plasmacytoma of the left paranasal sinus. Contrast-enhanced T1-weighted magnetic resonance image of the brain shows a mass in the left paranasal sinus (arrows), which has invaded the medial wall of the sinus.*

Plasmacytomas have been reported in several other sites, such as the parotid, the thyroid, the lungs, the breast, the testis, the skin, and the gastrointestinal tract. The most common site of SEP outside the head and neck area is the gastrointestinal tract. The symptoms produced are similar to those of the more common primary cancers at these sites.[43–52] The radiologic appearance of SEP is nonspecific. A CT scan and/or MRI of the affected area is necessary in order to delineate the extent of the lesion. In some patients with SEP, the adjacent lymph nodes or bone structures are involved by the tumor. Local bone destruction is quite usual in patients with SEP of the nasal cavity or the maxillary sinuses.[37] Patients with either bone or lymph node involvement can still be considered and treated as solitary tumors.

Treatment and response

RADIATION THERAPY

The treatment of choice is radiation therapy. These tumors are highly radiosensitive and, with a total radiation dose of at least 4000 cGy, the risk of local recurrence is less than 5%. Treatment techniques should be site-appropriate and should be designed to include the entire tumor with generous margins. Patients with disease of the nasal cavity or paranasal sinuses should be treated by a three-field technique, i.e. one anterior and two lateral wedged fields. For patients with tumors of the oral cavity, nasopharynx, oropharynx, and larynx, standard opposed lateral fields are used. Because the latter patients may progress with involvement of adjacent lymph nodes, some authors have suggested that elective neck irradiation should be added. Patients with SEP elsewhere should be treated with standard anterior-posterior and posterior-anterior fields.[37]

SURGERY

For most patients with head and neck SEP, the diagnosis can be established by fine-needle aspiration or by incisional biopsy, and thus an extensive surgical procedure is not required for diagnosis. Furthermore, radical surgery with curative intent in that area is usually a mutilating procedure and, as these tumors are highly radiosensitive, radical surgery is not necessary. For patients with non-head and neck plasmacytomas, complete surgical removal, if feasible, should be considered. For such patients with negative surgical margins, it is not clear whether adjuvant radiotherapy is needed.[35]

SYSTEMIC THERAPY

As with SBP, there is no evidence that administration of chemotherapy during or after radiation therapy is of benefit to patients with SEP.[42]

Prognostic factors and outcome

PATTERNS OF PROGRESSION

Sustained local tumor control is achieved in the overwhelming majority of patients. In most series, the probability of local relapse is 5% or less. Patients with SEP involving the head and neck area may progress with involvement of adjacent lymph nodes, and this complication is reduced significantly when the regional lymph nodes receive prophylactic irradiation.[11,20,37] Tsang et al.[14] reported that among six SEP patients with tumor size ≥ 5 cm, four patients developed local failure.

A proportion of patients with SEP develop distant failure. Most large series indicate that the probability of distant dissemination is less than 30% (Table 25.6). Progressive disease may present as typical multiple myeloma with bone lesions, bone marrow plasmacytosis, and rising levels of monoclonal protein. A recent review of the literature indicates that multiple myeloma occurs in approximately 15% of patients.[35] However, some patients develop multiple extramedullary lesions without intervening bone marrow plasmacytosis. The commonest site for soft-tissue involvement is the lymph nodes followed by the skin and subcutaneous tissues.[33] Other patients with SEP have developed solitary bone lesions several months or years after the original diagnosis.[42] In SBP and multiple myeloma, bone involvement is usually within the axial skeleton. In contrast, in SEP, bone lesions seem to be distributed in a random fashion throughout the skeleton.[33] When distant failure develops, this usually occurs within 2–3 years from diagnosis. Most series indicate that the probability of dissemination is lower in patients with SEP than in those with SBP (Table 25.6).

PROGNOSTIC FACTORS AND SURVIVAL

The small number of patients included in each series has prevented the clarification of prognostic variables associated with distant progression. Most recent series observed no significant difference in outcome when destruction of the adjacent bone was observed.[20,37,41] However, Harwood et al.[38] indicated a higher rate for distant failure for patients whose SEP involved adjacent bone. Galieni et al.[42] suggested a trend for more frequent

Table 25.6 *Progression and survival of patients with solitary extramedullary plasmacytoma*

Series	Number of patients	10 year disease free survival (%)	10 year survival (%)
Knowling et al.[9]	25	70	–
Brinch et al.[10]	18	80	76
Liebross et al.[37]	22	56	50
Galieni et al.[42]	46	78	80

dissemination for SEP arising outside the head and neck area. One series of 19 patients with pulmonary plasmacytoma indicated a low 5-year survival at 40%.[45] Susnerwala et al.[41] reported that, in their patients with SEP of the head and neck area, the probability of local control correlated with tumor grade: five of six patients with the asynchronous or plasmablastic type developed local failure after radiotherapy, whereas the probability of local control for low-grade tumors was 83%. The majority of patients die of unrelated causes and at least two-thirds of patients survive for more than 10 years.

KEY POINTS

- The diagnosis of solitary bone plasmacytoma (SBP) requires histologic evidence of a monoclonal plasma cell infiltrate in a single bone lesion and absence of myeloma elsewhere.
- When magnetic resonance imaging of the spine and pelvis is performed, approximately 30% of patients with presumed SBP show occult abnormal lesions.
- The recommended treatment plan for SBP is radical radiotherapy at a total dose of 4000–5000 cGy in 20–25 fractions.
- The 10-year disease-free survival rate of patients with SBP is approximately 30% and the median overall survival of these patients is about 10 years.
- The diagnosis of solitary extramedullary plasmacytoma (SEP) is based on histologic confirmation of a single extramedullary mass infiltrated by monoclonal plasma cells with no evidence of myeloma elsewhere.
- The recommended treatment of SEP is radiotherapy at a total dose of at least 4000 cGy and treatment techniques depend on the site of SEP.
- The 10-year disease-free survival and overall survival rates of patients with SEP are approximately 70%.

REFERENCES

● = Key primary paper
◆ = Major review article
* = Paper that represents the first formal publication of a management guideline

◆1. Dimopoulos MA, Moulopoulos LA, Maniatis A, Alexanian R. Solitary plasmacytoma of bone and asymptomatic multiple myeloma. Blood 2000; 96:2037–44.

2. Corwin J, Lindberg RD. Solitary plasmacytoma of bone vs. extramedullary plasmacytoma and their relationship to multiple myeloma. Cancer 1979; 43:1007–13.

3. Bataille R, Sany J. Solitary myeloma: clinical and prognostic features of a review of 114 cases. Cancer 1981; 48:845–51.

4. McLain RF, Weinstein JN. Solitary plasmacytomas of the spine: a review of 84 cases. J Spinal Disord 1989; 2:69–74.

●5. Moulopoulos LA, Dimopoulos MA, Weber D, Fuller L, Libshitz H, Alexanian R. Magnetic resonance imaging in the staging of solitary plasmacytoma of bone. J Clin Oncol 1993; 11:1311–15.

●6. Wilder RB, Ha CS, Cox JD, Webber D, Delasalle K, Alexanian R. Persistence of myeloma protein for more than one year after radiotherapy is an adverse prognostic factor in solitary plasmacytoma of bone. Cancer 2002; 94:1532–37.

7. Galieni P, Cavo M, Avvisati G, Pulsoni A, Falbo R, Bonelli MA. Solitary plasmacytoma of bone and extramedullary plasmacytoma: Two different entities? Ann Oncol 1995; 6:687–91.

●8. Frassica DA, Frassica FJ, Schray MF, Sim FH, Kyle RA. Solitary plasmacytoma of bone: Mayo Clinic experience. Int J Radiat Oncol Biol Phys 1989; 16:43–8.

●9. Knowling MA, Harwood AR, Bergsagel DE. Comparison of extramedullary plasmacytomas with solitary and multiple plasma cell tumors of bone. J Clin Oncol 1983; 1:255–62.

10. Brinch L, Hannisdal E, Foss Abrahamsen A, Kvaloy S, Langholm R. Extramedullary plasmacytomas and solitary plasma cell tumours of bone. EurJ Haematol 1990; 44:131–4.

●11. Bolek TW, Marcus RD, Mendenhall NP: Solitary plasmacytoma of bone and soft tissue. Int J Radiat Oncol Biol Phys 1996; 36:329–33.

12. Jackson A, Scarffe JH. Prognostic significance of osteopenia and immunoparesis at presentation in patients with solitary myeloma of bone. Eur J Cancer 1990; 26:363–71.

13. Holland J, Trenkner DA, Wasserman TH, Fineberg B. Plasmacytoma. Treatment results and conversion to myeloma. Cancer 1992; 69:1513–17.

●14. Tsang RW, Gospodarowicz MK, Pintilie M, Bezjak A, Wells W, Hodgson DC, et al. Solitary plasmacytoma treated with radiotherapy: impact of tumor size on outcome. Int J Radiat Oncol Biol Phys 2001; 50:113–20.

15. Schindler OS, Briggs TWR, Crillies SA. Bilateral demyelinating neuropathy in a solitary lytic and sclerotic myeloma of the proximal humerus: a case report. Int Orthop 1997; 21:59–61

◆16. Moulopoulos LA, Dimopoulos MA: Magnetic resonance imaging of the bone marrow in hematologic malignancies. Blood 1997; 90:2127–47.

17. Liebross RH, Ha CS, Cox JD, Weber D, Delasalle K, Alexanian R. Solitary bone plasmacytoma: outcome and prognostic factors following radiotherapy. Int J Radiat Oncol Biol Phys 1998; 441:1063–67.

●18. Dimopoulos MA, Goldstein J, Fuller L, Delasalle K, Alexanian R. Curability of solitary bone plasmacytoma. J Clin Oncol 1992; 10:587–90.

*19. Alexanian R. Localized and indolent myeloma. Blood 1980; 56:521–5.

20. Mayr, N, Wen BC, Hussey DH, Burns CP, Staples JJ, Vigliotti AP. The role of radiation therapy in the treatment of solitary plasmacytomas. Radiother Oncol 1990; 17:293–303.

21. Delauche-Cavallier MC, Laredo JD, Wybier M, Bard M, Ryckewalrt A. Solitary plasmacytoma of the spine. Long-term clinical course. *Cancer* 1988; **61**:1707–14.

*22. Chak LY, Cox RS, Bostwick DG, Hoppe TT. Solitary plasmacytoma of bone: treatment, progression and survival. *J Clin Oncol* 1987; **5**:1811–15.

23. Mendenhall CM, Thar TL, Million RR. Solitary plasmacytoma of bone and soft tissue. *Int J Radiat Biol Phys* 1980; **6**:1477–501.

*24. Mill W, Griffith R. The role of radiotherapy in the management of plasma cell tumors. *Cancer* 1980; **45**:647–52.

25. Ellis PA, Colls BM. Solitary plasmacytoma of bone: clinical features, treatment and survival. *Hematol Oncol* 1992; **10**:207–11.

26. Shih LY, Dunn P, Leung WM, Chen WJ, Wang PN. Localised plasmacytomas in Taiwan: comparison between extramedullary plasmacytoma and solitary plasmacytoma of bone. *Br J Cancer* 1995; **71**:128–33.

27. Jyothirmayi R, Gangadharan VP, Nair MK. Radiotherapy in the treatment of solitary plasmacytoma. *Br J Radiol* 1997; **70**:511–16.

28. Meis JM, Butler JJ, Osborne BM, Ordonez NG. Solitary plasmacytomas of bone and extramedullary plasmacytomas. A clinicopathologic and immunohistochemical study. *Cancer* 1987; **59**:1475–85.

29. Hotz MA, Schwaab G, Bosq J, Munck JN. Extramedullary solitary plasmacytoma of the head and neck. *Ann Otol Rhinol Laryngol* 1999; **108**:495–500.

30. Seider MJ, Cleary KR, Van Tassel P, Alexanian R, Schantz SP, Frias A, *et al.* Plasma cell granuloma of the nasal cavity treated by radiation therapy. *Cancer* 1991; **67**:929–32.

31. Kodana Y, Kawabata K, Yoshida S, Notohara K, Fujimori T, Chiba T. Malt lymphoma simulating an extramedullary plasmacytoma of the stomach. *Am J Med* 1999; **107**:530–2.

●32. Hussong JW, Perkins SL, Shnitzer B, Hargreaves H, Frizzerra G. Extramedullary plasmacytoma. A form of marginal zone cell lymphoma. *Am J Clin Pathol* 1999; **111**:111–16.

●33. Wiltshaw E. The natural history of extramedullary plasmacytoma and its relation to solitary myeloma of bone and myelomatosis. *Medicine* 1976; **55**:217–38.

34. Dimopoulos MA, Kiamouris C, Moulopoulos LA. Solitary plasmacytoma of bone and extramedullary plasmacytoma. *Hematol Oncol Clin North Am* 1999; **13**:1249–57.

◆35. Alexiou C, Kau R, Dietzfelbinger H, Kremor M, Spiess JC, Schratzenstaller B, *et al.* Extramedullary plasmacytoma. Tumor occurance and therapeutic concepts. *Cancer* 1999; **85**:2305–14.

36. Soesan M, Paccagnella A, Chiaron-Sileni V, Salvagno L, Fornasieno A, Sotti G, *et al.* Extramedullary plasmacytoma: clinical behaviour and response to treatment. *Ann Oncol* 1992; **3**:51–7.

●37. Liebross RH, Ha CS, Cox JD, Weber D, Delasalle K, Alexanian R. Clinical course of solitary extramedullary plasmacytoma. *Radiother Oncol* 1999; **52**:245–9.

38. Harwood AR, Knowling MA, Bergsagel DE. Radiotherapy of extramedullary plasmacytoma of the head and neck. *Clin Radiol* 1981; **32**:31–6.

39. Nofsinger YC, Mirza N, Rowan P, Lanza D, Weinstein G. Head and neck manifestations of plasma cell neoplasms. *Laryngoscope* 1997; **107**:741–6.

40. Miller FR, Laventu P, Wanamaker JR, Bonafede J. Plasmacytomas of the head and neck. *Otolaryngol Head Neck Surg* 1998; **119**:614–18.

●41. Susnerwala SS, Shanks JH, Banerjee SS, Scarffe JH, Farrington WT, Slevin NJ. Extramedullary plasmacytoma of the head and neck region: clinicopathological correlation in 25 cases. *Br J Cancer* 1997; **75**:921–7.

●42. Galieni P, Cavo M, Pulsoni A, Avvisati G, Bigazzi C, Neri S, *et al.* Clinical outcome of extramedullary plasmacytoma. *Haematologica* 2000; **85**:47–51.

43. Gonzalez-Garcia J, Ghufoor K, Sandhu G, Hadley TJ. Primary extramedullary plasmacytoma of the parotid gland: a case report and review of the literature. *J Laryngol Otol* 1998; **112**:179–81.

44. Rubin J, Johnson S, Killeen R. Extramedullary plasmacytoma of the thyroid associated with a serum monoclonal gammapathy. *Arch Otolaryngol Head Neck Surg* 1990; **116**:855–8.

45. Koss MH, Hochholzer L, Moran CA, Frizzera G. Pulmonary plasmacytomas: a clinico-pathologic and immunohistochemical study of five cases. *Ann Diagn Pathol* 1998; **2**:1–11.

46. Chim CS, Ng I, Tendell-Smith NJ, Liang R. Primary extramedullary plasmacytoma of the lacrimal gland. *Leuk Lymphoma* 2001; **42**:831–4.

47. De Chiara A, Losito S, Terracciano L, Di Giacomo R, Iaccarino G, Rubolotta MR. Primary plasmacytoma of the breast. *Arch Pathol Lab Med* 2001; **125**:1078–80.

48. Wan X, Tarantolo S, Orton DF, Greiner TC. Primary extramedullary plasmacytoma in the atria of the heart. *Cardiovasc Pathol* 2001; **10**:137–9.

49. Ramadan A, Naab T, Frederick W, Green W. Testicular plasmacytoma in a patient with the acquired immunodeficiency syndrome. *Tumori* 2000; **86**:480–2.

50. Holland AJ, Kubacz GJ, Warren JR. Plasmacytoma of the sigmoid colon associated with a diverticular stricture: case report and review of the literature. *J R Coll Surg Edinb* 1997; **42**:47–51.

51. Demirhan B, Sokmensuer C, Karakayali H, Gungen Y, Dogan A, Haberal M. Primary extramedullary plasmacytoma of the liver. *J Clin Pathol* 1997; **50**:74–6.

52. Tuting T, Bork K. Primary plasmacytoma of the skin. *J Am Acad Dermatol* 1996; **34**:386–90.

26

Plasma cell leukemia

XAVIER LELEU, IBRAHIM YAKOUB-AGHA AND THIERRY FACON

INTRODUCTION

Plasma cell leukemia (PCL) may occur as an unusual manifestation of multiple myeloma (MM) and/or as a rare form of leukemia. Most authors have credited Foa (1904) with the first description,[1] but this case report does not contain sufficient evidence for the diagnosis, and the first case may in fact be the patient reported by Gluzinski and Reichenstein in 1906.[2]

There are two forms of PCL: primary PCL (P-PCL), occurring *de novo* in patients without a pre-existing MM, first diagnosed in the leukemic phase (approximately 60% of the cases), and secondary PCL, arising as a late event in about 1% of patients previously diagnosed with MM and corresponding to a leukemic transformation.[3,4] In historical series, the incidence of PCL has been estimated at 1–2% of patients with MM.[3–5] In more recent series, the incidence of primary PCL has been estimated at between 2.6% and 4% of patients with MM,[5–8] 12% of patients with high tumor mass MM,[8] and 0.9% (8/847) of patients with acute leukemia.[6]

The disorder is defined as a malignant proliferation of plasma cells (PCs) involving the peripheral blood, with the presence of more than 20% of PCs in the peripheral blood and an absolute PC count of $>2 \times 10^9$/L. A diagnosis of PCL may also be considered when fewer PCs are present (e.g. between 1 and 1.9×10^9/L) as these patients have the same clinical and biological features, share the same cytogenetic abnormalities, and carry the same poor prognosis as classical P-PCL.[9,10] In typical MM, although the peripheral blood is usually not overtly contaminated with monoclonal PCs, several studies have documented small numbers of circulating PCs.[11] It is unknown why a small proportion of patients with plasma cell dyscrasia present with P-PCL and why some rare MM patients develop secondary PCL in the terminal phase.[12,13] Owing to the low frequency of this entity, most publications on PCL are based on case reports, and only five series with more than 15 patients can be found in the literature.[4,7–9,14]

CLINICAL FEATURES

In the five P-PCL series including at least 15 patients, the median age ranged between 51.5 and 65 years, possibly younger than the median age in MM series (Table 26.1).[4,7–9,14] The median interval from the first symptoms with the diagnosis of P-PCL is approximately 3 months compared with 12–16 months for MM and secondary PCL.[4,6,10]

P-PCL has a more aggressive clinical presentation than MM. In particular, there is a higher frequency of extramedullary involvement (liver, spleen, lymph node enlargement, extraosseous plasmacytomas) (Table 26.1).[4–10,12–14] Asthenia, bone pain, severe anemia, thrombocytopenia, and bleeding are common, as are renal failure and hypercalcemia. Bone pain is more frequent in secondary PCL (90%) than in P-PCL (25%).[10] Infections are reported in 35% of patients with P-PCL and 56% of patients with secondary PCL, and thus contribute significantly to the morbidity and mortality of PCL.

The proportion of P-PCL patients with extramedullary involvement has ranged from 23% to 100%.[4–8,14,15] Hepato-megaly and splenomegaly are the main sites involved, with an incidence of 52% and 44%, respectively, in P-PCL and 17% in secondary PCL.[4] Spontaneous rupture of the spleen has been reported.[16] The incidence of lymphadenopathy is not reported in all series, but it also

Table 26.1 *Clinical and laboratory features in three recent primary plasma cell leukemia series*

Characteristic	Dimopoulos[8]	Garcia-Sanz[7]	Costello[14]
Number of patients	27	26	18
Age (years, median)	57	65	51.5
Male (%)	–	46	61
Extramedullary disease (%)	37	23	28[a]
Central nervous system involvement (%)	0	4	5
Lytic lesions (%)	–	–	61
Hemoglobin <8.5 g/dL (%)	82	54	39
Leukocytes >20 × 10^9/L (%)	–	–	44
Platelets <100 × 10^9/L (%)	67	48	61
Bone marrow plasmacytosis (%, median)	–	–	76
Creatinine >180 μmol/L (%)	37	–	28
Calcium >2.86 mmol/L (%)	44	44	39

[a] Splenomegaly and/or hepatomegaly not reported.

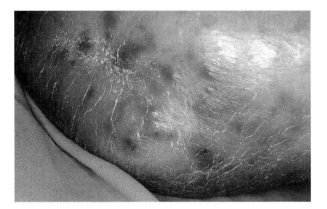

Figure 26.1 *Diffuse skin infiltrates from plasma cells.*

appears to differ between P-PCL and secondary PCL (12% vs. 6%).[4] Pleural effusions and pulmonary nodules,[14,17] extensive polypoid infiltration of the gastrointestinal tract,[18] and involvement of skeletal muscle,[19] testes,[20] and skin have all been described (Figs 26.1 and 26.2, Plates 9 and 10).[6,8,14,15,21]

Intracranial and meningeal involvement have been reported in both types of PCL at diagnosis[6,7,14,22–24] (Table 26.1) or as a form of localized relapse.[25] Myeloma of the central nervous system is more frequent in patients with high tumor mass, extramedullary disease, plasmablastic morphology, unfavorable cytogenetic abnormalities, and circulating PCs.[26] In a recent series of 18 MM patients with central nervous system involvement, four patients fulfilled the criteria for PCL.[26] Patients in whom PCs were detectable in the peripheral blood, albeit in insufficient quantities for the diagnosis of PCL, have also been considered at an increased risk of central nervous system involvement.[23]

The proportion of P-PCL patients with lytic bone lesions was 44%, 48% and 59% in three series including at least 25 patients,[4,7,9] and 51%, in a recent review,[5] lower than that usually observed in MM. Interestingly, MM

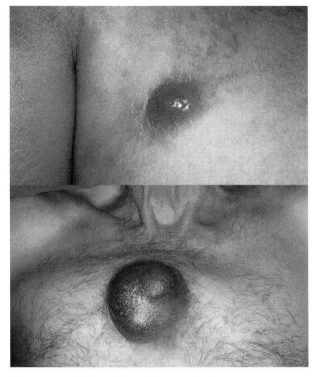

Figure 26.2 *Solitary skin nodules on the chest.*

patients with a high number of blood PCs were also less likely to have lytic bone disease.[11] As expected, lytic bone lesions were more frequent in secondary PCL with an incidence of approximately 70%, similar to that found in MM.[4,5] The presence of extensive osteosclerotic lesions has been reported on one occasion.[27] The presence of amyloidosis is very rare.[28]

LABORATORY FEATURES

The usual laboratory features found in large series of P-PCL are summarized in Table 26.1. The most frequent features are severe anemia and thrombocytopenia. This anemia is usually normocytic and normochromic, with rouleaux formation. The hemoglobin level was reported to be less than $10\,\mathrm{g/dL}$ in 45–87.5% of patients, with a median hemoglobin level of approximately $8.5\,\mathrm{g/dL}$ (Table 26.1)[4,7]. A platelet count less than $100 \times 10^9/\mathrm{L}$ was present in 50% of PCL compared with 10% in MM[10] and in 50% of P-PCL compared with 71% of secondary PCL.[6] In one series, the median platelet count was higher in P-PCL ($94 \times 10^9/\mathrm{L}$) than in secondary PCL ($26 \times 10^9/\mathrm{L}$).[4]

Examination of the bone marrow reveals a diffuse plasma cell infiltration varying from 50% to 100%, with the marrow infiltration usually exceeding the blood involvement. The PC are typically well-differentiated with eccentric nuclei, abundant basophilic cytoplasm, and a paranuclear clear zone. Atypical and binucleated PC are also usually present, as are plasmablasts with large immature nuclei and prominent nucleoli. In rare cases, the cells are lymphoid-like, or small and round with basophilic cytoplasm or with Russell bodies (Fig. 26.3, Plate 11).[6]

Hypercalcemia and impairment of renal function are observed more frequently in PCL than in MM.[7,8] In a recent series, calcium and creatinine serum levels greater than $2.86\,\mathrm{mmol/L}$ ($115\,\mathrm{mg/L}$) and $180\,\mu\mathrm{mol/L}$ ($2\,\mathrm{mg/dL}$) were reported in 44% and 37%, respectively, of PCL patients; this incidence was similar to that found in high tumor mass MM.[8] The serum β_2-microglobulin level was greater than $6\,\mathrm{mg/L}$ in 65% and 91% of P-PCL patients in two recent series,[7,8] and high serum lactate dehydrogenase (LDH) was also frequent, $>300\,\mathrm{IU/L}$ in 63% of patients[8] and $>460\,\mathrm{UI/L}$ in 48% of patients.[7]

Most patients with PCL have a monoclonal protein in the serum or urine, although non-secretory cases have been described.[4,6,8,14,29] PCL does not appear to be associated with secretion of any particular immunoglobulin or light-chain subclass, although it may be disproportionately common in the rare IgE MM.[30,31] In a report of IgE-related plasma cell disorders, five of the 19 cases were PCL.[32] The median serum monoclonal protein value at diagnosis is lower in P-PCL than secondary PCL, but it is comparable between MM and secondary PCL.[4,10]

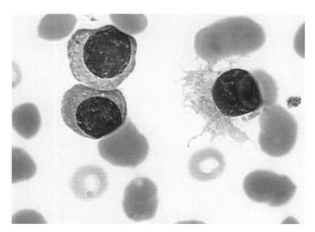

(a)

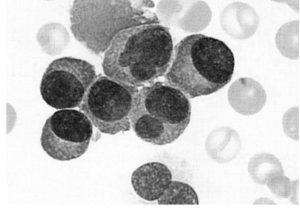

(b)

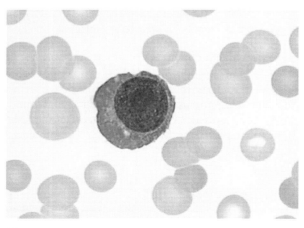

(c)

Figure 26.3 *Plasma cell leukemia (PCL): peripheral blood findings. (a) Plasma cells from an IgA κ primary PCL demonstrating coarse nuclear chromatin and moderately abundant cytoplasm. (b) Some cells from an IgG λ secondary PCL sustain classical morphology, whereas others demonstrate irregular nuclear shape. (c) This plasma cell (secondary IgA λ PCL) shows dispersed chromatin and a prominent nucleolus.*

Hyperviscosity has been reported with both IgG and IgA paraproteins.[33–35]

Immunophenotype

A few recent reports have analyzed the immunophenotypic profile of cases of PCL.[7,36,37] Some phenotypic differences exist between PCL and MM (Table 26.2), but these differences do not permit a complete discrimination between the two disorders.

Plasma cells from PCL showed the same immunophenotypic profile in the bone marrow and in the peripheral blood, and shared with MM a high expression of CD38 and CD138 antigens.[38] Fas/Apo-1 (CD95) expression was reported in the majority of plasma cell lines, in all PCL, and in the majority of MM patients, especially those with an extramedullary disease; this expression was correlated with an elevated level of serum LDH in serum.[39]

In one study,[7] immunophenotypic expression was similar in MM and PCL for CD2, CD3, CD16, CD10, CD13, and CD15. CD2, CD3, and CD16 were negative in all cases of PCL tested, while CD10, CD13, and CD15 were infrequently positive. PCL differed from MM in the expression of CD9, CD20, CD56, CD117, and HLA-DR antigens. Plasma cells from patients with P-PCL had a higher-expression of CD20 antigen than cells from patients with MM. In contrast, CD9, CD56, CD117, and HLA-DR were more frequently present in MM.[7]

The absence of CD56 (NCAM) on malignant PC has been considered as the hallmark of PCL and of a special subset of MM.[36] Patients with MM at diagnosis overexpress CD56 at diagnosis in 60–70% of cases.[7,36] In contrast, malignant PC from patients with either P-PCL or secondary PCL do not express CD56 at all in approximately 80% of cases. In secondary PCL evaluated serially, CD56 is lacking at diagnosis, demonstrating that CD56 is not downregulated at the endstage of the disease but rather not upregulated at diagnosis in this subset of patients.[7,36] The CD56−/weak MM subset at diagnosis has presenting features mimicking PCL, namely a low osteolytic potential and a more frequent leukemic phase.[36]

CD28 is associated with tumor expansion in MM and is able to discriminate secondary from primary PCL.[36,37] In a recent study, CD28 was detected in 92% of secondary PCL, more frequently in the peripheral blood than in the bone marrow, but in only 33% of P-PCL.[36]

Some rare studies have analyzed the expression of cytoadhesion molecules, considered important in anchoring PC to bone marrow stroma. Positivity for H-CAM (CD44),[40] LFA-1 (CD18),[41] LFA-3 (CD58),[42] VLA-5 (CD49e),[43,44] and cCD79 has been reported.[38]

Cytogenetic changes

At least in some patients, the development of PCL is the result of a multistep transformation process.[45] The major molecular genetic abnormalities in PCL in relation to MM (and sometimes MGUS) are summarized in Table 26.3.

The amplification of the c-myc oncogene and the concomitant overexpression of the c-myc protein has been reported, with no significant difference between PCL and MM.[46,47] p53 gene mutations are seen in PCL and in advanced and clinically aggressive MM.[48] MDM2 (murine double minute 2) overexpression was shown in all cases of PCL tested, while hypermethylation of the p16 gene was found in the majority of MM and PCL cases.[49–51] Expression of Bcl-2 was found in both MM and PCL, with an inverse correlation between the level of Bcl-2 and the proliferation rate.[52,53]

K- and N-ras genes are mutated in 30% of PCL and 9–31% of MM, with a predominance in advanced MM.[54] In another study, N-ras and/or K-ras2 mutations were found in 54.5% of MM, 50% of P-PCL, and 12.5% of MGUS and indolent MM.[55] Elevated telomerase activity has been found in all PCL and MM cell lines tested and in the majority of MM samples.[56]

Using conventional cytogenetics, the majority of PCL patients were found to have complex pseudodiploid or hypodiploid karyotypes, consisting of multiple numerical and structural changes. The most frequent abnormalities include gains or losses of material from chromosome 1 (see later), translocations involving 14q32, and deletions

Table 26.2 *Immunophenotypical differences between multiple myeloma and plasma cell leukemia (PCL) (Adapted from Garcia-Sanz et al.[7])*

Immunophenotype	Multiple myeloma (% of cases positive)	Primary plasma cell leukemia (% of cases positive)	Reference
CD9+	78	46	7
CD20+	17	50	7
CD28+	26	33 (secondary PCL 90–100%)	36, 37
CD56+	70	45	7
	67	25 (secondary PCL 13%)	36
CD117+	43	0	7
DR+	56	21	7

Table 26.3 *Molecular genetics in plasma cell dyscrasia*

Cytogenetic abnormality/ rearrangement	MGUS number (%)	SMM number (%)	MM number (%)	Primary PCL		
				Number (%)	P^a	Reference
14q32 rearrangement	69/143 (48)	18/38 (47)	477/653 (73)	38/45 (84)	NS	9
t(11;14)	19/147 (13)	9/39 (23)	105/669 (16)	15/46 (33)	0.006	
t(4;14)	3/147 (2)	1/39 (3)	68/669 (10)	6/46 (13)	NS	
t(14;16)	1/147	0/39	14/669 (2)	5/46 (11)	0.002	
del(13)	31/147 (21)	11/39 (28)	288/669 (43)	32/46 (70)	<0.001	62
c-*myc* rearrangement	2/65 (3)	1/24 (4)	82/529 (16)	3/23 (13)	NS	46
p53 mutations	–	0/12	0/24	3/10[b] (30)	–	48
Hypermethylation of *p16* gene	–	41/101 (40.5)		4/5 (80)	–	106
Expression of p16 protein	–	Present 4/4		Undetectable (3/13)	–	50
Bcl-2 expression	–	9/17 (53)		3/3[b] (100)	–	53
	–	High 40/40 (100) (PC from bone marrow) Weak 5/5 (100) (PC from extramedullary sites)		High 4/4 (100) (blood PC)	–	52
N- and K-*ras* mutations						
N-*ras*	0/30	28/164 (17)		8/31 (26)	–	54
K-*ras*	0/30	5/164 (3)		6/31 (19)	–	
N-*ras*	1/8 (12.5)[c]		7/30 (23)	3/10 (30)	–	55
K-*ras*	0/8		11/33 (33)	3/10 (30)	–	
Elevated level of telomerase activity	0/5	2/4 (50)	19/23 (83)	4/4 (100)	–	56

del(13), chromosome 13 deletion; MGUS, monoclonal gammopathy of undetermined significance; MM, multiple myeloma; NS, not significant; PC, plasma cell; PCL, plasma cell leukemia; SMM, smoldering multiple myeloma; –, not reported.

[a] For difference with MM.
[b] P-PCL and secondary PCL.
[c] MGUS and SMM.

of chromosome 13.[8,9,57–60] In a recent large study, patients with P-PCL were analyzed by cytogenetics or interphase and multicolor fluorescence *in situ* hybridization (FISH) and cytogenetic abnormalities were observed in 23 of 34 patients (68%) with usually complex hypodiploid or pseudodiploid karyotypes. Only three patients had hyperdiploidy, in contrast with published results in MM, where hyperdiploidy is observed in approximately 60% of patients.[9] These results were in accordance with a previous report where all except one patients were diploid (DNA index = 1) with the remaining case showing hypodiploidy.[7]

Comparative genomic hybridization (CGH) has also been used to demonstrate differences in genetic changes between MM and PCL. CGH showed a significantly higher proportion of losses of chromosome material (mean of 4.8 ± 3.4) in PCL than MM (mean of 1.2 ± 1.5).[61] In all five PCL patients tested, DNA copy number changes were identified by CGH analysis. Losses of chromosomal material are significantly more frequent in PCL, particularly

losses on 13q (four of five of PCL vs. 28% of MM patients) and 16 (four of five of PCL vs. 12% of MM patients). Losses involving 2q and 6p were only present in PCL.[61] However, all PCL patients showed gains in 1q (36% of MM patients). This characteristic and the fact that the short arm (1p) was preferentially involved in deletions had previously found using conventional cytogenetics.[58,59]

Interphase FISH experiments have focused on 14q32 and 13q14 abnormalities[7,9,62] (Table 26.3). An illegitimate rearrangement of the IgH gene is observed in approximately 80% of PCL patients, an incidence not significantly different from that found in MM (73%). The reciprocal translocation t(11;14)(q13;q32) is frequent in PCL with an higher incidence (33%) than in MM (16%).[62,63] The second most frequent translocation is t(4;14)(p16;q32) with a similar 10–15% incidence in PCL and MM.[9,62,64,65] The t(14;16)(q32;q23) was found in 11% of P-PCL, an incidence significantly higher than the 1% found in MM.[62–64,66] This translocation might, therefore, be associated with particular unidentified biological features allowing PC to disseminate within the peripheral blood.[62] Translocations of 8q24 are rare and complex. Translocation t(8;14)(q24;q32) has been rarely reported,[67,68] but no case was identified using FISH in a recent series of 46 P-PCL patients.[62] In a previous report of the same group, a translocation t(6;8)(q12-q15;q24) was found in two patients.[9]

Concerning numerical abnormalities, apart from the frequent gains in 1q, +18 has been reported, but the most striking feature was the lack of gains usually found in MM, such as +3, +6, +9, +11, and +15.[7] Numerical abnormalities of chromosome 8 have also been described.[69,70] A partial or complete deletion of chromosome 13 was found in 70% and 85% of P-PCL cases in two large series (Table 26.3).[7,62] Theses incidences were significantly higher than in MM (43% and 26%, respectively). Hypodiploidy (or pseudodiploidy) and monosomy 13 may explain, at least in part, the poor survival observed in PCL patients. Some other chromosome losses were reported in PCL, especially the loss of chromosome 16 (80% vs. 12% in MM),[61,71] 17 and 18,[71,72] 7,[8] and X.[7,73]

Cytokines in PCL

Interleukin-6 (IL-6) is the major cytokine implicated in growth of MM *in vitro* and may be important for progression *in vivo*.[74,75] Culture of PCs from PCL patients exhibited spontaneous growth after 5 days in culture and growth was stimulated by addition of exogenous IL-6.[75] In contrast, anti-IL-6 monoclonal antibody treatment resulted in a transient blockage of plasma cell proliferation.[76,77] Increased levels of soluble IL-6 receptor (sIL-6R) have been found in plasma cell dyscrasia, including PCL, compared with normal individuals.[78] In MM cell lines and PCL cells, IL-6 is able to exert an antiapoptotic effect by modulating the Ras-Raf-MAPK signaling cascades.[79]

Vascular endothelial growth factor (VEGF) is another key cytokine in the pathophysiology of MM and PCL. Besides stimulating angiogenesis and triggering IL-6 production from bone marrow stromal cells, it has direct effects on MM and PCL cells. Plasma cells from patients with PCL (and MM) both synthesize and secrete VEGF. VEGF triggers tumor cell proliferation of MM cells via the Raf-1-MEK-extracellular signal-regulated protein kinase (ERK) pathway, and migration of MM and PCL cells via a protein kinase C (PKC)-dependent pathway. The effects on the migration of MM and PCL cells suggest an important role in the transition of MM to PCL.[80] Insulin-like growth factor-1 (IGF-1) also promotes the proliferation of MM cells and protects them against apoptosis induced by dexamethasone or Apo2L/TRAIL (Apo2 ligand/TNF-related apoptosis-inducing ligand).[81] The IGF-1 receptor (IGF-1R) is expressed on MM cell lines and

MM samples and plays a major role in tumor growth and survival.[82]

PROGNOSIS AND TREATMENT

The prognosis in PCL is usually very poor. Interestingly, MM patients with a high number of blood PCs, albeit insufficient for the diagnosis of PCL, also have a poor prognosis.[11] The incidence of established adverse prognostic features, such as the serum β_2-microglobulin level, proportion of S-phase PC, renal function, and calcium and LDH serum levels, is significantly higher in PCL than in MM.[7] The vast majority of PCL patients fulfilled the criteria of high tumor mass MM, and the incidence of hypodiploid and pseudodiploid karyotypes is high.[7,9]

The short survival in patients with P-PCL is also related to the 20–30% proportion of patients dying of disease complications, especially infection, during the first 2 months of treatment.[8,9] Other patients died of complications owing to massive multiorgan tumor involvement.[14]

It appears that P-PCL with t(11;14) may be associated with a significantly better prognosis. In a recent series, P-PCL patients displaying t(11;14) had a significantly better survival at 12 months than patients lacking this translocation; however, this preliminary result deserves further evaluation.

The therapy of PCL is similar to that used for MM but no prospective studies have been performed in P-PCL, owing to the paucity of cases. In a recent series of 40 P-PCL patients diagnosed between 1992 and 2000, the median overall survival remained very short at 7 months (5 days to 38 months), although 13 of 40 patients received intensive treatment with stem cell support.[9] Patients with secondary PCL have usually received several lines of chemotherapy for MM, and they frequently have a reduced performance status and poor bone marrow function. As a consequence, their treatment has often been palliative and median survival times of 1.3 months[4] and 6.8 months[5] have been reported.

Conventional treatment

The most complete report of single alkylating agent treatment (with or without prednisone) is the review by Noel and Kyle,[3] which comprises 52 published cases. It was considered that 16 patients (31%) achieved a complete response to alkylating agents, 12 (23%) a partial response, and 24 (46%) had no response, although the definition of response was heterogeneous and unclear. The median survival was 1 year or more for patients with partial or complete responses, and less than 1 month for patients without a response; the median survival of all 52 patients was 3 months.

Among 17 patients from the Mayo Clinic, two achieved a response and five a partial response.[5] A response was defined as a decrease of more than 50% in the number of circulating PCs and a decrease of more than 50% in either the serum or the urine M-protein level; partial response was defined as a decrease of 25–50% of circulating PCs or a decrease of 25–50% in either the serum or the urine M-protein level. In a more recent series, there were no responders in ten patients receiving melphalan–prednisone (MP; or high-dose dexamethasone), and the median survival was only 2 months.[8] High-dose dexamethasone alone is not recommended.[8,14] Rare patients have achieved a prolonged response with a single alkylating agent.[4,72,83,84] Ifosfamide was given in two cases in PCL and one patient

showed a persistent response 8 months after completion of the treatment.[85] Gemcitabine induces a significant degree of apoptosis in MM and PCL lines tested *in vitro*, but there are no reports of its use in patients.[86]

Various combination chemotherapy regimens have been used: VAD (vincristine, doxorubicin, dexamethasone), modified VAD with liposomal doxorubicin, VAMP (vincristine, doxorubicin, methylprednisolone), VBAP (vincristine, BCNU, doxorubicin, prednisone), VMD (vincristine, mitoxantrone, dexamethasone), CVP (cyclophosphamide, vincristine, prednisone), and VMBCP (vincristine, BCNU, melphalan, cyclophosphamide, prednisone). These regimens have achieved response rates between 50 and 75% (Table 26.4).[4,6–8,10,14,21,87] In

Table 26.4 *Chemotherapy in primary plasma cell leukemia. Data refer to individual patients*

Regimen	Response	Duration (months)	Survival (months)	Reference
M and P; COAP; B, Chl, Mtx, Vdsn	CR	8	30	15
C, M, P	PR	7	10	6
CVP, COAP	NR	–	2	6
C, P, V, PTC, P	CR	15	18	6
CVP, M	CR	13	18	6
V, M, P	CR	44	51	6
CVP	PR	6	7	33
V, A, and P (induction), then monthly VAMP (maintenance)	CR	12+	12+	84
	CR	16+	16+	84
	CR	22+	22+	84
VMBCP	CR	8	11	107
CVP	CR	12+	22+	27
PTC, V, P	CR	23	57	108
PTC, V, P	CR	6	16	108
V Mitoxantrone D	NR	–	<3	109
	NR	–	<3	109
	NR	–	<3	109
CVP	CR	12	–	110
COAP; MP	PR	10	–	111
VAMP and Rbd	CR	4	4.5	112
CVP and M	PR	8	8	68
High-dose therapy				
HDM	NR	–	7	14
C2H2OP – allogeneic BMT	CR	27	27	14
VMCP/VBAP-HDM200	PR	18+	18+	7
VAD–ifosfamide–HDM200–rituximab	CR	22	26	93
VAD–HDM200	CR	10	20	113
VAD–cyclophosphamide–EDAP–HDM200	CR	3	3	94
	CR	14+	14+	94
	CR	26+	26+	94
VAD–allogeneic BMT	CR	8	22	25
VAD–HDM140	CR	13	22	25
HDM140 (and again at relapse)	CR	16	30+	92
VAD–HDM200–IFNα	PR	24	40+	88
VAMP–CHOP–HDM140 + TBI	CR	59+	59+	96

A, Adriamycin; B, BCNU (carmustine); BMT, bone marrow transplantation; C, cyclophosphamide; Chl, chlorambucil; CR, complete response; D, dexamethasone; E, etoposide; H, doxorubicin; HDM, high-dose melphalan; IFNα, interferon-α; M, melphalan; Mtx, methotrexate; NR, no response; P, prednisone; PR, partial response; PTC, peptichemio; Rbd, rubibomycin; TBI, total body irradiation; V, vincristine; Vdsn, vindesin.

P-PCL, two large retrospective series have demonstrated that overall survival was significantly better in patients treated with polychemotherapy than with MP (18 vs. 3 months and 20 vs. 2 months).[7,8] The inability to achieve a 50% clearing of blood plasma cell within 10 days after the initiation of treatment is predictive of a treatment failure with a median survival of 12 months, whereas in responding patients the response duration was similar to that of patients with high-tumor mass MM.[8]

There are a few reports of the use of interferon-α (IFNα) therapy and the results are controversial. In some studies, responding patients (after conventional or intensive treatment) were maintained on IFNα apparently without an adverse effect on disease progression.[8,88,89] By contrast, two reports clearly described patients who developed PCL triggered by IFNα therapy.[90,91] In one of these two patients, the leukemic evolution disappeared after discontinuation of IFNα.[90]

Intensive treatment

McElwain and Powles[92] pioneered the use of high-dose melphalan (HDM) for plasma-cell malignancies and their first patient suffered from P-PCL. An unmaintained complete remission following a first course of HDM 140 mg/m^2 lasted 16 months, and at the time of first relapse the patient received again HDM 140 mg/m^2 followed by an autologous bone marrow transplant (ABMT). The patient enjoyed a second complete remission and was alive 30 months from his first treatment.[92] Several other case reports have reported remissions lasting 1 year or more following autologous stem cell transplantation (ASCT)[7,25,88,92–96] (Table 26.4). In a European Group for Blood and Marrow Transplantation registry study, 135 patients with P-PCL undergoing ASCT were compared with 9887 MM patients.[97] The median survival of PCL patients post-ASCT was only 21 months, markedly inferior to that of the MM patients, which was 55 months, despite the facts that P-PCL were younger that MM patients, had an earlier transplant (median 6.6 months from diagnosis), and were probably pre-selected in surviving the early mortality and morbidity of initial chemotherapy.[97]

Very few patients with PCL have been treated with allogeneic bone marrow transplantation from an HLA identical sibling donor.[14,25,98] In MM, the use of allogeneic stem cell transplantation remains controversial owing to a high transplant-related mortality, but durable remissions exist, which have been attributed to a graft versus myeloma effect. In patients with relapsed or newly diagnosed high-risk MM, immunosuppressive non-myeloablative conditioning regimens (mini-allograft) induce an efficient disease control but are still associated with a significant graft versus host disease.[99] A combined procedure using an ASCT to reduce the tumor burden followed by a mini-allotransplantation would possibly be a promising approach for P-PCL patients. Other improvements may result from a better induction treatment before transplantation and maintenance treatments using novel agents (thalidomide, immunomodulatory drugs, bortezomid).

INNOVATIVE TREATMENTS

Treatment with monoclonal murine anti-IL-6 antibodies has been used in P-PCL based on results showing the involvement of IL-6 in the proliferation of MM cells *in vivo*, and an increased serum IL-6 level in patients with advanced MM and PCL.[76,77,100] Some patients had an objective antiproliferative effect associated with complete inhibition of C-reactive protein synthesis and low daily IL-6 production *in vivo* but none of the patients achieved a remission as judged by standard clinical criteria.[76]

Anti-CD20 antibody (rituximab) was used as consolidation treatment after autologous transplant in a patient with P-PCL but without a clear clinical benefit.[93]

PCL cells are sensible to lymphokine-activated killer (LAK) cells, especially when enhanced with rIL-2 or rIL-2+rIFNα.[101] A combined immunotherapy consisting of adoptive transfer of autologous tumor-specific T cells, low-dose IL-2, and a cellular vaccine of CD40-activated PCL cells has been shown to be feasible and safe, and was associated with a temporary decrease of PCL cells in the blood.[102]

Thalidomide has recently demonstrated a significant activity in refractory MM.[103] Although no specific evaluation of thalidomide in PCL has been performed, there is no doubt that thalidomide has a role in the treatment of PCL. In one patient with secondary PCL, thalidomide was associated with severe hepatic-related toxicity.[104] In the near future, other new drugs, including thalidomide analogs (Revimid, formerly CC5013) and the proteasome inhibitor bortezomid (formerly PS-341, Velcade), which seem very promising in refractory MM, will also be investigated. Preliminary *in vitro* results indicate that bortezomid causes activation of endogenous apoptotic routes in PCL.[105]

KEY POINTS

- Plasma cell leukemia (PCL) is a rare disorder, which may develop spontaneously (P-PCL) or evolve in patients with multiple myeloma (MM).
- The diagnosis is based on a relatively arbitrary definition consisting of a plasmacytosis exceeding 20% of the differential white cell count and an absolute value of 2×10^9/L.
- Nevertheless, P-PCL should also be considered when fewer plasma cells (PCs) are present because

these patients share many characteristics of true PCL and have a similar prognosis.

- Compared with MM patients, PCL patients have more extramedullary disease, anemia, thrombocytopenia, hypercalcemia, and renal failure, and a higher frequency of increased lactate dehydrogenase and β_2-microglobulin serum levels.
- They also have biological differences related to the intrinsic malignancy of the disease, higher frequency of adverse cytogenetic features (hypodiploidy, chromosome 13 deletions), low DNA cell content, and more immature phenotype.
- The former characteristics may explain the difference in chemosensitivity compared with MM and the poor outcome generally described for patients with P-PCL.
- Although the results remain poor, the survival of patients treated with combination chemotherapy has often been significantly longer than that of patients treated with melphalan and prednisone.
- In young patients, high-dose therapy followed by allogeneic or autologous stem cell rescue should be considered.
- Innovative treatments include non-myeloablative stem cell transplantation, thalidomide, thalidomide analog, and the proteasome inhibitor bortezomib.

REFERENCES

● = Key primary paper
◆ = Major review article

1. Foa P. Sulla produzione cellulare nell inflamazione ed inaltri procesi analoghi specialmente in cio che si riferisce alle plasmacellule. *Folia Haematol* 1904; **1**:166–7.
2. Gluzinski A, Reichenstein M. Myeloma and leucaemia lymphatica plasmocellularis. *Wien Klin Wochenschr* 1906; **19**:336–9.
◆3. Noel P, Kyle RA. Plasma cell leukemia: an evaluation of response to therapy. *Am J Med* 1987; **83**:1062–8.
●4. Pasqualetti P, Festuccia V, Collacciani A, Acitelli P, Casale R. Plasma cell leukemia. A report on 11 patients and review of the literature. *Panminerva Med* 1996; **38**:179–84.
◆5. Kyle RA, Maldonado JE, Bayrd ED. Plasma cell leukemia. Report on 17 cases. *Arch Intern Med* 1974; **133**:813–18.
◆6. Bernasconi C, Castelli G, Pagnucco G, Brusamolino E. Plasma cell leukemia: a report on 15 patients. *Eur J Haematol Suppl* 1989; **51**:76–83.
●7. Garcia-Sanz R, Orfao A, Gonzalez M, Tabernero MD, Blade J, Moro MJ, *et al.* Primary plasma cell leukemia: clinical, immunophenotypic, DNA ploidy, and cytogenetic characteristics. *Blood* 1999; **93**:1032–7.
◆8. Dimopoulos MA, Palumbo A, Delasalle KB, Alexanian R. Primary plasma cell leukaemia. *Br J Haematol* 1994; **88**:754–9.

◆9. Avet-Loiseau H, Daviet A, Brigaudeau C, Callet-Bauchu E, Terre C, Lafage-Pochitaloff M, *et al.* Cytogenetic, interphase, and multicolor fluorescence in situ hybridization analyses in primary plasma cell leukemia: a study of 40 patients at diagnosis, on behalf of the Intergroupe Francophone du Myelome and the Groupe Francais de Cytogenetique Hematologique. *Blood* 2001; **97**:822–5.
10. Kosmo MA, Gale RP. Plasma cell leukemia. *Semin Hematol* 1987; **24**:202–8.
11. Witzig TE, Gertz MA, Lust JA, Kyle RA, O'Fallon WM, Greipp PR. Peripheral blood monoclonal plasma cells as a predictor of survival in patients with multiple myeloma. *Blood* 1996; **88**:1780–7.
12. Blade J, Kyle RA. Non-secretory myeloma, immunoglobulin D myeloma, and plasma cell leukemia. *Hematol Oncol Clin North Am* 1999; **13**:1259–72.
◆13. Woodruff RK, Malpas JS, Paxton AM, Lister TA. Plasma cell leukemia (PCL): a report on 15 patients. *Blood* 1978; **52**:839–45.
●14. Costello R, Sainty D, Bouabdallah R, Fermand JP, Delmer A, Divine M, *et al.* Primary plasma cell leukaemia: a report of 18 cases. *Leuk Res* 2001; **25**:103–7.
15. Bareford D, Pamphilon DH, Barnard DL. Plasma cell leukaemia relapsing in the dermis. *Acta Haematol* 1984; **71**:359.
16. Stephens PJ, Hudson P. Spontaneous rupture of the spleen on plasma cell leukemia. *Can Med Assoc J* 1969; **100**:31–4.
17. Jean G, Lambertenghi-Deliliers G, Ranzi T, Polli E. Ultrastructural aspects of bone marrow and peripheral blood cells in a case of plasma cell leukemia. *Acta Haematol* 1971; **45**:36–49.
18. Sakai H, Sawamura M, Tamura J, Okamura S, Karasawa M, Murakami H, *et al.* A patient with primary plasma cell leukemia accompanied by an extensive polypoid infiltration of the gastrointestinal tract. *J Med* 1991; **22**:195–9.
19. Djaldetti M, Joshua H. Acute plasma cell leukemia: a case report. *Israel J Med Sci* 1961; **20**:109–13.
20. Andalaro VA Jr, Babott D. Testicular involvement in plasma-cell leukemia. *Urology* 1974; **3**:636–8.
21. Suzuki M, Kawauchi K, Sugiyama H, Yasuyama M, Watanabe H. Primary plasma cell leukemia: a case report of successful responder to a combination chemotherapy of vincristine, doxorubicin and dexamethasone. *Acta Haematol* 1989; **82**:95–7.
22. Bruyn GA, Zwetsloot CP, van Nieuwkoop JA, den Ottolander GJ, Padberg GW. Cranial nerve palsy as the presenting feature of secondary plasma cell leukemia. *Cancer* 1987; **60**:906–9.
23. Simons M, Cohn A, Miller K. Plasma cell leukemia with meningeal involvement. *N Y State J Med* 1986; **86**:539–40.
24. Turhal N, Henehan MD, Kaplan KL. Multiple myeloma: a patient with unusual features including intracranial and meningeal involvement, testicular involvement, organomegaly, and plasma cell leukemia. *Am J Hematol* 1998; **57**:51–6.
25. Leleu X, Jouet JP, Plantier I, Zandecki M, Lai JL, Mucha D, *et al.* Isolated neurological relapse following stem cell transplantation in plasma cell leukemia: a report of two cases. *Leukemia* 1999; **13**:307–9.

26. Fassas AB, Muwalla F, Berryman T, Benramdane R, Joseph L, Anaissie E, et al. Myeloma of the central nervous system: association with high-risk chromosomal abnormalities, plasmablastic morphology and extramedullary manifestations. Br J Haematol 2002; **117**:103–8.

27. Kuo MC, Shih LY. Primary plasma cell leukemia with extensive dense osteosclerosis: complete remission following combination chemotherapy. Ann Hematol 1995; **71**:147–51.

28. Kyle RA, Greipp PR. Amyloidosis (LA): clinical and laboratory features in 229 cases. Mayo Clin Proc 1983; **58**:665–8.

29. Pedraza MA. Plasma-cell leukemia with unusual immunoglobulin abnormalities. Am J Clin Pathol 1975; **64**:410–15.

30. Endo T, Okumura H, Kikuchi K, Munakata J, Otake M, Nomura T, et al. Immunoglobulin E (IgE) multiple myeloma: a case report and review of the literature. Am J Med 1981; **70**:1127–32.

31. Salmon SE, McIntyre OR, Ogawa M. IgE myeloma: total body tumor cell number and synthesis of IgE and DNA. Blood 1971; **37**:696–705.

32. West NC, Smith AM, Ward R. IgE myeloma associated with plasma cell leukaemia. Postgrad Med J 1983; **59**:784–5.

33. Douer D, Weinbergerr A, Djaldetti M, Asherov J, Pick I, Pinkhas J. Hyperviscosity syndrome in a patient with plasma cell leukemia. Acta Haematol 1979; **62**:81–5.

34. Geraci JM, Hansen RM, Kueck BD. Plasma cell leukemia and hyperviscosity syndrome. South Med J 1990; **83**:800–5.

35. Virella G, Preto RV, Graca F. Polymerized monoclonal IgA in two patients with myelomatosis and hyperviscosity syndrome. Br J Haematol 1975; **30**:479–87.

36. Pellat-Deceunynck C, Barille S, Jego G, Puthier D, Robillard N, Pineau D, et al. The absence of CD56 (NCAM) on malignant plasma cells is a hallmark of plasma cell leukemia and of a special subset of multiple myeloma. Leukemia 1998; **12**:1977–82.

37. Robillard N, Jego G, Pellat-Deceunynck C, Pineau D, Puthier D, Mellerin MP, et al. CD28, a marker associated with tumoral expansion in multiple myeloma. Clin Cancer Res 1998; **4**:1521–6.

38. Alonso ML, Rubiol E, Mateu R, Estivill C, Bellido M, Balmana J, et al. cCD79a expression in a case of plasma cell leukemia. Leuk Res 1998; **22**:649–53.

39. Hata H, Matsuzaki H, Takeya M, Yoshida M, Sonoki T, Nagasaki A, et al. Expression of Fas/Apo-1 (CD95) and apoptosis in tumor cells from patients with plasma cell disorders. Blood 1995; **86**:1939–45.

40. Tatsumi T, Shimazaki C, Goto H, Araki S, Sudo Y, Yamagata N, et al. Expression of adhesion molecules on myeloma cells. Jpn J Cancer Res 1996; **87**:837–42.

41. Van Riet I, De Waele M, Remels L, Lacor P, Schots R, Van Camp B. Expression of cytoadhesion molecules (CD56, CD54, CD18 and CD29) by myeloma plasma cells. Br J Haematol 1991; **79**:421–7.

42. Barker HF, Hamilton MS, Ball J, Drew M, Franklin IM. Expression of adhesion molecules LFA-3 and N-CAM on normal and malignant human plasma cells. Br J Haematol 1992; **81**:331–5.

43. Drew M, Barker HF, Ball J, Pearson C, Cook G, Franklin I. Very late antigen (VLA) expression by normal and neoplastic human plasma cells; including an assessment of antibodies submitted to the Vth International Workshop on Leucocyte Differentiation Antigens using human myeloma cell lines. Leuk Res 1996; **20**:619–24.

44. Kawano MM, Huang N, Harada H, Harada Y, Sakai A, Tanaka H, et al. Identification of immature and mature myeloma cells in the bone marrow of human myelomas. Blood 1993; **82**:564–70.

●45. Hallek M, Bergsagel PL, Anderson KC. Multiple myeloma: increasing evidence for a multistep transformation process. Blood 1998; **91**:3–21.

46. Avet-Loiseau H, Gerson F, Magrangeas F, Minvielle S, Harousseau JL, Bataille R. Rearrangements of the c-myc oncogene are present in 15% of primary human multiple myeloma tumors. Blood 2001; **98**:3082–6.

47. Sumegi J, Hedberg T, Bjorkholm M, Godal T, Mellstedt H, Nilsson MG, et al. Amplification of the c-myc oncogene in human plasma-cell leukemia. Int J Cancer 1985; **36**:367–71.

48. Neri A, Baldini L, Trecca D, Cro L, Polli E, Maiolo AT. p53 gene mutations in multiple myeloma are associated with advanced forms of malignancy. Blood 1993; **81**:128–35.

49. Quesnel B, Preudhomme C, Oscier D, Lepelley P, Collyn-d'Hooghe M, Facon T, et al. Over-expression of the MDM2 gene is found in some cases of haematological malignancies. Br J Haematol 1994; **88**:415–18.

50. Urashima M, Teoh G, Ogata A, Chauhan D, Treon SP, Hoshi Y, et al. Role of CDK4 and p16INK4A in interleukin-6-mediated growth of multiple myeloma. Leukemia 1997; **11**:1957–63.

51. Urashima M, Teoh G, Ogata A, Chauhan D, Treon SP, Sugimoto Y, et al. Characterization of p16(INK4A) expression in multiple myeloma and plasma cell leukemia. Clin Cancer Res 1997; **3**:2173–9.

52. Puthier D, Pellat-Deceunynck C, Barille S, Robillard N, Rapp MJ, Juge-Morineau N, et al. Differential expression of Bcl-2 in human plasma cell disorders according to proliferation status and malignancy. Leukemia 1999; **13**:289–94.

53. Harada N, Hata H, Yoshida M, Soniki T, Nagasaki A, Kuribayashi N, et al. Expression of Bcl-2 family of proteins in fresh myeloma cells. Leukemia 1998; **12**:1817–20.

54. Corradini P, Ladetto M, Inghirami G, Boccadoro M, Pileri A. N- and K-ras oncogenes in plasma cell dyscrasias. Leuk Lymphoma 1994; **15**:17–20.

55. Bezieau S, Devilder MC, Avet-Loiseau H, Mellerin MP, Puthier D, Pennarun E, et al. High incidence of N and K-Ras activating mutations in multiple myeloma and primary plasma cell leukemia at diagnosis. Hum Mutat 2001; **18**:212–24.

56. Xu D, Zheng C, Bergenbrant S, Holm G, Bjorkholm M, Yi Q, et al. Telomerase activity in plasma cell dyscrasias. Br J Cancer 2001; **84**:621–5.

◆57. Dewald GW, Kyle RA, Hicks GA, Greipp PR. The clinical significance of cytogenetic studies in 100 patients with multiple myeloma, plasma cell leukemia, or amyloidosis. Blood 1985; **66**:380–90.

58. Smadja N, Krulik M, Louvet C, de Gramont A, Gonzalez-Canali G, Mougeot-Martin M. Similar cytogenetic abnormalities in two cases of plasma cell leukemia. Cancer Genet Cytogenet 1991; **52**:123–9.

59. Taniwaki M, Nishida K, Takashima T, Nakagawa H, Fujii H, Tamaki T, et al. Nonrandom chromosomal rearrangements of 14q32.3 and 19p13.3 and preferential deletion of 1p in 21 patients with multiple myeloma and plasma cell leukemia. Blood 1994; **84**:2283–90.

60. Ueshima Y, Fukuhara S, Nagai K, Takatsuki K, Uchino H. Cytogenetic studies and clinical aspects of patients with plasma cell leukemia and leukemic macroglobulinemia. *Cancer Res* 1983; **43**:905–12.

61. Gutierrez NC, Hernandez JM, Garcia JL, Canizo MC, Gonzalez M, Hernandez J, et al. Differences in genetic changes between multiple myeloma and plasma cell leukemia demonstrated by comparative genomic hybridization. *Leukemia* 2001; **15**:840–5.

●62. Avet-Loiseau H, Facon T, Grosbois B, Magrangeas F, Rapp MJ, Harousseau JL, et al. Oncogenesis of multiple myeloma: 14q32 and 13q chromosomal abnormalities are not randomly distributed, but correlate with natural history, immunological features, and clinical presentation. *Blood* 2002; **99**:2185–91.

63. Avet-Loiseau H, Li JY, Facon T, Brigaudeau C, Morineau N, Maloisel F, et al. High incidence of translocations t(11;14)(q13;q32) and t(4;14)(p16;q32) in patients with plasma cell malignancies. *Cancer Res* 1998; **58**:5640–5.

64. Avet-Loiseau H, Brigaudeau C, Morineau N, Talmant P, Lai JL, Daviet A, et al. High incidence of cryptic translocations involving the Ig heavy chain gene in multiple myeloma, as shown by fluorescence in situ hybridization. *Genes Chromosomes Cancer* 1999; **24**:9–15.

65. Nakazawa N, Nishida K, Tamura A, Kobayashi M, Iwai T, Horiike S, et al. Interphase detection of t(4;14)(p16.3;q32.3) by in situ hybridization and FGFR3 overexpression in plasma cell malignancies. *Cancer Genet Cytogenet* 2000; **117**:89–96.

66. Chesi M, Bergsagel PL, Shonukan OO, Martelli ML, Brents LA, Chen T, et al. Frequent dysregulation of the c-maf proto-oncogene at 16q23 by translocation to an Ig locus in multiple myeloma. *Blood* 1998; **91**:4457–63.

67. Copplestone JA, Oscier DG, Johnson S. An 8;14 translocation in a case of plasma cell leukemia. *Leukemia Res* 1987; **11**:655–9.

68. Yamada K, Shionoya S, Amano M, Imamura Y. A Burkitt-type 8;14 translocation in a case of plasma cell leukemia. *Cancer Genet Cytogenet* 1983; **9**:67–70.

69. Perez Losada A, Woessner S, Sole F, Florensa L, Bonet C. Chromosomal and in vitro culture studies in a case of primary plasma cell leukemia. *Cancer Genet Cytogenet* 1994; **76**:36–8.

70. Shou Y, Martelli ML, Gabrea A, Qi Y, Brents LA, Roschke A, et al. Diverse karyotypic abnormalities of the c-myc locus associated with c- myc dysregulation and tumor progression in multiple myeloma. *Proc Natl Acad Sci USA* 2000; **97**:228–33.

◆71. Jonveaux P, Berger R. Chromosome studies in plasma cell leukemia and multiple myeloma in transformation. *Genes Chromosomes Cancer* 1992; **4**:321–5.

72. Wiernik PH, Sciortino D, Paietta E, Papenhausen P, Ciobanu N, Roberts M. Plasma cell leukemia with an unusual karyotype and prolonged survival with oral alkylating agent therapy. *J Cancer Res Clin Oncol* 1987; **113**:576–8.

◆73. Azar GM, Gogineni SK, Hyde P, Verma RS. Highly complex chromosomal abnormalities in plasma cell leukemia as detected by FISH technique. *Leukemia* 1997; **11**:772–4.

74. Zhang XG, Klein B, Bataille R. Interleukin-6 is a potent myeloma-cell growth factor in patients with aggressive multiple myeloma. *Blood* 1989; **74**:11–13.

75. Zhang XG, Bataille R, Widjenes J, Klein B. Interleukin-6 dependence of advanced malignant plasma cell dyscrasias. *Cancer* 1992; **69**:1373–6.

76. Bataille R, Barlogie B, Lu ZY, Rossi JF, Lavabre-Bertrand T, Beck T, et al. Biologic effects of anti-interleukin-6 murine monoclonal antibody in advanced multiple myeloma. *Blood* 1995; **86**:685–91.

77. Klein B, Wijdenes J, Zhang XG, Jourdan M, Boiron JM, Brochier J, et al. Murine anti-interleukin-6 monoclonal antibody therapy for a patient with plasma cell leukemia. *Blood* 1991; **78**:1198–204.

78. Ohtani K, Ninomiya H, Hasegawa Y, Kobayashi T, Kojima H, Nagasawa T, et al. Clinical significance of elevated soluble interleukin-6 receptor levels in the sera of patients with plasma cell dyscrasias. *Br J Haematol* 1995; **91**:116–20.

79. Chauhan D, Kharbanda S, Ogata A, Urashima M, Teoh G, Robertson M, et al. Interleukin-6 inhibits Fas-induced apoptosis and stress-activated protein kinase activation in multiple myeloma cells. *Blood* 1997; **89**:227–34.

80. Podar K, Tai YT, Davies FE, Lentzsch S, Sattler M, Hideshima T, et al. Vascular endothelial growth factor triggers signaling cascades mediating multiple myeloma cell growth and migration. *Blood* 2001; **98**:428–35.

81. Mitsiades CS, Mitsiades N, Poulaki V, Schlossman R, Akiyama M, Chauhan D, et al. Activation of NF-kappaB and upregulation of intracellular anti-apoptotic proteins via the IGF-1/Akt signaling in human multiple myeloma cells: therapeutic implications. *Oncogene* 2002; **21**:5673–83.

82. Mitsiades SC, Mitsiades N, Kung AL, Shringapurne R, Poulaki V, Richardson PG, et al. The IGF/IGF-1R system is a major therapeutic target for multiple myeloma, other hematologic malignancies and solid tumors. *Blood* 2002; **100**:170a.

83. Anderson I, Osgood EE. Acute plasmacytic leukemia responsive to cyclophosphamide. *J Am Med Assoc* 1965; **193**:188.

84. Gangadharan VP, Satishkumar K, Pillai R, Cherian V. Effective cytotoxic treatment of primary plasma cell leukaemia – a report of 3 cases. *Acta Oncol* 1994; **33**:714–15.

85. Malhotra H, Dhabhar BN, Saikia TK, Gopal R, Nadkarni KS, Nair CN, et al. Ifosfamide in plasma cell leukemia: a report of two cases and review of the literature. *Am J Hematol* 1992; **40**:226–8.

86. Gruber J, Geisen F, Sgonc R, Egle A, Villunger A, Boeck G, et al. 2′,2′-Difluorodeoxycytidine (gemcitabine) induces apoptosis in myeloma cell lines resistant to steroids and 2-chlorodeoxyadenosine (2-CdA). *Stem Cells* 1996; **14**:351–62.

87. Christou L, Hatzimichael E, Chaidos A, Tsiara S, Bourantas KL. Treatment of plasma cell leukemia with vincristine, liposomal doxorubicin and dexamethasone. *Eur J Haematol* 2001; **67**:51–3.

88. Panizo C, Rifon J, Rodriguez-Wilhelmi P, Cuesta B, Rocha E. Long-term survival in primary plasma cell leukemia after therapy with VAD, autologous blood stem cell transplantation and interferon-alpha. *Acta Haematol* 1999; **101**:193–6.

89. Yamagata N, Shimazaki C, Goto H, Hirata T, Ashihara E, Oku N, et al. IgE plasma cell leukemia successfully treated with combination VAD (vincristine, doxorubicin, dexamethasone) and MP (melphalan, prednisolone) followed by interferon-alpha. *Am J Hematol* 1994; **45**:262–4.

90. Blade J, Lopez-Guillermo A, Tassies D, Montserrat E, Rozman C. Development of aggressive plasma cell leukaemia under interferon-alpha therapy. *Br J Haematol* 1991; **79**:523–5.

91. Sawamura M, Murayama K, Ui G, Matsushima T, Tamura J, Murakami H, *et al*. Plasma cell leukaemia with alpha-interferon therapy in myeloma. *Br J Haematol* 1992; **82**:631.

●92. McElwain TJ, Powles RL. High-dose intravenous melphalan for plasma-cell leukaemia and myeloma. *Lancet* 1983; **2**:822–4.

93. Gemmel C, Cremer FW, Weis M, Witzens M, Moldenhauer G, Koniczek KH, *et al*. Anti-CD20 antibody as consolidation therapy in a patient with primary plasma cell leukemia after high-dose therapy and autologous stem cell transplantation. *Ann Hematol* 2002; **81**:119–23.

94. Hovenga S, de Wolf JT, Klip H, Vellenga E. Consolidation therapy with autologous stem cell transplantation in plasma cell leukemia after VAD, high-dose cyclophosphamide and EDAP courses: a report of three cases and a review of the literature. *Bone Marrow Transplant* 1997; **20**:901–4.

95. Sajeva MR, Greco MM, Cascavilla N, D'Arena G, Scalzulli P, Melillo L, *et al*. Effective autologous peripheral blood stem cell transplantation in plasma cell leukemia followed by T-large granular lymphocyte expansion: a case report. *Bone Marrow Transplant* 1996; **18**:225–7.

96. Yeh KH, Lin MT, Tang JL, Yang CH, Tsay W, Chen YC. Long-term disease-free survival after autologous bone marrow transplantation in a primary plasma cell leukaemia: detection of minimal residual disease in the transplant marrow by third- complementarity-determining region-specific probes. *Br J Haematol* 1995; **89**:914–16.

97. Drake M, Morris C, Hagman A, Lopponen T, Bjorkstrand B, Gahrton G, *et al*. Autologous transplantation in primary plasma cell leukaemia. *EBMT Meeting, Istanbul* 2003, abstract no. 836.

98. Russell N, Bessell E, Stainer C, Haynes A, Das-Gupta E, Byrne J. Allogeneic haemopoietic stem cell transplantation for multiple myeloma or plasma cell leukaemia using fractionated total body radiation and high-dose melphalan conditioning. *Acta Oncol* 2000; **39**:837–41.

99. Badros A, Barlogie B, Siegel E, Cottler-Fox M, Zangari M, Fassas A, *et al*. Improved outcome of allogeneic transplantation in high-risk multiple myeloma patients after non-myeloablative conditioning. *J Clin Oncol* 2002; **20**:1295–303.

100. Bataille R, Jourdan M, Zhang XG, Klein B. Serum levels of interleukin 6, a potent myeloma cell growth factor, as a reflect of disease severity in plasma cell dyscrasias. *J Clin Invest* 1989; **84**:2008–11.

101. Shimazaki C, Atzpodien J, Wisniewski D, Gulati SC, Kolitz JE, Fried J, *et al*. Cell-mediated toxicity of interleukin-2-activated lymphocytes against autologous and allogeneic human myeloma cells. *Acta Haematol* 1988; **80**:203–9.

102. Schultze JL, Anderson KC, Gilleece MH, Gribben JG, Nadler LM. A pilot study of combined immunotherapy with autologous adoptive tumour- specific T-cell transfer, vaccination with CD40-activated malignant B cells and interleukin 2. *Br J Haematol* 2001; **113**:455–60.

●103. Barlogie B, Zangari M, Spencer T, Fassas A, Anaissie E, Badros A, *et al*. Thalidomide in the management of multiple myeloma. *Semin Hematol* 2001; **38**:250–9.

104. Fowler R, Imrie K. Thalidomide-associated hepatitis: a case report. *Am J Hematol* 2001; **66**:300–2.

105. Pandiella A, Esparis-Ogando A, Gutierrez NC, San Miguel JF. Effect of proteasome inhibitor (PS341) in cells from primary plasma cell leukemia patients. *Blood* 2002; **100**:373b.

106. Gonzalez M, Mateos MV, Garcia-Sanz R, Balanzategui A, Lopez-Perez R, Chillon MC, *et al*. De novo methylation of tumor suppressor gene p16/INK4a is a frequent finding in multiple myeloma patients at diagnosis. *Leukemia* 2000; **14**:183–7.

107. Krsnik I, Penalver MA, Del Potro E, Diaz-Mediavilla J. Complete remission in plasma cell leukaemia. *Br J Haematol* 1987; **66**:145.

108. Montecucco C, Riccardi A, Merlini G, Ascari E. Complete remission in plasma cell leukaemia. *Br J Haematol* 1986; **62**:525–7.

109. Musto P, Greco MM, Falcone A, Carotenuto M. Treatment of plasma cell leukaemia and resistant/relapsed multiple myeloma with vincristine, mitoxantrone and dexamethasone (VMD protocol). *Br J Haematol* 1991; **79**:655–6.

110. Osanto S, Muller HP, Schuit HR, *et al*. Primary plasma cell leukaemia. A case report and a review of the literature. *Acta Haematol* 1983; **70**:122.

◆111. Shaw MT, Twele TW, Nordquist RE. Plasma cell leukemia: detailed studies and response to therapy. *Cancer* 1974; **33**:619–25.

112. Thijs LG, Hijmans W, Leene W, Muntinghe OG, Pietersz RN, Ploem JE. Blast cell leukaemia associated with IgA paraproteinaemia and Bence Jones protein. *Br J Haematol* 1970; **19**:485–92.

113. Ghosh K, Madkaikar M, Iyer Y, Pathare A, Jijina F, Mohanty D. Systemic capillary leak syndrome preceding plasma cell leukaemia. *Acta Haematol* 2001; **106**:118–21.

27

AL amyloidosis

RAYMOND L. COMENZO

INTRODUCTION

Amyloidosis is the term for a category of disease processes that share a common feature: the self-assembly of abnormal proteins to form extracellular deposits in tissues of insoluble, non-branching, linear fibrils that extend 7–10 nm in width, vary in length, and resist proteolysis.[1–3] It is likely that medical and forensic investigators recognized such deposits at autopsy over 350 years ago; some thought the material was a fatty substance, hence the term 'lardaceous disease'.[4] However, it was the pathologist Virchow who, in 1854, described the deposits in post mortem liver tissue with the botanical term 'amyloid' meaning 'starch' or 'cellulose', since they had a starch-like affinity for iodine. Virchow's misnomer has proven resilient.[5]

The deposits appear amorphous, hyaline, and fluffy under the light microscope, eosinophilic with hematoxylin–eosin stain. When stained with Congo red, however, the deposits change from eosinophilic in non-polarized light to the characteristic apple-green refrinrefringence in polarized light, an important observation first reported in 1927.[6] A century after Virchow's use of the term, the fibrillar nature of amyloid and its characteristic β-pleated-sheet configuration were described with the use of electron microscopy (Fig. 27.1, Plate 12).[7,8] But it was not until the 1970s that we learned that all of the variants of amyloidosis have fibril precursor proteins, i.e. normally soluble globular proteins that self-assemble and deposit as insoluble abnormal amyloid fibrils.[9–12] The fibril precursor proteins for the major varieties of amyloidosis are shown in Table 27.1.[13] The precursor

protein for light-chain-associated amyloidosis is a fragment of a monoclonal immunoglobulin protein, usually a portion of the free light chain. In the current paradigm, amyloidosis is considered to be a disease of protein misfolding or conformation.[14–17] At this time, a better understanding of the systemic amyloidoses and of the role of localized amyloidosis in degenerative neurological disorders (e.g. Alzheimer's disease, Parkinson's disease) has led to further basic research into the development of specific therapies for the different types of amyloidosis.[18–20]

AL amyloidosis is of particular interest to specialists in plasma cell diseases because clonal plasma cells secrete the monoclonal light chain proteins that form fibrils and deposits.[21,22] AL amyloidosis, then, is both a disorder of protein conformation *cum* deposition and a clonal plasma cell dyscrasia.[2] The 1990s ushered in an era of rapid progress in the implementation of new approaches to treatment, including stem cell transplantation and drugs to help the body resorb AL amyloid deposits.

PATHOGENESIS

The final pathway in the deposition process of amyloidosis involves the elaboration of amyloid fibrils in the extracellular matrix.[23–25] When the amyloid-subunit proteins are submitted to amino acid-sequencing studies, the main constituent of AL amyloid deposits is the light-chain variable region and less frequently part of the constant region or of the whole immunoglobulin.[26–32] Although the reasons why some immunoglobulin light chains form amyloid and others do not remain unknown,

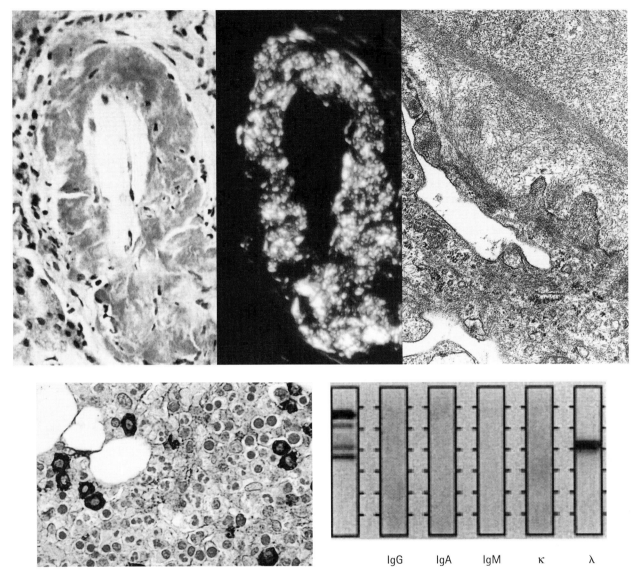

Figure 27.1 Top: *images of a Congo red-stained section of liver tissue in non-polarized light (left), the same tissue viewed in polarized light showing apple-green refringence (center), and an electron microscopy view of amyloid fibrils. Bottom: a section of bone marrow biopsy showing immunostained λ-restricted plasma cells (left, brown cells) and a urine immunofixation showing free monoclonal λ light chains (right). These findings are typical images of AL amyloidosis.*

Table 27.1 *Systemic amyloidosis variants*

Type	Fibril-precursor protein	Clinical syndrome
AL, AH	Immunoglobulin light or heavy chain	AL amyloidosis
ATTR	Mutant transthyretin	Hereditary amyloidoses
AA	Serum amyloid A (pre-albumin)	Secondary amyloidosis
AApoA1	Apolipoprotein A1	Familial amyloidotic polyneuropathy (Iowa)
AGel	Gelsolin	Familial amyloidotic polyneuropathy (Finnish)
Aβ2m	β_2-microglobulin	Dialysis-associated
AFib	Fibrinogen A α-chain	Renal amyloid, hypertension

comparisons of the primary structures of normal and abnormal light chains have shed light on why some light chains may form fibrils.[33,34] Another major constituent of amyloid deposits of all types is the plasma glycoprotein serum amyloid P component (SAP), one of the pentraxin family of proteins.[35] Of note, SAP may be a pathologic chaperone for amyloid fibrils because it is very resistant to proteolysis. Amyloid fibrils studded with SAP molecules *in vitro* are protected from phagocytosis and proteolytic degradation.[36]

Equally as relevant as why fibrils form is why they form where they do. One of the curious hallmarks of AL amyloidosis is the variety of organs that may be symptomatically involved.[2,37] A third of patients, for example, present with dominant renal amyloidosis in the form of nephrotic syndrome, often with few symptoms associated with other organs of involvement. Although the mechanistic basis of this tropism remains unknown, evaluations of the immunoglobulin light-chain genetics underlying AL amyloidosis have suggested that some light-chain variable region germline or donor genes are more likely to give one pattern of organ involvement than another.[38–40]

The effects of primary structure on the conformation of immunoglobulin light chains appear to be the basis for amyloid.[41–43] Purified urinary light chains from AL amyloidosis patients reproduce the disease when injected into mice, while purified urinary proteins from myeloma patients who do not have AL amyloidosis do not cause amyloid deposits.[44] Primary-structure analyses have emphasized the contribution of critical uncommon amino-acid substitutions to the stability and interactive properties of misfolded or partially folded light chains.[33] Such partially folded intermediate forms may be prone to self-assemble aberrantly.[16,17] The identification of potentially destabilizing uncommon amino-acid substitutions at unique positions in the variable regions of AL amyloidosis light chains has supported this hypothesis.[45,46] Also, atomic force microscopy has been used to analyze the *in vitro* formation of amyloid fibrils from light-chain proteins produced by recombinant technology.[47] Studies performed at different time points in the process identified a pattern of assemblage in which filaments associated mutually to form fibrils that similarly formed thicker units. This model differs from the alternative proposal that fibrils grow by extension as soluble light-chain monomers or oligomers stack one upon another.[43]

In addition, the interactions between AL amyloidosis light chains and passenger constituents of amyloid deposits, such as glycosaminoglycans, may be related to these critical amino-acid variations and may influence the course of AL amyloidosis disease by stabilizing filament and fibril formation, and by enhancing the resistance of AL amyloid deposits to proteolysis.[48] SAP, as noted above, is particularly interesting in this regard but employs a calcium-dependent binding mechanism in its interactions with amyloid fibrils. Other modifications of light chain conformation, such as post-translational glycosylation, may be related to critical amino-acid substitutions and may predispose light chains to self-assemble.[49]

In the majority of patients with AL amyloidosis, free monoclonal light chains and minimal bone marrow plasmacytosis are detected, often in association with suppression of non-involved immunoglobulin production.[2] Sixty percent of patients have marrow biopsies showing 10% or fewer clonal plasma cells.[37] The levels of monoclonal protein and the plasma cell infiltrates in the marrow do not increase over time, as is the case in multiple myeloma. Over the past decade, a more complete understanding of the genetic endowment of AL amyloidosis clones has opened new research vistas.[50] The clones that cause AL amyloidosis are distinctly different from myeloma clones with respect to their repertoire of immunoglobulin light-chain variable germline (Ig V_L) genes but similar in that their immunoglobulin genes are highly mutated (i.e. antigen-driven or post-germinal center clones), and surprisingly similar to myeloma clones with respect to their cytogenetics.[38–40,51–55]

The repertoire of Ig V_L genes in AL amyloidosis is skewed, unlike that in myeloma, which is similar to the normal expressed repertoire.[54,55] Nearly half of AL amyloidosis clones employ two particular immunoglobulin λ light-chain variable region germline genes, the 3r (λIII) and 6a (λVI) germline donors. There are curious differences between the degree of homology with germline in both instances: AL amyloidosis clones using genes derived from the 3r germline have a significantly higher divergence from the germline sequence than those using the 6a donor.[38,40] This difference may be related to antigen selection or to the inherent amyloid-forming propensity of 6a light chains.[56]

Interestingly, the cytogenetic abnormalities commonly seen in myeloma clones are also found in AL amyloidosis. Aneuploidy is common, with trisomies of chromosome 7, 9, 11, 15, and 18 seen in a significant fraction of cases. Translocations of chromosome 14 including t(4;14) are common and abnormalities of chromosome 13 frequent by florescence *in situ* hybridization (FISH).[57,58] These studies are technically challenging because of the sparsity of plasma cells in this disease and have been conducted with small sample sizes; there is no evidence of prognostic significance with cytogenetic or FISH abnormalities. AL amyloidosis is, then, equivalent to monoclonal gammopathy or early myeloma with minimal marrow infiltration with respect to plasma cell number and cytogenetic and FISH findings. The natural history of the disease, however, is dominated by the progressive deposits and the relentless advance to endstage organ dysfunction and death.

With respect to a basis for the organ tropism of AL amyloidosis, using the reverse-transcriptase polymerase chain reaction to clone AL amyloidosis light chain genes and available databases for germline gene identification, we and others sought to test the hypothesis that the Ig V_L genes used by AL amyloidosis clones influenced organ tropism. In one series, Ig V_L germline genes were identified from 60 patients with AL amyloidosis and it was found that those with clones derived from the 6a germline gene were more likely to present with dominant renal involvement, while those with clones derived from the 1c, 2a2, and 3r genes were more likely to present with dominant cardiac and multisystem disease.[38] In addition, in a renal mesangial cell model of *in vitro* amyloidosis, 6a light chains formed more amyloid more rapidly and without the benefit of amyloid enhancing factor than did other λ light chains. Furthermore, patients with Vκ clones were more likely to have dominant hepatic involvement. In another series, Ig V_L germline genes were identified from 58 patients with AL amyloidosis, and 6a light chains were again significantly more frequent in patients with major kidney involvement, while 3r light chains appeared able to infiltrate all amyloid target organs.[40]

Despite these suggestive data, what remains utterly unexplained is how the self-assembly of misfolded light chain proteins causes progressive organ dysfunction and clinical disease at a tempo more rapid than that seen in hereditary variants of amyloidosis. An attractive hypothesis is that partially folded light-chain intermediates formed in the early stages of assemblage are directly or indirectly more toxic to cellular metabolism than the deposits themselves.[59]

EPIDEMIOLOGY

The epidemiology of amyloidosis is difficult to define precisely, since the disease is likely often undiagnosed and the data from tertiary referral centers are unrepresentative. AL amyloidosis is a rare disorder with an age-adjusted incidence estimated to be 5.1–12.8 per million person-years, resulting in approximately 1275–3200 new cases annually in the USA and, by projection from the US incidence, 255–640 cases in the UK, an incidence similar to that of chronic myelogenous leukemia and Hodgkin's disease.[60] AL amyloidosis appears to be more common in men based on data from tertiary centers, but the difference may be due to self-selection and referral bias. Sixty percent of patients with AL amyloidosis are between 50 and 70 years of age at diagnosis, and only 10% are younger than 50.[37] The median age at diagnosis is 63 years, the same as for multiple myeloma. AL amyloidosis is approximately one-fifth as common as multiple myeloma but confers a worse prognosis because the median survival of patients seen within 1 month of diagnosis is 13.2 months.[37]

Survival is poor due to progressive organ failure. Patients who present with congestive heart failure survive a median of 4 to 8 months; fewer than 5% of AL amyloidosis patients survive 10 years from diagnosis.[61,62] The presence or absence of symptomatic amyloid cardiac involvement is the most important prognostic factor with respect to survival. Historically, the time from onset of symptoms to the diagnosis of AL amyloidosis has varied depending on the dominant symptomatic organ system. In patients presenting with congestive heart failure or nephrotic syndrome, symptoms usually have been present for a median of 3 months.[37] Patients with neuropathy or slowly progressive hepatomegaly may be symptomatic for a year prior to diagnosis.

The incidence of mutant transthyretin (ATTR) amyloidosis is unknown, but it is less common than AL amyloidosis, with the number of diagnosed cases in referral centers representing 10–20% of the number of cases of AL amyloidosis.[63–66] An exception is the variant-sequence transthyretin associated with late-onset cardiac amyloidosis in blacks, which is caused by the substitution of isoleucine for valine in codon 122 of the transthyretin gene (Ile 122).[67] AA amyloidosis secondary amyloidosis is uncommon in the developed world but is reportedly more common than AL amyloidosis in less developed countries.[68]

CLINICAL PRESENTATION

The presenting features of AL amyloidosis are protean. Specific symptoms reflect the organ or organs most prominently involved, although examination of biopsy material will reveal some amyloid deposition in the vasculature of virtually every organ system except the central nervous system. Presenting symptoms are commonly fatigue, weakness, decreased libido, and weight loss, although the diagnosis is rarely made until symptoms referable to a specific organ appear.[1,2,37]

Since the kidneys and the heart are most often involved, nephrotic syndrome and/or congestive cardiac failure are common modes of presentation. However, AL amyloidosis can present in a wide variety of ways, often causing diagnostic difficulty until the possibility of the disorder is considered. Criteria of amyloid-related organ involvement are shown in Table 27.2.

Renal amyloidosis

A third of AL amyloidosis patients have dominant renal amyloid at diagnosis, half of whom excrete 10 g or more of protein daily. A significant number of patients with dominant renal amyloidosis are asymptomatic and are diagnosed only after proteinuria is revealed as part of a

Table 27.2 *Non-invasive criteria of amyloid-related major organ involvement[a]*

Heart
- Echocardiogram showing increased mean ventricular wall thickness and thickened valves with no history of hypertension or valvular heart disease
- Electrocardiogram showing unexplained low voltage
- New York Heart Association functional capacity class 2 or higher without ischemic heart disease

Kidneys
- 24-hour albuminuria greater than 500 mg

Liver
- Right upper quadrant discomfort
- Early satiety
- Hepatomegaly

Peripheral nervous system
- Orthostatic hypotension
- Lower extremity sensory or polyneuropathy
- Impotence, diarrhea, or constipation

[a] In all instances, a positive biopsy remains the gold standard.

routine examination. Typically amyloid deposited in the glomeruli leads to proteinuria and nephrotic syndrome and, when discovered, such findings usually lead to renal biopsy, securing the diagnosis. Massive proteinuria with profound edema and hypoalbuminemia may occur with normal serum creatinine and blood urea nitrogen concentrations, although evidence of mild renal dysfunction is frequently found. AL amyloidosis rarely presents as progressive renal failure and, even in the presence of a markedly elevated serum creatinine, systemic hypertension is uncommon. Renal failure requiring dialysis develops in about a third of patients after 2 years despite standard oral therapy but only in about 10% of patients after dose-intensive therapy with stem cell support.[69,70]

The signs and symptoms of nephrotic syndrome include peripheral edema, frothy urine, low serum albumin, and hypercholesterolemia. The associated fatigue and listlessness can be debilitating; in addition, the presence of occult effusions, pleural and pericardial, can give the picture of heart failure. Patients are salt-avid but may be volume-depleted at times, causing nausea and vomiting, and complicating attempts at diuresis. Volume-depletion can also cause orthostasis, mimicking autonomic neuropathy.[71]

Cardiac amyloidosis

A quarter of AL amyloidosis patients have dominant symptomatic cardiac involvement at diagnosis. Right-sided heart dysfunction is a common finding in these patients and, early on, they have relatively preserved left ventricular function despite ventricular thickening due to deposits of amyloid. Patients complain of dyspnea on exertion, and frequently have prominent jugular venous distension, a right-sided third heart-sound, congestive hepatomegaly, and lower extremity edema. Coronary angiography, if performed, usually shows clean coronary arteries. Advanced cardiac amyloid causes a restrictive cardiomyopathy, resulting in diminished cardiac output, sometimes exacerbated by an increase in the heart rate. Frank congestive heart failure, usually rapid in onset and progressive, may be preceded by asymptomatic electrocardiographic abnormalities. In severe cases, atrial thrombi may be present even in sinus rhythm, and the onset of atrial fibrillation is associated with a high risk of thromboembolism.[72] Sudden death, often subsequent to symptomatic bradycardia or micturition syncope, is common in patients with cardiac amyloidosis.[73] A role for anti-arrhythmic agents or implanted defibrillators has not been defined.

Cardiac amyloidosis can also lead to conduction disturbances and arrhythmias. Premature ventricular contractions are most common, but supraventricular arrhythmias also occur and may have life-threatening hemodynamic consequences. Other manifestations include sinus arrest and atrioventricular block. Electrocardiographic findings frequently include low voltage and a pseudoinfarct pattern with Q waves in the anterior leads in the absence of coronary artery disease. This pattern may lead to the incorrect diagnosis of atherosclerotic heart disease, particularly in patients who have cardiac amyloidosis associated with typical angina. The echocardiogram remains the most practical method for assessing cardiac amyloid. A common echocardiographic finding is concentric ventricular hypertrophy with measurable thickening of the posterior wall and septum in diastole, mimicking that seen with hypertensive heart disease or hypertrophic cardiomyopathy.[74] Unlike the electrocardiograms of patients with bona fide ventricular hypertrophy, however, the electrocardiograms of patients with cardiac amyloid often show low voltage with left-axis deviation as well as the pseudoinfarct pattern noted above.

Hepatic and gastrointestinal amyloidosis

A quarter of AL amyloidosis patients present with symptomatic hepatic or gastrointestinal involvement with amyloid; these syndromes can occur simultaneously or separately.[75] The gastrointestinal tract may become infiltrated with amyloid but only rarely to the extent that malabsorption or pseudo-obstruction occur.[76] Symptoms of hepatic involvement may include early satiety, weight loss, nausea, dyspepsia, and right upper quadrant fullness or discomfort.[77] Gastrointestinal involvement can present with frank rectal bleeding as well as symptoms of nausea, food intolerance, and weight loss. Many gastrointestinal symptoms may be a function of autonomic neuropathy interfering with gastric motility. Symptoms due to involvement of the gastrointestinal tract usually are linked to the location and extent of amyloid deposits.[71] The entire length of the gastrointestinal tract may be involved; macroglossia can be massive and produce difficulty eating or drinking despite minimal difficulty with swallowing. Airway obstruction, sleep apnea, achalasia, hematemesis, and gastroparesis are among the many possible manifestations of gastrointestinal amyloid. Rarely, bowel perforation or hepatic rupture due to amyloid occurs; the decision to allow surgical management of such problems should be based on the presence or absence of co-morbid organ involvement.[78] If symptomatic heart or renal amyloid disease is also present, conservative non-surgical management is preferable.

Peripheral and autonomic neuropathy due to amyloidosis

Up to a fifth of AL amyloidosis patients have peripheral neuropathy.[79] There may be exquisitely painful sensory symptoms. Patients usually have a symmetric lower extremity neuropathy, as opposed to the asymmetric picture seen in chronic inflammatory demyelinating polyneuropathies. Autonomic involvement is frequent and linked to a variety of symptoms, notably orthostatic hypotension, disturbances in gastrointestinal motility causing chronic impairment of the gustatory sense (dysgeusia), nausea, recurrent constipation or diarrhea, and impotence. Motor neuropathy is uncommon, and sensory neuropathy usually has a distal to proximal and symmetric pattern. Profound postural hypotension can occur without concomitant tachycardia because of cardiac dysautonomia and the heart's inability to respond appropriately. The occurrence of orthostatic hypotension and cardiac failure or nephrotic syndrome in the same patient limits the use of angiotensin-converting enzyme inhibitors and other drugs that may worsen hypotension.

Amyloidosis involving other organ systems

Many other organ systems can be involved with amyloid, including connective tissue, skin, and muscles, the respiratory tract, and the genitourinary system (Fig. 27.2). A history of carpal tunnel syndrome is frequently elicited and may precede other features of the disease by a year or more. An erosive arthritis may occur. Periorbital ecchymoses ('raccoon eyes') occur in about one-fifth of patients and are pathognomonic for AL amyloidosis (Fig. 27.2).[2] In some cases, the process is truly localized in association with a limited infiltrate of monoclonal plasma cells, or

low-grade or mucosal-associated non-Hodgkin's lymphoma.[80] Localized AL amyloidosis of the larynx, tracheobronchial tree, duodenum, and bladder usually does not progress to systemic disease and generally carries a favorable prognosis.[81]

DIAGNOSIS

Tissue diagnosis

The diagnosis of AL amyloidosis should be considered in patients with monoclonal gammopathies who have constitutional or neurologic symptoms, and in young patients who present with unexplained congestive heart failure, new-onset nephrotic syndrome, peripheral polyneuropathy, or symptomatic non-infectious hepatomegaly. The presentations detailed above can serve as a guide for thought because obtaining a tissue diagnosis is the critical second step after first thinking of the diagnosis. Occasionally, the diagnosis is missed despite obtaining tissue because the deposits are not always easily appreciated with hematoxolin–eosin staining and neither the primary physician nor the pathologist requests Congo red staining. A tissue diagnosis can usually be established by Congo red staining of biopsies of subcutaneous abdominal fat (80% sensitivity), of the rectum or of involved organs.[82,83]

Having established the diagnosis of amyloid, immunohistochemistry is sometimes performed to determine the type of amyloid, although the sensitivity and specificity of immunostaining remain controversial.[84–91] Potassium permanganate ($KMnO_4$) treatment prior to Congo red staining distinguishes AA (secondary) from other types of amyloidosis because the apple-green birefringence of AA amyloid is lost with $KMnO_4$ treatment, while that of other types of amyloidosis is usually not. Immunohistochemical staining for κ or λ light-chain amyloidosis, however, is technically challenging and often unreliable. Therefore, the histological diagnosis of AL amyloidosis usually rests on the presence of amyloid noted on Congo red-stained tissue in association with a clonal plasma cell dyscrasia.

Assessing the plasma cell dyscrasia

The clonal plasma cell dyscrasia is usually identified by immunofixation of urine and serum revealing a monoclonal protein (M-protein), and by bone marrow biopsy with immunohistochemical staining for plasma cell antigens (e.g. CD138) and light-chain isotypes demonstrating the clonal dominance of λ (κ/λ ratio < 1) or κ (κ/λ ratio > 3) staining plasma cells; marrow biopsies should

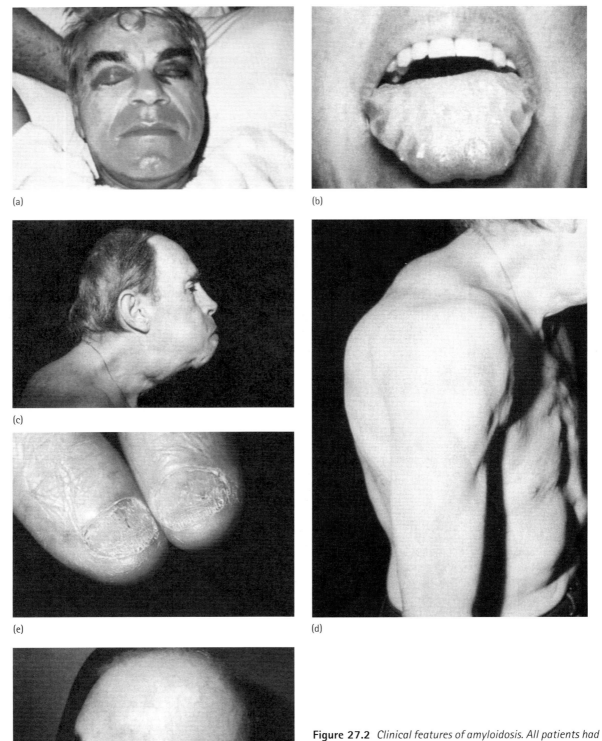

(a)

(b)

(c)

(d)

(e)

(f)

Figure 27.2 *Clinical features of amyloidosis. All patients had AL amyloidosis. (a) Ecchymoses around the eyes with a characteristic absence of soft-tissue swelling; (b) an enlarged tongue (macroglossia) with prominent indentations caused by the teeth; (c, d) soft-tissue deposits of amyloid in the submandibular glands and synovial tissues, the 'shoulder-pad sign;' (e) nail dystrophy; and (f) total alopecia of the scalp. (Reprinted with permission from Falk et al., N Engl J Med 1997; **337**:898–909.[2] Copyright © 1997 Massachusetts Medical Society.)*

also be stained with Congo red for the presence of amyloid.[2] Immunofixation of urine and serum are specifically indicated after a tissue diagnosis of amyloidosis has been made. Indeed, it is important to perform immunofixation even if routine protein electrophoresis is negative, because the paraprotein in AL amyloidosis is often present at a very low level and protein electrophoresis often fails to reveal the presence of an M-protein.[92] The κ to λ ratio in AL amyloidosis is 1:3 in contrast to the 3:2 ratio in myeloma and in the normal B-cell repertoire.

The recent availability of a reliable and highly sensitive serum free light-chain assay may significantly change the way that AL amyloidosis patients and others, such as those with non-secretory myeloma, are both diagnosed and monitored during therapy.[93,94] Historically, 5–10% of AL amyloidosis patients presented with no evidence by immunofixation of a monoclonal gammopathy, although careful inspection of immunohistochemically stained marrow specimens would allow one to infer the presence of clonal disease in some instances. In a study of 18 patients with AL amyloidosis, and negative serum and urine immunofixation studies, two-thirds were found to have abnormal serum free light-chain concentrations.[95] These results are particularly striking because the free light-chain assay is quantitative, unlike immunofixation studies, and is approximately ≥50 times more sensitive for the presence of clonal free light chains than immunofixation. A series of free light-chain values in newly diagnosed patients with AL amyloidosis is depicted in Fig. 27.3. The importance of the free light-chain assay in AL amyloidosis highlights the conundrum one faces in a patient with amyloidosis, but without clear-cut evidence of a monoclonal gammopathy or clonal plasma cell dyscrasia.

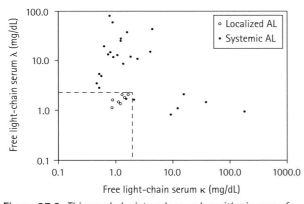

Figure 27.3 *This graph depicts values on logarithmic axes of κ and λ serum free light chains from 33 newly diagnosed patients with AL amyloidosis, seven of whom had localized disease. The box about the origin depicts the upper limit of normal values for κ and λ light chains in our laboratory at Memorial Sloan-Kettering Cancer Center. Of interest, the patients with localized amyloidosis had no evidence of elevated serum free light chains.*

The free light-chain assay will add useful data to the evaluation of such patients.

Distinguishing AL from hereditary variants of amyloidosis

Concerns about whether amyloid is AL amyloidosis or another type are warranted because myelotoxic chemotherapies have no place in the treatment of hereditary or secondary amyloidoses; such concerns are most appropriate in three situations. In black patients, particularly those over the age of 60, the concern of misdiagnosing AL amyloidosis is raised because of the increased frequency of both hereditary (ATTR, isoleucine 122) amyloid and monoclonal gammopathy of undetermined significance (MGUS).[67] In patients with hypertension, renal amyloidosis, and low-level monoclonal proteins, the concern is warranted based on a recent report of patients with the fibrinogen A α-chain variant of hereditary amyloid and low-level monoclonal proteins being misdiagnosed, and undergoing dose-intensive chemotherapy and autologous stem cell transplant.[96] In elderly patients with cardiac amyloid only and monoclonal gammopathies, the concern of misdiagnosis is based on the possible presence of MGUS and senile cardiac amyloidosis, a disease entity that remains poorly understood and involves the deposition of normal transthyretin in the myocardium. MGUS is found in 5% of normal individuals over the age of 70.[97] The most practical guides to keep in mind when dealing with these situations are that (1) amyloidosis in the bone marrow is characteristic of AL amyloidosis (hence, the importance of Congo red staining of marrow biopsy specimens); (2) 'vitreal floaters' on ophthalmologic examination are characteristic of ATTR variants; and (3) the deposits in the fibrinogen A α-chain variant often obliterate the glomeruli and, importantly, stain immunohistochemically for fibrinogen.[65,96] In cases requiring further diagnostic clarification with respect to mutant transthyretin or fibrinogen A α-chain variants versus AL amyloidosis, polymerase chain reaction (PCR) assays can be performed for the transthyretin or fibrinogen A α-chain genes employing DNA from patient blood or marrow cells. DNA sequence and translational analysis of PCR amplicons compared with wild-type remain the gold standard for confirming the presence of a mutant gene.

SAP scintiscan

As noted above, SAP is a normal serum protein that specifically binds to all types of amyloid fibrils. When SAP is labeled with ^{123}I it can be used for whole-body scintigraphic imaging to confirm the presence of amyloid.[98,99] In addition, the distribution of the radiolabel can provide an indication as to the type of amyloid. Bone marrow involvement and heterogeneous organ involvement are much more characteristic of AL amyloidosis amyloid than of other types. The SAP scan is helpful in depicting organ involvement and in monitoring response to therapy. The SAP scan is not helpful in evaluating cardiac involvement because of the background signal from blood moving in the chambers of the heart. Recently, it has been reported that radiolabeled aprotinin (an anti-serine protease) targets amyloid deposits with particular sensitivity for cardiac amyloid. Until such scans become widely available, however, cardiac involvement of the heart is best diagnosed and evaluated by echocardiography as discussed earlier. Magnetic resonance imaging (MRI) may be useful in evaluating amyloid in some organs, such as the gastrointestinal tract, lung and bones.

Routine laboratory evaluation

Routine testing in all patients should include a full blood count, coagulation screen, renal and hepatic blood chemistries, a 24-hour urine for total protein, chest X-ray, electrocardiogram, and echocardiogram. Chest X-ray may show prominent vascular markings and pleural effusions, although the latter are more often associated with left-heart failure or nephrotic syndrome with hypoalbuminemia. In patients with relevant findings, a gastric emptying scan, nerve conduction studies, and pulmonary function tests may be useful.

The peripheral blood picture is usually normal. Anemia is rare; if present, it is usually due to other causes unless there is evidence of amyloidosis associated with myeloma, gastrointestinal bleeding and consequent iron loss, massive marrow deposits of amyloid, or advanced renal dysfunction causing low levels of erythropoietin. Coagulation tests may reveal abnormalities of the international normalized ratio (INR) or the partial thromboplastin test (APTT) and, when they do, should be further evaluated for the presence of thrombin inhibitors (about 30% of patients) and factor X deficiency (about 5% of patients).[100,101] Proteinuria is common; levels that exceed 150 mg/day are abnormal and those that exceed 3 g/day are considered nephrotic. In nephrotic syndrome, serum cholesterol level may be elevated and the serum albumin level decreased. Abnormalities of liver function tests related to hepatic amyloid are often limited to an elevated alkaline phosphatase; a rising bilirubin level is a poor prognostic sign and usually a terminal event.

Because of the protean manifestations and its rarity, AL amyloidosis may go undiagnosed until the patient has become morbidly ill owing to failure of several major organ systems. The median survival of patients with AL amyloidosis is 1–2 years but prognosis is linked to dominant organ involvement. In one series of AL amyloidosis

patients, those with heart failure survived a median of 8 months and only 2.5% of them survived 5 years.[102] In a multivariate analysis of 168 patients with AL amyloidosis amyloid, the presence of heart failure, Bence Jones proteinuria, hepatomegaly, and multiple myeloma negatively affected survival during the first year.[103] Thereafter, the predictors of poor survival were increased serum creatinine, multiple myeloma, orthostatic hypotension, and serum monoclonal protein. Few studies have specifically addressed the prognostic variables.

In patients with dominant or symptomatic cardiac involvement, the progression of restrictive disease, bi-ventricular failure, and arrhythmias go hand in hand with a decline in performance status. Survival is negatively influenced by diminution of left ventricular function and by increased mean left ventricular wall thickness. For patients with symptomatic polyneuropathy in association with orthostasis, gastroparesis, nausea, and chronic diarrhea, performance status and survival are also severely compromised. Peripheral neuropathy rarely improves with treatment and is an indicator of poor prognosis.[79] Of note, the performance status of patients with dominant renal involvement (i.e. nephrotic syndrome) often improves after treatment with gentle use of diuretics and salt restriction (<1500 mg/day). Other supportive care measures that may be useful include albumin infusions, antidiarrheals, and the use of agents such as midodrine or fludrocortisone to treat postural hypotension; such measures may contribute significantly to the improved well-being of AL amyloidosis patients.[71]

If a tissue diagnosis of amyloidosis has been obtained, AL amyloidosis diagnosed, and the extent of clinically relevant organ involvement determined, the next step is defining the options for therapy. There is not a validated staging system for AL amyloidosis; nevertheless, a crude system of sorts has developed because the toxicities of stem cell transplant in AL amyloidosis patients forced the issue of patient selection to the fore. The criteria for organ involvement have been reviewed above (Table 27.2, p. 404) and the options for therapy at this time are based in part on the number of organ systems involved and the extent of cardiac involvement if present.

THERAPY

Standard chemotherapy

The primary approach to therapy is to reduce the production of the light-chain fibril precursor protein by treating the plasma cell dyscrasia. This is an indirect therapy with respect to tissue deposits of amyloid; there are currently no effective ways to dissolve the deposits directly.

However, decreased production of the light-chain fibril precursor protein has been shown to result in stabilization and even regression of deposits.

To reduce light-chain production, the same therapeutic approaches used for multiple myeloma are used to treat AL amyloidosis (Table 27.3). These include low-dose oral chemotherapy regimens such as melphalan and prednisone (MP), single-agent dexamethasone, and combination regimens such as VBMCP (vincristine, BCNU, melphalan, cyclophosphamide, and prednisone). These therapies, however, are unsatisfactory. The conundrum of therapy is that a less toxic treatment that works gradually may be ineffective because death may occur before there is time for the amyloid deposits to regress. Because deposits in key viscera such as the heart or liver may progress rapidly, AL amyloidosis can be an acutely fatal disease with death occurring soon after diagnosis, although most patients do not succumb quite so quickly. There is, therefore, an argument that patients with a higher amyloid load would benefit from more aggressive treatment, such as stem cell transplantation; however, these are the patients at highest risk of regimen-related toxicities, which are a far greater problem in AL amyloidosis patients than in other autologous stem cell transplant patients, as we discuss later. To add to the difficulty of selecting appropriate treatment, there have been very few randomized controlled trials in AL amyloidosis.

Melphalan and prednisone was the first effective treatment for amyloidosis, and has been shown in randomized controlled trials to improve the outlook for patients with AL amyloidosis.[104,105] Overall median survival was prolonged from 12 months in controls to 18 months in patients receiving MP (Fig. 27.4a). Although MP results in a response (defined as greater than 50% reduction in M-protein) in only one-quarter of AL amyloidosis patients, with a median time to response of 12 months, responders do survive significantly longer than non-responders (median 89 vs. 14 months).[104] Patients with nephrotic syndrome fare better than those with cardiac involvement, of whom only 15–20% experience a response. This partly reflects the fact that MP takes approximately a year to produce maximum benefit. The side effects of melphalan include myelotoxicity and, in patients who survive for more than 3.5 years, there is a

20% of risk of myelodysplasia, often leading to secondary leukemia.[106]

A prospective randomized trial of MP versus the VBMCP combination chemotherapy regimen showed no difference in response rate or survival; both resulted in median survivals of about 2 years.[107] VAD (vincristine, Adriamycin, and dexamethasone) induces remission in 70% of patients with myeloma, and the response is very

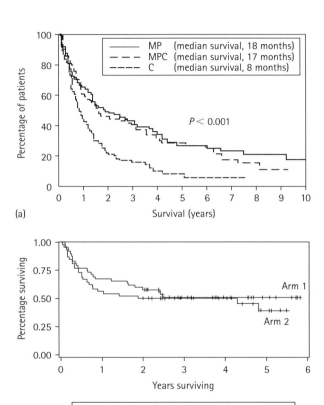

(a)

(b)

Figure 27.4 *Survival with therapies. (a) The survival curve of 222 AL patients treated on a clinical trial with melphalan and prednisone (MP). Newly diagnosed untreated patients were stratified based on organ involvement, and randomized to receive MP, MP with colchicine (MPC), or colchicine (C) alone. Median survival is significantly extended to 18 months in patients receiving MP-containing regimens. (Reprinted with permission from Kyle et al., N Engl J Med 1997;**336**:1202–7.[104] Copyright © 1997 Massachusetts Medical Society.) (b) The survival curve of 100 AL patients treated on a clinical trial using high-dose melphalan and autologous stem cell transplantation (SCT). Newly diagnosed untreated patients were stratified based on organ involvement, and randomized to receive immediate SCT (Arm 1) or two cycles of MP followed by SCT (Arm 2). There was no difference in overall survival between the two arms; median survival had not been reached with 45 months median follow-up.[129] (Based on Sanchorawala V, Comenzo RL, unpublished data.)*

Table 27.3 *Standard treatments for AL amyloidosis*

Therapy (references)	Response rate	Level of evidence
MP (104, 105, 107)	~30%	Phase III trials
VBMCP (107)	29%	Phase III trial
VAD (108)	Unknown	Anecdotal
Dexamethasone (109)	30%	Phase II trial

MP, melphalan and prednisone; VAD, vincristine, Adriamycin, and dexamethasone; VBMCP, vincristine, BCNU, melphalan, cyclophosphamide, and prednisone.

rapid, with maximum response reached after 2 or 3 months in most patients. This rapidity of response could prove particularly advantageous in treating AL amyloidosis. There are several anecdotal reports showing improved organ function and reduction of amyloid load in patients treated with VAD, but there have been no formal clinical trials.[108] It is important to note that patients with amyloid are more vulnerable than myeloma patients to some of the side effects of this regimen, including neuropathy, fluid retention, and cardiac toxicity. Dexamethasone also produces responses in 30% of patients.[109] Neither dexamethasone nor combination chemotherapy significantly improves the outcomes or prolongs survival beyond that seen with MP. Approximately 5% of patients treated with alkylating agents survive for 10 years or more.[62] These long-term survivors are predominantly patients without symptomatic cardiac involvement or peripheral neuropathy and with relatively normal renal function. Of note, thalidomide is currently being investigated in several clinical trials for patients with AL amyloidosis; preliminary results indicate that it is a difficult treatment for patients to tolerate, requiring frequent dose reductions and discontinuation of therapy (A. Dispenzieri, personal communication).

Autologous stem cell transplantation

Minimal progress had been made in reversing AL amyloidosis until the mid-1990s when patients first received dose-intensive intravenous melphalan and autologous hematopoietic stem cell transplantation (SCT).[110–112] The effectiveness of SCT in reversing the amyloid deposits in nearly two-thirds of surviving patients has been documented at numerous centers, and amyloid scans have demonstrated resorption of amyloid deposits subsequent to the reduction or elimination of the clonal plasma cell dyscrasia that is their root cause.[113,114] Such reversals result from 'turning off' the clonal plasma cell factory, making the fibril precursor protein. As the deposit process is halted and the deposits resorbed, both the performance status and the quality of life of AL amyloidosis patients can improve.[115]

The experience with SCT in AL amyloidosis is evolving and remains to some degree controversial.[116,117] Only 20% or so of newly diagnosed AL amyloidosis patients are eligible for SCT using standard cardiac and pulmonary criteria, and the increased selectivity required by the toxicity of SCT may reduce that number. With respect to treatment-related deaths, the average 100-day mortality of SCT in four single-center studies was 21% and in two multicenter studies 39%, so the risks of SCT in this population are considerable.[113,115,118–121] In addition, numerous deaths have been reported during stem cell mobilization, highlighting AL amyloidosis SCT

patients as unusually prone to adverse events.[115,119,120] Transplant-related mortality was high in these early studies because the visceral reserve of AL amyloidosis patients is compromised by deposition disease. AL amyloidosis patients commonly have renal, cardiac, hepatic, gastrointestinal, or neuropathic problems that make them distinct from other transplant candidates. That is, the majority of autologous transplant patients have hematologic malignancies but no visceral organ dysfunction, whereas the majority of AL amyloidosis SCT patients present with the opposite findings. Therefore, refinement of patient selection has become a priority.[116,117]

Transplant–related toxicities

The extent of amyloid organ involvement clearly accounts for much of the transplant-related mortality. In two similar single-center trials, those with two or fewer organ systems involved had significantly superior 100-day survival (81%, 25 of 31) compared with those who had more than two systems involved (25%, four of 12; $P < 0.01$, Fisher's exact test).[115,118] Similar results can be appreciated in an examination of the multicenter studies reported.[113,121] The causes of death included cardiac arrhythmias, the development of intractable hypotension and multiorgan failure, and gastrointestinal bleeding. Toxic responses to transplantation occur more frequently in patients with amyloidosis than in those who receive transplants for other indications. In our experience, the peri-transplant mortality in patients with cardiac amyloid and congestive heart failure, or a history of arrhythmias, syncope, or recurrent pleural effusions, approaches 100%, while patients with uncomplicated or well-compensated dominant cardiac amyloid and no other symptomatic organ involvement have a 50% peri-transplant mortality and 33% 1-year survival; whether this represents an improvement on standard therapy awaits randomized trials.

The frequency and grade of regimen-related toxicities (RRTs) are to some degree a function of the dose of intravenous melphalan, as indicated by the lower-grade toxicities experienced by AL amyloidosis SCT patients treated at 100 as opposed to 200 mg/m^2 of melphalan.[115,120] Of particular note, the gastrointestinal toxicity with 200 mg/m^2 of melphalan is striking, as are the higher rates of edema and bleeding. Indeed, as previously noted, gastrointestinal bleeding has been a significant cause of early mortality with SCT.[122] Gastrointestinal bleeding particularly is unusual after autologous transplant and, in frequency and severity, is unique to patients with AL amyloidosis. If amyloid extensively infiltrates the submucosa of the stomach or lower tract, the potential for severe mucositis with hemorrhage clearly must be anticipated, while neuropathic compromise of the enteric plexus often results in atony, persistent post-transplant nausea, and failure to thrive. For these reasons, pre-transplant planning and peri-transplant supportive care become essential. Recommendations with respect to peri-transplant management have recently been described in detail.[117] Pre-transplant patient evaluation should include a detailed review of gastrointestinal signs and symptoms, serial stool guaiacs, endoscopic studies to define pathology when indicated by symptoms or other findings, and a complete assessment of coagulation status.

Risk–adapted intravenous melphalan

At this time, it is reasonably clear that patients with more than two major organs involved or with advanced cardiomyopathy are at high risk of dying within the peri-transplant period and, therefore, are poor-risk candidates for SCT on high-dose regimens. At the same time, patients with one or two organs involved, and those with uncomplicated cardiac disease, remain candidates for stem cell transplantation on clinical trials. We recommend that the dose of intravenous melphalan be attenuated based on age and organ involvement. We call this a risk-adapted approach, based on the dose-related differences in toxicity observed in clinical trials (at 100 and 200 mg/m^2 of intravenous melphalan) and on age-related differences in survival.

A suggested risk-adapted schema is described in Table 27.4. Patients with one or two organs involved without dominant cardiac amyloid are considered 'good risk' and would receive 200 (if < 61 years old), 140 (if 61–71 years), or 100 mg/m^2 of intravenous melphalan (if >71 years). Patients with one or two organs involved and cardiac amyloid that is uncomplicated are considered 'intermediate risk', and would receive either 140 or 100 mg/m^2 based on age with a cut-off at 61 years of age. It is also reasonable to provide more intensive management for patients in this category, as some have done, in a monitored setting. Patients with more than two organs involved or advanced cardiomyopathy are considered

Table 27.4 *A suggested risk-adapted approach to stem cell transplantation for AL amyloidosis*

Good risk (any age; all criteria met)
- No cardiac involvement
- Only one or two major organs involved
- Creatinine clearance ⩾51 mL/minute

Intermediate risk (age <71)
- One or two organs involved
- May have compensated cardiac involvement
- May have renal involvement with creatinine clearance <51 mL/minute

Poor risk (either criteria)
- More than two major organs involved
- Advanced cardiac amyloid

'poor risk' (i.e. not SCT candidates) and would be treated with therapies such as MP. There will be patients whose disease defies these simple categories, for example patients with renal insufficiency only but with creatinine clearances less than 50 mL/minute, or those with dominant hepatic disease and a rising bilirubin. Such patients are at higher than average risk for organ failure with SCT and our recommendations will make the decision to offer SCT no less difficult.

Blood stem cell mobilization

Owing to the ease of collection and quicker engraftment observed with blood stem cells over autologous bone marrow, most of the high-dose chemotherapy experience in AL amyloidosis is with blood stem cells. Contamination with clonotypic plasma cells has been demonstrated in the components from patients with amyloidosis undergoing leukapheresis after growth factor priming.[123,124] CD34+ cell selection is possible in these patients with adequate yields for successful engraftment, but the effect of having a positively purged apheresis product on the disease course remains unknown.[124] Two-thirds of patients had amyloid identified in the bone marrow by Congo red staining, and AL amyloidosis depositions did not obviously impair stem cell mobilization.[115] Currently, granulocyte colony-stimulating factor (G-CSF) mobilization is used at the majority of centers transplanting AL amyloidosis patients regularly and can be considered the standard approach to mobilization in this population; in addition, because of the advantages associated with prompt myeloid and thrombopoietic recovery, we recommend that the optimal dose of CD34+ cells in AL amyloidosis SCT patients be 5–10 × 10^6 CD34+ cells/kg.[117]

Given the impaired visceral reserve, vasculopathy, and coagulopathies associated with AL amyloidosis, it was predictable that RRT would be more prominent in AL amyloidosis SCT patients. It was not expected, however, that there would be significant toxicity associated with stem cell mobilization and collection.[115,119] Deaths have been reported during mobilization of patients with symptomatic cardiac amyloid or multisystem disease, at centers employing both moderate doses of cyclophosphamide (e.g. 2.5 g/m^2) and using growth factors alone. During mobilization with G-CSF (16 μg/kg per day × 5 days), we and others on rare occasions observed a sometimes fatal though unexplained syndrome associated with progressive hypoxia and hypotension unresponsive to supportive measures. It can occur in patients without cardiac involvement and may be due to a combination of the effects of G-CSF, activated platelets returned during leukapheresis, pulmonary shunting, cytokines, or mediators of septic hemodynamics.[125] Currently, to minimize the risk of such toxicities, we recommend that G-CSF dosing for mobilization be given twice a day in lower doses (6 μg/kg every 12 hours) with collection beginning on day 5, 2–4 hours after the morning dose of G-CSF.[126]

Immune recovery post–SCT

The immune recovery after autologous SCT for AL amyloidosis has been studied in a small number of patients.[127] Peripheral blood counts of T-helper cells (CD4+) were found to be significantly decreased and T-cell function depressed at 3 months following SCT in patients with AL amyloidosis amyloidosis, unlike T-suppressor (CD8+) cell, monocyte, B-cell, and natural killer (NK) cell counts as well as levels of B-cell functional activity, which return to baseline. These outcomes are similar to those reported for other patients with hematologic diseases after autologous SCT, although the promptness of the recovery of humoral immunity is somewhat atypical.[128]

Current clinical research

It is apparent that continued efforts to treat AL amyloidosis with SCT will depend on clinical trials that evaluate approaches designed to make SCT less morbid or to answer specific questions of interest. The risk-adapted approach we suggest may expand the pool of AL amyloidosis SCT candidates, and reduce the morbidity and mortality associated with SCT for AL amyloidosis. Currently, there is a multicenter phase III trial under way under the aegis of a French myeloma intergroup, and AL amyloidosis patients are being randomized to receive high-dose melphalan with SCT or oral melphalan and dexamethasone. There are also phase II trials looking at tandem transplant under way at several American centers, and there are phase II Eastern Clinical Oncology Group (ECOG) and Food and Drug Administration (FDA) orphan-drug sponsored SCT trials that have just been completed but have yet to be reported fully. The preliminary report of the latter, a randomized prospective phase II trial in which newly diagnosed patients received either two cycles of MP then SCT, or SCT immediately, has recently been presented. The trial demonstrates that such patients, eligible by minimal criteria for SCT, did not appear to benefit from initial therapy with MP and that, for patients with cardiac involvement, there was a survival advantage to receiving prompt SCT with intravenous melphalan. The caveat is that the overall treatment-related mortality and 1-year mortality attributed to progression of disease was nearly 40%. Median survivals for both groups had not been reached with nearly 4 years median follow-up, indicating that the median survival for newly diagnosed AL patients well enough to undergo autologous SCT probably exceeds 5 years (Fig. 27.4b).

Stem cell transplantation for AL amyloidosis is effective in a minority of patients, such as those with limited organ disease and no significant cardiac involvement. The response rates of the plasma cell dyscrasia and amyloid-related organ involvement with SCT are higher than those seen in patients treated with traditional MP, and patients achieving complete remissions of the plasma cell dyscrasia can experience marked functional improvement and usually survive more than 5 years. However, the morbidity and mortality are clearly higher than in patients with multiple myeloma or other hematologic malignancies undergoing autologous SCT. We anticipate that improved patient selection and peri-transplant management, and adoption of a risk-adapted approach to melphalan dosing based on age and distribution of disease, will accelerate the acquisition of the generalized expertise needed for the conduct of multicenter phase II SCT trials and eventually phase III trials.

Solid organ transplantation

It is perhaps the least noted irony of systemic amyloidosis that patients with hereditary variants in most developed countries are deemed useful candidates for curative solid organ (i.e. liver) transplantation in part because of the potential for 'domino' transplants.[130,131] That is, the patient's native ATTR-producing liver is used as a graft in another recipient. Ironically, at the same time, the use of solid organ transplantation (liver, heart, and kidney) in patients with AL amyloidosis is usually deemed poor risk because of the likely accumulation of amyloid in the grafted organ.[132] There have been numerous patients who have successfully undergone cardiac allograft and then SCT; the feasibility of this approach is established and a phase II trial needs to be performed to demonstrate safety and efficacy in a systematic fashion.[133–135] On the other hand, renal transplantation has been shown to be effective and renal allografts survive for lengthy periods in many recipients especially after SCT.[136] A relevant question in AL amyloidosis patients who present with dialysis-dependent renal failure is whether simultaneous renal allograft and autologous SCT might permit a reduction in the need for immunosuppressive medications and also reduce the incidence of renal graft rejection. Such a phase I trial would be appropriate and answer a question relevant to renal transplant in general.

New approaches

All chemotherapeutic approaches to AL amyloidosis treat the disease by attacking the source of production of the precursor protein, i.e. the clonal plasma cells, and by seeking to reduce their number. New approaches currently under investigation include treatments aimed at mobilizing or inhibiting amyloid deposits, such as amyloid-reactive antibodies, iodinated doxorubicin, and competitive inhibitors of SAP-binding to amyloid fibrils.[137–140]

The development of amyloid-reactive antibodies was based on the premise that an immune reaction to amyloid deposits might help to stimulate fibril disassembly.[137,141] Amyloid tumors formed by injection of human AL amyloid extracts into the skin of healthy mice were resolved within several weeks by an immune-mediated mechanism involving the generation of antiamyloid antibodies that recognized antigenic determinants common to AL amyloid fibrils. Mice were then immunized with human amyloid fibrils to generate such antibodies. The antiamyloid reagent generated recognized a β-pleated structure common to AL amyloidosis fibrils. The therapeutic potential of this antibody was demonstrated by injecting it into mice in which human amyloid tumors had been induced and confirming the occurrence of 'amyloidolysis' as compared with untreated animals. The antibody localized within the amyloid tumors and caused rapid resolution of this material by an infiltration of neutrophils. The manufacture of a human chimeric form of the antibody is currently under way, but the propensity for causing neutrophilic infiltrates and inflammation will likely raise concerns among those designing the phase I trial for its use.

Serendipitously an amyloid physician in Italy noted that administration of a new anthracycline anticancer drug, 4-iodo-4-deoxydoxorubicin (I-DOX), to a patient with AL amyloidosis amyloidosis resulted in rapid clinical improvement.[138,139] Subsequently, Dr Merlini led the investigation into the mechanism of action of I-DOX and further tested its activity clinically. A phase I trial was conducted, and significant responses were seen in a small number of patients, unrelated to the cytotoxicity of I-DOX or its effect on the underlying plasma cell dyscrasia and M-protein. The most impressive responses were seen in patients with soft-tissue or muscular bulky amyloid deposits; no significant recovery of amyloid-related organ dysfunction was observed. Of note, I-DOX was cleared from the plasma faster in amyloid patients than in those receiving the drug in clinical trials for cancer, a phenomenon consistent with I-DOX binding to amyloid deposits. Subsequent experiments confirmed the specific targeting to AL amyloidosis types of amyloid fibrils *in vitro* and *in vivo*. In initial phase II trials, I-DOX had limited activity and a phase I–II dose-finding trial is currently under way.[142,143]

The search for inhibitors of amyloid fibril formation continues. Some have studied the interaction of compounds with constituents of amyloid deposits in order to stimulate protelytic breakdown and resorption. In the murine model for AA amyloidosis, several small molecule anionic sulfates and sulfonates, such as polyvinylsulfonate, were shown to inhibit fibril formation and lead to resorption of amyloid deposits.[20] Also, the effects of SAP on amyloid fibrils have been evaluated in numerous ways; for example, mice with targeted deletion of the SAP gene showed reduced induction of AA amyloidosis and, in other experiments, the displacement of SAP from fibrils enhanced proteolytic degradation. Hence, Drs Pepys and Hawkins proposed that such molecular dissection of the deposits might be a useful therapeutic target.[36] Using a *tour de force* of modern pharmacologic methods, a palindromic compound Ro 63-3300 was identified that literally turned the SAP dimer inside out, depleting serum SAP, and making it unavailable sterically and quantitatively for binding to amyloid fibrils.[140] Recently, preliminary results of the first phase I trial of continuous infusion of a congener of this molecule (Ro 63-8695 or R-1-[6-[R-2-carboxypyrrolidin-1-y1]-6-oxohexanoyl]pyrrolidin-2-carboxylic acid (CPHPC)) were reported and CPHPC infusion was well tolerated and without toxicity.[140] Further work with CPHPC is awaited with great anticipation.

Monitoring the responses to therapy

The primary endpoint of clinical trials in this disease should remain survival from diagnosis. It will not benefit AL amyloidosis patients if an effective therapy is found – even one that accelerates resorption of amyloid from tissue depots – if the process of resorption itself is excessively morbid and frequently causes sudden death, e.g. because of intractable arrhythmias. Therefore, one cannot overemphasize the importance of designing and conducting phase II trials with explicit criteria of treatment-related mortality and stopping rules, and phase III trials that include patients representative of the population of AL amyloidosis patients. In such instances, the endpoint of survival should maintain primacy.

Other important endpoints in clinical trials have also usually included the response of amyloid-related organ disease and the response of the plasma cell dyscrasia.[104,105,115,118] The criteria for organ-disease response to therapy have been based on non-invasive testing and have usually been described as improved, stable, or worsened. Biopsy-based criteria do not exist and the SAP scan, although likely an ideal way to monitor response to therapy, is of limited availability. Although scans using radiolabeled aprotinin have been shown in pilot studies to provide useful information regarding amyloid-related cardiac disease, such scans have not become widely available.[144] Therefore, we are left with non-invasive measures to evaluate response of amyloid-disease to therapy. Interestingly, a direct link between organ-system improvement and survival has been described in numerous series, but a statistical algorithm for correlating improvement in specific organs with improvement in quality of life or survival has yet to be completely defined.

For patients with cardiac involvement, an improvement or response to therapy is defined as a decrease of ≥ 2 mm in mean left ventricular wall thickness in patients with baseline wall thickness >11 mm, or a decrease in two classes in NYHA class (i.e. from 3 to 1). Stable disease is defined as no evidence of clinical response and no progressive disease by clinical, electrocardiographic, and echocardiographic evaluation. Progression of cardiac involvement post-therapy is defined by worsening clinical signs or symptoms, worsening NYHA class (i.e. from 1 to 3), or an increase of ≥ 2 mm in mean left ventricular wall thickness in a patient with baseline wall thickness ≤ 11 mm. For patients with renal involvement, an improvement or response to therapy is defined as a 50% decrease in daily proteinuria without progressive renal insufficiency, and for those with hepatic involvement improvement was defined as a decrease in liver span of ≥ 2 cm with a concomitant decrease of alkaline phosphatase by 50%. For patients with neuropathic involvement, improvement is defined as normalization of orthostatic vital signs and symptoms, and resolution of gastric atony and of abnormal findings on neurologic examination. Stabilization or worsening of renal, hepatic, and neuropathic involvement at most centers is defined by consensus based upon clinical evaluation and appropriate non-invasive tests.[115]

Scoring the response of the clonal plasma cell disease to therapy has recently become more complicated owing to the availability of the free light-chain assay. This assay is likely several logs more sensitive than immunofixation in clinical practice. Hence, the definition of a complete hematologic response measured objectively by negative immunofixation electrophoresis of serum and urine has been challenged. After stem cell transplantation, for example, it has frequently been observed that some patients experience worsening of amyloid-related organ disease despite apparent elimination of the monoclonal protein by immunofixation, and vice versa.[145] Most but not all of the patients who experience complete hematologic responses also manifest improvement of amyloid. It is now reasonably obvious that the resolution of amyloid disease in AL amyloidosis patients after therapy is a function of at least two variables: the serum free light-chain concentration and the 'amyloidogenicity' of the free light chain. As a rule of thumb, reductions of the free light chain that exceed 50% of baseline are likely to lead to improvements in amyloid disease and probably prolong survival.

Standard criteria for hematologic responses have been modeled after myeloma response scoring. Patients whose clonal plasma disease becomes undetectable by immunofixation and whose marrow normalizes with immunostaining for plasma cell antigens have been considered complete responders; they have no evidence of the previously identified clonal monoclonal bands on immunofixation and normal bone marrow biopsies. Patients achieving at least a 50% reduction in baseline measures of plasma cell activity have been considered partial responders. Patients not achieving either of these categories of response have been considered nonresponders from a plasma cell dyscrasia viewpoint, no matter the degree of response from an organ-involvement viewpoint. Patients who were either complete or partial responders at prior follow-up evaluation(s) but who show evidence of recurrent clonal plasma cell activity at a subsequent follow-up visit are considered in relapse.

With these standard criteria, the possibility existed, then, for some patients to respond with remission of amyloid disease but with only a partial or no response in detectable plasma cell activity. This possibility could occur if a subclone of the plasma cell clone were responsible for making the fibril precursor light chain, and the treatment eliminates the subclone, leaving the parent clone only modestly reduced. The possibility also exists, as previously noted, that small numbers of clonal plasma cells could persist below the level of detection by immunofixation, making a strongly 'amyloidogenic' precursor light chain, and could lead to progression of amyloid-related disease despite apparent complete hematologic response. Therefore, in order to be confident in the monitoring of response to therapy, what are needed are two sensitive tools to be used at diagnosis: the free light-chain assay and an *in vitro* 'amyloidogenicity assay' quantifying the propensity of a patient's light chain to self-assemble and cause *in vivo* disease. We now have one tool, the free light-chain assay, and can use it to monitor therapy. We need to develop and validate the second tool.[146,147]

CONCLUSION

AL amyloidosis remains a disease for which our tests, treatments, and knowledge continue to be deficient in critical ways. The recent availability of the free light-chain assay promises to improve diagnostic testing and the ability to monitor response to therapy. In other respects, our approaches to evaluating amyloid-related organ disease and following patients in therapy have not significantly and extensively changed for years. Developing tests for grading the amyloid-forming potential of specific light chains as well as nuclear or other scans for assessing all of the multiple organs involved with amyloid disease are goals for the future. Nevertheless, survival remains the primary endpoint for patients as well as clinical investigators. Stem cell transplant for AL amyloidosis remains effective in younger patients and those with limited disease; hopefully, it can be risk-adapted in order to optimize benefit and limit mortality. It will remain a controversial therapy until there is a phase II trial showing low transplant-related mortality or a phase III trial defining greater benefit. Solid organ transplantation is no less controversial in this rare disorder; hopefully, the combined use of stem cell and solid organ transplantation will be developed for systematic assessment in a clinical trial. New drugs to inhibit deposits from forming or to mobilize them from organs provide exciting prospects and are entering clinical trials at this time. Finally, as we come to understand more fully the basis of the cellular and organ-specific toxicities of the intermediate forms of fibril precursor light chains, we hope that novel cytoprotective pathways are discerned and that the promise of a simple effective drug treatment is fulfilled. The ideal treatment of AL amyloidosis in the future will likely involve a combination of drugs aimed at eliminating the supply of fibril precursor light chains, inhibiting light chain self-assembly into fibrils, and safely enhancing resorption of existing fibrillar deposits.

KEY POINTS

- The clinical manifestations of AL amyloidosis are protean.
- AL amyloidosis is both a plasma cell dyscrasia and a deposition disease.
- The fibril precursor protein is usually immunoglobulin light chain, more often λ than κ (λ:κ 3:1).
- Median survival is about 2 years with standard therapy.
- Survival is a function of cardiac involvement.
- Selected patients are eligible for stem cell transplant.
- Stem cell transplant is the most effective therapy but has high treatment-related toxicity.
- New therapies now in clinical trials may reverse amyloid deposits.

REFERENCES

● = Key primary paper
◆ = Major review article
* = Paper that represents the first formal publication of a management guideline

◆1. Gillmore JD, Hawkins PN, Pepys MB. Amyloidosis: a review of recent diagnostic and therapeutic developments. *Br J Haematol* 1997; **99**:245–56.

◆2. Falk RH, Comenzo RL, Skinner M. The systemic amyloidoses. *N Engl J Med* 1997; **337**:898–909.

3. Merlini G, Bellotti. Mechanisms of disease: molecular mechanisms of amyloidosis. *N Engl J Med 2003*; **339**:583–96.

4. Kyle RA. Amyloidosis: a convoluted story. *Br J Haematol* 2001; **114**:529–38.

●5. Virchow VR. Über eine im Gehirn and Rückenmark des Menschen auf gefund eine Substanz mit chemischen Reaction der Cellulose. *Virchows Arch Pathol Anat* 1854; **6**:135–8.

●6. Divry P, Florkin M. Sur les propréés optiques de l'amyloïde. *C R Seances Soc Biol* 1927; **97**:1808–10.

●7. Cohen AS, Calkins E. Electron microscopic observations on a fibrous component in amyloid of diverse origins. *Nature* 1959; **183**:1202–3.

8. Shirahama T, Cohen AS. High resolution electron microscopic analysis of the amyloid fibril. *J Cell Biol* 1967; **33**:679–708.

9. Bonar L, Cohen AS, Skinner MM. Characterization of the amyloid fibril as a cross-beta protein. *Proc Soc Exp Biol Med* 1969; **131**:1373–5.

●10. Glenner GG, Terry W, Harada M, Isersky C, Page D. Amyloid fibril proteins: proof of homology with immunoglobulin light chains by sequence analyses. *Science* 1971; **172**:1150–1.

11. Benditt EP, Eriksen N, Hermodson MA, Ericsson LH. The major proteins of human and monkey amyloid substance: common properties including unusual N-terminal amino acid sequences. *FEBS Lett* 1971; **19**:169–73.

12. Costa PP, Figueira AS, Bravo FR. Amyloid fibril protein related to prealbumin in familial amyloidotic polyneuropathy. *Proc Natl Acad Sci USA* 1978; **75**:4499–503.

13. Westermark P, Araki S, Benson MD, Cohen AS, Frangione B, Masters CL, *et al.* Nomenclature of amyloid fibril proteins: report from the meeting of the International Nomenclature Committee on Amyloidosis, August 8–9, 1998, part 1. *Amyloid* 1999; **6**:63–6.

14. Kelly JW. Towards an understanding of amyloidosis. *Nat Struct Biol* 2002; **9**:323–5.

15. Ferreira ST, De Felice FG. Protein dynamics, folding and misfolding: from basic chemistry to human conformational diseases. *FEBS Lett* 2001; **498**:129–34.

◆16. Wetzel R. Domain stability in immunoglobulin light chain deposition disorders. *Adv Protein Chem* 1997; **50**:183–242.

●17. Stevens F, Pokkuluri PR, Schiffer M. Protein conformation and disease: pathological consequences of analogous mutations in homologous proteins. *Biochemistry* 2000; **39**:15 291–6.

18. Eliezer D, Kutluay E, Bussell R, Browne G. Conformational properties of α-Synuclein in its free and lipid-associated states. *J Mol Biol* 2001; **307**:1061–73.

●19. Klabunde T, Petrassi HM, Oza VB, Raman P, Kelly JW, Sacchettini JC. Rational design of potent human transthyretin amyloid disease inhibitors. *Nat Struct Biol* 2000; **7**:312–21.

20. Kisilevsky R, Lemieux LJ, Fraser PE, Kong X, Hultin P, Szarek W. Arresting amyloidosis in vivo using small-molecule anionic sulphonates or sulphates: implication for Alzheimer's disease. *Nat Med* 1995; **1**:143–8.

◆21. Dhodapkar MV, Merlini G, Solomon A. Biology and therapy of immunoglobulin deposition diseases. *Hematol Oncol Clin North Am* 1997; **11**:89–110.

◆22. Gertz MA, Lacy MQ, Dispenzieri A. Amyloidosis. *Hematol Oncol Clin North Am* 1999; **13**:1211–33.

23. Buxbaum J. Mechanisms of disease: monoclonal immunoglobulin deposition. *Hematol Oncol Clin North Am* 1992; **6**:323–46.

24. Benson MD. Amyloidosis. In: Scriver CR, Beaudet AL, Sly WS, Valle D (eds) *The metabolic and molecular bases of inherited disease*, 7th edn, Vol. 3. New York: McGraw-Hill, 1995:4159–91.

◆25. Bellotti V, Mangione P, Merlini G. Review: immunoglobulin light chain amyloidosis is the archetype of structural and pathogenic variability. *J Struct Biol* 2000; **130**:280–9.

26. Putnam FW, Whitley EJ, Paul C, Davidson JN. Amino acid sequence of a kappa Bence-Jones protein from a case of primary amyloidosis. *Biochemistry* 1973; **12**:3763–80.

27. Omtvedt LA, Haavik S, Hounsell EF, Barsett H, Slette K. The carbohydrate structure of the amyloid immunoglobulin light chain protein EPS. *Int J Exp Clin Invest* 1995; **2**:150–8.

28. Ramstad HM, Sletten K, Husby G. The amino acid sequence and carbohydrate composition of an immunoglobulin kappa light chain amyloid fibril protein (AL) of variable subgroup I. *Amyloid* 1995; **2**:223–8.

29. Westmark P, Sletten K, Natvig JB. Structure and antigenic behavior of kappa immunoglobulin light-chain amyloid proteins. *Acta Pathol Microbiol Scand* 1981; **89**:99–203.

30. Liepnieks JJ, Benson MD, Dulet FE. Comparison of the amino acid sequences of ten kappa I amyloid proteins. In: Natvig JB, Forre O, Husby G, Husebekk A, Skogen B, Sletten K, *et al.* (eds) *Amyloid and amyloidosis*. Boston: Dordrecht, 1990:153–6.

31. Pick AI, Kratzin HD, Barnikol-Watanabe S, Hilschmann N. Complete amino acid sequence of AL amyloidosis Bence Jones protein POL of the lambda I subclass. In: Natvig JB, Forre O, Husby G, Husebekk A, Skogen B, Sletten K, *et al.* (eds) *Amyloid and amyloidosis*. Boston: Dordrecht, 1990:177–80.

32. Wally J, Kica G, Zhang Y, Ericsson T, Connors L, Benson M, *et al.* Identification of a novel substitution in the constant region of a gene coding for an amyloidogenic kappa 1 light chain. *Biochim Biophys Acta Molec Basis Dis* 1999; **1454**:49–57.

33. Hurle MR, Helms LR, Li L, Chan W, Wetzel R. A role for destabilizing amino acid replacements in light chain amyloidosis. *Proc Natl Acad Sci USA* 1994; **91**:5446–50.

◆34. Stevens FJ, Myatt EA, Chang CH, Westholm F, Eulitz M, Weiss D, *et al.* A molecular model for self-assembly of amyloid fibrils from immunoglobulin light chains. *Biochemistry* 1995; **34**:10697–702.

●35. Skinner M, Cohen AS, Shirahama T, Cathcart ES. P-component (pentagonal unit) of amyloid: isolation, characterization and sequence analysis. *J Lab Clin Med* 1974; **84**:604–14.

36. Tennent GA, Lovat LB, Pepys MB. Serum amyloid P component prevents proteolysis of the amyloid fibrils of Alzheimer disease and systemic amyloidosis. *Proc Natl Acad Sci USA* 1995; **92**:4299–303.

●37. Kyle RA, Gertz MA. Primary systemic amyloidosis: clinical and laboratory features in 474 cases. *Semin Hematol* 1995; **32**:45–59.

●38. Comenzo RL, Zhang Y, Martinez C, Osman K, Herrera G. The tropism of organ involvement in primary systemic amyloidosis: contributions of Ig V_L germline gene use and plasma cell burden. *Blood* 2001; **98**:714–20.

39. Abraham RS, Price-Troska DL, Gertz MA, Kyle RA, Fonseca R. Association of rearranged light chain variable region genes with organ tropism and light chain associated (AL) amyloidosis. *Blood* 2001; **98**:151b.

●40. Perfetti V, Casarini S, Palladini G, Vignarelli M, Klersy C, Diegoli M, *et al.* Analysis of V-J expression in plasma cells from primary (AL) amyloidosis and normal bone marrow identifies 3r (III) as a new amyloid-associated germline gene segment. *Blood* 2002; **100**:948–53.

41. Stevens PW, Raffen R, Hanson DK, Deng Y, Berrios-Hammond M, Westholm F, *et al.* Recombinant immunoglobulin variable domains generated from synthetic genes provide a system for in vitro characterization of light-chain amyloid proteins. *Protein Sci* 1995; **4**:421–32.

42. Schiffer M. Molecular anatomy and pathologic expression of antibody light chains. *Am J Pathol* 1996; **148**:1339–44.

43. Schormann N, Murell JR, Liepnieks JJ, Benson MD. Tertiary structure of an amyloid immunoglobulin light chain protein: a proposed model for amyloid fibril formation. *Proc Natl Acad Sci USA* 1995; **92**:9490–9.

●44. Solomon A, Weiss DT, Kattine AA. Nephrotoxic potential of Bence Jones proteins. *N Engl J Med* 1991; **324**:1845–51.

45. Stevens FJ. Four structural risk factors identify most fibril-forming light chains. *Amyloid* 2000; **7**:200–7.

46. Raffen R, Dieckman LJ, Szpunar M, Wunschl C, Pokkuluri P, Dave P, *et al.* Physicochemical consequences of amino acid variations that contribute to fibril formation by immunoglobulin light chains. *Protein Sci* 1999; **8**:509–17.

47. Ionescu-Zanetti C, Khurana R, Gillespie JR, Petrick J, Trabachino L, Minert L, *et al.* Monitoring the assembly of Ig light-chain amyloid fibrils by atomic force microscopy. *Proc Natl Acad Sci USA* 1999; **96**:13 175–9.

48. Stevens FJ, Kiselevsky R. Immunoglobulin light chains, glycosaminoglycans, and amyloid. *Cell Mol Life Sci* 2000; **57**:441–9.

49. Buxbaum J. Mechanisms of disease: monoclonal immunoglobulin deposition. Amyloidosis, light chain deposition disease, and light and heavy chain deposition disease. *Hematol Oncol Clin North Am* 1992; **6**:323–46.

50. Perfetti V, Vignarelli MC, Casarini S, Ascari E, Merlini G. Biological features of the clone involved in primary amyloidosis (AL). *Leukemia* 2001; **15**:196–202.

51. MacLennan IC, Liu YJ, Oldfield S, Zhang J, Lane PJ. The evolution of B-cell clones. *Curr Top Microbiol Immunol* 1990; **159**:37–63.

52. Perfetti V, Ubbiali P, Vignarelli MC, Diegoli M, Fasani R, Stoppini M, *et al.* Evidence that amyloidogenic light chains undergo antigen-driven selection. *Blood* 1998; **91**:2948–54.

53. Sahota S, Leo R, Hamblin T, Stevenson FK. Myeloma VL and VH gene sequences reveal a complementary imprint of antigen selection in tumor cells. *Blood* 1997; **89**:219–26.

54. Kosmas C, Stamatopoulos K, Stavroyianni N, Zoi K, Belessi C, Vinion N, *et al.* Origin and diversification of the clonogenic cell in multiple myeloma: lessons from the immunoglobulin repertoire. *Leukemia* 2000; **14**:1718–26.

55. Kosmas C, Viniou N-A, Stamatopoulos K, Courtenay-Luck N, Papadaki T, Kollia P, *et al.* Analysis of the light chain variable region in multiple myeloma. *Br J Haematol* 1996; **94**:306–17.

●56. Solomon A, Frangione B, Franklin EC. Bence-Jones proteins and light chains of immunoglobulins. Preferential association of the VλVI subgroup of human light chains with amyloidosis (AL). *J Clin Invest* 1982; **70**:453–60.

57. Hayman SR, Bailey RJ, Jalal SM, Ahmann G, Dispenzieri A, Gertz M, *et al.* Translocations involving the immunoglobulin heavy-chain locus are possible early genetic events in patients with primary systemic amyloidosis. *Blood* 2001; **98**:2266–8.

58. Harrison CJ, Mazzullo H, Ross FM, Cheung K, Gerrard G, Harewood L, *et al.* Translocations of 14q32 and deletions of 13q14 are common chromosomal abnormalities in systemic amyloidosis. *Br J Haematol* 2002; **117**:427–35.

59. Khurana R, Gillespie JR, Talapatra A, Minert L, Ionescu-Zanetti C, Millett I, *et al.* Partially folded intermediates as critical precursors of light chain amyloid fibrils and amorphous aggregates. *Biochemistry* 2001; **40**:3525–35.

●60. Kyle RA, Linos A, Beard CM, Linke R, Gertz M, O'Fallon W, *et al.* Incidence and natural history of primary systemic amyloidosis in Olmstead County, Minnesota, 1950 through 1989. *Blood* 1992; **79**:1817–22.

●61. Cueto-Garcia L, Reeder GS, Kyle RA, Wood D, Seward J, Naessens J, *et al.* Echocardiographic findings in systemic amyloidosis: spectrum of cardiac involvement and relation to survival. *J Am Coll Cardiol* 1985; **6**:737–43.

62. Kyle RA, Gertz MA, Greipp PR, Witzig T, Lust J, Lacy M, *et al.* Long-term survival (10 years or more) in 30 patients with primary amyloidosis. *Blood* 1999; **93**:1062–6.

63. Tawara S, Nakazato M, Kangawa K, Matsuo H, Araki S. Identification of amyloid prealbumin variant in familial amyloidotic polyneuropathy (Japanese type). *Biochem Biophys Res Commun* 1983; **116**:880–8.

64. Saraiva MJM, Birken S, Costa PP, Goodman DS. Amyloid fibril protein in familial amyloidotic polyneuropathy, Portuguese type: definition of molecular abnormality in transthyretin (prealbumin). *J Clin Invest* 1984; **74**:104–19.

65. Benson MD, Clemicki T. Transthyretin amyloidosis. *Amyloid* 1996; **3**:44–56.

66. Skinner M. Amyloidosis. In: Lichtenstein LM, Fauci AS (eds) *Current therapy in allergy, immunology, and rheumatology*, 5th edn. St Louis: Mosby-Year Book, 1996:235–40.

●67. Jacobson DR, Pastore RD, Yaghoubian R, Kane I, Gallo G, Buck FS, *et al.* Variant-sequence transthyretin (isoleucine 122) in late-onset cardiac amyloidosis in black Americans. *N Engl J Med* 1997; **336**:466–73.

68. Gertz MA, Kyle RA. Secondary systemic amyloidosis: response and survival in 64 patients. *Medicine (Baltimore)* 1991; **70**:246–56.

69. Gertz MA, Kyle RA, O'Fallon WM. Dialysis support of patients with primary systemic amyloidosis. A study of 211 patients. *Arch Intern Med* 1992; **152**:2245–50.

70. Dember LM, Sanchorawala V, Seldin DC, Wright G, LaValley M, Berk J, *et al.* Effect of dose-intensive intravenous melphalan and autologous blood stem-cell transplantation on AL amyloidosis-associated renal disease. *Ann Intern Med* 2001; **134**:746–53.

◆71. Merlini G. Treatment of primary amyloidosis. *Semin Hematol* 1995; **32**:60–79.

72. Dubrey S, Pollak A, Skinner M, Falk RH. Atrial thrombi occurring during sinus rhythm in cardiac amyloidosis: evidence for atrial electromechanical dissociation. *Br Heart J* 1995; **74**:541–4.

73. Chamarthi B, Dubrey SW, Cha K, Skinner M, Falk RH. Features and prognosis of exertional syncope in light-chain associated AL amyloidosis cardiac amyloidosis. *Am J Cardiol* 1997; **80**:242–5.

74. Falk RH, Plehn JF, Deering T, Schick EC Jr, Boinay P, Rubinow A, *et al.* Sensitivity and specificity of the echocardiographic features of cardiac amyloidosis. *Am J Cardiol* 1987; **59**:418–22.

75. Friedman S, Janowitz HD. Systemic amyloidosis and the gastrointestinal tract. *Gastroenterol Clin North Am* 1998; **27**:595–614.

76. Tada S, Iida M, Yao T, Kitamoto T, Yao T, Fujishima M. Intestinal pseudo-obstruction in patients with amyloidosis: clinicopathologic differences between chemical types of amyloid protein. *Gut* 1993; **34**:1412–17.

77. Gertz MA, Kyle RA. Hepatic amyloidosis: clinical appraisal in 77 patients. *Hepatology* 1997; **25**:118–21.

78. Sandberg-Gertz'en H, Ericzon BG, Blombert B. Primary amyloidosis with spontaneous splenic rupture, cholestasis, and liver failure treated with emergency liver transplantation. *Am J Gastroenterol* 1998; **93**:2254–8.

79. Rajkumar SV, Gertz MA, Kyle RA. Prognosis of patients with primary systemic amyloidosis who present with dominant neuropathy. *Am J Med* 1998; **104**:232–7.

80. Lim JK, Lacy MQ, Kurtin PJ, Kyle RA, Gertz MA. Pulmonary marginal zone lymphoma of MALT type as a cause of localized pulmonary amyloidosis. *J Clin Pathol* 2001; **54**:642–6.

81. Gillmore JD, Hawkins PN. Amyloidosis and the respiratory tract. *Thorax* 1999; **54**:444–51.

82. Libbey CA, Skinner M, Cohen AS. Use of abdominal fat tissue aspirate in the diagnosis of systemic amyloidosis. *Arch Intern Med* 1983; **143**:1549–52.

83. Duston MA, Skinner M, Shirahama T, Cohen AS. Diagnosis of amyloidosis by abdominal fat aspiration: analysis of four years' experience. *Am J Med* 1987; **82**:412–14.

84. Westermark GT, Johnson KH, Westermark P. Staining methods for identification of amyloid in tissue. *Meth Enzymol* 1999; **309**:3–25.

85. Linke RP. Immunochemical typing of amyloid deposits after microextraction from biopsies. *Appl Pathol* 1985; **3**:18–28.

86. Van de Kaa CA, Hol PR, Huber J, Linke R, Kooiker C, Grays E. Diagnosis of the type of amyloid in paraffin wax embedded tissue sections using antisera against human and animal amyloid proteins. *Virchows Arch A Pathol Anat Histopathol* 1986; **408**:649–64.

87. Picken MM, Pelton K, Frangione B, Gallo G. Primary amyloidosis A: immunohistochemical and biochemical characterization. *Am J Pathol* 1987; **129**:536–42.

88. Ršcken C, Schwotzer EB, Linke RP, Saeger W. The classification of amyloid deposits in clinicopathological practice. *Histopathology* 1996; **29**:325–35.

89. Kaplan B, Yakar S, Kumar A. Immunochemical characterization of amyloid in diagnostic biopsy tissue. *Amyloid* 1997; **4**:80–6.

90. Kaplan B, Vidal R, Kumar A, Ghiso J, Gallo G. Immunochemical microanalysis of amyloid proteins in fine-needle aspirates of abdominal fat. *Am J Clin Pathol* 1999; **112**:403–7.

91. Olsen KE, Sletten K, Westermark P. The use of subcutaneous fat tissue for amyloid typing by enzyme linked immunosorbent assay. *Am J Clin Pathol* 1999; **111**:355–62.

92. Kyle RA, Katzmann JA. Immunochemical characterization of immunoglobulins. In: Roos NR, de Macario EC, Folds JD, Lane HC, Nakamura RM (eds) *Manual of clinical laboratory immunology*. Washington, DC: ASM Press, 1997:156–78.

●93. Bradwell A, Carr-Smith HD, Mead GP, Tang L, Showell P, Drayson M, *et al.* Highly sensitive automated immunoassay for immunoglobulin free light chains in serum and urine. *Clin Chem* 2001; **47**:673–80.

94. Drayson M, Tang LX, Drew R, Mead G, Carr-Smith H, Bradwell A. Serum free light-chain measurements for identifying and monitoring patients with nonsecretory multiple myeloma. *Blood* 2001; **97**:2900–2.

●95. Hawkins PN, Gallimore R, Bradwell AR, Smith L, Lachmann HJ. Highly sensitive automated immunoassay for free immunoglobulin light-chains in diagnosis and follow-up of AL amyloidosis. In: Bely M, Apathy A (eds) *Amyloid and amyloidosis: Proceedings of the IXth International Symposium on Amyloidosis*, Budapest, Hungary. David Apathy, 2001:227–9.

●96. Lachmann HL, Booth DR, Booth SE, Bybee A, Gilbertson J, Gillmore J, *et al.* Misdiagnosis of hereditary amyloidosis as AL (primary) amyloidosis. *N Engl J Med* 2002; **346**:1786–91.

∗97. Kyle RA, Therneau TM, Rajkumar SV, Offord J, Larson D, Plevak M, *et al.* A long-term study of prognosis in monoclonal gammopathy of undetermined significance. *N Engl J Med* 2002; **346**:564–9.

●98. Hawkins PN, Lavender JP, Pepys MB. Evaluation of systemic amyloidosis by scintigraphy with ^{123}I-labeled serum amyloid P component. *N Engl J Med* 1990; **323**:508–13.

99. Hawkins PN, Aprile C, Capri G. Scintigraphic imaging and turnover studies with iodine-131 labeled serum amyloid P component in systemic amyloidosis. *Eur J Nucl Med* 1998; **25**:701.

●100. Greipp PR, Kyle RA, Bowie EJ. Factor X deficiency in amyloidosis: a critical review. *Am J Hematol* 1981; **11**:443–50.

101. Choufani EB, Sanchorawala V, Ernst T, Quillen K, Skinner M, Wright DG, *et al.* Acquired factor X deficiency in patients with amyloid light-chain amyloidosis: incidence, bleeding manifestations, and response to high-dose chemotherapy. *Blood* 2001; **97**:1885–7.

102. Gertz MA, Kyle RA. Primary systemic amyloidosis: A diagnostic primer. *Mayo Clin Proc* 1989; **64**:1505–19.

103. Kyle RA, Greipp PR, O'Fallon WM. Primary systemic amyloidosis: multivariate analysis for prognostic factors in 168 cases. *Blood* 1986; **68**:220–4.

∗104. Kyle R, Gertz M, Greipp P, Witzig T, Lust J, Lacy M, *et al.* A trial of three regimes for primary amyloidosis: colchicine alone, melphalan and prednisolone, and melphalan, prednisolone and colchicine. *N Engl J Med* 1997; **336**:1202–7.

∗105. Skinner M, Anderson JJ, Simms R, Falk R, Wang M, Libbey C, *et al.* Treatment of 100 patients with primary amyloidosis: a randomized trial of melphalan, prednisone, and colchicine versus colchicine alone. *Am J Med* 1996; **100**:290–8.

106. Gertz MA, Kyle RA. Acute leukemia and cytogenetic abnormalities complicating melphalan treatment of primary systemic amyloidosis. *Arch Intern Med* 1990; **150**:629–33.

107. Gertz MA, Lacy MQ, Lust JA, Greipp PR, Witzig TE, Kyle RA. Prospective randomized trial of melphalan and prednisone versus vincristine, carmustine, melphalan,

cyclophosphamide, and prednisone in the treatment of primary systemic amyloidosis. *J Clin Oncol* 1999; **17**:262–7.

108. Sezer O, Schmid P, Shweigert M, Heider U, Eucker J, Harder H, *et al.* Rapid reversal of nephritic syndrome due to primary systemic AL amyloidosis after VAD and subsequent high-dose chemotherapy with autologous stem cell support. *Bone Marrow Transplant* 1999; **23**:967–9.

∗109. Gertz MA, Lacy MQ, Lust JA, Greipp PR, Witzig TE, Kyle RA. Phase II trial of high-dose dexamethasone for untreated patients with primary systemic amyloidosis. *Med Oncol* 1999; **16**:104–9.

110. Comenzo RL, Vosburgh E, Simms RW, Bergethon P, Sarnacki D, Finn K, *et al.* Dose-intensive melphalan with blood stem cell support for the treatment of AL amyloidosis amyloidosis: one-year follow-up in five patients. *Blood* 1996; **88**:2801–6.

111. Moreau P, Milpied N, de Faucal P, Petit T, Herboullier P, Bataille R, *et al.* High-dose melphalan and autologous bone marrow transplantation for systemic AL amyloidosis with cardiac involvement. *Blood* 1996; **87**:3063–4.

112. Van Buren M, Hene RJ, Verdonck LF, Verzijlbergen FJ, Lokhorst HM. Clinical remission after syngeneic bone marrow transplantation in a patient with AL amyloidosis. *Ann Intern Med* 1995; **122**:508–10.

113. Gillmore JD, Apperley JF, Craddock C, Madhoo S, Pepys MB, Hawkins PN. High dose melphalan and stem cell rescue for AL amyloidosis. In: Kyle RA, Gertz MA (eds) *Amyloid and amyloidosis*. Pearl River, NY: Parthenon Publishing, 1999:60–3.

114. Comenzo RL. Autologous hematopoietic cell transplantation for AL amyloidosis. In: Forman SJ, Blume KG, Thomas ED (eds) *Hematopoietic cell transplantation*, 2nd edn. New York: Blackwell, 1999:1014–28.

∗115. Comenzo RL, Vosburgh E, Falk RH, Sanchorawala V, Reisinger J, Dubrey S, *et al.* Dose-intensive melphalan with blood stem-cell support for the treatment of AL amyloidosis: survival and responses in 25 patients. *Blood* 1998; **91**:3662–70.

116. Kyle RA. High-dose therapy in multiple myeloma and primary amyloidosis: an overview. *Semin Oncol* 1999; **26**:74–83.

∗117. Comenzo RL, Gertz MA. Autologous stem cell transplantation for primary systemic amyloidosis. *Blood* 2002; **99**:4276–82.

118. Gertz MA, Lacy MQ, Gastineau DA, Inwards D, Chen M, Tefferi A, *et al.* Blood stem cell transplantation as therapy for primary systemic amyloidosis (AL). *Bone Marrow Transplant* 2000; **26**:963–9.

119. Saba N, Sutton D, Ross H, Siu S, Crump R, Keating A, *et al.* High treatment-related mortality in cardiac amyloid patients undergoing autologous stem cell transplant. *Bone Marrow Transplant* 1999; **24**:853–5.

120. Comenzo RL, Sanchorawala V, Fisher C, Akpek G, Farhat M, Cerda S, *et al.* Intermediate-dose intravenous melphalan and blood stem cells mobilized with sequential GM + G-CFS or G-CSF alone to treat AL (amyloid light chain) amyloidosis. *Br J Haematol* 1999; **104**:553–9.

121. Moreau P, Leblond V, Baurquelot P. Prognostic factors of survival and response after high-dose therapy and autologous stem cell transplantation in systemic AL amyloidosis: a report on 21 patients. *Br J Haematol* 1998; **101**:766–9.

122. Kumar S, Dispenzieri A, Lacy MQ, Litzow MR, Gertz MA. High incidence of gastrointestinal bleeding after autologous stem cell transplant for primary systemic amyloidosis. *Bone Marrow Transplant* 2001; **28**:381–5.

123. Perfetti V, Ubbiali P, Magni M, Colli Vignarelli M, Casarini S, Matteucci P, et al. Cells with clonal light chains are present in peripheral blood at diagnosis and in apheretic stem cell harvests of primary amyloidosis. *Bone Marrow Transplant* 1999; **23**:323–7.

124. Comenzo RL, Michelle D, LeBlanc M, Wally J, Zhang Y, Kica G, et al. Mobilized CD34+ cells selected as autografts in patients with primary light-chain amyloidosis: rationale and application. *Transfusion* 1998; **38**:60–9.

125. Gertz MA, Lacy MQ, Bjornsson J, Litzow MR. Fatal pulmonary toxicity related to the administration of granulocyte-colony stimulating factor in amyloidosis: a report and review of growth factor-induced pulmonary toxicity. *J Hematother Stem Cell Res* 2000; **9**:635–43.

126. Arbona C, Prosper F, Benet I, Mena F, Solano C, Garcia-Conde J. Comparison between once a day vs twice a day G-CSF for mobilization of peripheral blood progenitor cells (PBPC) in normal donors for allogeneic PBPC transplantation. *Bone Marrow Transplant* 1998; **22**:39–45.

127. Akpek G, Lenz G, Lee SM, Sanchorawala V, Wright D, Colarusso T, et al. Immunologic recovery after autologous blood stem cell transplantation in patients with AL amyloidosis. *Bone Marrow Transplant* 2001; **28**:1105–10.

128. Guillaume T, Rubinstein DB, Symann M. Immune reconstitution and immunotherapy after autologous hematopoietic stem cell transplantation. *Blood* 1998; **92**:1471–90.

129. Sanchorawala V, Wright DG, Seldin DC, Falk RH, Finn KT, Dember LM, et al. High-dose intravenous melphalan and autologous stem cell transplantation as initial therapy or following two cycles of oral therapy for the treatment of AL amyloidosis: results of a randomized prospective trial. *Blood* 2001; **98**:815a.

130. Lewis WD, Skinner M, Simms RW, Jones LA, Cohen AS, Jenkins RL. Orthotopic liver transplantation for familial amyloidotic polyneuropathy. *Clin Transplant* 1994; **8**:107–10.

131. Holmgren G, Ericzon BG, Groth CG, Steen L, Suhr O, Andersen O, et al. Clinical improvement and amyloid regression after liver transplantation in hereditary transthyretin amyloidosis. *Lancet* 1993; **341**:1113–16.

132. Hosenpud JD, DeMarco T, Frazier OH, Griffith B, Uretsky B, Menkis A, et al. Progression of systemic disease and reduced long-term survival in patients with cardiac amyloidosis undergoing heart transplantation: follow-up results of a multicenter survey. *Circulation* 1991; **84**:III338–43.

133. Hall R, Hawkins PN. Cardiac transplantation for AL amyloidosis. *Br Med Journal* 1994; **309**:1135–7.

134. Dubrey S, Falk RH. Heart transplantation in AL amyloidosis. *Amyloid* 1995; **2**:284–7.

135. Pelosi F, Capehart J, Roberts WC. Effectiveness of cardiac transplantation for primary (AL) cardiac amyloidosis. *Am J Cardiol* 1997; **79**:532–5.

136. Isoniemi H, Kyll Anen L, Ahonen J, Hackerstedt K, Salmela K, Pasternack A. Improved outcome of renal transplantation in amyloidosis. *Transpl Int* 1994; **7**:S298–300.

137. Hrncic R, Wall J, Wolfenbarger DA, Murphy C, Schell M, Weiss D, et al. Antibody-mediated resolution of light chain-associated amyloid deposits. *Am J Pathol* 2000; **157**:1239–46.

138. Gianni L, Bellotti V, Gianni M, Merlini G. New drug therapy for amyloidoses: resorption of AL amyloidosis type deposits with 4-iodo-4-deoxydoxorubicin. *Blood* 1995; **86**:855–61.

139. Merlini G, Ascari E, Amboldi N, Bellotti V, Arbustini E, Perpetti V, et al. Interaction of the anthracycline 4-iodo-4-deoxydoxorubicin with amyloid fibrils: inhibition of amyloidogenesis. *Proc Natl Acad Sci USA* 1995; **92**:2959–63.

140. Pepys M, Herbert J, Hutchinson WL, Tennent G, Lachmann H, Gallimore J, et al. Targeted pharmacological depletion of serum amyloid P component for treatment of human amyloidosis. *Nature* 2002; **417**:254–9.

141. O'Nuallain B, Wetzel R. Conformational Abs recognizing a generic amyloid fibril epitope. *Proc Natl Acad Sci USA* 2002; **99**:1485–90.

142. Merlini G, Anesi E, Garini P, Perpetti V, Obici L, Ascari E, et al. Treatment of AL amyloidosis amyloidosis with 4'-iodo-4'-deoxydoxorubicin: an update. *Blood* 1999; **93**:1112–3.

143. Gertz MA, Lacy MQ, Dispenzieri A, Cheson B, Barlogie B, Kyle R, et al. A multicenter phase II trial of 4'-iodo-4'-deoxydoxorubicin (IDOX) in primary amyloidosis (AL). *Amyloid* 2002; **9**:24–30.

144. Aprile C, Marinone G, Saponaro R, Bonino C, Merlini G. Cardiac and pleuropulmonary AL amyloid imaging with technetium-99m labelled aprotinin. *Eur J Nucl Med* 1995; **22**:1393.

145. Comenzo RL. Hematopoietic cell transplantation for primary systemic amyloidosis: what have we learned. *Leuk Lymphoma* 2000; **37**:245–58.

146. Myatt EA, Westholm FA, Weiss DT, Solomon A, Schiffer M, Stevens FJ. Pathogenic potential of human monoclonal immunoglobulin light chains: relationship of in vitro aggregation to in vivo organ deposition. *Proc Natl Acad Sci USA* 1994; **91**:3034–8.

147. Merlini G, Bellotti V, Andreola A, Palladini G, Obici L, Casarini S, et al. Protein aggregation. *Clin Chem Lab Med* 2001; **39**:1065–75.

28

Heavy-chain diseases

JEAN-PAUL FERMAND AND JEAN-CLAUDE BROUET

INTRODUCTION

Heavy-chain diseases (HCDs) are lymphoproliferative disorders of B cells, which are characterized by the production of a monoclonal immunoglobulin (Ig) molecule composed of truncated heavy (H) chains with no associated light (L) chains. The diagnosis of these conditions depends on the detection of the structurally abnormal immunoglobulin molecules in the patient's serum or urine. Heavy-chain diseases involving the three main immunoglobulin classes have been described: α-HCD is the most frequent, μ-HCD is rare, and γ-HCD is of intermediate incidence.

HCD PROTEINS: STRUCTURAL AND GENETIC ASPECTS

HCD proteins

Most γ-HCD proteins are dimers, whereas most α- and μ-HCD proteins appear to consist primarily of multiple polymers of different sizes. The molecular weight of the monomeric unit varies between 27 000 and 49 000 for γ-HCD proteins, 29 000 and 35 000 for α-HCD proteins, and 35 000 and 55 000 for μ-HCD proteins. Allowance is usually made in these figures for carbohydrates, since the carbohydrate content of many of these HCD proteins is high.

HCD proteins consist primarily of the Fc region of the heavy chain with a normal carboxy-terminal end. The missing portion of the chain in most instances involves both the VH and C1 regions. Frangione and Milstein were the first to demonstrate that the structural defect in one

particular γ-HCD protein is an internal deletion.[1,2] Such internal deletions have since been recorded for several other, but not all, HCD proteins.

More than 25 HCD proteins have been sequenced[3,4] (unpublished data). They fall into five groups, which are illustrated in Fig. 28.1. The first group consists of proteins with a sequence that starts with the hinge region. The sequence of this protein is identical to that of the corresponding constant part of the γ, α, or μ chain. In the second group, the alteration consists of an entire deletion of the CH1 domain. In the third group, only the VH domain is missing. In the fourth group, there is a double deletion within the variable domain, and the sequence of the protein begins with a small number of amino-acid

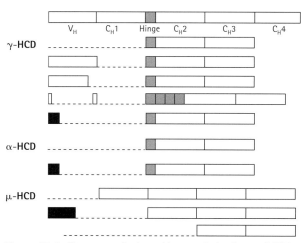

Figure 28.1 *Structure of selected heavy-chain disease (HCD) proteins. Shaded bars represent the hinge region, solid bars represent regions of unknown origin, and dashed lines represent gaps.*

residues derived from the VH genes followed by the portion of the sequence coded by the JH segment. The normal sequence resumes within the hinge region or CH2 constant domain. In the last group, the amino sequence of the HCD protein begins with an unusual sequence that has no homology with immunoglobulin sequences.

Immunoglobulin genes in HCD

The study of nucleic acids coding for the truncated Ig heavy chain has shed some light on the mechanism leading to the production of these abnormal Ig. Sequencing of the productively rearranged Ig genes from cells producing HCD proteins has been achieved in six cases.[4–9] Figure 28.2 summarizes the structure of DNA, RNA, and HCD protein in five HCD cases. Common features include a high level of somatic mutation, deletions, and insertions of sequences of unknown origin in rearranged genes. In most cases, the VDJ region displays a high level of mutation in both coding and non-coding regions. Homology to the germinal sequence ranges from 70% to 90%, increasing with increasing distance from the V region, as occurs for rearranged normal VDJ regions. No mutations are

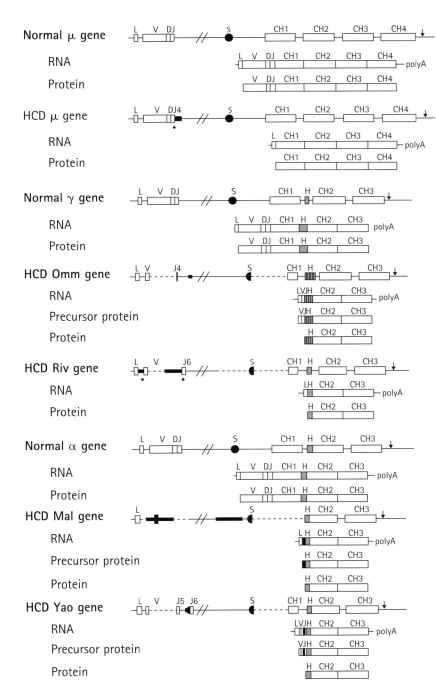

Figure 28.2 *Structure of different heavy-chain disease (HCD) productive genes, and associated RNA transcript and protein compared with their normal rearranged counterpart. CH, constant region; D, diversity; H, hinge; J, joining; L, leader; S, switch region; V, variable region. Asterisks indicate altered splice sites; solid bars represent insertions in coding (large bar) or non-coding (small bars) regions; dashed lines indicate deletion.*

found beyond the J-C intron. There are also extensive deletions in the VDJ segments, and deletions may also comprise all or part of the CH1 gene. Lastly, DNA insertions hundreds of base pairs long are found, which show no homology with any known human sequence, including immunoglobulin gene sequences. Similarly, there is no homology between insertions observed in immunoglobulin genes from different patients. In one case, however, a DNA insertion contained two stretches that were homologous to a satellite-I DNA and to a leader peptide-VH intron.

Three conclusions may be drawn from these data:

1 Unusual end-terminal sequences of some HCD proteins derive from the insertion of nucleotides of unknown origin.[10] Of note, in most cases of α-HCD the intracellular precursor protein contains an amino-terminal sequence that is cleaved before secretion of the HCD protein. The HCD protein, therefore, begins with the hinge sequence.
2 The alterations within the VH and JH regions, and the high number of mutations, result in unusual splicing, using alternative sites, and eliminating a large part or all of the VH and JH segments.
3 The isotypic distribution of HCD proteins differs from that of normal immunoglobulins with a strong under-representation of isotypes coded by most 3′ genes, such as γ2 , γ4, and a total lack of α2-HCD. The latter observation is striking, because α-HCD is the most common type of HCD.

Interestingly, alterations of immunoglobulin genes in HCD are not limited to productive rearrangements. A non-functional α1 gene implicated in a t(9;14) translocation in a case of α-HCD exhibited similar abnormalities, including a high number of mutations and a deletion of the 3′ end of a VH rearranged gene.[11] Moreover, a nucleotide sequence established for a rearranged κ-light-chain gene in cells from a patient with γ-HCD exhibited similar features.[12] With respect to α-HCD, in all eight cases studied, the presence of rearranged κ genes and of non-productive κ mRNA was observed (unpublished results). Normal κ light chains are found, however, in at least one-half of the cases of μ-HCD and in rare cases of γ- or α-HCD.[13]

The absence of the CH1 domain in nearly all cases of HCD probably explains the secretion of these abnormal proteins that otherwise would be retained in the endoplasmic reticulum in the absence of light chains (which normally would displace heavy chains from their chaperones in the reticulum). The absence of CH1 also explains the lack of covalent association between truncated heavy chains and light chains when the latter are produced, for instance, in μ-HCD.

Of note, deletions and insertions have been recently observed in normal germinal B cells, which are the target of the normal process of somatic mutations within the follicule.[14] Although only minor alterations have been recorded for these normal germinal-center B cells, it is conceivable that rare B cells with extensive alterations in Ig genes may arise during the process of hypermutation, perhaps because of a survival advantage. The latter could be related, for instance, to bcl-6 alterations, since this oncogene is also a target of the hypermutation process.[15]

Diagnostic analysis of HCD proteins

PROTEIN ANALYSIS IN SERUM AND OTHER FLUIDS

The demonstration by immunochemical methods of the presence of immunoglobulin heavy chains and absence of light chains in the serum (or jejunal fluid, in the case of α-HCD) is mandatory for the diagnosis of HCD.

The abnormal immunoglobulin chains are not evidenced by serum electrophoresis in nearly one-half the cases of α-HCD, one-third of the cases of γ-HCD, and two-thirds of the cases of μ-HCD. When detectable by electrophoresis, the pathologic protein does not always show the discrete narrow spike suggestive of a monoclonal immunoglobulin abnormality. Instead, HCD proteins may feature a broad band that often extends from the α2 to the β2 region in α-HCD (Fig. 28.3a). This remarkable electrophoretic behavior of α-HCD may be related to the tendency of these chains to polymerize or to their high carbohydrate content.[16]

The identification of the HCD proteins, therefore, relies on serum immunoelectrophoresis, immunoselection, or immunofixation (Figs 28.3 and 28.4). The pathologic protein may escape detection by immunoelectrophoresis when its concentration is low. Immunoselection combined with immunoelectrophoresis usually allows the detection of HCD proteins.[17] This technique, however, requires rather large amounts of highly selected antisera to κ and λ light chains, capable of precipitating completely all the monoclonal and polyclonal immunoglobulin molecules (see Chapter 9). Immunofixation is an easier process to perform, is sensitive, and allows the detection of HCD when the level of polyclonal immunoglobulin is low or when the migration of the pathologic protein extends beyond the α, γ, or β region.

Of note, other serum immunoglobulin abnormalities may be found in HCD. Serum levels of normal polyclonal immunoglobulin molecules of all classes may be reduced or, more rarely, increased.[18,19] Serum monoclonal IgG or IgM were also disclosed in several cases of α-, γ, and μ-HCD.[18–21]

Because of its low molecular weight, γ-HCD protein is often present in urine. In μ-HCD, sizeable amounts of free monoclonal κ light-chain immunoglobulins are found in two-thirds of cases.[16]

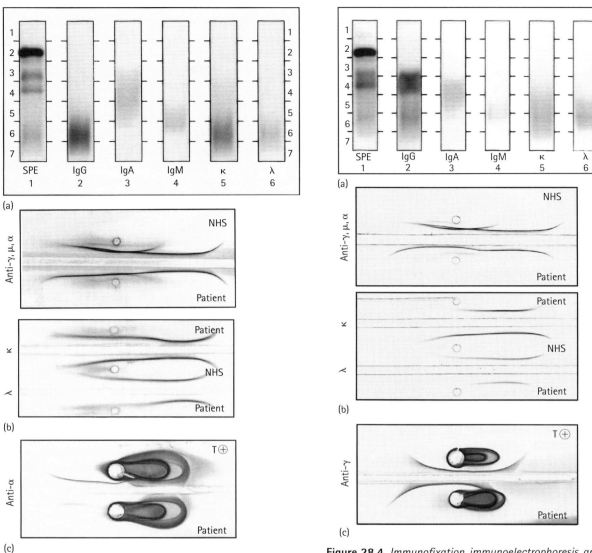

(a)

(b)

(c)

Figure 28.3 *Immunofixation, immunoelectrophoresis, and immunoselection in a case of α-heavy-chain disease (HCD). (a) The pathological protein migrates in the β globulin area and is revealed only by the anti-α (IgA) antiserum. (b) Immunoelectrophoresis of normal serum (NHS) and α-HCD-containing serum. Normal serum Ig are revealed by both anti-heavy-chain and light-chain antisera, while the abnormal Ig is not reactive with antisera to light chains. (c) Immunoselection, the free precipiting line is revealed by anti-α antiserum. T+, control serum containing an α-HCD protein.*

Figure 28.4 *Immunofixation, immunoelectrophoresis, and immunoselection in a case of γ-heavy-chain disease (HCD). (a) The pathological protein migrates in the β globulin area and is revealed only by the anti-γ?(IgG) antiserum. (b) Immunoelectrophoresis of normal serum or γ-HCD-containing serum. Normal serum Ig are revealed by both anti-heavy-chain and light-chain antisera, while the abnormal Ig is not reactive with antisera to light chains. (c) Immunoselection, the free precipiting line is revealed by anti-α antiserum. T+, control serum containing an γ-HCD protein.*

The α-HCD protein, bound to the secretory fragment, is present in significant amounts in the jejunal fluid of patients with the digestive form of α-HCD. The immunochemical techniques used for the detection of α-HCD protein are the same as for serum; however, jejunal fluid must be collected carefully and concentrated to avoid protein degradation.[22] In some patients with the clinicopathologic features of α-HCD, the pathologic protein can be found in the jejunal fluid but cannot be detected in serum.[23]

Intracellular HCD proteins

Intracytoplasmic heavy chains in the absence of light chains can usually be demonstrated in proliferating lymphocytes, lymphoplasmacytic or plasma cells, or immunoblasts by conventional immunofluorescence or immunoperoxidase techniques using cell suspensions or histological sections.[24] Exceptions to this pattern do exist, however, because κ light chains have been found in the cytoplasm or at the surface of the proliferating plasma cells in three cases of α- or γ-HCD.[13] Immunochemical studies permit the detection of the rare cases of non-secretory α-HCD in patients who have the characteristic clinicopathologic pattern but do not have detectable α-HCD protein in the serum or jejunal fluid.[25] In one such patient, molecular studies identified the mechanism responsible for the absence of secretion: a deletion had occurred of the polyadenylation site for secretory α1-chain mRNA; however, the membrane form of the abnormally short α heavy chain was produced.[7]

Of note, immunological studies performed in γ-HCD showed that a γ-HCD protein may be detected in the serum of patients with various B- or T-cell malignancies that are not directly involved in the production of the abnormal immunoglobulin.[18]

CLINICAL, EPIDEMIOLOGICAL, AND PATHOLOGICAL FEATURES AND TREATMENT OF SPECIFIC HEAVY-CHAIN DISEASES

α–Heavy-chain disease

α-HCD was first described in 1968 by Seligmann et al.[26] It primarily involves the IgA secretory system and manifests as a disease of the gastrointestinal tract in almost all patients.[21]

PATHOLOGY

In most cases, α-HCD involves the whole length of the small intestine without intervening normal mucosa. Three grades of increasing malignancy are usually distinguished.[27] At stage A, a mature plasmacytic or lymphoplasmacytic infiltrate invades the mucosal lamina propria, and may be associated with a variable degree of villous atrophy. Stage B is intermediate, the infiltrate, containing dystrophic plasma cells and atypical immunoblast-like cells, invading at least the submucosa. Stage C corresponds to an immunoblastic lymphoma, either forming discrete ulcerated tumors or extensively infiltrating long segments of the intestine wall. Three similar histological stages can be identified in the mesenteric lymph nodes, which are usually (but not always in stage A) involved in the pathological process. Involvement of other lymph nodes, bone marrow, liver, and spleen is uncommon, except when the enteric lesions are stage C. In contrast, localization of the disease in gastric and colorectal mucosa is not rare, even in stage A disease. At any given site, the histologic lesions may progress from stage A to B or from stage B to C. Different stages can be found at the same time in different organs or even at different sites in the same organ, and this heterogeneity should be kept in mind when performing pre-therapeutic staging.

The pattern of α-HCD pathological lesions often includes clear lymphoepithelial lesions made of centro-cytic-like cells. Therefore, Isaacson[28] considers α-HCD as a subtype of the lymphomas, which arise from mucosa-associated lymphoid tissue (MALT). α-HCD has the characteristic histopathological findings of the so-called immunoproliferative small-intestinal disease (IPSID) of which it is the most frequent form. IPSIDs are part of the heterogeneous group of formerly called 'Mediterranean' lymphoma, which indicated a common clinical pattern and a peculiar epidemiology.[29]

EPIDEMIOLOGY

Most reports of α-HCD have concerned patients from the Mediterranean area or from the Middle East. In addition, numerous cases have been described in inhabitants of sub-Saharan Africa, Central and South America, Southern and Eastern Europe, the Indian subcontinent, and the Far East, whatever their racial and ethnic origin. In developed countries, α-HCD may occur among developing-world immigrants and underprivileged native populations. Indeed, the main common denominator for these patients is a low socioeconomic status and poor hygiene conditions resulting in recurrent infectious diarrhea and chronic par-asitic infestation.[21] The age distribution in α-HCD is also striking, since most patients are between 15 and 35 years of age. The disease predominates slightly in males.

These epidemiological features strongly suggest that environmental factors operating since early infancy could play a major role in the pathogenesis of α-HCD. A potential specific microorganism remains to be identified and the mechanisms leading to the emergence of a clonal population synthesizing the structurally abnormal IgA are still speculative, as previously discussed. The postulated environmental antigenic stimulation might be associated with an underlying immunodeficiency, for example, due to malnutrition, or with predisposing genetic factors not clearly identified by the familial studies performed so far.

CLINICAL FEATURES

In the great majority of cases, α-HCD is an enteric disease.[21] Non-digestive forms involving the respiratory tract, lymph nodes, or the thyroid have been reported in rare patients.[30–32]

The usual clinical presentation is chronic diarrhea with abdominal pain, vomiting, weight loss, and evidence of malabsorption. In addition to signs of malnutrition, clubbed fingers are a frequent physical finding. Digestive tumors, abdominal lymphadenopathy, and their complications, including obstruction and perforation, may also lead to diagnosis, usually at stage C, and after a neglected or misdiagnosed period of chronic diarrhea. Presentation with tumor localization in the liver, spleen, peripheral lymphadenopathy, or bone marrow is uncommon.

Usual biological investigations confirm malabsorption and protein-losing enteropathy. Radiographic manifestations include hypertrophic and pseudo-polypoid mucosal folds in the small intestine, sometimes associated with stenosis of extrinsic or intrinsic origin, ulcerations, or fistulas. Endoscopic examination of duodenum and jejunum, combined with biopsies, is a sensitive diagnostic approach, an infiltrated pattern being the most suggestive endoscopic finding.[33]

COURSE AND TREATMENT

The spontaneous course of α-HCD may include periods of improvement, often following antibiotic treatment. A single case of clinical and immunologic complete remission was observed in the absence of therapy after the patient was removed from an unfavorable environment.[34]

The modalities of treatment depend on a precise knowledge of the extent and histologic stage of the disease.[21] This requires computed tomography of the abdomen, gastrojejunoscopy, and ileocolonoscopy, including systematic biopsies. In addition, because of the frequent asynchrony of stage of the histopathological lesions at different sites, staging laparotomy should be considered, except in patients with previous evidence of stage C lesions.[35]

Patients with stage A lesions limited to the gut and mesenteric lymph nodes should be initially treated with oral antibiotics selected by the sensitivity pattern of the intestinal bacteria. Alternatively, tetracycline, metronidazole, and ampicillin are good choices. Any documented parasite should be treated. A minimum 6-month trial is required for establishing responsiveness and about 40% of patients may achieve complete clinical, histological, and immunological remission with antibiotic therapy alone. Maintenance treatment is unnecessary, but close surveillance for the early detection of overt transformation to lymphoma is mandatory. Of note, a persistently abnormal α-chain mRNA was still detected in one patient who otherwise appeared to be in complete clinical and pathologic remission after tetracycline therapy but who subsequently relapsed.[25]

For patients with stage B or C, antibiotic and antiparasitic treatments are also useful in improving the malabsorption syndrome. In these patients (and in patients with stage A without marked improvement after a 6-month course of antibiotic), combination chemotherapy must also be given. A doxorubicin-based regimen is usually recommended. Patients with disseminated stage C disease achieving a good response to conventional or salvage chemotherapy could be candidates for intensification with autologous stem cell transplantation.

The long-term prognosis of α-HCD remains imprecise because of the lack of large series with prolonged follow-up. In the Tunisian series, including six, two and 13 patients with stage A, stage B, and stage C disease, respectively, the complete remission rate was 52% (64% for stages B and C) and the 3-year overall survival was 67%.[36]

γ–Heavy-chain disease

Since the first description of γ-HCD in 1964, by Franklin and Osserman,[37,38] approximately 100 cases have been reported in the literature (reviewed in Fermand et al.[18] and Wahner-Roedler and Kyle[19]). In contrast to the uniform clinicopathological pattern of α-HCD, γ-HCD can present with a great variety of clinical and pathological features that are difficult to integrate into a unified disease concept. Indeed, γ-heavy-chain 'disease' represents a heterogeneous condition that may not justify designation of a single disease process.[18,39]

CLINICAL FEATURES

γ-HCD has been described throughout the world and no epidemiological pattern has been recognized. It occurs equally in males and females, most often in the sixth decade of life or beyond, although the disease has been observed in children and young adults.

γ-HCD most often presents as a lymphoproliferative disorder featured by lymphadenopathy, splenomegaly and constitutional symptoms. Generalized peripheral lymphadenopathy is present at the time of diagnosis in about two-thirds of patients and fever is present in about one-fourth. Waxing and waning of lymph nodes can be observed. Palatal edema and swelling of the uvula related to involvement of Waldeyer's ring, which was initially thought to be a hallmark of the disease, actually occurs in less than 15% of cases. Splenomegaly is frequent and γ-HCD may present with an isolated large spleen. Mediastinal and/or abdominal lymphadenopathies may also occur.

Skeletal involvement has been described in only rare cases and γ-HCD almost never mimics multiple myeloma. Various extrahematopoietic tumor localizations may occur, particularly in cutaneous and subcutaneous tissues, in the thyroid, parotid and salivary glands, and in the stomach.[18,19]

HEMATOPATHOLOGIC FINDINGS

In contrast to α-HCD, γ-HCD has no specific histological pattern.[18,40] The most frequent is a pleomorphic malignant lymphoplasmacytic proliferation mainly seen in bone marrow and lymph nodes. This may be associated with unusual pathologic features, such as the presence of eosinophils, epithelioid, and multinucleated giant cells, suggesting atypical granulomatous lesions. It may also be intermingled with large immunoblasts with atypical nuclei resembling Reed–Sternberg cells. These associated features, in addition to some degree of vascular proliferation, may lead to histologic patterns suggesting angio-immunoblastic lymphadenopathy or Hodgkin's disease. A γ-heavy-chain protein was detected in the course of a classical Hodgkin's disease in a single patient, in whom it persisted during a long-lasting remission.[41,42]

In some cases, γ-HCD may be featured by a predominantly plasmacytic proliferation or may present as a chronic lymphocytic leukemia. The plasmacytic pattern, which usually includes malignant plasma cells, is more frequently found in extranodal localizations, such as thyroid and salivary glands. It may express as plasma cell leukemia, which was reported in two patients at onset or as a terminal event. The occurrence of a large-cell lymphoma supervening on the lymphoplasmacytic chronic proliferation appears unusual in γ-HCD. In contrast, non-Hodgkin's lymphoma of various histologic types, and of low or intermediate grade of malignancy, may be observed.

In several reported cases, the histological appearance of the enlarged lymphoid organs only showed a moderate lymphoplasmacytic infiltration without evidence of an overt malignant process. In 5–10% of patients with a γ-HCD protein, there is no evidence of any underlying lymphoproliferative disorder, including after extensive evaluations repeated during prolonged follow-up. Such negative findings are especially observed in patients with autoimmune disorders and, in some, the γ-HCD protein may disappear spontaneously.

Cytogenetic studies have been seldom reported. Unique abnormality or characteristic cytogenetic features of the various types of lymphomas were not found.

ASSOCIATED DISORDERS

The occurrence of autoimmune disorders is frequent in patients with γ-HCD.[18,19] Indeed, autoimmune diseases are found in about one-fourth of patients, without taking into account the presence of serum autoantibodies that have no clinical relevance. Rheumatoid arthritis and autoimmune cytopenias (hemolytic anemia and/or thrombocytopenic purpura) are the most frequent. Both may precede the discovery of the γ-HCD protein by several years. Other autoimmune or related conditions associated with γ-HCD include lupus erythematosus, Sjögren's syndrome, myasthenia gravis, thyroiditis, and vasculitis. All may be observed with or without associated underlying lymphoid disorder of proven or uncertain malignancy and, in some patients, the occurrence of a malignant proliferation was diagnosed only several years after the development of the autoimmune disorder.

Neurological manifestations of uncertain mechanism have been reported in several patients with γ-HCD. Various solid tumors have been diagnosed before, simultaneously with, or after the discovery of the γ-HCD protein. A myeloid disorder has been documented in a few patients.[43]

COURSE AND TREATMENT

As expected from its diverse picture, the clinical course of γ-HCD varies from an asymptomatic state to a rapidly progressive malignancy. Accordingly, therapeutic decisions should depend on the underlying clinicopathological features, without taking into account the presence of the abnormal Ig.[18,19]

In an asymptomatic patient without overt lymphoid proliferation, no therapy is indicated and the spontaneous disappearance of the γ-HCD protein may occur, as reported in several cases. In patients with a low-grade lymphoplasmacytic, immunocytoma-like malignancy, a trial of chlorambucil may be recommended. Alternatively, cyclophosphamide can be used, alone or in combination with vincristine and prednisone. Courses of melphalan and prednisone may be preferred when the proliferation is predominantly plasmacytic. The efficacy of fludarabine was reported in one patient.[44] In patients with an aggressive non-Hodgkin's lymphoma, doxorubicin-containing regimens should be used.

The serum amount of the γ-HCD protein usually varies in parallel with the evolution of the associated malignant process. However, relapses without reappearance of the abnormal Ig have been observed. In addition, the appearance of the γ-HCD protein during the course of a treated lymphoid malignancy has been reported. Such dissociated evolution may traduce a mutational event or the emergence of a new clone.

μ–Heavy-chain disease

μ-HCD is a rare disease. Indeed, since the first case was described in 1969,[45] only 30 documented cases have been published in the literature (reviewed in Preud'homme et al.,[46] Wahner-Roedler and Kyle,[47] and Witzens et al.[48]). Of the 31 reported patients, 17 were men, 27 were Caucasians, three were African-American, and one was Asian. Age at diagnosis varied from 15 to 80 years (median 60 years). Most patients presented with splenomegaly, hepatomegaly, and, less frequently, peripheral lymphadenopathies, in conjunction with an associated lymphoproliferative disorder. Some patients had other pathological conditions, such as systemic lupus erythematosus, hepatic cirrhosis, or myelodysplasia.[48]

The lymphoid disorder is usually characterized by a lymphoplasmacytic proliferation. It may mimic chronic lymphocytic leukemia (CLL), whereas the secretion of a μ-HCD protein is rare in the usual forms of CLL. μ-HCD may also have features of Waldenström's macroglobulinemia or multiple myeloma. Lytic bone lesions were present in three of 15 reported patients. μ-HCD protein may also be detected in the absence of any overt immunoproliferative disease.

In patients with an associated lymphoid disorder, examination of the bone marrow usually shows an increase in plasma cells and in lymphocytes, which may include vacuolated plasma cells. This is seen in about two-thirds of patients with bone marrow plasmacytosis and warrants a search for μ-HCD, particularly when a Bence Jones proteinuria is also detected. As already mentioned, Bence Jones proteinuria is not rare in μ-HCD (in contrast to α- and γ-HCD, in which monoclonal light chains are usually not detectable in the serum and urine) and may lead to the occurrence of cast nephropathy.[46]

Survival of reported patients with μ-HCD ranged from less than 1 month to more than 10 years. Therapeutic indications and modalities depend on the underlying lymphoid disorder.

KEY POINTS

- Heavy-chain diseases (HCDs) are lymphoproliferative disorders of B cells producing immunoglobulin molecules consisting of incomplete heavy chains devoid of light chains.
- There are three types of heavy-chain disease, i.e. α-HCD, γ-HCD, and μ-HCD, α-HCD being the most frequent and μ-HCD the most rare.
- α-HCD usually presents as a gastrointestinal disorder, while γ-HCD and μ-HCD have more varied clinical manifestations, usually including lymphadenopathy, splenomegaly, and constitutional symptoms.
- Early-stage α-HCD may resolve with appropriate antibiotic treatment.
- For later-stage α-HCD and for μ-HCD and γ-HCD where there is evidence of underlying lymphoma, chemotherapy is appropriate, with drugs used for lymphoproliferative disorders, such as cyclophosphamide, doxorubicine, and fludarabine.

REFERENCES

● = Key primary paper
◆ = Major review article

1. Frangione B, Franklin EC. Heavy chain diseases: clinical features and molecular significance of the disordered immunoglobulin structure. *Semin Hematol* 1973; **10**:53–64.

2. Frangione B, Milstein C. Partial deletion in the heavy chain disease protein ZUC. *Nature* 1969; **224**:57–9.
3. Cogné M, Silvain C, Khamlichi AA, Preud'homme JL. Structurally abnormal immunoglobulins in human immunoproliferative disorders. *Blood* 1992; **79**:2181–95.
4. Prelli F, Frangione B. Franklin's disease: Ig gamma 2H chain mutant BUR. *J Immunol* 1992; **148**:949–52.
5. Alexander A, Anicito I, Buxbaum J. Gamma heavy chain disease in man: genomic sequence reveals two non-contiguous deletions in a single case. *J Clin Invest* 1988; **82**:1244–52.
6. Bentaboulet M, Mihaesco E, Gendron MC, Brouet JC, Tsapis A. Genomic alterations in a case of alpha chain disease leading to the generation of composite exons from the JH region. *Eur J Immunol* 1989; **19**:2093–8.
7. Cogné M, Preud'homme JL. Gene deletions force nonsecretory alpha chain disease plasma cells to produce membrane-form alpha chain only. *J Immunol* 1990; **145**:2455–8.
8. Guglielmi P, Bakhshi A, Cogné M, Seligmann M, Korsmeyer SJ. Multiple genomic defects result in an alternative RNA splice creating a human gamma H chain disease protein. *J Immunol* 1988; **141**:1762–8.
9. Tsapis A, Bentaboulet M, Pellet P, Mihaesco E, Thierry D, Seligmann M, Brouet JC. The productive gene for alpha-H chain disease protein MAL is highly modified by insertion-deletion processes. *J Immunol* 1989; **143**:3821–7.
10. Fakhfakh F, Dellagi K, Ayadi H, Bouguerra A, Fourati R, Ben-Ayed F, Brouet JC, Tsapis A. Alpha heavy chain disease alpha mRNA contain nucleotide sequences of unknown origins. *Eur J Immunol* 1992; **22**:3037–40.
11. Pellet P, Berger R, Bernheim A, Bouret JC, Tsapis A. Molecular analysis of a t(9;14) (p11;q32) translocation occurring in a case of human alpha heavy chain disease. *Oncogene* 1989; **4**:653–7.
12. Cogné M, Bakhshi A, Korsmeyer SJ, Guglielmi P. Gene mutations and alternate RNA slicing result in truncated Ig light chains in human gamma heavy chain disease. *J Immunol* 1988; **141**:1738–44.
13. Preud'homme JL, Brouet JC, Seligmann M. Cellular immunoglobulins in human gamma and alpha heavy chain diseases. *Clin Exp Immunol* 1979; **37**:283–91.
14. Goossens T, Klein U, Küppers R. Frequent occurrence of deletions and duplications during somatic hypermutation: implications for oncogene translocations and heavy chain disease. *Proc Natl Acad Sci USA* 1998; **95**:2463–8.
15. Shen HM, Peters A, Baron B, Zhu X, Storb U. Mutation of bcl-6 gene in normal B cells by the process of somatic hypermutation of Ig genes. *Science* 1998; **280**:1750–2.
◆16. Seligmann M, Mihaesco E, Preud'homme JL, Danon F, Brouet JC. Heavy chain diseases: Current findings and concepts. *Immunol Rev* 1979; **48**:145–67.
◆17. Doe WF, Danon F, Seligmann M. Immunodiagnosis of alpha chain disease. *Clin Exp Immunol* 1979; **36**:189–97.
◆18. Fermand JP, Brouet JC, Danon F, Seligmann M. Gamma heavy chain disease : heterogeneity of the clinicopathologic features. *Medicine* 1989; **68**:321–35.
◆19. Wahner-Roedler DL, Kyle RA. Heavy chain diseases. In: Wiernik PH, Canellos GP, Dutcher JP, Kyle RA (eds) *Neoplastic diseases of the blood*, 3rd edn. Edinburgh: Churchill Livingstone, 1996:613.

20. Presti BC, Sciotto CG, Marsh SG. Lymphocytic lymphoma with associated gamma heavy chain and IgM-lambda paraprotein: an unusual biclonal gammopathy. *Am J Clin Pathol* 1990; **93**:137–41.

◆21. Rambaud JC, Brouet JC, Seligmann M. Alpha chain disease and related lymphoproliferative disorders. In: Ogra P, Mestecky J, Lamm ME, Strober W, Bienenstock J, McGhee JR (eds) *Handbook of mucosal immunology*. London: Academic Press, 1994:425–33.

22. Lucidarme D, Colombel JF, Brandtzaeg P, Tulliez M, Chaussade S, Marteau P, *et al.* Alpha-chain disease: analysis of alpha-chain protein and secretory component in jejunal fluid. *Gastroenterology* 1993; **104**:278–85.

23. Rambaud JC, Galian A, Danon F, Preud'homme JL, Brandtzaeg P, Wasseff M, *et al.* Alpha-chain disease without qualitative serum IgA abnormality: report of two cases, including a 'nonsecretory' form. *Cancer* 1983; **51**:686–93.

24. Buxbaum JN, Preud'homme JL. Alpha and gamma heavy chain diseases in man: intracellular origin of the aberrant polypeptides. *J Immunol* 1972; **109**:1131–7.

25. Matuchansky C, Cogné M, Lemaire M, Babin P, Touchard G, Chamaret S, *et al.* Nonsecretory alpha chain disease with immunoproliferative small-intestinal disease. *N Engl J Med* 1989; **320**:1534–9.

26. Seligmann M, Danon F, Hurez D, Mihaesco E, Preud'homme JL. Alpha chain disease: a new immunoglobulin abnormality. *Science* 1968; **162**:1396–7.

◆27. Galian A, Lecestre MJ, Scotto J, Bognel C, Matuchansky C, Rambaud JC. Pathological study of alpha chain disease with special emphasis on evolution. *Cancer* 1977; **39**:2081–101.

◆28. Isaacson PG. Gastrointestinal lymphoma. *Hum Pathol* 1994; **25**:1020–9.

◆29. Fine KD, Stone MJ. α-HCD, mediterranean lymphoma and immunoproliferative small intestinal disease: a review of clinicopathological features, pathogenesis and differential diagnosis. *Am J Gastroenterol* 1999; **9**:1139–52.

30. Florin-Christensen A, Doniach D, Newcomb PB. Alpha-chain disease with pulmonary manifestations. *Br Med J* 1974; **2**:413–15.

31. Takahashi K, Naito M, Matsuoka Y, Takatsuki K. A new form of alpha-chain disease with generalized lymph node involvement. *Pathol Res Pract* 1988; **183**:717–23.

32. Tracy RP, Kyle RA, Leitch JM. Alpha heavy-chain disease presenting as goiter. *Am J Clin Pathol* 1984; **2**:336–9.

33. Halphen M, Najjar T, Jaafoura H, Cammoun M, and Group Tufrali. Diagnostic value of upper intestinal fiber endoscopy in primary small intestinal lymphoma. A prospective study by the Tunisian-French Intestinal Lymphoma Group. *Cancer* 1986; **58**:2140–5.

34. Sala P, Tonutti E, Mazzolini S, Antonutto G, Bamezza M. Alpha-heavy chain disease: report of a case with spontaneous regression. *Scand J Haematol* 1983; **31**:149–54.

35. Tabbane F, Mourali N, Cammoun M, Naijar T. Results of laparotomy in immuno-proliferative small intestinal disease. *Cancer* 1988; **61**:1699–706.

36. Ben-Ayed F, Halphen M, Najjar T. Treatment of alpha chain disease. Results of a prospective study in 21 Tunisian patients by the Tunisian-French Intestinal Lymphoma Study Group. *Cancer* 1989; **63**:1251–6.

37. Franklin EC, Lowenstein J, Bigelow B, Meltzer M. Heavy chain disease – new disorder of serum γ-globulins: report of first case. *Am J Med* 1964; **37**:332–50.

38. Osserman EF, Takatsuki K. Clinical and immunochemical studies of four cases of heavy (Hγ2) chain disease. *Am J Med* 1964; **37**:351–73.

◆39. Kyle RA, Greipp PR, Banks PM. The diverse picture of gamma heavy chain disease: report of seven cases and review of literature. *Mayo Clin Proc* 1981; **56**:439–51.

◆40. Wester SM, Banks PM, Li CY. The histopathology of gamma heavy-chain disease. *Am J Clin Pathol* 1982; **78**:427–36.

41. Cozzolino F, Vercelli D, Castigli E, Becucci A, Di Guglielmo R. A new case of gamma heavy chain disease. Clinical and immunochemical studies. *Scand J Haematol* 1982; **28**:145–50.

42. Hudnall SD, Alperin JB, Petersen JR. Composite nodular lymphocyte-predominance Hodgkin disease and gamma heavy-chain disease: a case report and review of the literature. *Arch Pathol Lab Med* 2001; **125**:803–7.

43. Ellis VM, Cowley DM, Taylor KM, Marlton P. Gamma heavy chain disease developing in association with myelodysplastic syndrome. *Br J Haematol* 1992; **81**:125–6.

44. Agrawal S, Abboudi Z, Matutes E, Catovsky D. First report of fludarabine in gamma heavy-chain disease. *Br J Haematol* 1994; **88**:653–5.

45. Forte FA, Prelli F, Yount WJ, Jerry LM, Kochwa S, Franklin EC, Kunkel HG. Heavy chain disease of the μtype: report of the first case. *Blood* 1970; **36**:137–44.

46. Preud'homme JL, Bauwens M, Dumont G, Goujon JM, Dreyfus B, Touchard G. Cast nephropathy in μ heavy chain disease. *Clin Nephrol* 1997; **48**:118–21.

47. Wahner-Roedler DL, Kyle RA. Mu-heavy chain disease: Presentation as a benign monoclonal gammopathy. *Am J Hematol* 1992; **40**:56–60.

48. Witzens M, Egerer G, Stahl D, Werle E, Goldschmidt H, Haas R. A case of μ heavy-chain disease associated with hyperglobulinaemia, anaemia, and a positive Coombs test. *Ann Hematol* 1998; **77**:231–4.

29

Waldenström's disease

GIAMPAOLO MERLINI AND STEVEN P. TREON

INTRODUCTION

Waldenström's macroglobulinemia (WM) is a distinct clinicopathological entity resulting from the proliferation of B lymphocytes that show maturation to plasma cells, constituting a pathognomonic bone marrow lymphoplasmacytic infiltrate, and that synthesize monoclonal IgM.[1] This condition is considered to correspond to the lymphoplasmacytic lymphoma as defined by the Revised European American lymphoma (REAL) and World Health Organisation classification systems.[2–4] The disease was first reported by Jan Waldenström (Fig. 29.1), who described two patients with a high level of macroglobulin, i.e. pentameric immunoglobulin M (IgM), marked hyperviscosity with typical funduscopic picture, and lymphocytoid bone marrow infiltration.[5]

EPIDEMIOLOGY AND ETIOLOGY

Waldenström's macroglobulinemia is a rare disease, with an incidence that is ten times less frequent than multiple myeloma, accounting for approximately 2% of all hematologic malignancies. The age-adjusted incidence rate is 3.4 per million among males and 1.7 per million among females in the USA, with a geometrical increase with age.[6] The incidence rate for WM is higher among Caucasians, with African descendants representing only 5% of all patients. A previous study had reported an age-standardized annual incidence rate of 6.1 per million in white men and 2.5 per million in white women.[7]

Genetic factors may contribute to the pathogenesis of WM, as suggested by several reports of familiar disease, including involvement of monozygotic twins,[8] as well as frequent familiar association with other lymphoproliferative and immunological disorders in healthy relatives, including hypogammaglobulinemia, autoantibodies (especially rheumatoid factors), increased serum immunoglobulin levels, and hyperreactive B cells.[9,10] Increased expression of the *bcl-2* gene with enhanced B-cell survival may underlie the increased immunoglobulin synthesis in familial WM.[11] The role of environmental factors in WM is undetermined. There is no clear association with chronic antigenic stimulation from infections, autoimmune diseases, or allergy or with specific occupational exposure.[12] The relevance of viral infection remains to be established. Data regarding a possible link between hepatitis C virus (HCV) and WM are inconclusive and limited to small patient populations.[13–16] The role of human herpesvirus-8 remains undetermined in the pathogenesis of WM.[17–19]

BIOLOGY

Cytogenetic findings

Several studies, usually performed on limited series of patients, have been published on cytogenetic findings in WM. A great variety of numerical and structural chromosome abnormalities have been reported (reviewed by Merlini[20]), but none of these is specific. Complex

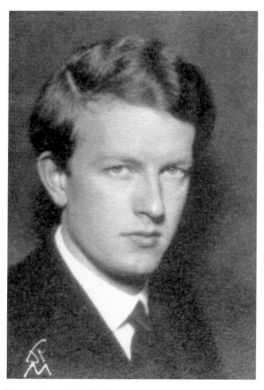

Acta Medica Scandinavica. Vol. CXVII, fasc. III—IV, 1944.

(From Med. Clin. Akad. Hospital, Upsala (Sweden). Chief: Prof. G. Bergmark).

Incipient myelomatosis or «essential« hyperglobulinemia with fibrinogenopenia — a new syndrome?

By

JAN WALDENSTRÖM.

Submitted for publication September 2, 1943.

Figure 29.1 *Jan Waldenström at the age of 38, when he described the two prototypic cases of macroglobulinemia in* Acta Medica Scandinavica.

karyotypes are usually associated with more aggressive disease.[21,22] Notable, however, is the absence of IgH switch region rearrangements.[23]

NATURE OF THE CLONAL CELLS

The WM bone marrow B-cell clone shows intraclonal differentiation from small lymphocytes with large focal deposits of surface immunoglobulins, to lymphoplasmacytic cells, to mature plasma cells that contain intracytoplasmic immunoglobulins.[24] Clonal B cells are detectable among blood B lymphocytes, and their number increases in patients who fail to respond to therapy or who progress.[25] These clonal blood cells present the peculiar capacity to differentiate spontaneously, in *in vitro* culture, to plasma cells. This is through an interleukin-6 (IL-6)-dependent process in IgM monoclonal gammopathy of undetermined significance (MGUS) and mostly an IL-6-independent process in WM patients.[26] All these cells express the monoclonal IgM present in the blood and a variable percentage of them also express surface IgD. The characteristic immunophenotypic profile of the lymphoplasmacytic cells in WM includes the expression of the pan B-cell markers CD19, CD20, CD22, CD79, and FMC7.[2,27–30] The majority of cases do not express CD10 or CD23. Expression of CD5 and CD23, the hallmarks of CLL, is detectable in 5–20% of cases; however,

co-expression of these two markers is rare, probably occurring in less than 5%.[27]

This is a post-germinal center phenotype and suggests that the disorder may arise from memory B cells.[20] This indication is further strengthened by the results of the analysis of the nature (silent or amino-acid replacing) and distribution (in framework or CDR regions) of somatic mutations in Ig heavy- and light-chain variable regions performed in patients with WM.[31,32] This analysis showed a high rate of replacement mutations, compared with the closest germline genes, clustering in the CDR regions and without intraclonal variation. Subsequent studies confirmed that tumor V_H genes present somatic mutations and a complete lack of intraclonal variation, and no evidence for any isotype-switched transcripts.[33,34] These data indicate that WM may originate from a IgM$^+$ and/or IgM$^+$IgD$^+$ memory B cell. Normal IgM$^+$ memory B cells localize in bone marrow, where they mature to IgM-secreting cells.[35]

CLINICAL FEATURES

Waldenström's macroglobulinemia is a disease of the elderly with a median age of 63 years (range 25–92), with a slight predominance of males over females.[36] The symptoms are usually vague and non-specific, the most common being weakness, anorexia, and weight loss. Raynaud's phenomenon and symptoms due to peripheral neuropathy may precede more serious manifestations by many years. Symptoms and physical findings at diagnosis are summarized in Table 29.1. Hepatosplenomegaly and lymphadenopathy are prominent in a minority of patients. Purpura is frequently associated with cryoglobulinemia and more rarely with AL amyloidosis,

Table 29.1 *Presenting features and physical findings at diagnosis in 215 patients with Waldenström's macroglobulinemia*

	Frequency (%)
Symptoms	
Weakness	66
Anorexia	25
Peripheral neuropathy	24
Weight loss	17
Fever	15
Raynaud's phenomenon	11
Physical findings	
Hepatomegaly (>2 cm from the costal margin)	20
Splenomegaly	19
Lymphadenopathy	15
Purpura	9
Hemorrhagic manifestations	7

while hemorrhagic manifestations and neuropathies are multifactorial (see later). The morbidity associated with WM is caused by the concurrence of two main components: tissue infiltration by neoplastic cells and, more importantly, the physicochemical and immunological properties of the monoclonal IgM (Fig. 29.2).

As shown in Table 29.2, the monoclonal IgM can produce clinical manifestations through several different mechanisms related to its physicochemical properties, non-specific interactions with other proteins, antibody activity, and tendency to deposit in tissues.[37–39]

Physicochemical effects of the IgM

HYPERVISCOSITY SYNDROME

Blood hyperviscosity is the most common complication of circulating IgM, occurring in 17% patients.[36] The mechanisms behind the marked increase in the resistance to blood flow and the resulting impaired transit through the microcirculatory system are rather complex.[40–42] The main determinants are: (1) a high concentration of monoclonal IgMs, which may form aggregates and may bind water through their carbohydrate component; and (2) their interaction with blood cells. Monoclonal IgMs increase red cell aggregation (*rouleaux* formation) and red cell internal viscosity while also reducing deformability. The possible presence of cryoglobulins can contribute to increasing blood viscosity as well as to

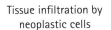
Tissue infiltration by
neoplastic cells

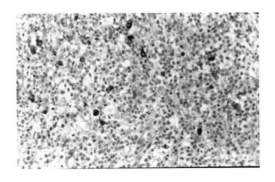

Bone marrow	Lungs
Liver	GI tract
Spleen	Kidneys
Lymph nodes	Skin
	Eyes
	CNS

Biologic properties of
the monoclonal IgM

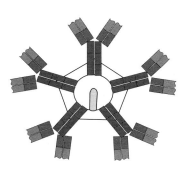

Hyperviscosity syndrome	Polyneuropathies
Cryoglobulinemia I	Cryoglobulinemia II
Hemostatic abnormalities	Cold agglutinin disease
AL amyloidosis	
Tissue deposits of amorphous IgM	

Figure 29.2 *The morbidity associated with Waldenström's macroglobulinemia is caused by the concurrence of two main components: tissue infiltration by neoplastic cells and, more importantly, the physicochemical and immunological properties of the monoclonal IgM. CNS, central nervous system; GI, gastrointestinal.*

Table 29.2 *Clinical manifestations caused by monoclonal IgM (from Merlini G. Waldenström's macroglobulinemia – clinical manifestations and prognosis. In: Schechter GP, Hoffman R, Schrier SL (eds) Hematology 1999. Washington, DC: American Society of Hematology, 1999:358–69. Copyright American Society of Hematology, used with permission)*

Properties of monoclonal IgM	Resulting condition	Clinical manifestations
Physicochemical		
Intrinsic viscosity	Hyperviscosity syndrome	Fatigue, headache, blurred vision, easy mucosal bleeding, impaired mentation up to coma
Precipitation on cooling	Cryoglobulinemia type I	Raynaud's phenomenon, acrocyanosis, necrosis, ulcers, purpura, cold urticaria
Protein–protein interaction	Hemostatic abnormalities	Bleeding diathesis: bruising, purpura, mucosal bleeding; rarely, brain hemorrhages
Antibody activity versus:		
Nerve constituents	Polyneuropathies	Anti-MAG-related: symmetric, distal, progressive, sensorimotor neuropathy, ataxic gait, bilateral foot drop IgM with other specificities: – symmetric, distal, progressive painful sensory neuropathy – prominent motor neuropathy
IgG	Cryoglobulinemia type II	Weakness, purpura, arthralgias, proteinuria, renal failure, progressive, symmetric distal sensorimotor neuropathy combined with mononeuropathies (e.g. foot or wrist drop)
RBC antigens	Cold agglutinin hemolytic anemia	Mild, chronic hemolytic anemia exacerbated after cold exposure; Raynaud's phenomenon, acrocyanosis, and livedo reticularis
Tendency to deposit into tissues		
As amorphous aggregates in skin, GI tract, kidney	Specific organ dysfunction	Skin: bullous skin disease, papules on extremities GI: diarrhea, malabsorption, bleeding Kidney: mild, reversible proteinuria, mostly asymptomatic
As amyloid fibrils (light chains)	AL amyloidosis	Fatigue, weight loss, periorbital purpura, edema, hepatomegaly, macroglossia Dysfunction of organs involved: kidneys, heart, liver, peripheral sensory and autonomic neuropathies

GI, gastrointestinal; MAG, myelin-associated glycoprotein; RBC, red blood cell.

the tendency to induce erythrocyte aggregation. Serum viscosity is proportional to IgM concentration up to 30 g/L, then increases sharply at higher levels.[42] Plasma viscosity and hematocrit are directly regulated by the body. Increased plasma viscosity may also contribute to inappropriately low erythropoietin production, which is the major reason for anemia in these patients.[43] Clinical manifestations are related to circulatory disturbances that can be best appreciated by ophthalmoscopy, which shows distended and tortuous retinal veins, hemorrhages and papilledema (Fig. 29.3, Plate 13). Symptoms usually occur when the monoclonal IgM concentration exceeds 50 g/L[38] or when serum viscosity is >4 centipoises (cp),[44] but there is a great individual variability, with some patients showing no evidence of hyperviscosity even at 10 cp. The most common symptoms are oronasal bleeding, visual disturbances due to retinal bleeding, and dizziness that may rarely lead to coma.[45] Heart failure can be aggravated, particularly in the elderly, owing to increased blood viscosity, expanded plasma volume, and anemia. Inappropriate transfusion can exacerbate hyperviscosity and may precipitate cardiac failure.

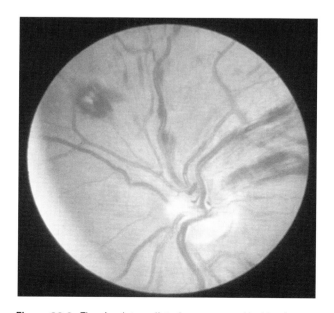

Figure 29.3 *The circulatory disturbances caused by blood hyperviscosity are best appreciated by ophthalmoscopy, which shows distended and tortuous retinal veins, hemorrhages, and papilledema.*

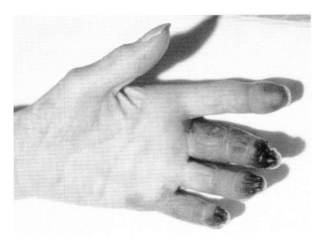

Figure 29.4 *Necrosis of the tip of the fingers in a patient with Waldenström's macroglobulinemia and type I cryoglobulinemia.*

TYPE I CRYOGLOBULINEMIA

In 7–20% of WM patients, the monoclonal IgM can behave as a cryoglobulin (type I), but it is symptomatic in 5% or less of the cases.[28,46] Cryoprecipitation is mainly dependent on the concentration of monoclonal IgM; for this reason plasmapheresis or plasma exchange are commonly effective in this condition. Symptoms result from impaired blood flow in small vessels and include Raynaud's phenomenon, acrocyanosis, and necrosis of the regions most exposed to cold (tip of the nose, ears, fingers, toes; see Fig. 29.4 and Plate 14), malleolar ulcers, purpura, and cold urticaria. Renal manifestations may occur but are infrequent.

Protein–protein interactions

Monoclonal IgM can interact (with low affinity) with circulating proteins or with proteins associated with cell membrane including the coagulation factors fibrinogen, and factors V, VII, and VIII, resulting in prolonged clotting times.[38] Platelet function (adhesion and aggregation) is also impaired, probably due to platelet coating by macroglobulins, and results in prolonged bleeding time.[38] These abnormalities are IgM-concentration-dependent and are reversible following therapy.

Antibody activity

Monoclonal IgM may exert its pathogenic effects through specific recognition of autologous antigens, the most notable being nerve constituents, immunoglobulin determinants, and red blood cell antigens (Table 29.2).

NEUROPATHY

In a series of 215 patients with WM, Merlini *et al.*[36] reported the clinical presence of peripheral neuropathy in 24% of WM patients (Table 29.1), although prevalence rates ranging from 5 to 38% have been reported in other series.[47,48] An estimated 6.5–10% of idiopathic neuropathies are associated with a monoclonal gammopathy, with a preponderance of IgM (60%) followed by IgG (30%) and IgA (10%) (reviewed in Nemni *et al.*[49] and Ropper and Gorson[50]) (see also Chapter 23). In WM patients, the nerve damage is mediated by diverse pathogenetic mechanisms: IgM antibody activity toward nerve constituents causing demyelinating polyneuropathies; endoneurial granulofibrillar deposits of IgM without antibody activity, associated with axonal polyneuropathy; occasionally by tubular deposits in the endoneurium associated with IgM cryoglobulin and, rarely, by amyloid deposits or by neoplastic cell infiltration of nerve structures.[51]

Half of the patients with IgM neuropathy have a distinctive clinical syndrome that is associated with antibodies against a minor 100-kDa glycoprotein component of nerve, myelin-associated glycoprotein (MAG). Anti-MAG antibodies are generally monoclonal IgMκ, and usually also exhibit reactivity with other glycoproteins or glycolipids that share antigenic determinants with MAG.[52–54] The anti-MAG-related neuropathy is typically distal and symmetrical, affecting both motor and sensory functions; it is slowly progressive with a long period of stability.[48,55] Most patients present with sensory complaints (paresthesias, aching discomfort, dysesthesias, or lancinating pains), imbalance and gait ataxia, owing to lack proprioception, and leg muscles atrophy in advanced stage.

Patients with predominantly demyelinating sensory neuropathy in association with monoclonal IgM to gangliosides with disialosyl moieties, such as GD1b, GD3, GD2, GT1b, and GQ1b, have also been reported.[56,57] Anti-GD1b and anti-GQ1b antibodies were significantly associated with predominantly sensory ataxic neuropathy.[57] These antiganglioside monoclonal IgMs present core clinical features of chronic ataxic neuropathy with variably present ophthalmoplegia and/or red blood cell cold agglutinating activity. The disialosyl epitope is also present on red blood cell glycophorins, thereby accounting for the red cell cold agglutinin activity of anti-Pr_2 specificity.[58,59]

Monoclonal IgM proteins that bind to gangliosides with a terminal trisaccharide moiety, including GM2 and GalNac-GD1A, are associated with chronic demyelinating neuropathy and severe sensory ataxia, unresponsive to corticosteroids.[60] Antiganglioside IgM proteins may also cross-react with lipopolysaccharides of *Campylobacter jejuni*, whose infection is known to precipitate the Miller Fisher syndrome, a variant of the Guillain–Barré syndrome.[61] This finding indicates that molecular mimicry may play a role in this condition.

Antisulfatide monoclonal IgM proteins, associated with sensory/sensorimotor neuropathy, have been detected in 5% of patients with IgM monoclonal gammopathy and neuropathy.[62] Motor neuron disease has been reported in patients with WM, and monoclonal IgM with anti-GM1 and sulfoglucuronyl paragloboside activity.[63] POEMS (polyneuropathy, organomegaly, endocrinopathy, M-protein, and skin changes) syndrome is rarely associated with WM.[64]

TYPE II CRYOGLOBULINEMIA

The antibody activity of the monoclonal IgM to immunoglobulin (rheumatoid factors) is at the basis of type II cryoglobulinemia. This is an immune complex disease characterized by vasculitis affecting small vessels that is associated with HCV infection.[65] The clinical manifestations are those of immune complex-mediated vasculitis of small vessels and range from benign purpura to life-threatening severe systemic vasculitis. The main clinical features are weakness, purpura (87%), arthralgias (60–70%), Raynaud's phenomenon (20%), and renal (35–50%), hepatic (40–70%), and peripheral nerve involvement (30–40%). Renal involvement represents one of the most serious complications of type II cryoglobulinemia and is characterized by a membranoproliferative glomerulonephritis with a particular monocyte infiltration.[66] Clinically, this involvement may range from isolated proteinuria to overt nephritic syndrome with periods of remission and exacerbation, and, if not appropriately treated, may eventually end in renal failure.

COLD AGGLUTININ HEMOLYTIC ANEMIA

Monoclonal IgM may present cold agglutinin activity, i.e. it recognizes specific red cell antigens at temperatures below physiological, producing chronic hemolytic anemia. This disorder occurs in approximately 10% of patients[67] and is associated with cold agglutinin titers >1:1000 in most cases. The monoclonal component is usually an IgMk and reacts most commonly with I/i antigens, with complement fixation and activation.[68,69] Specificity for other red blood cell antigens has been described.[37] Mild chronic hemolytic anemia can be exacerbated after cold exposure but rarely does hemoglobin drop below 70 g/L. The hemolysis is usually extravascular (removal of C3b opsonized cells by the reticuloendotelial system, primarily in the liver) and rarely intravascular from complement destruction of red blood cell (RBC) membrane. The agglutination of RBCs in the cooler peripheral circulation also causes Raynaud's syndrome, acrocyanosis, and livedo reticularis. Macroglobulins with the properties of both cryoglobulins and cold agglutinins with anti-Pr specificity have been reported. These properties may have as a common basis the immune binding of the sialic acid-containing carbohydrate present on red blood cell glycophorins and on Ig molecules.[70] Several other macroglobulins with various antibody activity toward autologous antigens (i.e. phospholipids, tissue and plasma proteins, etc.) and foreign ligands have also been reported.[37–39]

Tissue deposition

The monoclonal protein can deposit in several tissues as amorphous aggregates. Linear deposition of monoclonal IgM along the skin basement membrane is associated with bullous skin disease.[71] Amorphous IgM deposits in the dermis determine the so-called IgM storage papules on the extensor surface of the extremities – macroglobulinemia cutis.[72] Deposition of monoclonal IgM in the lamina propria and/or submucosa of the intestine may be associated with diarrhea, malabsorption, and gastrointestinal bleeding.[73,74] It is well known that kidney involvement is less common and less severe in WM than in multiple myeloma, probably because the amount of light chain excreted in the urine is generally lower in WM than in myeloma and because of the absence of contributing factors, such as hypercalcemia, although cast nephropathy has also been described in WM.[75] On the other hand, the IgM macromolecule is more susceptible to being trapped in the glomerular loops where ultrafiltration presumably contributes to its precipitation, forming subendothelial deposits of aggregated IgM proteins that occlude the glomerular capillaries.[76] Mild and reversible proteinuria may result and most patients are asymptomatic.

The deposition of monoclonal light chain as fibrillar amyloid deposits (AL amyloidosis) is uncommon in patients with WM.[77] Clinical expression and prognosis are similar to those of other AL patients with involvement of heart (44%), kidneys (32%), liver (14%), lungs (10%), peripheral/autonomic nerves (38%), and soft tissues (18%). However, the incidence of cardiac and pulmonary involvement is higher in patients with monoclonal IgM than with other immunoglobulin isotypes. The association of WM with reactive amyloidosis (AA) has been documented rarely.[78,79] Simultaneous occurrence of fibrillary glomerulopathy, characterized by glomerular deposits of wide non-congophilic fibrils and amyloid deposits, has been reported in WM.[80]

Manifestations related to tissue infiltration by neoplastic cells

Tissue infiltration by neoplastic cells is rare and can involve various organs and tissues, from the bone marrow (described later) to the liver, spleen, lymph nodes, and possibly the lungs, gastrointestinal tract, kidneys, skin, eyes, and central nervous system. Pulmonary involvement in the form of masses, nodules, diffuse infiltrate, or pleural effusions is relatively rare, since the overall incidence of pulmonary and pleural findings reported for WM is only 3–5%.[81–83] Cough is the most common presenting symptom, followed by dyspnea and chest pain. Chest radiographic findings include parenchymal infiltrates, confluent masses, and effusions. Malabsorption, diarrhea,

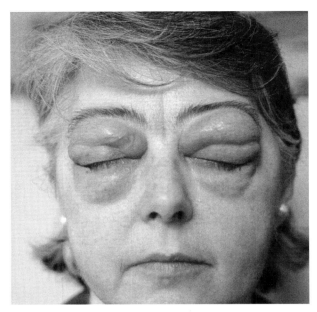

Figure 29.5 *Involvement of the periorbital structures by neoplastic cells in a patient with Waldenström's macroglobulinemia.*

Table 29.3a *Values of the main laboratory parameters in 215 patients with Waldenström's macroglobulinemia*

Parameter	Value, median (range)
Hemoglobin (g/L)	109 (40–157)
WBC ($\times 10^9$/L)	6.9 (1.5–12.3)
Platelets ($\times 10^9$/L)	192 (18–534)
IgM monoclonal component (g/L)	23.3 (10.5–98.7)
Serum viscosity (relative to water)	1.9 (1.75–5.0)

Table 29.3b *Frequencies of abnormal hematology parameters in 215 patients with Waldenström's macroglobulinemia*

Parameter	Frequency (%)
Hemoglobin <120 g/L	63
WBC <3 $\times 10^9$/L	4
Platelets <100 $\times 10^9$/L	16
IgM monoclonal component:	
κ/λ	80/20
>30 g/L	35
Bence Jones proteinuria	38
Serum β_2-microglobulin >3 mg/L	62
Relative serum viscosity >4	17

WBC, white blood cells.

bleeding, or obstruction indicate involvement of the gastrointestinal tract at the level of the stomach, duodenum, or small intestine.[84–87] In contrast to multiple myeloma, infiltration of the kidney interstitium with lymphoplasmacytoid cells is not a rare event in WM,[76,88] while renal or perirenal masses are unusual.[89] The skin can be the site of dense lymphoplasmacytic infiltrates, similar to that seen in the liver, spleen, and lymph nodes, forming cutaneous plaques and, rarely, nodules.[72,90] Chronic urticaria and IgM gammopathy are the two cardinal features of the Schnitzler syndrome, which is not usually associated initially with clinical features of WM,[91] although evolution to WM is not uncommon.[72] Thus, close follow-up of these patients is warranted. Invasion of articular and periarticular structures by WM malignant cells is rarely reported.[92] The neoplastic cells can infiltrate the periorbital structures (Fig. 29.5, Plate 15), lacrimal gland, and retro-orbital lymphoid tissues, resulting in ocular nerve palsies.[93,94] Direct infiltration of the central nervous system by monoclonal lymphoplasmacytic cells as infiltrates or as tumors constitutes the rarely observed Bing–Neel syndrome, characterized clinically by confusion, memory loss, disorientation, and motor dysfunction (reviewed in Civit *et al.*[95]).

LABORATORY INVESTIGATIONS AND FINDINGS

Laboratory findings are summarized in Tables 29.3a and b.

Hematological abnormalities

Anemia is the most common finding in patients with symptomatic WM and is caused by a combination of factors: mild decrease in red cell survival, impaired erythropoiesis, hemolysis, moderate plasma volume expansion, and blood loss from the gastrointestinal tract. Blood smears are usually normocytic and normochromic, and rouleaux formation is often pronounced. Electronically measured mean corpuscular volume may be elevated spuriously owing to erythrocyte aggregation. In addition, the hemoglobin estimate can be inaccurate, i.e. falsely high, because of interaction between the monoclonal protein and the diluent used in some automated analyzers.[96] Leukocyte and platelet counts are usually within the reference range at presentation, although patients may occasionally present with severe thrombocytopenia. As reported above, monoclonal B lymphocytes expressing surface IgM and late-differentiation B-cell markers can be detected in blood by flow cytometry.

A raised erythrocyte sedimentation rate is almost constantly observed in WM and may be the first clue to the presence of the macroglobulin.[5] The clotting abnormality detected most frequently is prolongation of thrombin time. AL amyloidosis should be suspected in all patients with nephrotic syndrome, cardiomyopathy, hepatomegaly, or peripheral neuropathy. Diagnosis requires the demonstration of green birefringence under polarized light of amyloid deposits stained with Congo red.

Biochemical investigations

High-resolution electrophoresis combined with immunofixation of serum and urine are recommended for identification and characterization of the IgM monoclonal protein (Fig. 29.6).[97] The light chain of the monoclonal IgM is κ in 75–80% of patients.[36,44] A few WM patients have more than one M-component. The concentration of the serum monoclonal protein is very variable but in most cases lies within the range of 15–45 g/L. Densitometry should be adopted to determine IgM levels for serial evaluations because nephelometry is unreliable and shows large intralaboratory as well as interlaboratory variation (see Chapter 9).[97] The presence of cold agglutinins or cryoglobulins may affect determination of IgM levels and, therefore, testing for cold agglutinins and cryoglobulins should be performed at diagnosis. If present, subsequent serum samples should be analyzed under warm conditions for determination of serum monoclonal IgM level. Although Bence Jones proteinuria is frequently present, it exceeds 1 g/24 hours in only 3% of cases.[98]

Serum β_2-microglobulin was above the upper limit of the reference range (3 mg/L) in approximately 60% of WM patients at diagnosis in our study population (Table 29.3b).

Blood viscosity

Blood viscosity should be measured if the patient has signs or symptoms of hyperviscosity syndrome. Measurement of viscosity in whole blood at low shear rates may be the best indicator of hemorheological changes in patients with WM.[99] In practice, a correlation between level of M-protein and symptoms may be used to anticipate repeat plasma exchanges as the M-protein approaches the level associated with hyperviscosity. Fundoscopy remains an excellent indicator of clinically relevant hyperviscosity. Cryoglobulins should be searched for

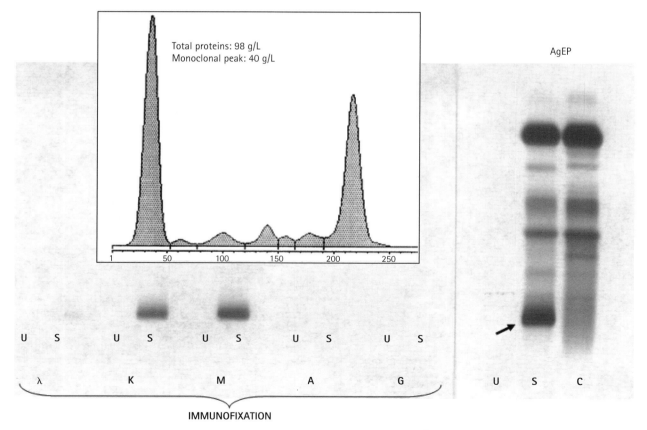

Figure 29.6 Right: *high-resolution agarose gel electrophoresis (AgEP) of control serum (C) and of serum (S) and urine (U) from a patient with Waldenström's macroglobulinemia (anode above). An important monoclonal component is present in the serum, in the gamma region (arrow).* Left: *By immunofixation using anti-IgG (G), anti-IgA (A), anti-IgM (M), anti-κ (K), and anti-λ (λ) antisera the serum monoclonal band is typed as IgMκ, while no monoclonal protein is detectable by immunofixation in the urine.* Inset: *The monoclonal IgMk is quantified by densitometry as being 40 g/L.*

(following the method indicated in the guidelines of the College of American Pathologists[100]) in the presence of suggestive clinical features. Rheumatoid factor activity and low C4 levels (<8 mg/dL) are common findings in type II cryoglobulinemia.

Bone marrow findings

The bone marrow is always involved in WM. Bone marrow biopsy is necessary since aspiration frequently yields a 'dry tap.' Three cytological subtypes have been identified in conjunction with patterns of bone marrow infiltration: lymphoplasmacytoid, constituted by small lymphocytes and plasmacytoid cells characterized by a nodular pattern (47% of all patients); lymphoplasmacytic, in which small lymphocytes and mature plasma cells predominate and mast cells may be conspicuous, associated mainly with an interstitial/nodular pattern (42%); and polymorphous, with a packed marrow and characterized by a wide spectrum of cells, including small lymphocytes, plasmacytoid cells, plasma cells, large transformed cells, and immunoblasts with mitotic figures (11%).[101] 'Intranuclear' periodic acid-Schiff (PAS)-positive inclusions (Dutcher-Fahey bodies; see Fig. 29.7 and Plate 16)[102] consisting of IgM deposits in the perinuclear space, and sometimes in intranuclear vacuoles, may be seen occasionally in lymphoid cells.

Other investigations

Magnetic resonance imaging (MRI) of the spine in conjunction with computed tomography (CT) of the abdomen and pelvis are useful in evaluating the disease status in WM.[103] Bone marrow involvement can be documented by MRI studies of the spine in over 90% of patients, while CT of the abdomen and pelvis demonstrated

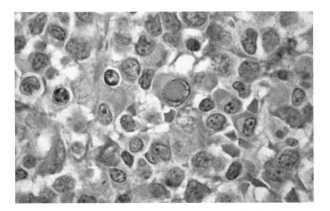

Figure 29.7 *Lymphoplasmacytic population with abundant plasma cell component and presence of a Dutcher–Fahey body in a lymph node. (Courtesy of Professor Umberto Magrini, Department of Human Pathology, University of Pavia, Italy.)*

enlarged nodes in 43% of WM patients.[103] Lymph node biopsy may show preserved architecture or replacement by infiltration of neoplastic cells with lymphoplasmacytoid, lymphoplasmacytic, or polymorphous cytological patterns. The residual disease after high-dose chemotherapy with allogeneic or autologous stem-cell rescue can be monitored by polymerase chain reaction (PCR)-based methods using primers specific for the monoclonal Ig variable regions.

DIAGNOSTIC CRITERIA AND DIFFERENTIAL DIAGNOSIS

A monoclonal IgM may be seen in most forms of B-cell lymphoproliferative disorder as well as in IgM-MGUS.[44,104] Recent papers have focused on the necessity to develop diagnostic criteria,[28,105] and the lack of accepted criteria for the diagnosis of WM has triggered an international initiative to define such criteria.[4] There is a wide consensus that the diagnosis should rely on the following three main criteria:

1   Central to the diagnosis of WM is the demonstration, by trephine biopsy, of *bone marrow infiltration by a lymphoplasmacytic cell population* constituted by small lymphocytes with evidence of plasmacytoid/ plasma cell differentiation constituting more than 20% of the total bone marrow cells. The pattern of bone marrow infiltration may be diffuse, interstitial, or nodular, showing usually an intertrabecular pattern of infiltration. A solely paratrabecular pattern of infiltration is unusual and should raise the possibility of follicular lymphoma.[4]

2   The bone marrow infiltration should routinely be confirmed by *immunophenotypic studies* (flow cytometry and/or immunohistochemistry) showing the following profile: sIgM+CD19+CD20+CD22+ CD79+. The majority of cases will not express CD10 or CD23, while a proportion of patients (5–20%) appear to express the CD5 antigen. In these cases, care should be taken to exclude chronic lymphocytic leukemia and mantle cell lymphoma satisfactorily.[4]

3   A *serum monoclonal IgM* is present by definition and usually at significant concentration (>20 g/L).[1,20,106] However, most experts agree that a diagnosis of WM could be made irrespective of IgM concentration in the presence of bone marrow infiltration by a lymphoplasmacytic cell population with characteristic immunophenotype.[4] Patients with a serum IgG and IgA monoclonal protein, or without a monoclonal component (non-secretory lymphoplasmacytic lymphoma), have been reported, and they present similar clinical problems to those seen in WM

patients. However, their relationship to WM is unclear at present.

These criteria identify a large group of patients diagnosed as WM who may be asymptomatic, and most probably not in need of treatment, as well as those who are symptomatic and in need of treatment.

It is also well recognized that a population of patients exist who have clinically overt manifestations owing to the biological effects of the monoclonal IgM but in whom there is no evidence of bone marrow infiltration by lymphoplasmacytic lymphoma, and in whom the central diagnostic criteria for WM are not therefore fulfilled. Such patients will usually have peripheral neuropathy, cryoglobulins, cold agglutinin disease, AL amyloidosis, or any of the other rare clinical manifestations listed in Table 29.2. It is appropriate to consider these patients as having an IgM-related disorder.[4,97,107]

Patients with asymptomatic monoclonal IgM without bone marrow infiltration, or with a bone marrow infiltrate <20%, can be classified as having IgM-MGUS. This condition is by far the most common among individuals with a monoclonal IgM.[44,108] Differentiation of a patient with IgM-MGUS from one with asymptomatic WM may be difficult.[109] For instance, some patients may have a detectable bone marrow clonal B cells by flow cytometry but without morphological evidence of bone marrow infiltration at trephine biopsy. These patients should be classified as IgM-MGUS until further outcome data become available.

The clinicopathological correlates of monoclonal IgMs constitute a broad spectrum, including chronic lymphocytic leukemia (CLL), diffuse large B-cell lymphoma, extranodal marginal-zone lymphoma, follicular lymphoma, and mantle-cell lymphoma.[104] A monoclonal IgM may be present in virtually all subtypes of peripheral B-cell disorders and, although monoclonal protein concentrations are generally higher in WM, there is considerable overlap. Immunophenotypic criteria are, therefore, essential for the accurate diagnosis of WM.[104] A differential diagnosis between WM, CLL, and small lymphocytic lymphoma may be difficult sometimes.[110] Patients with chronic lymphocytic leukemia generally have a monoclonal B-cell lymphocytosis of more than 5×10^9/L and leukemic B cells with the following markers: co-expression of CD5 and pan-B-cell antigens CD19, CD20, and CD23, weak surface immunoglobulin (most often IgM or IgM and IgD with either κ or λ light chain), weak/negative CD22, and negative FMC7 and CD79B.[111] Guidelines for subtyping small B-cell lymphomas in bone marrow biopsies have been established,[112] and molecular biology techniques are increasingly being used in the differential diagnosis of these lymphomas.[113] In patients with μ heavy-chain disease, immunofixation or immunoselection studies are necessary to confirm the presence of Ig heavy-chain fragment without the corresponding light chain.[97,114] A lymphoplasmacytic bone marrow infiltration producing a significant serum monoclonal IgM could occur in association with some small B-cell lymphomas, such as MALT lymphoma,[115,116] marginal zone lymphoma, nodal monocytoid B-cell lymphoma, and a variant of chronic lymphocytic leukemia.[117,118]

Patients with bone marrow infiltrate consisting entirely of IgM-producing plasma cells (cytoplasmic IgM+, CD20−, CD138+) possibly associated with lytic skeletal lesions and hypercalcemia should be considered as having IgM myeloma.[119–122] Although IgM myeloma and WM can have overlapping clinical features,[44] with tumor cells showing a hybrid multiple myeloma-WM phenotype,[119] demonstration of a t(11;14) cytogenetic abnormality helps in distinguishing IgM myeloma from MM, since t(11;14) has been seen in most (seven of eight) cases of IgM myeloma, but not in WM.[123]

These differential diagnoses are summarized in Table 29.4.

Table 29.4 *Classification of Waldenström's macroglobulinemia (WM) and related disorders*

Disorder	Laboratory features	Clinical features
WM	Lymphoplasmacytic infiltrate in marrow Specific immunophenotype[a] Serum monoclonal IgM	May be symptomatic or asymptomatic
IgM-related disorder	No marrow infiltration	Symptomatic, e.g. peripheral neuropathy, cryoglobulins, cold agglutinin disease, AL amyloidosis
IgM-MGUS	No marrow infiltrate	Asymptomatic
Other B-cell lymphoproliferative disorders[b]	Differentiate by immunophenotype	
μ-HCD	Heavy-chain fragment with no associated light chain	
IgM myeloma	IgM-producing plasma cells (cytoplasmic IgM+, CD20−, CD138+, t(11;14)+)	Possibly associated with lytic skeletal lesions and hypercalcemia

[a] sIg+CD19+CD20+CD22+CD79+CD5±CD10−CD23−.
[b] Chronic lymphocytic leukemia (CLL), diffuse large B-cell lymphoma, extranodal marginal-zone lymphoma, follicular lymphoma, and mantle-cell lymphoma.
HCD, heavy-chain disease; MGUS, monoclonal gammopathy of undetermined significance.

TREATMENT OF WALDENSTRÖM'S MACROGLOBULINEMIA

As part of the 2nd International Workshop on Waldenström's macroglobulinemia, a consensus panel was organized to recommend criteria for the initiation of therapy in patients with WM. The panel recommended that initiation of therapy should not be based on the IgM level *per se*, since this may not correlate with the clinical manifestations of WM. The consensus panel, however, agreed that initiation of therapy was appropriate for patients with constitutional symptoms, such as recurrent fever, night sweats, fatigue due to anemia, or weight loss. The presence of progressive symptomatic lymphadenopathy or splenomegaly provides additional reasons to begin therapy. The presence of anemia with a hemoglobin value of ≤ 10 g/dL or a platelet count $< 100 \times 10^9$/L owing to marrow infiltration also justifies treatment. Certain complications, such as hyperviscosity syndrome, symptomatic sensorimotor peripheral neuropathy, systemic amyloidosis, renal insufficiency, or symptomatic cryoglobulinemia, may also be indications for therapy.[124]

Options for initial therapy

A precise therapeutic algorithm for the upfront treatment of WM remains to be defined given a paucity of randomized clinical trials in this uncommon disorder. In view of this situation, a consensus panel composed of experts who treat WM was recently organized as part of the 2nd International Workshop on Waldenström's macroglobulinemia, which considered alkylator agents (e.g. chlorambucil), nucleoside analogs (cladribine or fludarabine), and the monoclonal antibody rituximab as reasonable choices for upfront therapy of WM.[125] Importantly, the panel felt that individual patient considerations, including the presence of cytopenias, need for more rapid disease control, age, and candidacy for autologous transplant therapy, should be taken into account in making the choice of a first-line agent. For patients who are candidates for autologous transplant therapy, and in whom such therapy is seriously considered, the panel recommended that exposure to alkylator or nucleoside analog therapy should be limited.

ALKYLATOR–BASED THERAPY

Oral alkylating drugs, alone and in combination therapy with steroids, have been extensively evaluated in the upfront treatment of WM. The greatest experience with oral alkylator therapy has been with chlorambucil, which has been administered on both a continuous (i.e. daily dose schedule) as well as an intermittent schedule. Patients receiving chlorambucil on a continuous schedule typically receive 0.1 mg/kg per day, whilst on the intermittent schedule patients will typically receive 0.3 mg/kg for 7 days, every 6 weeks. In a prospective randomized study, Kyle *et al.*[126] reported no significant difference in the overall response rate between these schedules (Table 29.5), although interestingly the median response duration was greater for patients receiving intermittent versus continuously dosed chlorambucil (46 vs. 26 months). Despite the favorable median response duration in this study for use of the intermittent schedule, no difference in the median overall survival was observed. Moreover, an increased incidence for development of myelodysplasia and acute myelogenous leukemia with the intermittent (three of 22 patients) versus the continuous (none of 24 patients) chlorambucil schedule prompted the authors of this study to express preference for use of continuous chlorambucil dosing.

The use of steroids in combination with alkylator therapy has also been explored. Dimopoulos and Alexanian[98] evaluated chlorambucil (8 mg/m^2) along with prednisone (40 mg/m^2) given orally for 10 days, every 6 weeks, and reported a major response (i.e. reduction of IgM by greater than 50%) in 72% of patients. Non-chlorambucil-based alkylator regimens employing melphalan and cyclophosphamide in combination with steroids have also been examined by Petrucci *et al.*[127] and

Table 29.5 *Alkylator-based therapy in Waldenström's macroglobulinemia*

Study	Number of patients	Setting	Regimen	Major RR[a] (%)	Median response duration
Facon[129]	110	UnRx	Chlorambucil (continuous)	31	NA
Kyle[126]	24	UnRx	Chlorambucil (continuous)	75	26 months
	22	UnRx	Chlorambucil (intermittent)	64	46 months
Dimopoulos[98]	77	UnRx	Chlorambucil, prednisone	72	NA
Petrucci[127]	31	UnRx	Melphalan, cyclophosphamide, prednisone→cyclophosphamide, prednisone (continuous)	74	66 months
Case[128]	33	UnRx and Rx	M-2 (BCNU, cyclophosphamide, vincristine, melphalan, prednisone)	82	43 months (CR), 39 months (PR)

[a] ≥ 50% reduction in serum IgM levels.
CR, complete response; NA, not applicable; PR, partial response; RR, response rate; Rx, previously treated; UnRx, previously untreated.

Case *et al.*[128] producing slightly higher overall response rates and response durations, although the benefit of these more complex regimens over chlorambucil remains to be demonstrated.

Facon *et al.*[129] have evaluated parameters predicting for response to alkylator therapy. Their studies in patients receiving single-agent chlorambucil demonstrated that age ≥60, male sex, symptomatic status, and cytopenias (but, interestingly, not high tumor burden and serum IgM levels) were associated with poor response to alkylator therapy. Additional factors to be taken into account in considering alkylator therapy for patients with WM include necessity for more rapid disease control given the slow nature of response to alkylator therapy, as well as consideration for preserving stem cells in patients who are candidates for autologous transplant therapy.

NUCLEOSIDE ANALOG THERAPY

Both cladribine and fludarabine have been extensively evaluated in untreated as well as previously treated WM patients. Cladribine administered as a single agent by continuous intravenous infusion, by 2-hour daily infusion, or by subcutaneous bolus injections for 5–7 days has resulted in major responses in 40–90% of patients who received primary therapy,[130–134] whilst in the salvage setting responses have ranged from 38% to 54% (Tables 29.6 and 29.7).[130,131,133–135] Median time to achievement of response in responding patients following cladribine ranged from 1.2 to 5 months.[130,133] The overall response rate with daily infusional fludarabine therapy administered mainly on 5-day schedules in previously untreated and treated WM patients has ranged from 38 to 100%[136–139] and 30–40%,[136,139–141] respectively, which are on par with the response data for cladribine (Tables 29.6 and 29.7). Median time to achievement of response for fludarabine was also on par with cladribine at 3–6 months. In general, response rates and durations of responses have been greater for patients receiving nucleoside analogs as first-line agents, although in four studies wherein both untreated and previously treated patients were enrolled, no substantial difference in the overall response rate was reported.[131,132,134,139] Myelo-suppression commonly occurred following prolonged exposure to either of the nucleoside analogs, as did lymphopenia with sustained depletion of both $CD4^+$ and $CD8^+$ T-lymphocytes observed in WM patients 1 year following initiation of therapy.[130,132] Treatment-related mortality due to myelosuppression and/or opportunistic infections attributable to immunosuppression occurred in up to 5% of all treated patients in some series with either nucleoside analog.

Factors predicting for response to nucleoside analogs in WM included age at start of treatment (<70 years), pre-treatment hemoglobin >95 g/L, platelets >75 000/mm³, disease relapsing off therapy, patients with resistant disease within the first year of diagnosis, and a long interval between first-line therapy and initiation of a nucleoside analog in relapsing patients.[130,136,142] There are limited data on the use of an alternate nucleoside analog to salvage patients whose disease relapsed or demonstrated resistance off cladribine or fludarabine therapy. Three of four (75%) patients responded to cladribine to salvage patients who progressed following an unmaintained remission to fludarabine, whereas only one of ten (10%) with disease resistant to fludarabine responded to cladribine.[143] However, Lewandowski *et al.*[144] recently reported a response in two of six patients (33%) and disease stabilization in the remaining patients to fludarabine, in spite of an inadequate response or progressive disease following cladribine therapy.

MONOCLONAL ANTIBODY THERAPY

Monoclonal antibody therapy has been extensively evaluated as upfront therapy in patients with WM. Rituximab,

Table 29.6 *Nucleoside analogs in untreated Waldenström's macroglobulinemia*

Study	Number of patients	Median number of courses	Major RR[a] (%)	Median response duration
Cladribine				
Dimopoulos[130]	26	2	85	2+ to 39+ months
Delannoy[131]	5	2	40	NA
Fridrik[132]	10	4	90	NA
Liu[133]	7	3	57	NA
Hellman[134]	9	4	44	NA
Fludarabine				
Dimopoulos[137]	2	3	100	NA
Foran[138]	15	5.2[b]	79	40 months
Thalhammer–Scherrer[139]	7	6	85	44+ months
Dhodapkar[140]	118	4–8	38	59 months

[a] ≥50% reduction in serum IgM levels.
[b] Mean number of infusions.
NA, not applicable; RR, response rate.

a chimeric antibody that targets CD20, was reported by Treon et al.[145] to induce a remission, and reverse anemia in a patient with WM that lasted over 19 months. Byrd et al.[146] subsequently demonstrated a 57% response rate (all partial response; PR) for seven heavily pre-treated WM patients who received four infusions of rituximab ($375 \, mg/m^2$ per week). The median progression-free survival for patients in this series was 6.6+ months. In a preliminary report, Weber et al.[147] reported a 75% response rate (two complete response (CR), four PR) for patients who received 4 weekly infusions of rituximab, with a median time to remission of 2 months and an unmaintained remission duration of 9 months. In addition to these studies, Foran et al.[148] demonstrated responses (both PR) in two of seven (29%) heavily pre-treated WM patients who received 4 weekly infusions of rituximab. Analysis of data pertaining to those WM patients who responded in the Foran et al.[148] study could not be distinguished because WM patients were grouped together and analyzed with B-CLL patients under the Kiel classification of immunocytomas. In a larger experience of single-agent rituximab use in WM, Treon et al.[149] reported on the outcome of 30 WM patients who had a median of one prior therapy and received treatment with rituximab (median 4; range 1–11.3 weekly infusions). Overall, 18 of 30 (60%) WM patients who were treated in this study

had a response, with eight (27%) patients achieving a PR and ten (33%) patients achieving a minor response (MR). Moreover, nine (30%) patients in this series had stable disease (SD) following treatment with rituximab. The time to treatment failure (TTF) for responding patients in this study was 8.9 months (3–20+ months) and 6.1 months (3–12+ months) for patients with SD. In addition, 19 of 30 (63%) and 15 of 30 (50%) patients had an increase in their hematocrit (HCT) and platelet (PLT) counts, respectively. Pre-rituximab therapy, seven of 30 (23.3%) patients were either transfusion or erythropoietin dependent, whereas only one of 30 (3.3%) patients required transfusions (no erythropoietin) after rituximab.

The use of an extended schedule of rituximab (i.e. four infusions of weekly rituximab followed by four additional weekly infusions at week 12) has also been explored in WM with improvements in response duration suggested by the outcome of two studies (Table 29.8). In a study involving 27 patients, Dimopoulos et al.[150] demonstrated an overall response rate (ORR) of 56%, with 44% of patients achieving a major response. The median time to progression in this study was not reached with a median follow-up of 16 months. In a study conducted by Waldenström's Macroglobulinemia Clinical Trials Group, 29 patients received extended rituximab therapy.[151]

Table 29.7 *Nucleoside analogs in previously treated Waldenström's macroglobulinemia*

Study	Number of patients	Median number of courses	Major RR[a] (%)	Median response duration
Cladribine				
Dimopoulos[136]	46	2	43	12 months
Delannoy[131]	13	2	38	NA
Betticher[135]	25	3	40	8 months
Liu[133]	13	3	54	NA
Hellman[134]	13	4	38	NA
Fludarabine				
Dimopoulos[137]	26	3	31	NA
Zinzani[141]	12	6	41	10+ months
Leblond[142]	71	6	30	32 months
Dhodapkar[140]	64	4–8	33	30 months

[a] ≥50% reduction in serum IgM levels.
NA, not applicable; RR, response rate.

Table 29.8 *Rituximab therapy in Waldenström's macroglobulinemia*

Study	Number of patients	Median number of courses	Major RR[a] (%)	Median response duration
Byrd[146]	6	4	57	6.6+ months
Weber[147]	7	4	75	9.0 months
Foran[148]	7	4	29	NA
Treon[149]	30	4	27	8.0 months
Dimopoulos[150]	27	8	56	16+ months
Treon[151]	29	8	48	20+ months

[a] ≥50% reduction in serum IgM levels.
NA, not applicable; RR, response rate.

Nineteen patients attained a response, with 14 patients (48.3%) achieving a major response. The time to best response was 17 months. Only 2 of 19 patients demonstrated progressive disease with a median follow-up of 29 months. Improvements in haematological function were again observed. Prior to therapy anemia (Hct <30%) and thrombocytopenia (<100 000/mm^3) were observed in 34.6% and 30.7% of patients, respectively. Post-rituximab therapy, anemia, and thrombocytopenia were present in 15.4% and 3.8% of patients.

The level of circulating IgM may predict those patients who are more likely to benefit from rituximab therapy. Dimopoulos et al.,[150] in their study of extended rituximab therapy in WM patients, observed a response rate of 58% for those patients who had a serum IgM level of <4000 mg/dL versus 13% in those who had a serum IgM level of >4000 mg/dL. Similarly, Treon et al.,[151] in their study of extended rituximab therapy, observed that the overall response rate was 75% for patients who had a serum IgM level of <6000 mg/dL, whilst only 20% of patients with a serum IgM level of >6000 mg/dL demonstrated a response. Importantly, no correlation between bone marrow involvement and response to rituximab was observed in the study by Treon et al.,[151] suggesting that serum IgM levels per se may modulate response to rituximab. The mechanism for this finding remains to be clarified.

The genetic background of patients may also be important for determining response to rituximab. In particular, a correlation between polymorphisms at position 158 in the Fc gamma RIIIa receptor (CD16), an activating Fc receptor on important effector cells that mediate antibody-dependent cell-mediated cytotoxicity (ADCC), and rituximab response was observed in WM patients. Individuals may encode either the amino acid valine or phenylalanine at position 158 in the Fcγ RIIIa receptor. WM patients who carried the valine amino acid (either in a homozygous or heterozygous pattern) had a fourfold higher major response rate (i.e. ≥50% decline in serum IgM levels) to rituximab versus those patients who expressed phenylalanine in a homozygous pattern.[152]

The combination of rituximab therapy in conjunction with chemotherapy has also been explored. Weber et al.[153] examined the combination of cladribine and cytoxan in combination with rituximab in 17 patients with newly diagnosed WM. Patients received two cycles, which were administered 6 weeks apart of cladribine (1.5 mg/m^2 subcutaneous thrice daily × 7 days), cytoxan (40 mg/m^2 orally twice daily × 7 days), and rituximab (375 mg/m^2 intravenously weekly × 4 weeks). A greater than 75% reduction in serum IgM levels, which defined a partial response, was observed in 94% of patients who received combination therapy with cladribine, cytoxan, and rituximab. While the response rate appeared to be on par with the outcomes of historical controls who had received treatment with cladribine alone (93%), and cladribine plus cytoxan (92%), median response durations appeared to have been greatly extended with the addition of cytoxan and rituxan to cladribine therapy. Treon et al.[154] have also examined the combination of rituximab with fludarabine. Patients received six cycles of fludarabine along with eight infusions of rituximab over 31 weeks. An overall response rate, defined as ≥25% reduction in serum IgM levels, was observed in 90% of patients. Delays in therapy due to cytopenias were common, however, and the impact on response duration remains to be defined.

While therapy with rituximab has been well tolerated in the above series, abrupt increases in serum IgM levels have been observed in certain patients following treatment with rituximab, including in one patient who experienced a central nervous system bleed after her serum viscosity level tripled following rituximab therapy. The cause for this finding remains to be defined, and close monitoring of serum IgM and serum viscosity levels (if IgM levels climb) appears reasonable while patients are receiving therapy with rituximab.

While the experience with monoclonal antibody therapy in WM has largely been confined to rituximab, the use of radioconjugated serotherapy targeting CD20, as well as the use of monoclonal antibodies directed at other serotherapy target antigens, is being explored. Emmanouilides[155] reported a response in a WM patient who received the yttrium-90-conjugated CD20-directed monoclonal antibody Zevalin. More recently, Crowley-Nowick et al.[156] have recently reported activity of the CD52 monoclonal antibody Campath-1H in several WM patients with advanced disease. Serotherapies directed at other target antigens, including CD22 and CD40, are being contemplated in view of the expression of these antigens on WM tumor cells.[157]

Treatment options for relapsed and refractory disease

A consensus panel on therapeutics for WM also considered options for patients with relapsed and refractory disease.[125] For patients in relapse or who have refractory disease, the use of an alternative first-line agent as defined above was considered as a reasonable choice, with the caveat that for those patients for whom autologous transplantation was being considered seriously, further exposure to stem-cell-damaging agents (i.e. many alkylator agents and nucleoside analogue drugs) should be avoided, and a non-stem-cell-toxic agent such as rituximab should be considered if stem cells have not been previously harvested.

THALIDOMIDE

Thalidomide as a single agent, and in combination with dexamethasone and clarithromycin, has also been examined in patients with WM, in view of the success of these regimens in patients with advanced multiple myeloma. Dimopoulos et al.[158] demonstrated a major response in five of 20 (25%) previously untreated and treated patients who received single-agent thalidomide. Dose escalation from the thalidomide start dose of 200 mg daily was hindered by development of side effects, including the development of peripheral neuropathy in five patients obligating discontinuation or dose reduction. Low doses of thalidomide (50 mg orally daily) in combination with dexamethasone (40 mg orally once a week) and clarithromycin (250 mg orally twice a day) have also been examined, with 10 of 12 (83%) previously treated patients demonstrating at least a major response.[159] However, in a follow-up study by Dimopoulos et al.[160] using a higher thalidomide dose (200 mg orally daily) along with dexamathasone (40 g orally once a week) and clarithromycin (500 mg orally twice a day), only two of ten (20%) previously treated patients responded.

INTERFERON-α

The activity of interferon-α (IFNα) has been examined in WM patients. Rotoli et al.[161] used IFNα (3 million IU daily for 1 month, then thrice weekly) to treat 38 WM patients with a high paraprotein (>3000 mg/dL) and observed a 50% ORR (12 PR, 6 MR). Patients tolerated therapy well, and disappearance of hyperviscosity, along with increases in hemoglobin levels and reduction in bone marrow lymphoplasmacytosis, was observed in responding patients. Legouffe et al.[162] treated 14 WM patients with progressive disease with very low doses of IFNα (1 million IU thrice weekly) for a median duration of 10.3 (range 2–44) months and noted increases in hemoglobin levels in six of 14 (42%) of patients, while four of 14 (28%) demonstrated a decrease of >20% in paraprotein levels following therapy. Treatment was stopped for three patients owing to flu-like symptoms, and in one patient due to thrombocytopenia. De Rosa et al.[163] reported the outcome of three WM patients who received IFNα (3 million IU daily or thrice weekly) and reported one PR and two MR following 4 months of therapy. Lastly, Bhavnani et al.[164] described a WM patient with symptomatic cryoglobulinemia who received INFα (3 million IU thrice weekly) and demonstrated a PR and resolution of symptoms attributable to cryoglobulinemia following INFα therapy. Interestingly, this patient's paraprotein, cryoglobulin levels, and attributable symptoms increased after cessation of IFNα therapy, which subsequently subsided following re-introduction of IFNα.

HIGH–DOSE THERAPY AND STEM CELL TRANSPLANTATION

The use of transplant therapy has also been explored in patients WM. Desikan et al.[165] reported their initial experience of high-dose chemotherapy and autologous stem cell transplant, which has more recently been updated by Munshi et al.[166] Their studies involved eight previously treated WM patients between the ages of 45 and 69 years, who received either melphalan at 200 mg/m^2 ($n = 7$) or melphalan at 140 mg/m^2 along with total body irradiation. Stem cells were successfully collected in all eight patients, although a second collection procedure was required for two patients who had extensive previous nucleoside analog exposure. There were no transplant-related mortalities and toxicities were manageable. All eight patients responded, with seven of eight patients achieving a major response, and one patient achieving a complete response with durations of response ranging from 5+ to 77+ months. Dreger et al.[167] investigated the use of the DEXA-BEAM (dexamethasone, BCNU, etoposide, cytarabine, melphalan) regimen followed by myeloablative therapy with cyclophosphamide, and total body irradiation and autologous stem cell transplantation in seven WM patients, which included four untreated patients. Serum IgM levels declined by >50% following DEXA-BEAM and myeloablative therapy for six of seven patients, with progression-free survival ranging from 4+ to 30+ months. All three evaluable patients, who were previously treated, also attained a major response in a study by Anagnostopoulos et al.[168] in which WM patients received various preparative regimens and showed event-free survivals of 26+, 31, and 108+ months. Tournilhac et al.[169] recently reported the outcome of 18 WM patients in France who received high-dose chemotherapy followed by autologous stem cell transplantation. All patients were previously treated with a median of three (range 1–5) prior regimens. Therapy was well tolerated with an improvement in response status observed for seven patients (six PR to CR; one SD to PR), while only one patient demonstrated progressive disease. The median event-free survival for all non-progressing patients was 12 months. There have also been other reports of WM patients achieving durable responses to high-dose chemotherapy and autologous transplant.[170,171] Reports on the use of high-dose chemotherapy and allogeneic transplantation in WM are limited. Martino et al.[172] reported event-free survivals of 3 and 9 years for two young patients (ages 34 and 39) with progressive disease, including one patient who progressed after high-dose chemotherapy and autologous stem cell transplantation. Tournilhac et al.[169] reported the outcome of allogeneic transplantation in ten previously treated WM patients (ages 35–46) who received a median of three prior therapies, including three patients with progressive disease despite therapy. Two of three patients with progressive disease responded, and an improvement in response status was observed in five patients. The median event-free survival for non-progressing, evaluable patients was 31 months. Concerning in this series was the death of three patients owing to transplantation-related toxicity. Similarly, Anagnostopoulos and Giralt.[173] reported that two of three patients in their series who underwent allogeneic transplantation experienced an early death or death from complicating graft versus host disease. The third patient in this series did not respond to therapy. In view of the high rate of mortality associated with high-dose chemotherapy and allogeneic transplantation, Maloney *et al.*[174] have evaluated the use of non-myeloablative allogeneic transplantation in five patients with refractory WM. In this series, three of three evaluable patients (all of whom had matched sibling donors) responded with two CR and one in PR at 1–3 years post-transplant.

PROGNOSIS

Waldenström's macroglobulinemia presents with a chronic, indolent course and with a highly variable prognosis. The median survival reported in large series ranges from 5 to 7 years (Fig. 29.8), [28,36,44,98,129,140,175–177] although an observed survival of 9 years[46] and a 10-year projected overall survival of 55%[178] have been reported. Because WM is a rare disease, relatively few studies on prognosis have been conducted on large patient populations.[36,97,129,140,175–178] Advanced age, anemia, and thrombocytopenia were correlated by univariate analysis with a poorer outcome in virtually all studies. Neutropenia and male sex,[129] weight loss and cryoglobulinemia,[177] albumin level[36,176] and blood cell counts,[176] serum β_2-microglobulin level[36,140,178] and IgM level less than 40 g/L,[140] and hyperviscosity and β_2-microglobulin level[178] were also significantly correlated with survival. A few scoring systems have been proposed based on these analyses:

- age $\geqslant$70 years, hemoglobin $<$90 g/L, weight loss, cryoglobulinemia;[177]
- age $<$65 years, serum albumin $<$40 g/L, hemoglobin $<$120 g/L, cytopenias (platelets $<$150, leukocytes $<$4.0, neutrophils $<$1.5 $\times$ 10^9/L);[176]
- serum β_2-microglobulin $\geqslant$3 mg/L, hemoglobin $<$120 g/L, serum IgM $<$40 g/L.[140]

An update of the study of the Italian group, which included 274 patients, indicated that serum β_2-microglobulin, hemoglobin, albumin, and age defined prognosis of patients with WM thoroughly.[36] In agreement with other studies, serum β_2-microglobulin and hemoglobin level appeared to be the most consistent prognostic determinants.[36,140,178] It is possible that with validation from future studies, both prognostic stratification and decision to start treatment may result from serum β_2-microglobulin level and hemoglobin. Asymptomatic patients with low serum β_2-microglobulin levels and

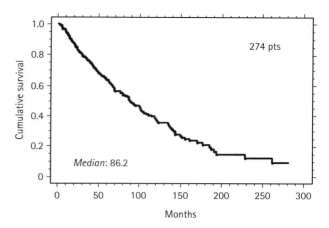

Figure 29.8 *Overall survival of 274 Waldenström's macroglobulinemia patients (Kaplan–Meier analysis). Unpublished data, courtesy of Professor Paolo Gobbi.*

preserved hemoglobin can be observed over long periods without therapy.[175]

Since WM is a disease of the elderly, up to 32% of patients die of unrelated causes[176] and the association with malignancy, both before therapy and during follow-up, is common (39% of patients in a series[175]).[44,98,175,177] The most common causes of death in these patients are progression of the lymphoproliferative process (in about 50%),[176] infections, and cardiac failure.[44] Few patients die of cerebrovascular accidents, renal failure, or gastrointestinal bleeding.[44] In the pre-terminal stage of the disease, the development of aggressive large-cell lymphomas, usually of the immunoblastic type (Richter's syndrome),[179,180] have been reported in 6% of patients treated for WM.[180,181] This transformation is characterized by unexplained fever, weight loss, rapidly enlarging lymph nodes, extranodal extension, and reduction of the level of monoclonal IgM. Rarely, WM may be complicated by acute[182,183] or chronic myeloid leukemia,[184] in most cases after treatment with alkylating agents, although patients who had not been previously treated have also been reported.

KEY POINTS

- Waldenström's macroglobulinemia (WM) is a distinct clinicopathological entity of monoclonal B lymphocytes that show maturation to plasma cells constituting a pathognomonic bone marrow lymphoplasmacytic infiltrate and synthesizing IgM.
- Several lines of evidence indicate that WM may originate from a IgM$^+$ and/or IgM$^+$IgD$^+$ memory B cell.

- The morbidity associated with WM is caused by the concurrence of two main components: tissue infiltration by neoplastic cells and, more importantly, the physicochemical and immunological properties of the monoclonal IgM.
- Blood hyperviscosity is the most common complication of circulating IgM.
- Monoclonal IgM may exert its pathogenic effects through specific recognition of autologous antigens, the most notable being nerve constituents (causing peripheral neuropathy), immunoglobulin determinants (causing type II cryoglobulinemia), and red blood cell antigens (causing cold agglutinin chronic hemolytic anemia).
- Diagnosis of WM requires demonstration, by trephine biopsy, of bone marrow infiltration by a lymphoplasmacytic cell population constituted by small lymphocytes with immunophenotypical evidence of plasmacytoid/plasma cell differentiation constituting more than 20% of the total bone marrow cells, associated with the presence of a serum IgM monoclonal protein.
- Initiation of therapy should not be based on IgM level *per se*, since this may not correlate with the clinical manifestations of WM.
- Initiation of therapy is appropriate for patients with constitutional symptoms, such as recurrent fever, night sweats, fatigue due to anemia, or weight loss, presence of progressive, symptomatic lymphadenopathy, or splenomegaly. Anemia or a platelet count $<100 \times 10^9$/L due to marrow infiltration also justifies treatment. Certain complications, such as hyperviscosity syndrome, symptomatic sensorimotor peripheral neuropathy, systemic amyloidosis, renal insufficiency, or symptomatic cryoglobulinemia, may also be indications for therapy.
- Alkylating agents, nucleoside analogs, and rituximab are reasonable choices for first-line therapy of WM. For relapsed disease, it is reasonable to use an alternative first-line agent or re-use of the same agent. However, since autologous stem cell transplantation may have a role in treating patients with relapsed disease, it is recommended that patients in whom autologous transplantation is seriously being considered should have limited exposure to alkylator or nucleoside analog drugs. Combination chemotherapy for patients who can tolerate myelotoxic therapy or thalidomide alone or with dexamethasone are reasonable choices for relapsed patients.

- Autologous stem cell transplantation may be considered for patients with refractory or relapsing disease. Allogeneic transplantation should only be undertaken in the context of a clinical trial.
- Prognosis depends on age, hemoglobin level, serum β_2-microglobulin level, and cytopenias.

ACKNOWLEDGMENTS

Professor Paolo G. Gobbi and Dr Chiara Broglia kindly provided the data from the Italian collaborative WM study group.

REFERENCES

● = Key primary paper
◆ = Major review article
* = Paper that represents the first formal publication of a management guideline

◆1. Waldenström JG. Macroglobulinemia – a review. *Haematologica* 1986; **71**:437–40.
◆2. Harris NL, Jaffe ES, Stein H, Banks PM, Chan JK, Cleary ML, *et al.* A revised European-American classification of lymphoid neoplasms: a proposal from the International Lymphoma Study Group. *Blood* 1994; **84**:1361–92.
◆3. Harris NL, Jaffe ES, Diebold J, Flandrin G, Muller-Hermelink HK, Vardiman J, *et al.* The World Health Organization classification of neoplastic diseases of the hematopoietic and lymphoid tissues. Report of the Clinical Advisory Committee meeting, Airlie House, Virginia, November, 1997. *Ann Oncol* 1999; **10**:1419–32.
◆4. Owen RG, Treon SP, Al-Katib A, Fonseca R, Greipp PR, McMaster ML, *et al.* Clinicopathological definition of Waldenström's macroglobulinemia: Consensus Panel Recommendations from the Second International Workshop on Waldenström's macroglobulinemia. *Semin Oncol* 2003; **30**:110–15.
●5. Waldenström J. Incipient myelomatosis or 'essential' hyperglobulinemia with fibrinogenopenia – a new syndrome? *Acta Med Scand* 1944; **117**:216–47.
●6. Groves FD, Travis LB, Devesa SS, Ries LA, Fraumeni JF Jr. Waldenström's macroglobulinemia: incidence patterns in the United States, 1988–1994. *Cancer* 1998; **82**:1078–81.
7. Herrinton LJ, Weiss NS. Incidence of Waldenström's macroglobulinemia. *Blood* 1993; **82**:3148–50.
8. Fine JM, Muller JY, Rochu D, Marneux M, Gorin NC, Fine A, Lambin P. Waldenström's macroglobulinemia in monozygotic twins. *Acta Med Scand* 1986; **220**:369–73.
9. Bjornsson OG, Arnason A, Gudmunosson S, Jensson O, Olafsson S, Valimarsson H. Macroglobulinaemia in an Icelandic family. *Acta Med Scand* 1978; **203**:283–8.

10. Renier G, Ifrah N, Chevailler A, Saint-Andre JP, Boasson M, Hurez D. Four brothers with Waldenström's macroglobulinemia. *Cancer* 1989; **64**:1554–9.

11. Ogmundsdottir HM, Sveinsdottir S, Sigfusson A, Skaftadottir I, Jonasson JG, Agnarsson BA. Enhanced B cell survival in familial macroglobulinaemia is associated with increased expression of Bcl-2. *Clin Exp Immunol* 1999; **117**:252–60.

12. Linet MS, Humphrey RL, Mehl ES, Brown LM, Pottern LM, Bias WB, et al. A case-control and family study of Waldenström's macroglobulinemia. *Leukemia* 1993; **7**:1363–9.

13. Santini GF, Crovatto M, Modolo ML, Martelli P, Silvia C, Mazzi G, et al. Waldenström macroglobulinemia: a role of HCV infection? *Blood* 1993; **82**:2932.

14. De Rosa G, Gobbo ML, De Renzo A, Notaro R, Garofalo S, Grimaldi M, et al. High prevalence of hepatitis C virus infection in patients with B-cell lymphoproliferative disorders in Italy. *Am J Hematol* 1997; **55**:77–82.

15. Mussini C, Ghini M, Mascia MT, Giovanardi P, Zanni G, Lattuada I, et al. Monoclonal gammopathies and hepatitis C virus infection. *Blood* 1995; **85**:1144–5.

16. Silvestri F, Barillari G, Fanin R, Zaja F, Infanti L, Patriarca F, et al. Risk of hepatitis C virus infection, Waldenström's macroglobulinemia, and monoclonal gammopathies. *Blood* 1996; **88**:1125–6.

17. Brousset P, Theriault C, Roda D, Attal M, Delsol G. Kaposi's sarcoma-associated herpesvirus (KSHV) in bone marrow biopsies of patients with Waldenström's macroglobulinaemia. *Br J Haematol* 1998; **102**:795–7.

18. Agbalika F, Mariette X, Marolleau JP, Fermand JP, Brouet JC. Detection of human herpesvirus-8 DNA in bone marrow biopsies from patients with multiple myeloma and Waldenström's macroglobulinemia. *Blood* 1998; **91**:4393–4.

19. Stone SA, Lennette ET, Newman JT, Burfoot A, Stone MJ. Serologic prevalence of antibody to human herpesvirus type 8 in patients with various monoclonal gammopathies. *Leuk Lymphoma* 2000; **37**:197–203.

◆20. Merlini G. Waldenström's macroglobulinemia – clinical manifestations and prognosis. In: Schechter GP, Hoffman R, Schrier SL (eds) *Hematology 1999*. Washington, DC: American Society of Hematology, 1999:358–69.

21. Mansoor A, Medeiros LJ, Weber DM, Alexanian R, Hayes K, Jones D, et al. Cytogenetic findings in lymphoplasmacytic lymphoma/Waldenström macroglobulinemia. Chromosomal abnormalities are associated with the polymorphous subtype and an aggressive clinical course. *Am J Clin Pathol* 2001; **116**:543–9.

22. Schop RF, Jalal SM, Van Wier SA, Ahmann GJ, Bailey RJ, Kyle RA, et al. Deletions of 17p13.1 and 13q14 are uncommon in Waldenström macroglobulinemia clonal cells and mostly seen at the time of disease progression. *Cancer Genet Cytogenet* 2002; **132**:55–60.

23. Schop RF, Kuehl WM, Van Wier SA, Ahmann GJ, Price-Troska T, Bailey RJ, et al. Waldenström macroglobulinemia neoplastic cells lack immunoglobulin heavy chain locus translocations but have frequent 6q deletions. *Blood* 2002; **100**:2996–3001.

●24. Preud'homme JL, Seligmann M. Immunoglobulins on the surface of lymphoid cells in Waldenström's macroglobulinemia. *J Clin Invest* 1972; **51**:701–5.

25. Smith BR, Robert NJ, Ault KA. In Waldenström's macroglobulinemia the quantity of detectable circulating monoclonal B lymphocytes correlates with clinical course. *Blood* 1983; **61**:911–14.

●26. Levy Y, Fermand JP, Navarro S, Schmitt C, Vainchenker W, Seligmann M, et al. Interleukin 6 dependence of spontaneous in vitro differentiation of B cells from patients with IgM gammapathy. *Proc Natl Acad Sci USA* 1990; **87**:3309–13.

◆27. Matutes E, Owusu-Ankomah K, Morilla R, Garcia MJ, Houlihan A, Que TH, et al. The immunological profile of B-cell disorders and proposal of a scoring system for the diagnosis of CLL. *Leukemia* 1994; **8**:1640–5.

◆28. Owen RG, Barrans SL, Richards SJ, O'Connor SJ, Child JA, Parapia LA, Morgan GJ, et al. Waldenström macroglobulinemia. Development of diagnostic criteria and identification of prognostic factors. *Am J Clin Pathol* 2001; **116**:420–8.

◆29. Johnson S, Oscier D, Leblond V. Waldenström's macroglobulinaemia. *Blood Rev* 2002; **16**:175.

30. Feiner HD, Rizk CC, Finfer MD, Bannan M, Gottesman SR, Chuba JV, et al. IgM monoclonal gammopathy/Waldenström's macroglobulinemia: a morphological and immunophenotypic study of the bone marrow. *Mod Pathol* 1990; **3**:348–56.

●31. Wagner SD, Martinelli V, Luzzatto L. Similar patterns of V kappa gene usage but different degrees of somatic mutation in hairy cell leukemia, prolymphocytic leukemia, Waldenström's macroglobulinemia, and myeloma. *Blood* 1994; **83**:3647–53.

32. Aoki H, Takishita M, Kosaka M, Saito S. Frequent somatic mutations in D and/or JH segments of Ig gene in Waldenström's macroglobulinemia and chronic lymphocytic leukemia (CLL) with Richter's syndrome but not in common CLL. *Blood* 1995; **85**:1913–19.

33. Shiokawa S, Suehiro Y, Uike N, Muta K, Nishimura J. Sequence and expression analyses of mu and delta transcripts in patients with Waldenström's macroglobulinemia. *Am J Hematol* 2001; **68**:139–43.

●34. Sahota SS, Forconi F, Ottensmeier CH, Provan D, Oscier DG, Hamblin TJ, et al. Typical Waldenström macroglobulinemia is derived from a B-cell arrested after cessation of somatic mutation but prior to isotype switch events. *Blood* 2002; **100**:1505–7.

●35. Paramithiotis E, Cooper MD. Memory B lymphocytes migrate to bone marrow in humans. *Proc Natl Acad Sci USA* 1997; **94**:208–12.

●36. Merlini G, Baldini L, Broglia C, Comelli M, Goldaniga M, Palladini G, et al. Prognostic factors in symptomatic Waldenström's macroglobulinemia. *Semin Oncol* 2003; **30**:211–15.

◆37. Merlini G, Farhangi M, Osserman EF. Monoclonal immunoglobulins with antibody activity in myeloma, macroglobulinemia and related plasma cell dyscrasias. *Semin Oncol* 1986; **13**:350–65.

◆38. Farhangi M, Merlini G. The clinical implications of monoclonal immunoglobulins. *Semin Oncol* 1986; **13**:366–79.

39. Marmont AM, Merlini G. Monoclonal autoimmunity in hematology. *Haematologica* 1991; **76**:449–59.

●40. Mackenzie MR, Babcock J. Studies of the hyperviscosity syndrome. II. Macroglobulinemia. *J Lab Clin Med* 1975; **85**:227–34.

◆41. Gertz MA, Kyle RA. Hyperviscosity syndrome. *J Intens Care Med* 1995; **10**:128-41.

◆42. Kwaan HC, Bongu A. The hyperviscosity syndromes. *Semin Thromb Hemost* 1999; **25**:199-208.

●43. Singh A, Eckardt KU, Zimmermann A, Gotz KH, Hamann M, Ratcliffe PJ, *et al*. Increased plasma viscosity as a reason for inappropriate erythropoietin formation. *J Clin Invest* 1993; **91**:251-6.

◆44. Kyle RA, Garton JP. The spectrum of IgM monoclonal gammopathy in 430 cases. *Mayo Clin Proc* 1987; **62**:719-31.

45. Gertz MA, Fonseca R, Rajkumar SV. Waldenström's macroglobulinemia. *Oncologist* 2000; **5**:63-7.

46. Kyrtsonis MC, Vassilakopoulos TP, Angelopoulou MK, Siakantaris P, Kontopidou FN, Dimopoulou MN, *et al*. Waldenström's macroglobulinemia: clinical course and prognostic factors in 60 patients. Experience from a single hematology unit. *Ann Hematol* 2001; **80**:722-7.

●47. Dellagi K, Dupouey P, Brouet JC, Billecocq A, Gomez D, Clauvel JP, *et al*. Waldenström's macroglobulinemia and peripheral neuropathy: a clinical and immunologic study of 25 patients. *Blood* 1983; **62**:280-5.

◆48. Nobile-Orazio E, Marmiroli P, Baldini L, Spagnol G, Barbieri S, Moggio M, *et al*. Peripheral neuropathy in macroglobulinemia: incidence and antigen-specificity of M proteins. *Neurology* 1987; **37**:1506-14.

49. Nemni R, Gerosa E, Piccolo G, Merlini G. Neuropathies associated with monoclonal gammapathies. *Haematologica* 1994; **79**:557-66.

◆50. Ropper AH, Gorson KC. Neuropathies associated with paraproteinemia. *N Engl J Med* 1998; **338**:1601-7.

◆51. Vital A. Paraproteinemic neuropathies. *Brain Pathol* 2001; **11**:399-407.

◆52. Latov N, Braun PE, Gross RB, Sherman WH, Penn AS, Chess L. Plasma cell dyscrasia and peripheral neuropathy: identification of the myelin antigens that react with human paraproteins. *Proc Natl Acad Sci USA* 1981; **78**:7139-42.

●53. Chassande B, Leger JM, Younes-Chennoufi AB, Bengoufa D, Maisonobe T, Bouche P, *et al*. Peripheral neuropathy associated with IgM monoclonal gammopathy: correlations between M-protein antibody activity and clinical/electrophysiological features in 40 cases. *Muscle Nerve* 1998; **21**:55-62.

54. Weiss MD, Dalakas MC, Lauter CJ, Willison HJ, Quarles RH. Variability in the binding of anti-MAG and anti-SGPG antibodies to target antigens in demyelinating neuropathy and IgM paraproteinemia. *J Neuroimmunol* 1999; **95**:174-84.

◆55. Latov N, Hays AP, Sherman WH. Peripheral neuropathy and anti-MAG antibodies. *Crit Rev Neurobiol* 1988; **3**:301-32.

56. Dalakas MC, Quarles RH. Autoimmune ataxic neuropathies (sensory ganglionopathies): are glycolipids the responsible autoantigens? *Ann Neurol* 1996; **39**:419-22.

●57. Eurelings M, Ang CW, Notermans NC, Van Doorn PA, Jacobs BC, Van den Berg LH. Antiganglioside antibodies in polyneuropathy associated with monoclonal gammopathy. *Neurology* 2001; **57**:1909-12.

●58. Ilyas AA, Quarles RH, Dalakas MC, Fishman PH, Brady RO. Monoclonal IgM in a patient with paraproteinemic polyneuropathy binds to gangliosides containing disialosyl groups. *Ann Neurol* 1985; **18**:655-9.

◆59. Willison HJ, O'Leary CP, Veitch J, Blumhardt LD, Busby M, Donaghy M, *et al*. The clinical and laboratory features of chronic sensory ataxic neuropathy with anti-disialosyl IgM antibodies. *Brain* 2001; **124**:1968-77.

60. Lopate G, Choksi R, Pestronk A. Severe sensory ataxia and demyelinating polyneuropathy with IgM anti-GM2 and GalNAc-GD1A antibodies. *Muscle Nerve* 2002; **25**:828-36.

●61. Jacobs BC, O'Hanlon GM, Breedland EG, Veitch J, Van Doorn PA, Willison HJ. Human IgM paraproteins demonstrate shared reactivity between Campylobacter jejuni lipopolysaccharides and human peripheral nerve disialylated gangliosides. *J Neuroimmunol* 1997; **80**:23-30.

●62. Nobile-Orazio E, Manfredini E, Carpo M, Meucci N, Monaco S, Ferrari S, *et al*. Frequency and clinical correlates of anti-neural IgM antibodies in neuropathy associated with IgM monoclonal gammopathy. *Ann Neurol* 1994; **36**:416-24.

◆63. Gordon PH, Rowland LP, Younger DS, Sherman WH, Hays AP, Louis ED, *et al*. Lymphoproliferative disorders and motor neuron disease: an update. *Neurology* 1997; **48**:1671-8.

64. Pavord SR, Murphy PT, Mitchell VE. POEMS syndrome and Waldenström's macroglobulinaemia. *J Clin Pathol* 1996; **49**:181-2.

65. Ferri C, Greco F, Longombardo G, Palla P, Moretti A, Marzo E, *et al*. Antibodies against hepatitis C virus in mixed cryoglobulinemia patients. *Infection* 1991; **19**:417-20.

66. D'Amico G. Renal involvement in hepatitis C infection: cryoglobulinemic glomerulonephritis. *Kidney Int* 1998; **54**:650-71.

●67. Crisp D, Pruzanski W. B-cell neoplasms with homogeneous cold-reacting antibodies (cold agglutinins). *Am J Med* 1982; **72**:915-22.

●68. Pruzanski W, Shumak KH. Biologic activity of cold-reacting autoantibodies (first of two parts). *N Engl J Med* 1977; **297**:538-42.

●69. Pruzanski W, Shumak KH. Biologic activity of cold-reacting autoantibodies (second of two parts). *N Engl J Med* 1977; **297**:583-9.

●70. Tsai CM, Zopf DA, Yu RK, Wistar R Jr, Ginsburg V. A Waldenström macroglobulin that is both a cold agglutinin and a cryoglobulin because it binds N-acetylneuraminosyl residues. *Proc Natl Acad Sci USA* 1977; **74**:4591-4.

71. Whittaker SJ, Bhogal BS, Black MM. Acquired immunobullous disease: a cutaneous manifestation of IgM macroglobulinaemia. *Br J Dermatol* 1996; **135**:283-6.

◆72. Daoud MS, Lust JA, Kyle RA, Pittelkow MR. Monoclonal gammopathies and associated skin disorders. *J Am Acad Dermatol* 1999; **40**:507-35.

73. Gad A, Willen R, Carlen B, Gyland F, Wickander M. Duodenal involvement in Waldenström's macroglobulinemia. *J Clin Gastroenterol* 1995; **20**:174-6.

74. Case records of the Massachusetts General Hospital. Weekly clinicopathological exercises. Case 3-1990. A 66-year-old woman with Waldenström's macroglobulinemia, diarrhea, anemia, and persistent gastrointestinal bleeding. *N Engl J Med* 1990; **322**:183-92.

75. Isaac J, Herrera GA. Cast nephropathy in a case of Waldenström's macroglobulinemia. *Nephron* 2002; **91**:512-15.

●76. Morel-Maroger L, Basch A, Danon F, Verroust P, Richet G. Pathology of the kidney in Waldenström's macroglobulinemia. Study of sixteen cases. *N Engl J Med* 1970; **283**:123–9.

77. Gertz MA, Kyle RA, Noel P. Primary systemic amyloidosis: a rare complication of immunoglobulin M monoclonal gammopathies and Waldenström's macroglobulinemia. *J Clin Oncol* 1993; **11**:914–20.

78. Moyner K, Sletten K, Husby G, Natvig JB. An unusually l arge (83 amino acid residues) amyloid fibril protein AA from a patient with Waldenström's macroglobulinaemia and amyloidosis. *Scand J Immunol* 1980; **11**:549–54.

79. Gardyn J, Schwartz A, Gal R, Lewinski U, Kristt D, Cohen AM. Waldenström's macroglobulinemia associated with AA amyloidosis. *Int J Hematol* 2001; **74**:76–8.

80. Dussol B, Kaplanski G, Daniel L, Brunet P, Pellissier JF, Berland Y. Simultaneous occurrence of fibrillary glomerulopathy and AL amyloid. *Nephrol Dial Transplant* 1998; **13**:2630–2.

●81. Rausch PG, Herion JC. Pulmonary manifestations of Waldenström macroglobulinemia. *Am J Hematol* 1980; **9**:201–9.

82. Fadil A, Taylor DE. The lung and Waldenström's macroglobulinemia. *South Med J* 1998; **91**:681–5.

83. Kyrtsonis MC, Angelopoulou MK, Kontopidou FN, Siakantaris MP, Dimopoulou MN, Mitropoulos F, *et al.* Primary lung involvement in Waldenström's macroglobulinaemia: report of two cases and review of the literature. *Acta Haematol* 2001; **105**:92–6.

84. Kaila VL, el Newihi HM, Dreiling BJ, Lynch CA, Mihas AA. Waldenström's macroglobulinemia of the stomach presenting with upper gastrointestinal hemorrhage. *Gastrointest Endosc* 1996; **44**:73–5.

85. Yasui O, Tukamoto F, Sasaki N, Saito T, Yagisawa H, Uno A, Nanjo H. Malignant lymphoma of the transverse colon associated with macroglobulinemia. *Am J Gastroenterol* 1997; **92**:2299–301.

86. Rosenthal JA, Curran WJ Jr, Schuster SJ. Waldenström's macroglobulinemia resulting from localized gastric lymphoplasmacytoid lymphoma. *Am J Hematol* 1998; **58**:244–5.

87. Recine MA, Perez MT, Cabello-Inchausti B, Lilenbaum RC, Robinson MJ. Extranodal lymphoplasmacytoid lymphoma (immunocytoma) presenting as small intestinal obstruction. *Arch Pathol Lab Med* 2001; **125**:677–9.

88. Veltman GA, van Veen S, Kluin-Nelemans JC, Bruijn JA, van Es LA. Renal disease in Waldenström's macroglobulinaemia. *Nephrol Dial Transplant* 1997; **12**:1256–9.

89. Moore DF Jr, Moulopoulos LA, Dimopoulos MA. Waldenström macroglobulinemia presenting as a renal or perirenal mass: clinical and radiographic features. *Leuk Lymphoma* 1995; **17**:331–4.

90. Mascaro JM, Montserrat E, Estrach T, Feliu E, Ferrando J, Castel T, *et al.* Specific cutaneous manifestations of Waldenström's macroglobulinaemia. A report of two cases. *Br J Dermatol* 1982; **106**:17–22.

●91. Schnitzler L, Schubert B, Boasson M, Gardais J, Tourmen A. Urticaire chronique, lésions osseuses, macroglobulinémie IgM: Maladie de Waldenström? *Bull Soc Fr Dermatol Syphiligr* 1974; **81**:363–8.

92. Roux S, Fermand JP, Brechignac S, Mariette X, Kahn MF, Brouet JC. Tumoral joint involvement in multiple myeloma and Waldenström's macroglobulinemia – report of 4 cases. *J Rheumatol* 1996; **23**:2175–8.

93. Orellana J, Friedman AH. Ocular manifestations of multiple myeloma, Waldenström's macroglobulinemia and benign monoclonal gammopathy. *Surv Ophthalmol* 1981; **26**:157–69.

94. Ettl AR, Birbamer GG, Philipp W. Orbital involvement in Waldenström's macroglobulinemia: ultrasound, computed tomography and magnetic resonance findings. *Ophthalmologica* 1992; **205**:40–5.

95. Civit T, Coulbois S, Baylac F, Taillandier L, Auque J. [Waldenström's macroglobulinemia and cerebral lymphoplasmocytic proliferation: Bing and Neel syndrome. Apropos of a new case.] *Neurochirurgie* 1997; **43**:245–9.

96. McMullin MF, Wilkin HJ, Elder E. Inaccurate haemoglobin estimation in Waldenström's macroglobulinaemia. *J Clin Pathol* 1995; **48**:787.

97. Merlini G, Aguzzi F, Whicher J. Monoclonal gammapathies. *J Int Fed Clin Chem* 1997; **9**:171–6.

98. Dimopoulos MA, Alexanian R. Waldenström's macroglobulinemia. *Blood* 1994; **83**:1452–9.

99. Persson SU, Larsson H, Odeberg H. How should blood rheology be measured in macroglobulinaemia? *Scand J Clin Lab Invest* 1998; **58**:669–76.

100. Kallemuchikkal U, Gorevic PD. Evaluation of cryoglobulins. *Arch Pathol Lab Med* 1999; **123**:119–25.

●101. Bartl R, Frisch B, Mahl G, Burkhardt R, Fateh-Moghadam A, Pappenberger R, *et al.* Bone marrow histology in Waldenström's macroglobulinaemia. Clinical relevance of subtype recognition. *Scand J Haematol* 1983; **31**:359–75.

●102. Dutcher TF, Fahey JL. The histopathology of macroglobulinemia of Waldenström. *J Natl Cancer Inst* 1959; **22**:887–917.

●103. Moulopoulos LA, Dimopoulos MA, Varma DG, Manning JT, Johnston DA, Leeds NE, *et al.* Waldenström macroglobulinemia: MR imaging of the spine and CT of the abdomen and pelvis. *Radiology* 1993; **188**:669–73.

●104. Owen RG, Parapia LA, Higginson J, Misbah SA, Child JA, Morgan GJ, *et al.* Clinicopathological correlates of IgM paraproteinemias. *Clin Lymphoma* 2000; **1**:39–43.

105. Stone MJ. Myeloma and macroglobulinemia: what are the criteria for diagnosis? *Clin Lymphoma* 2002; **3**:23–5.

◆106. Bennett JM, Catovsky D, Daniel MT, Flandrin G, Galton DA, Gralnick HR, *et al.* Proposals for the classification of chronic (mature) B and T lymphoid leukaemias. French-American-British (FAB) Cooperative Group. *J Clin Pathol* 1989; **42**:567–84.

◆107. Osserman EF, Merlini G, Butler VP Jr. Multiple myeloma and related plasma cell dyscrasias. *J Am Med Assoc* 1987; **258**:2930–7.

108. Roberts-Thomson PJ, Nikoloutsopoulos T, Smith AJ. IgM paraproteinaemia: disease associations and laboratory features. *Pathology* 2002; **34**:356–61.

◆109. Kyle RA. Monoclonal gammopathy of undetermined significance and solitary plasmacytoma. Implications for progression to overt multiple myeloma. *Hematol Oncol Clin North Am* 1997; **11**:71–87.

◆110. Pangalis GA, Angelopoulou MK, Vassilakopoulos TP, Siakantaris MP, Kittas C. B-chronic lymphocytic leukemia, small lymphocytic lymphoma, and lymphoplasmacytic lymphoma, including Waldenström's macroglobulinemia: a clinical, morphologic, and biologic spectrum of similar disorders. *Semin Hematol* 1999; **36**:104–14.

111. Cheson BD, Bennett JM, Grever M, Kay N, Keating MJ, O'Brien S, et al. National Cancer Institute-sponsored Working Group guidelines for chronic lymphocytic leukemia: revised guidelines for diagnosis and treatment. *Blood* 1996; **87**:4990–7.

112. Henrique R, Achten R, Maes B, Verhoef G, Wolf-Peeters C. Guidelines for subtyping small B-cell lymphomas in bone marrow biopsies. *Virchows Arch* 1999; **435**:549–58.

113. Frater JL, Tsiftsakis EK, Hsi ED, Pettay J, Tubbs RR. Use of novel t(11;14) and t(14;18) dual-fusion fluorescence in situ hybridization probes in the differential diagnosis of lymphomas of small lymphocytes. *Diagn Mol Pathol* 2001; **10**:214–22.

*114. Keren DF. Procedures for the evaluation of monoclonal immunoglobulins. *Arch Pathol Lab Med* 1999; **123**:126–32.

115. Allez M, Mariette X, Linares G, Bertheau P, Jian R, Brouet JC. Low-grade MALT lymphoma mimicking Waldenström's macroglobulinemia. *Leukemia* 1999; **13**:484–5.

116. Valdez R, Finn WG, Ross CW, Singleton TP, Tworek JA, Schnitzer B. Waldenström macroglobulinemia caused by extranodal marginal zone B-cell lymphoma: a report of six cases. *Am J Clin Pathol* 2001; **116**:683–90.

117. Diebold J, Molina T, Tissier F, Le Tourneau A, Audouin J. Waldenström's macroglobulinemia is a biological syndrome which may occur during the evolution of different types of low grade B cell lymphoma. *Leukemia* 1999; **13**:1637–8.

118. Nakata M, Matsuno Y, Takenaka T, Kobayashi Y, Takeyama K, Yokozawa T, et al. B-cell lymphoma accompanying monoclonal macroglobulinemia with features suggesting marginal zone B-cell lymphoma. *Int J Hematol* 1997; **65**:405–11.

119. Haghighi B, Yanagihara R, Cornbleet PJ. IgM myeloma: case report with immunophenotypic profile. *Am J Hematol* 1998; **59**:302–8.

120. Dierlamm T, Laack E, Dierlamm J, Fiedler W, Hossfeld DK. IgM myeloma: a report of four cases. *Ann Hematol* 2002; **81**:136–9.

121. Zarrabi MH, Stark RS, Kane P, Dannaher CL, Chandor S. IgM myeloma, a distinct entity in the spectrum of B-cell neoplasia. *Am J Clin Pathol* 1981; **75**:1–10.

122. Takahashi K, Yamamura F, Motoyama H. IgM myeloma – its distinction from Waldenström's macroglobulinemia. *Acta Pathol Jpn* 1986; **36**:1553–63.

123. Avet-Loiseau H, Garand R, Lode L, Robillard N, Bataille R. 14q32 translocations discriminate IgM multiple myeloma from Waldenström's macroglobulinemia. *Semin Oncol* 2003; **30**:153–5.

*124. Kyle RA, Treon SP, Alexanian R, Barlogie B, Bjorkholm M, Dhodapkar M, et al. Prognostic markers and criteria to initiate therapy in Waldenström's macroglobulinemia: Consensus Panel Recommendations from the Second International Workshop on Waldenström's macroglobulinemia. *Semin Oncol* 2003; **30**:116–120.

*125. Gertz M, Anagnostopoulos A, Anderson KC, Branagan AR, Coleman M, Frankel S, et al. Treatment recommendations in Waldenström's macroglobulinemia: Consensus Panel Recommendations from the Second International Workshop on Waldenström's macroglobulinemia. *Semin Oncol* 2003; **30**:121–6.

●126. Kyle RA, Greipp PR, Gertz MA, Witzig TE, Lust JA, Lacy MQ, et al. Waldenström's macroglobulinaemia: a prospective study comparing daily with intermittent oral chlorambucil. *Br J Haematol* 2000; **108**:737–42.

127. Petrucci MT, Avvisati G, Tribalto M, Giovangrossi P, Mandelli F. Waldenström's macroglobulinaemia: results of a combined oral treatment in 34 newly diagnosed patients. *J Intern Med* 1989; **226**:443–7.

128. Case DC Jr, Ervin TJ, Boyd MA, Redfield DL. Waldenström's macroglobulinemia: long-term results with the M-2 protocol. *Cancer Invest* 1991; **9**:1–7.

●129. Facon T, Brouillard M, Duhamel A, Morel P, Simon M, Jouet JP, et al. Prognostic factors in Waldenström's macroglobulinemia: a report of 167 cases. *J Clin Oncol* 1993; **11**:1553–8.

●130. Dimopoulos MA, Kantarjian H, Weber D, O'Brien S, Estey E, Delasalle K, et al. Primary therapy of Waldenström's macroglobulinemia with 2-chlorodeoxyadenosine. *J Clin Oncol* 1994; **12**:2694–8.

131. Delannoy A, Ferrant A, Martiat P, Bosly A, Zenebergh A, Michaux JL. 2-Chlorodeoxyadenosine therapy in Waldenström's macroglobulinaemia. *Nouv Rev Fr Hematol* 1994; **36**:317–20.

132. Fridrik MA, Jager G, Baldinger C, Krieger O, Chott A, Bettelheim P. First-line treatment of Waldenström's disease with cladribine. Arbeitsgemeinschaft Medikamentose Tumortherapie. *Ann Hematol* 1997; **74**:7–10.

133. Liu ES, Burian C, Miller WE, Saven A. Bolus administration of cladribine in the treatment of Waldenström macroglobulinaemia. *Br J Haematol* 1998; **103**:690–5.

134. Hellmann A, Lewandowski K, Zaucha JM, Bieniaszewska M, Halaburda K, Robak T. Effect of a 2-hour infusion of 2-chlorodeoxyadenosine in the treatment of refractory or previously untreated Waldenström's macroglobulinemia. *Eur J Haematol* 1999; **63**:35–41.

135. Betticher DC, Hsu Schmitz SF, Ratschiller D, von Rohr A, Egger T, Pugin P, et al. Cladribine (2-CDA) given as subcutaneous bolus injections is active in pretreated Waldenström's macroglobulinaemia. Swiss Group for Clinical Cancer Research (SAKK). *Br J Haematol* 1997; **99**:358–63.

136. Dimopoulos MA, Weber D, Delasalle KB, Keating M, Alexanian R. Treatment of Waldenström's macroglobulinemia resistant to standard therapy with 2-chlorodeoxyadenosine: identification of prognostic factors. *Ann Oncol* 1995; **6**:49–52.

137. Dimopoulos MA, O'Brien S, Kantarjian H, Pierce S, Delasalle K, Barlogie B, et al. Fludarabine therapy in Waldenström's macroglobulinemia. *Am J Med* 1993; **95**:49–52.

●138. Foran JM, Rohatiner AZ, Coiffier B, Barbui T, Johnson SA, Hiddemann W, et al. Multicenter phase II study of fludarabine phosphate for patients with newly diagnosed lymphoplasmacytoid lymphoma, Waldenström's macroglobulinemia, and mantle-cell lymphoma. *J Clin Oncol* 1999; **17**:546–53.

139. Thalhammer-Scherrer R, Geissler K, Schwarzinger I, Chott A, Gisslinger H, Knobl P, et al. Fludarabine therapy in Waldenström's macroglobulinemia. Ann Hematol 2000; **79**:556–9.

140. Dhodapkar MV, Jacobson JL, Gertz MA, Rivkin SE, Roodman GD, Tuscano JM, et al. Prognostic factors and response to fludarabine therapy in patients with Waldenström macroglobulinemia: results of United States intergroup trial (Southwest Oncology Group S9003). Blood 2001; **98**:41–8.

141. Zinzani PL, Gherlinzoni F, Bendandi M, Zaccaria A, Aitini E, Salvucci M, et al. Fludarabine treatment in resistant Waldenström's macroglobulinemia. Eur J Haematol 1995; **54**:120–3.

●142. Leblond V, Ben Othman T, Deconinck E, Taksin AL, Harousseau JL, Delgado MA, et al. Activity of fludarabine in previously treated Waldenström's macroglobulinemia: a report of 71 cases. Groupe Cooperatif Macroglobulinemie. J Clin Oncol 1998; **16**:2060–4.

143. Dimopoulos MA, Weber DM, Kantarjian H, Keating M, Alexanian R. 2Chlorodeoxyadenosine therapy of patients with Waldenström macroglobulinemia previously treated with fludarabine. Ann Oncol 1994; **5**:288–9.

144. Lewandowski K, Halaburda K, Hellmann A. Fludarabine therapy in Waldenström's macroglobulinemia patients treated previously with 2-chlorodeoxyadenosine. Leuk Lymphoma 2002; **43**:361–3.

145. Treon SP, Shima Y, Preffer FI, Doss DS, Ellman L, Schlossman RL, et al. Treatment of plasma cell dyscrasias by antibody immunotherapy. Semin Oncol 1999; **26**:97–106.

146. Byrd JC, White CA, Link B, Lucas MS, Velasquez WS, Rosenberg J, et al. Rituximab therapy in Waldenström's macroglobulinemia: preliminary evidence of clinical activity. Ann Oncol 1999; **10**:1525–7.

●147. Weber DM, Gavino M, Huh Y, Cabanillas F, Alexanian R. Phenotypic and clinical evidence supports rituximab for Waldenström's macroglobulinemia. Blood 1999; **94**:125.

●148. Foran JM, Gupta RK, Cunningham D, Popescu RA, Goldstone AH, Sweetenham JW, et al. A UK multicentre phase II study of rituximab (chimaeric anti-CD20 monoclonal antibody) in patients with follicular lymphoma, with PCR monitoring of molecular response. Br J Haematol 2000; **109**:81–8.

●149. Treon SP, Agus DB, Link B, Rodrigues G, Molina A, Lacy MQ, et al. CD20-Directed antibody-mediated immunotherapy induces responses and facilitates hematologic recovery in patients with Waldenström's macroglobulinemia. J Immunother 2001; **24**:272–9.

●150. Dimopoulos MA, Zervas C, Zomas A, Kiamouris C, Viniou NA, Grigoraki V, et al. Treatment of Waldenström's macroglobulinemia with rituximab. J Clin Oncol 2002; **20**:2327–33.

●151. Treon SP, Emmanouilides CA, Kimby E, Branagan A, Mitsiades C, Anderson KC, et al. Pre-therapy serum IgM levels predict clinical response to extended rituximab in Waldenström's macroglobulinemia. Blood 2002; **100**:813a.

●152. Treon SP, Fox EA, Hansen MM, Verselis S, Branagan A, Touroutoglou N, et al. Polymorphism in Fc gamma RIIIa (CD16) receptor expression are associated with clinical responses in Waldenström's macroglobulinemia. Blood 2002; **100**:773a.

●153. Weber DM, Dimopoulos MA, Delasalle K, Rankin K, Gavino M, Alexanian R. 2-Chlorodeoxyadenosine (2-CdA) alone or in combination for previously untreated Waldenström's macroglobulinemia. Semin Oncol 2003; **30**:243–7.

●154. Treon SP, Wasi P, Emmanouilides CA, Frankel SR, Kimby E, Lister A, et al. Combination therapy with rituximab and fludarabine is highly active in Waldenström's macroglobulinemia. Blood 2002; **100**:211a.

155. Emmanouilides C. Radioimmunotherapy for Waldenström's macroglobulinemia. Semin Oncol 2003; **30**:258–61.

156. Crowley-Nowick P, Preffer FI, Kelliher A, Treon SP. Campath-1H for treatment of Waldenström's macroglobulinemia. Proceedings of the Second International Workshop on Waldenström's Macroglobulinemia, 2002, Athens, Greece.

157. Treon SP, Kelliher A, Keele B, Frankel S, Emmanouilides C, et al. Expression of serotherapy target antigens in Waldenström's macroglobulinemia: therapeutic considerations and conmsiderations. Semin Oncol 2003; **30**:248–52.

●158. Dimopoulos MA, Zomas A, Viniou NA, Grigoraki V, Galani E, Matsouka C, et al. Treatment of Waldenström's macroglobulinemia with thalidomide. J Clin Oncol 2001; **19**:3596–601.

159. Coleman C, Leonard J, Lyons L, Szelenyi H, Niesvizky R. Treatment of Waldenström's macroglobulinemia with clarithromycin, low-dose thalidomide and dexamethasone. Semin Oncol **30**:270–4.

160. Dimopoulos MA, Zomas K, Tsatalas K, Hamilos G, Efstathiou E, Gika D, et al. Treatment of Waldenström's macroglobulinemia with single agent thalidomide or with combination of clarithromycin, thalidomide and dexamethasone. Semin Oncol 2003; **30**:265–9.

●161. Rotoli B, De Renzo A, Frigeri F, Buffardi S, Marceno R, Cavallaro AM, et al. A phase II trial on alpha-interferon (alpha IFN) effect in patients with monoclonal IgM gammopathy. Leuk Lymphoma 1994; **13**:463–9.

●162. Legouffe E, Rossi JF, Laporte JP, Isnard F, Oziol E, Fabbro M, et al. Treatment of Waldenström's macroglobulinemia with very low doses of alpha interferon. Leuk Lymphoma 1995; **19**:337–42.

163. De Rosa G, De Renzo A, Buffardi S, Rotoli B. Treatment of Waldenström's macroglobulinemia with interferon. Haematologica 1989; **74**:313–15.

164. Bhavnani M, Marples J, Yin JA. Treatment of Waldenström's macroglobulinemia with alpha interferon. J Clin Pathol 1990; **43**:437.

●165. Desikan R, Dhodapkar M, Siegel D, Fassas A, Singh J, Singhal S, et al. High-dose therapy with autologous haemopoietic stem cell support for Waldenström's macroglobulinaemia. Br J Haematol 1999; **105**:993–6.

166. Munshi NC, Barlogie B. Role for high dose therapy with autologous hematopoietic stem cell support in Waldenström's macroglobulinemia. Semin Oncol 2003; **30**:282–5.

167. Dreger P, Glass B, Kuse R, Sonnen R, von Neuhoff N, Bolouri H, et al. Myeloablative radiochemotherapy followed by reinfusion of purged autologous stem cells for

Waldenström's macroglobulinaemia. *Br J Haematol* 1999; **106**:115–18.

●168. Anagnostopoulos A, Dimopoulos MA, Aleman A, Weber D, Alexanian R, Champlin R, *et al.* High-dose chemotherapy followed by stem cell transplantation in patients with resistant Waldenström's macroglobulinemia. *Bone Marrow Transplant* 2001; **27**:1027–9.

●169. Tournilhac O, Leblond V, Tabrizi R, Gressin R, Colombat P, Milpied N, *et al.* Transplantation in Waldenström's macroglobulinemia – the French Experience. *Semin Oncol* 2003; **30**:291–6.

170. Yang L, Wen B, Li H, Yang M, Jin Y, Yang S, *et al.* Autologous peripheral blood stem cell transplantation for Waldenström's macroglobulinemia. *Bone Marrow Transplant* 1999; **24**:929–30.

171. Mustafa M, Powles R, Treleaven J. Total therapy with VAMP/CVAMP plus high dose melphalan and autograft for IgM lymphoplasmacytoid disease. *Blood* 1998; **92**:281b.

172. Martino R, Shah A, Romero P, Brunet S, Sierra J, Domingo-Albos A, *et al.* Allogeneic bone marrow transplantation for advanced Waldenström's macroglobulinemia. *Bone Marrow Transplant* 1999; **23**:747–9.

173. Anagnostopoulos A, Giralt S. Autologous and allogeneic stem cell transplantation in Waldenström's macroglobulinemia: review of the literature and future directions. *Semin Oncol* 2003; **30**:286–90.

174. Maloney DG, Sandmaier B, Maris M, Storb R. The use of non-myeloablative allogeneic hematopoietic cell transplantation for patients with refractory Waldenström's macroglobulinemia: replacing high-dose cytotoxic therapy with graft versus tumor effects. *Proceedings of the Second International Workshop on Waldenström's Macroglobulinemia*, 2002, Athens, Greece.

◆175. Desikan KR, Dhodapkar MV, Barlogie B. Waldenström's macroglobulinemia. *Curr Treat Options Oncol* 2000; **1**:97–103.

●176. Morel P, Monconduit M, Jacomy D, Lenain P, Grosbois B, Bateli C, *et al.* Prognostic factors in Waldenström macroglobulinemia: a report on 232 patients with the description of a new scoring system and its validation on 253 other patients. *Blood* 2000; **96**:852–8.

●177. Gobbi PG, Bettini R, Montecucco C, Cavanna L, Morandi S, Pieresca C, *et al.* Study of prognosis in Waldenström's macroglobulinemia: a proposal for a simple binary classification with clinical and investigational utility. *Blood* 1994; **83**:2939–45.

●178. Garcia-Sanz R, Montoto S, Torrequebrada A, de Coca AG, Petit J, Sureda A, *et al.* Waldenström macroglobulinaemia: presenting features and outcome in a series with 217 cases. *Br J Haematol* 2001; **115**:575–82.

179. Beaudreuil J, Lortholary O, Martin A, Feuillard J, Guillevin L, Lortholary P, *et al.* Hypercalcemia may indicate Richter's syndrome: report of four cases and review. *Cancer* 1997; **79**:1211–5.

180. Garcia R, Hernandez JM, Caballero MD, Gonzalez M, San Miguel JF. Immunoblastic lymphoma and associated non-lymphoid malignancies following two cases of Waldenström's macroglobulinemia. A review of the literature. *Eur J Haematol* 1993; **50**:299–301.

181. Harousseau JL, Flandrin G, Tricot G, Brouet JC, Seligmann M, Bernard J. Malignant lymphoma supervening in chronic lymphocytic leukemia and related disorders. Richter's syndrome: a study of 25 cases. *Cancer* 1981; **48**:1302–8.

182. Rodriguez JN, Fernandez-Jurado A, Martino ML, Prados D. Waldenström's macroglobulinemia complicated with acute myeloid leukemia. Report of a case and review of the literature. *Haematologica* 1998; **83**:91–2.

183. Pagano L, Larocca LM. Simultaneous presentation of Waldenström's macroglobulinemia and acute myeloid leukemia. *Haematologica* 2002; **87**:EIM07.

184. Vitali C, Bombardieri S, Spremolla G. Chronic myeloid leukemia in Waldenström's macroglobulinemia. *Arch Intern Med* 1981; **141**:1349–51.

Index